Essential Practical Prescribing

This title is also available as an e-book.

For more details, please see

www.wiley.com/buy/ 9781118837733

or scan this QR code:

Essential Practical Prescribing

Georgia Woodfield MBChB MRCP
Specialist Registrar in Gastrointestinal Medicine, London

Benedict Lyle Phillips MBChB BSc (Hons) MRCS MSc
Specialist Registrar in General Surgery, NE London Deanery

Victoria Taylor MBChB BSc MRCP
Specialist Registrar in Respiratory Medicine, London

Amy Hawkins BA (Hons) MBChB (Hons) MRCP MSc
Specialist Registrar in Palliative Medicine, London

Andrew Stanton MD FRCP
Consultant Respiratory Physician
The Great Western Hospital, Swindon;
Honorary Senior Clinical Lecturer, University of Bristol

With contribution from Marie O'Sullivan MB ChB
Specialist Registrar in Obstetrics & Gynaecology, Severn Deanery

WILEY Blackwell

This edition first published 2016 © 2016 by John Wiley & Sons, Ltd

Registered office: John Wiley & Sons, Ltd, The Atrium, Southern Gate, Chichester, West Sussex, PO19 8SQ, UK

Editorial offices: 9600 Garsington Road, Oxford, OX4 2DQ, UK
The Atrium, Southern Gate, Chichester, West Sussex, PO19 8SQ, UK
111 River Street, Hoboken, NJ 07030-5774, USA

For details of our global editorial offices, for customer services and for information about how to apply for permission to reuse the copyright material in this book please see our website at www.wiley.com/wiley-blackwell

Library of Congress Cataloging-in-Publication Data
Names: Woodfield, Georgia, author. | Phillips, Benedict Lyle, author. |
   Taylor, Victoria, MBChB, author. | Hawkins, Amy, MBChB, author. | Stanton,
   Andrew, MD, author. | O'Sullivan, Marie, active 2015, contributor.
Title: Essential practical prescribing / Georgia Woodfield, Benedict Lyle
   Phillips, Victoria Taylor, Amy Hawkins, Andrew Stanton ; with contribution from Marie O'Sullivan.
Description: Chichester, West Sussex ; Hoboken, NJ : John Wiley & Sons, Inc.,
   2016. | Includes bibliographical references and index.
Identifiers: LCCN 2015046044 (print) | LCCN 2015048186 (ebook) |
   ISBN 9781118837733 (pbk.) | ISBN 9781118837702 (pdf) | ISBN 9781118837696 (epub)
Subjects: | MESH: Drug Prescriptions
Classification: LCC RM139 (print) | LCC RM139 (ebook) | NLM QV 748 | DDC
   615.1/4—dc23
LC record available at http://lccn.loc.gov/2015046044

A catalogue record for this book is available from the British Library.

Wiley also publishes its books in a variety of electronic formats. Some content that appears in print may not be available in electronic books.

Set in 10/12 Adobe Garamond Pro by Aptara
Printed and bound in Singapore by Markono Print Media Pte Ltd

1   2016

Contents

Preface

This textbook was inspired by the need for a practical prescribing textbook for medical students and junior doctors. In a 2009 General Medical Council (GMC) report, 9% of hospital prescriptions contained errors, where 18.7% of these were made by junior doctors (Dornan *et al.*, 2009). A 2008 GMC report of newly qualified UK doctors showed that prescribing was the 'main area of practice in which errors were reported by respondents, indicating a significant potential risk' (Illing *et al.*, 2008). Aside from these figures, the initial inspiration for the book came from my own and others' personal experiences of being a doctor training in busy UK hospitals. Starting as a doctor is daunting, particularly due to the sudden weight of responsibility, much of which lies in prescribing medications. A National Patient Safety Agency study in 2007 found that 32% of the most serious UK drug error incidents were caused by prescribing (NPSA, 2009). When I (GW) started I would have certainly found a practical prescribing book beneficial, as common prescriptions do not become embedded in your memory until you have had the experience to draw back on.

Later on, whilst teaching medical students in the Great Western Hospital Swindon, it became clear that many were worried about becoming junior doctors, where prescribing was a major theme. I and the co-authors (working as clinical teaching fellows or with regular teaching roles) therefore ran prescribing tutorials for medical students, and received hugely positive feedback from them. This encouraged us to publish the data from the tutorials, present at conferences and ultimately write this textbook.

We believe our textbook fills a gap in a critical subject area by relating to medical students and junior doctors in a practical and accessible way. We have tried to ensure this by basing it on our own experiences as junior doctors. It is concise enough to be used as a ward guide, particularly as the DRUGS Checklists provide a quick summary of how to write prescriptions. The book also contains MCQs on a companion website (see the link at the end of each chapter) for those revising for the Prescribing Skills Assessment or wanting to test their knowledge. The website also has easily accessible DRUGS Checklist boxes, where important information is condensed for ease of reference.

We hope this book helps you to avoid mistakes, learn tips from doctors who have gone before you and be the best doctor you can be. Good Luck!

Georgia Woodfield
Benedict Lyle Phillips
Victoria Taylor
Amy Hawkins
Andrew Stanton

References

Dornan T, Ashcroft D, Heathfield H *et al.* (2009). *Final report. An in Depth Investigation into Causes of Prescribing Errors by Foundation Trainees in Relation to their Medical Education. Equip Study.* Available at: www.gmc-uk.org/FINAL_Report_prevalence_and_causes_of_prescribing_errors.pdf_28935150.pdf (accessed Dec. 2015).

Illing J, Morrow G, Kergon C *et al.* (2008). *How Prepared are Medical Graduates to Begin Practice? A Comparison of Three Diverse UK Medical Schools.* Available at: www.gmc-uk.org/FINAL_How_prepared_are_medical_graduates_to_begin_practice_September_08.pdf_29697834.pdf (accessed Dec. 2015).

NHS National Patient Safety Agency (NPSA) (2009). National Reporting and Learning Service. *Safety in Doses Improving the Use of Medicines in the NHS. Learning from National Reporting 2007.* Available at: www.nrls.npsa.nhs.uk/resources/?entryid45=61625 (accessed Dec. 2015).

Acknowledgements

We are most grateful to a number of our colleagues from the Great Western Hospital, the University of Bristol and London for their time and expertise in reviewing and providing valuable comments and suggestions to improve sections of the book.

Chapter 2 Emergency Department: Dr Clare Taylor, Emergency Medicine Consultant at the Royal United Hospitals, Bath

Chapter 3 Cardiology: Dr Andrianos Kontogeorgis, Senior Clinical Fellow in Cardiology and Electrophysiology at the Royal Brompton Hospital, London

Chapter 5 Gastroenterology: Dr Ajeya Shetty, Gastroenterology Consultant at the Great Western Hospital, Swindon

Chapter 6 Neurology: Dr Stephan Hinze, Neurology Consultant at the Great Western Hospital, Swindon

Chapter 7 Surgery: Dr Tony Pickworth, Consultant Anaesthetist at the Great Western Hospital Swindon

Chapter 8 Care of the Elderly: Dr Sameer Maini, Care of the Elderly Consultant at the Great Western Hospital, Swindon

Chapter 9 Anticipatory Prescribing at the End of Life: Professor Karen Forbes, Palliative Medicine Consultant at the University Hospitals, Bristol

Chapter 10 Renal: Dr Gavin Dreyer, Specialist Registrar in Nephrology in the NE London Deanery, Dr Rhys Evans, Specialist Registrar in Nephrology in the NE London Deanery and Dr Ulla Hemmilä, Specialist Registrar in Nephrology in the NE London Deanery

Chapter 11 Microbiology: Dr Robert Baker, Microbiology Consultant at the Musgrove Park Hospital, Taunton

Chapter 12 Rheumatology: Dr Lyn Williamson, Rheumatology Consultant at the Great Western Hospital, Swindon

Chapter 13 Dermatology: Dr Sam Gibbs, Dermatology Consultant at the Great Western Hospital, Swindon

Chapter 14 Obstetrics and Gynaecology: Mr Kevin Jones, Obstetrics and Gynaecology Consultant at the Great Western Hospital, Swindon

Chapter 15 Diabetes: Professor Andy Levy, Consultant Endocrinologist, University Hospitals, Bristol

Thank you also to Dr Stanton for believing in us and supporting us every step of the way.

How to use your textbook

Features contained within your textbook

Every chapter begins with **key topics** of the chapter and the **learning objectives** to the topic.

◀ **Key topics** give a summary of the topics covered in a chapter.

Learning objectives describe the main learning points in a chapter.

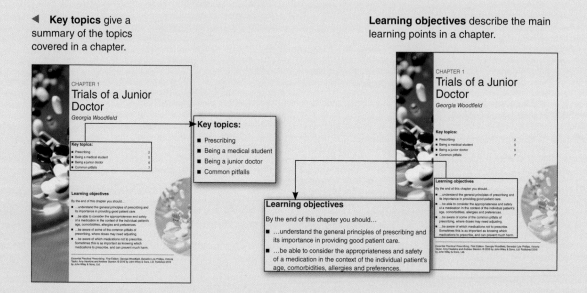

Case studies give practical clinical examples of prescribing for each key topic

DRUGS checklists give the Dose/Route/Units/Given/Special Situations for each drug discussed in the book. These are also available on the companion website.

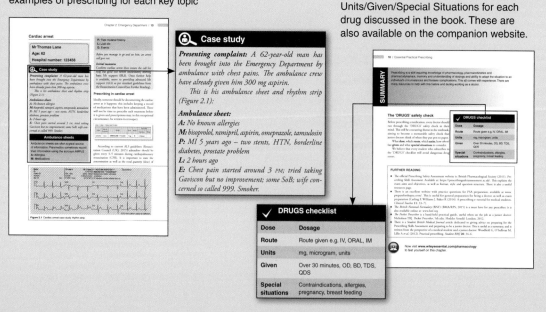

▶ **Top tip boxes** give inside information on a topic.

[TOP TIP] Adrenaline and other emergency medication often come pre-made-up in a special device, such as a 'mini-jet'. It's a good idea to learn how to use these before you need to use one in an emergency. You could ask your local Resus Officer or one of the emergency medicine physicians to show you.

▶ **Guidelines boxes** direct you to the latest online guidance on a topic.

① Guidelines

NICE provides the following guidance for post-acute management of suspected anaphylaxis (NICE, 2011):
Prior to discharge, all patients should
- Be observed for 6–12 hours
- Be offered an adrenaline autoinjector (these usually contain 300 micrograms of adrenaline) and be taught how to use it
- Be offered a referral to a specialist allergy clinic
- Be advised how to avoid the allergen, if known

Evidence boxes direct you to the key evidence and drug trials on a topic.

🔍 Evidence

Evidence is difficult to obtain in arrest situations but some studies have been carried out which suggest that adrenaline improves the chances of return of spontaneous circulation (ROSC). No study has determined the optimal dose or number of doses that should be used. There is no good evidence that the use of adrenaline during cardiac arrest improves the chances of survival to discharge and, worryingly, more recent reviews of the available evidence suggest that the use of adrenaline may be associated with poorer long-term outcomes (Callaway, 2013; Miller, 2013). Further studies are underway, including a randomised control trial (RCT).

Key learning points boxes give a summary of the topics covered in a section.

🔑 Key learning points

Cardiac arrest
- Currently recommended medication is: 1:10000 adrenaline, 1 mg IV every 3–5 minutes.
- Adrenaline should be given as soon as possible in non-shockable cardiac arrest situations. Shocks should not be delayed to give adrenaline in shockable rhythms.

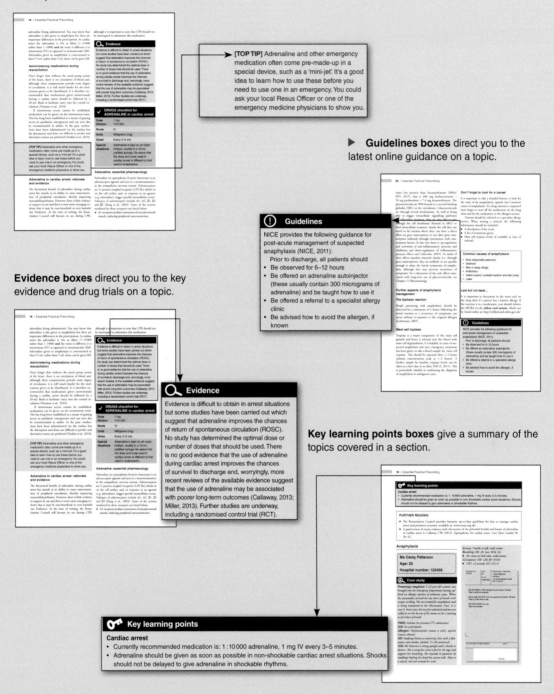

About the companion website

Don't forget to visit the companion website for this book:

www.wileyessential.com/prescribing

There you will find valuable material designed to enhance your learning, including:

- MCQs
- Downloadable DRUGS checklists

Scan this QR code to visit the companion website

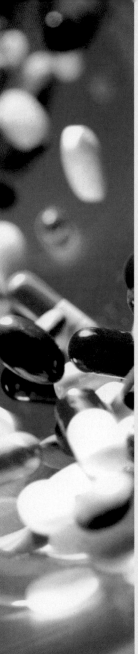

CHAPTER 1
Trials of a Junior Doctor

Georgia Woodfield

Key topics:

Learning objectives

By the end of this chapter you should…

- …understand the general principles of prescribing and its importance in providing good patient care.

- …be able to consider the appropriateness and safety of a medication in the context of the individual patient's age, comorbidities, allergies and preferences.

- …be aware of some of the common pitfalls of prescribing, where doses may need adjusting.

- …be aware of which medications *not* to prescribe. Sometimes this is as important as knowing which medications to prescribe, and can prevent much harm.

Essential Practical Prescribing, First Edition. Georgia Woodfield, Benedict Lyle Phillips, Victoria Taylor, Amy Hawkins and Andrew Stanton. © 2016 by John Wiley & Sons, Ltd. Published 2016 by John Wiley & Sons, Ltd.

Prescribing

Introduction

Prescribing is a daunting task as a junior doctor. No pharmacology textbook can prepare you for the responsibility of signing your name to a drug and giving it to your patient. The best preparation is practice but there are a few key principles that will prevent major errors being made. It is well recognised that drug errors are a major cause of patient morbidity and mortality, hence prescribing was a key area targeted by the National Patient Safety Agency (NPSA, 2007). In a 2009 GMC report, 9% of hospital prescriptions contained errors, with FY1 doctors making 8.4% of prescription errors and FY2 doctors making 10.3% of errors (highest error rate) in 19 UK hospitals on 7 days. In addition, a 2008 GMC report of medical students moving to FY1 showed prescribing was the 'main area of practice in which errors were reported, indicating a significant potential risk' (GMC, 2008). One conclusion for the 2012 review of Tomorrow's Doctors guidance (GMC, 2009a) was that development of ward-based teaching of prescribing should be supported.

General prescribing principles

A few basic rules go a long way with regards to writing a drug on a drug chart. With every prescription, all of the following need to be clearly specified; then there can be no mistake with the prescription side of things:

- Correctly identify the patient with at least three identifiers on the drug chart: full name, date of birth, NHS number (these three are the legal minimum) and hospital number.
- Write the date and time.
- All allergies must be written clearly at the front of the drug chart.
- Write the drug in the correct section of the chart: once-only drugs, regular, as required, variable prescriptions, infusions and fluids section; some charts have a dedicated thromboprophylaxis section, insulin section and antibiotic section.
- Write the drug name clearly, with its formulation if required (e.g. insulin is not enough, the formulation has to be specified, e.g. NovoRapid insulin) and ideally in capital letters for clarity.
- Choose the correct dose with clear units. Milligrams can be abbreviated to mg and millilitres to mL, whereas 'units' must be written in full, as must 'microgram' or 'microlitre' to prevent confusion with a mu (μ) abbreviation.
- The route must be specified. Oral can be abbreviated to PO, intravenous to IV, intramuscular to IM, subcutaneous to SC and topical to TOP (Table 1.1).
- The timing must be specified. Once daily can be abbreviated to OD, twice daily can be abbreviated to BD, three times daily can be abbreviated to TDS, four times daily can be abbreviated to QDS. 'As required' can be abbreviated to PRN but the maximum frequency has to be specified. Any other frequencies should be written in full for clarity, e.g. 'every Monday, Wednesday and Friday'. Don't forget to cross through days where the drug is not required to ensure it is not administered by accident. The frequency and specific hour is clarified by circling the corresponding time on the prescription chart.
- A start and stop date (if applicable) must be specified.

Table 1.1 Abbreviations used to indicate drug timings.

Abbreviation	Latin	English translation
OD	Omne die	Once daily
BD	Bis die	Twice daily
TDS	Ter die sumendus	Three time per day
QDS	Quarta die sumendus	Four times per day
OM	Omne mane	Every morning
ON	Omne nocte	Every evening
PRN	Pro re nata	As needed
Stat	Statim	Immediately

- The indication must be specified for all antibiotics and unusual or important drugs that must not be stopped, e.g. trimethoprim for urinary tract infection, tacrolimus for renal transplant. The more information the better.
- Any further instructions go into the 'additional information' box, e.g. alendronate requires the patient to stay upright for 30 minutes following ingestion. Often the pharmacist will add this specific information.
- The prescriber's signature and printed name must accompany every prescription, as well as a contact number or bleep.

Navigating a drug chart

Most drug charts follow a set pattern and layout. There is a dedicated section for once-only drugs, regular, as required and variable prescription (Figure 1.1). There is usually an infusion and fluids section, but this can be on a separate chart. Some charts have a dedicated thromboprophylaxis section, antibiotic section and insulin section.

Calculating drug doses

There are number of drugs that require weight-specific prescriptions. For instance, enoxaparin at a therapeutic dose for treatment of deep vein thrombosis/pulmonary embolism (DVT/PE) has to be given at 1.5 mg per kg. This may be reduced to 1 mg per kg in renal impairment. Many drugs need half-dose reduction in renal failure; see Common pitfalls section.

However, the most confusing drug dosings to calculate are the infusion rates, as medics are so used to prescribing in mg rather than mL per hour. This involves checking the concentration of the drug (e.g. 1 mg per mL), then prescribing both the number of mg but also the corresponding number of mL per hour. One tip for this is using the drug administrations guide that nurses will have on every ward. This specifies the different available preparations of drugs, their concentration, which crystalloid they should be mixed with and the speed of administration. Always check calculations, and ask pharmacists to help with unfamiliar drugs.

Using the British National Formulary

The *British National Formulary* (BNF) (BMA/RPS, 2015) can be hard to use at first, but is a great resource which is nationally recognised and updated every 6 months. A common initial difficulty with the BNF is that it works strictly by drug and classes of drug, rather than by conditions. It therefore relies on you knowing which drug you require and the indication. It will not tell you alternate drugs to use for a certain condition. Sometimes the clinical situation, therefore, does not tally with the situation in the BNF, leaving the inexperienced prescriber unsure how to proceed. One solution to this are books such as the *Pocket Prescriber* (Nicholson, 2012). This is small, portable and easy to use for common prescriptions. The BNF app on the iPhone is also free of charge and very handy, needing no internet connection. Also, do not be afraid to ask a pharmacist.

Importantly, the BNF has a subsection for each drug detailing indications, cautions, contraindications, considerations in hepatic and renal impairment, pregnancy and breastfeeding, as well as a pretty exhaustive list of side effects. There is also an entire section (appendix 1) detailing possible drug interactions (BMA/RPS, 2015).

Prescribing blood products

Prescribing blood is similar to prescribing any other medication, except that there is usually a dedicated prescribing chart for blood products, which is also separate from the fluid prescribing chart. The specific blood component must be specified, for example packed red cells (what is conventionally thought of as a blood transfusion), platelets, fresh frozen plasma (FFP), cryoprecipitate and factor VIII. Blood products are prescribed by number of units (or number of pools in the case of platelets) rather than as a volume. This is because the volume varies each time. The time over which the unit is run is important, as the maximum time over which 1 unit of packed red calls can run is 4 hours. This is to prevent the blood spending too long at an ambient temperature, which could allow bacterial proliferation and clots to form. Platelets generally consist of a lower volume and are run through quickly, as is FFP as this is usually given in large

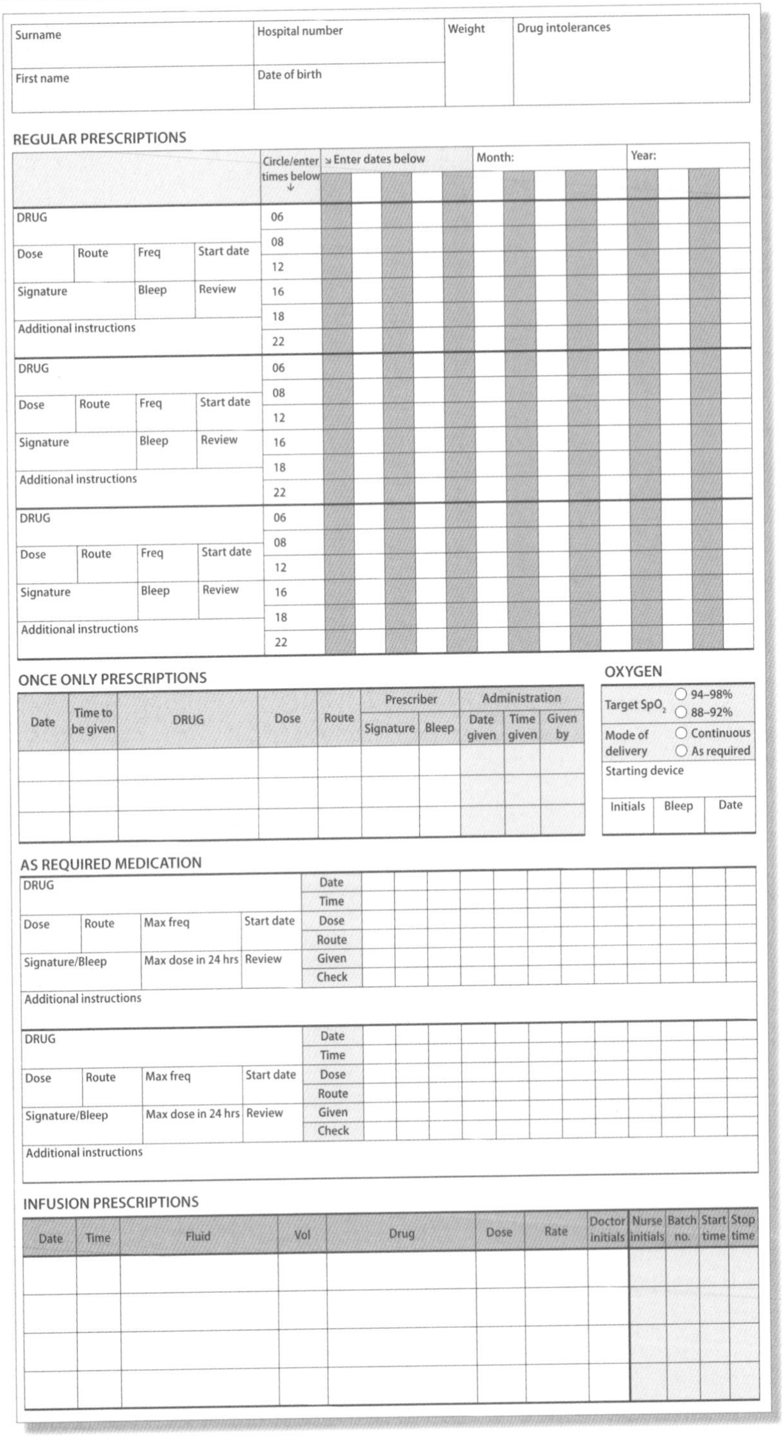

Surname	Hospital number	Weight	Drug intolerances
First name	Date of birth		

REGULAR PRESCRIPTIONS

	Circle/enter times below ↓	⌄ Enter dates below	Month:	Year:

DRUG				06
Dose	Route	Freq	Start date	08
				12
Signature		Bleep	Review	16
				18
Additional instructions				22

DRUG				06
Dose	Route	Freq	Start date	08
				12
Signature		Bleep	Review	16
				18
Additional instructions				22

DRUG				06
Dose	Route	Freq	Start date	08
				12
Signature		Bleep	Review	16
				18
Additional instructions				22

ONCE ONLY PRESCRIPTIONS

Date	Time to be given	DRUG	Dose	Route	Prescriber		Administration		
					Signature	Bleep	Date given	Time given	Given by

OXYGEN

Target SpO₂	○ 94–98% ○ 88–92%
Mode of delivery	○ Continuous ○ As required
Starting device	

Initials	Bleep	Date

AS REQUIRED MEDICATION

DRUG				Date	
				Time	
Dose	Route	Max freq	Start date	Dose	
				Route	
Signature/Bleep		Max dose in 24 hrs	Review	Given	
				Check	
Additional instructions					

DRUG				Date	
				Time	
Dose	Route	Max freq	Start date	Dose	
				Route	
Signature/Bleep		Max dose in 24 hrs	Review	Given	
				Check	
Additional instructions					

INFUSION PRESCRIPTIONS

Date	Time	Fluid	Vol	Drug	Dose	Rate	Doctor initials	Nurse initials	Batch no.	Start time	Stop time

Figure 1.1 A blank drug chart showing typical sections for regular, once-only, as-required and infusion medications.

bleed situations. Please see Chapter 7 Surgery to understand blood product prescribing more fully.

Prescribing fluids

All UK hospitals will have a section of the drug chart or a separate prescription form for IV fluids. The type of fluid, volume, speed of administration and any additives need to be specified. Please see the Fluid Management section of Chapter 7 Surgery for more detailed information about fluid prescribing.

Factors to consider when prescribing

There are a few other factors to consider when prescribing, apart from the correctness and clarity of the prescription itself. These start with patient choice and preferences. Sometimes patients have ideas and opinions regarding preferences for drug formulations and drug classes. For instance, some patients find ranitidine a more effective treatment for acid reflux than omeprazole, even though omeprazole has more evidence for its use. As the aim of this treatment is relief of symptoms, patient preference is the most important factor here.

Another important consideration is the legality surrounding prescribing. The prescription is a legal record of drug administration and hence needs to be a clear document providing factual evidence of what occurred, as well as recording the accountable parties. These parties would include the prescriber (mainly) but also the professional who administered the drug. It is therefore in your interest as a doctor to make all prescriptions as clear and informative as possible, as any mistakes could be directly attributed to you however good the intention. This is crucial in the age of increasing litigation and where dangerous agents are being administered to patients who are putting their faith in the medical profession.

Some drugs come in multiple formulations, where some may be more effective for certain conditions. For example, mesalazine for inflammatory bowel disease comes in numerous preparations such as Pentasa, which is occasionally used for Crohn's disease, whereas Asacol is commonly used for ulcerative colitis. In a similar way, morphine preparations vary in their speed of onset, duration and tolerance between patients.

Cost of medications is also a consideration, but not generally for a junior doctor. Cheapest options are generally tried first, for example omeprazole, before changing to more expensive products in the drug class such as esomeprazole if effectiveness or tolerability is an issue.

Being a medical student

Preparing for the prescribing skills assessment

Prescribing is a daunting task as a junior doctor. No pharmacology textbook can prepare you for the responsibility of signing your name to a drug and giving it to your patient. However, despite the immediate need for junior doctors to prescribe drugs safely and effectively upon qualification (GMC, 2009b), there is variation in how this is taught at universities. For this reason the Prescribing Skills Assessment (PSA) has been developed to ensure a basic level of understanding and experience in prescribing before graduation.

In order to practise as a foundation doctor in some deaneries (from August 2015), this examination must be passed, and has been adopted by many medical schools as a component of finals examinations.

The content of the exam is designed to represent common scenarios and test essential knowledge. The majority of questions therefore focus on medical emergencies such as chronic obstructive pulmonary disease (COPD) exacerbations, asthma attacks, pulmonary oedema and acute coronary syndrome. The questions that many find most difficult are about side effects and interactions of commonly prescribed drugs. These can be looked up in the BNF (BMA/RPS, 2015), but this is time consuming and stressful in an exam situation, particularly because the BNF tends to list every side effect without discussing the most important. It is therefore worth knowing side effects of commonly prescribed drugs such as statins and beta blockers before the exam. The best way to prepare for the PSA is therefore to revise medical emergency prescribing and common drugs, rather than trying to learn long lists of side effects of less common drugs. Useful books are therefore those that focus in on these common scenarios and are perhaps less detailed, such as the *Pocket Prescriber*. This has a section on medical emergencies, which includes information on side effects and interactions of specific drugs (Nicholson, 2012). Other useful resources are the BNF, NICE guidelines on common treatment regimens, as well as pharmacology text books.

Preparing to be an FY1

The PSA is based on scenarios that junior doctors prescribe for, so preparing for the PSA is excellent practice for FY1. However, theory of prescribing is one thing, but problems can be highlighted when put in a specific patient situation with the responsibility of writing out the prescription. Practical skills such as catheterisation are taught using simulation and models, yet prescribing is often taught with a more theoretical approach. It is therefore really useful to practise writing on real drug charts. This can be done by practising prescribing scenarios with other students using specific patient examples, or writing mock prescriptions for patients after seeing them on the ward. This is an excellent way of practising because when presenting the history and examination to a senior or presenting on the post take ward round, the mock drug chart can also be checked. This gives valuable feedback to the student and highlights common and easy to make mistakes. It is much better to learn this way than to make the mistakes in real life. Of course, it is imperative that the mock drug chart is not confused with the real drug chart. This could be avoided by writing 'Student Practice Drug Chart: Not for Ward Use' on the front and doing it away from the bedside.

Simulation tutorials can also be useful for learning about prescribing. These consist of students being given a simulated patient case (which could be a written case) and being asked to prescribe on drug charts for the first 5 to 30 minutes of the patient's care. This simulates the situation that occurs when seeing any new patient as a junior doctor, with the focus being to stabilise the patient before a senior can come to help (Woodfield *et al.*, 2014).

Being a junior doctor

Common bleeps relating to prescribing

Many of the common bleeps that a new doctor receives involve aspects of prescribing. Most common

requests include prescriptions for analgesia, antiemetics, laxatives, IV fluids, warfarin and sedation for agitated/aggressive patients. Medication review may also be requested for confused patients or those with new renal impairment. Medications may also be implicated in other requests, such as requests to review a patient with new confusion, a rash, diarrhoea, low blood pressure or high/low heart rate.

Things I wish I had known

Six things I wish I had done on Week 1 to help with prescribing:

1. Printed out the protocols for common presentations for quick reference: Diabetes Ketoacidosis (DKA) Insulin Chart, Acute Coronary Syndrome Protocol, Antibiotic Guidelines. Each hospital has slightly different guidelines.
2. Bought a clipboard for storage and instant access to spare blood forms, X-ray request forms, blood gas syringes, endoscopy request forms and blank sheets of paper.
3. Always had more than one pen.
4. Put out gentamicin level blood forms for the phlebotomist the day before with the time specified, so that the prescription can be reviewed effectively the following day.
5. Included patient's allergies on the ward handover list – particularly if there is history of anaphylaxis.
6. Written down the bleep numbers of all key people that I might need, rather than wasting time going through the switch board – this includes the pharmacist, physiotherapist, occupational therapist, microbiologist, biochemistry, haematology, transfusion and radiology departments.

What to do when you don't know

- **Ask** – it is always best to check prescriptions, as the potential damage is huge. This includes patient safety considerations, patient harm/death, breach of trust, upset, as well as legal and litigation considerations.
- Ask your senior if there is any misunderstanding about the indication or preparation of an intended

drug, and check with the pharmacy the dosing, always ensuring that they have taken into account other factors such as allergies and renal function. This is both of your responsibilities, but you are likely to know the patent better and are in a good position to give this vital information.

- The microbiology registrar/consultant are frequently the go-to individuals for advice regarding antibiotics and antivirals.
- If there is doubt about a person's regular medication, or dosing at home, the GP practice should have an up-to-date prescription list that they can fax to you. GP surgery secretaries will sometimes read these out over the phone, but a fax is a much more reliable written record. Family members are often also very useful for this, but care must be taken not to rely on the word of a non-qualified individual, particularly if you have no written record of the medications they are recommending.
- Part of the pharmacist's job for every new admission is medicine reconciliation. This means checking that all the medications that a patient is taking at home have been accounted for and that the doses are correct. This is a safety net where the drug history is unclear.

Common pitfalls

Poor renal function

Renally excreted drugs will accumulate in the body if renal function is impaired. This means that less of the drug is required to have the same effect. If the usual medication dose is given to someone with renal failure, the medication may become toxic or may over-exert its effects, as the concentration in the blood will be much higher than anticipated. Renally excreted drugs therefore must have their doses adjusted before being given to renally impaired patients. This is explained fully in Chapter 10 Renal.

The BNF has a section on renal impairment, with corrected doses depending on the creatinine clearance (BMA/RPS, 2015). There is also a renal handbook, which is very useful and freely available online, endorsed by the UK Renal Pharmacy Group (Ashley *et al.*, 2009).

However, it is essential that junior doctors are aware of the commonly prescribed drugs that need adjusting in renal failure (please see Chapter 10 Renal for full information):

1. Metformin causes lactic acidosis in renal failure. Consider sliding scale insulin as a replacement if blood sugar needs controlling in this situation.
2. Angiotensin-converting enzyme (ACE) inhibitors, angiotensin receptor blockers (ARBs), spironolactone and furosemide all worsen renal failure and should be withheld in acute kidney injury (although furosemide is sometimes used in acute kidney impairment [AKI]).
3. Antibiotic (in particular gentamicin and vancomycin) levels must be taken to guide dosing to avoid severe nephrotoxicity and ototoxicity. Augmentin IV and Tazocin also have renal dosing regimes (BD rather than TDS).
4. Low molecular weight heparin is usually given at half the dose for people with an estimated glomerular filtration rate (eGFR) <30.
5. Digoxin is renally excreted and will therefore accumulate in renal failure. This is very important to be aware of as it also has a narrow therapeutic index, meaning it will cause toxicity at a relatively low level. Digoxin levels must therefore be taken and digoxin withheld if there is any suspicion of toxicity.

Pregnancy

In any pregnant person, the risk versus benefits must be considered of any medication, as any drug in the mother's blood stream has a risk of affecting the fetus. The BNF has a section on pregnancy (BMA/RPS, 2015). For many common drugs there is enough evidence of their use in pregnancy to be confident that there is little risk to the fetus (e.g. laxatives, paracetamol, some antiemetics and omeprazole). However, there are very few trials on pregnant women, and this tends to be a relatively healthy group, so there is often limited evidence regarding safety of drugs. It is therefore always best to look up all intended prescriptions in the BNF or potentially ask a member of the obstetrics and gynaecology team, as they have the most experience of prescribing in pregnancy. Please see Chapter 14 Obstetrics and Gynaecology.

The elderly

Elderly patients bring a further set of prescribing considerations (see Chapter 8 Care of the Elderly). The prescription itself may need to be altered as body weight may be <50 kg; however, the formulation of the medication may also need alteration. Some tablets are large and may be difficult to swallow, hence liquid preparations may be more appropriate, or a person may find capsules easier than tablets. Pill burden may also be a consideration and combination tablets may reduce this (e.g. co-codamol rather than codeine and paracetamol separately). Tablets may also need to be spaced throughout the day to make the regimen more manageable, as a difficult and troublesome regimen will increase the chances of poor compliance.

Polypharmacy is also a concern from the perspective of drug interactions, possibility of harm from side effects as well as increased chance of poor compliance. The ability to rationalise medications is very important, and often falls to GPs and care-of-the-elderly physicians, but it should be every doctor's job. Rationalising medications involves weighing up the potential benefit of the medication versus the harm, and thereby stopping non-essential drugs with the aim of prioritising the patient's main health problems and quality of life. One example could be stopping a statin in an elderly man who is struggling to swallow tablets, as a statin has a long-term benefit which the patient may not receive. This rationale could stand for any primary or secondary preventative medication in an elderly or very unwell patient.

Allergies

Beware of allergies to specific drugs, particularly serious allergies, as the patient may well be allergic to other medications in that group. For example, an allergy to ramipril is likely to infer an allergy to lisinopril. There are also cross-over allergies. For example, a percentage of patients who are allergic to penicillins are also allergic to cephalosporins, thought to be because they share a common betalactam ring. This should only influence prescribing if the allergy is a serious anaphylactic reaction, as otherwise this would rule out a whole class of antibiotics to a lot of patients unnecessarily. Also, the rate of serious reactions is only around 0.04–0.08% (Herbert *et al.*, 2000) (see Chapter 11 Microbiology). However, it is also true that patient with serious penicillin allergies are more likely to be allergic to any class of antibiotic, hence caution is required with all antibiotic prescriptions.

Morphine preparations

Morphine must be prescribed with its brand name as well as its route, as this greatly affects its absorption, speed of onset and duration of action. Morphine can be given IV, SC, topically, as an IV or SC infusion, orally in tablets or orally in liquid. Please see Chapter 7 Surgery on analgesia, as well as Chapter 9 Anticipatory prescribing at the end of life on prescribing in palliative care. The route and formulation are greatly affected by the type of pain, potential for reversibility and co-morbidities of the patient.

Hyponatraemia

Hyponatraemia can lead to confusion and drowsiness and may contribute to poor quality of life and falls. Low sodium levels can be iatrogenic, hence this must be considered in patients with a persistently low sodium.

Drugs that worsen hyponatraemia are:

1. Non-steroidal-anti-inflammatory drugs (NSAIDs) cause increased total body water, therefore have a dilutional effect. They lead to euvolaemic hyponatraemia, and have no effect on total body sodium.
2. Thiazide and loop diuretics increase renal water losses and cause the excretion of urine that is sodium and potassium-rich (Sterns, 2011). Loop diuretics are less likely than thiazides to cause hyponatraemia, unless they cause severe volume depletion (Agrawal *et al.*, 2008).
3. Antidepressants, including tricyclics and selective serotonin reuptake inhibitors (SSRIs), can lead to the syndrome of inappropriate secretion of antidiuretic hormone (SIADH). This is thought to be because serotonin is involved

in regulating ADH secretion (Kadowaki *et al.*, 1983). SIADH can be managed by fluid restriction, but consultation with a psychiatrist may be required to consider alternative antidepressants (such as a monoamine oxidase inhibitor).

4. Morphine and other opioids can have an antidiuretic action, leading to euvolaemic hyponatraemia (Porter and Kaplan, 2011).

5. Carbamazepine increases total body water with whole-body sodium levels unaffected, causing euvolaemic hyponatraemia (Porter and Kaplan, 2011).

Cardiac failure

Any drug that slows heart rate or reduces myocardial contractility may potentially exacerbate heart failure in someone with a chronically failing heart. Please see Chapter 3 Cardiology.

Drugs to be aware of in heart failure are:

1. Beta blockers slow heart rate and depress myocardium, hence are contraindicated in acute cardiac failure as they are likely to worsen pulmonary oedema. However, low-dose beta blockers have prognostic benefits for chronic cardiac failure (CCF), but high doses can precipitate acute deterioration. The dose therefore needs titration. Bisoprolol and carvedilol have the most evidence in CCF. Patients with CCF should therefore be on a beta blocker unless it cannot be tolerated (see Chapter 3 Cardiology).

2. Dihydropyridine Ca channel blockers (amlodipine, nifedipine) are negatively ionotropic and reduce myocardial contractility.

3. Phenylalkylamine Ca channel blockers (verapamil and diltiazem) are highly negatively ionotropic, and depress cardiac function, more than the Dihydropyridine Ca channel blockers (see BNF [BMA/RPS, 2015]).

4. Flecainide can have proarrhythmic effects in CCF (see BNF [BMA/RPS, 2015]). Do not give if there is a history of myocardial infarction.

5. Fast IV fluid/blood has an increased risk of fluid overload in CCF, therefore caution and reassessment are needed. The solution is slow maintenance fluid replacement and giving 1 unit blood over the maximum time (4 hours) with furosemide cover.

Compliance

Even with the best prescribing knowledge, no benefit will be transferred to the patient without compliance to the intended medication regimen. This is a complex area as there are many reasons why patients do not take their medications. The key reasons that doctors can ensure are eliminated are lack of adequate explanation and poor understanding of the rationale. It is the doctor's and pharmacist's job to explain why medications will be useful and what the expected effects will be. If there is a lag before the drug will become effective the patient must know about this so that they don't give up on the drug too early. They also must be advised about what to do in the event of side effects, as many of these can be easily managed without withdrawing the drug.

The patient must also have faith in the medical professional and trust that the medication may help them. Without this, it is unlikely that they will take it.

Other factors may be social stigma, such as in a young diabetic having to inject insulin at meal times, or an HIV-positive patient having to take antiretrovirals. This can be addressed by exploring the patient's ideas, concerns and expectations and trying to find a solution.

Side effects, or perceived side effects, are of course a large reason for poor compliance. A large pill burden or necessity for frequent medication throughout the day may also influence compliance. Some drugs also require frequent monitoring, such as warfarin requiring regular INR blood tests. These factors may culminate in patients missing appointments and missing medications.

The patient must also have a desire to improve their symptoms. Some individuals have given up hope and may have very low mood, meaning that they no longer have the will to improve their condition. Alternatively, patients may feel they can help themselves without the need for medical input, and may prefer to take homeopathic or alternative therapies first.

SUMMARY

Prescribing is a skill requiring knowledge of pharmacology, pharmacokinetics and pharmacodynamics, memory and understanding of dosings and ability to adapt the situation to an individual's circumstances and foresee complications. This all comes with experience. There are many resources to help with this before and during working as a doctor.

The 'DRUGS' safety check

Before prescribing a medication, every doctor should run through the 'DRUGS' safety check in their mind. This will be a recurring theme in the textbook, aiming to become a memorable safety check that junior doctors think of when they put pen to paper.

What **dose**, which **route**, which **units**, how often/fast **given** and what **special situations** to consider.

We believe that every student who subscribes to the 'DRUGS' checklist will avoid dangerous drug errors.

✓ DRUGS checklist	
Dose	Dosage
Route	Route given e.g. IV, ORAL, IM
Units	mg, microgram, units
Given	Over 30 minutes, OD, BD, TDS, QDS
Special situations	Contraindications, allergies, pregnancy, breast feeding

---

FURTHER READING

- The official Prescribing Safety Assessment website is: British Pharmacological Society (2011). *Prescribing Skills Assessment*. Available at: https://prescribingsafetyassessment.ac.uk/. This explains the exam aims and objectives, as well as format, style and question structure. There is also a useful resources page.
- There is an excellent website with practice questions for PSA preparation, available at www.prepareforthepsa.com/. This is useful for general preparation for being a doctor, as well as exam preparation (Catling F, Williams J, Baker R (2014). A prescribing e–tutorial for medical students. *Clinical Teache*r **11**: 33–7).
- The *British National Formulary* (BNF) (BMA/RPS, 2015) is a must have for any prescriber; it is also available online at: www.bnf.org
- *The Pocket Prescriber* is a hand-held practical guide, useful when on the job as a junior doctor: Nicholson TRJ. *Pocket Prescriber*, 5th edn. Hodder Arnold: London, 2012.
- There is a *Student British Medical Journal* article dedicated to giving advice on preparing for the Prescribing Skills Assessment and preparing to be a junior doctor. This is useful as a summary, and is written from the perspective of a medical student and a junior doctor: Woodfield G, O'Sullivan M, Lillie A *et al.* (2012). Practical prescribing. *Student BMJ* **20**: 34–6.

 Now visit **www.wileyessential.com/pharmacology** to test yourself on this chapter.

References

Agrawal V, Agarwal M, Joshi S *et al.* (2008). Hyponatremia and hypernatremia: disorders of water balance. *J Assoc Physicians India* **56**, 956–64.

Ashley C, Currie A: UK Renal Pharmacy Group (2009). *The Renal Drug Handbook*, 3rd edn. Radcliffe Publishing, Oxford.

British Medical Association and Royal Pharmaceutical Society of Great Britain (BMA/RPS) (2015). *British National Formulary 69*, 69th edn. BMJ group and Pharmaceutical Press, London. Available at: www.bnf.org (accessed Dec. 2015).

General Medical Council (GMC) (2009a). *Tomorrow's Doctors*. Available at: www.gmc-uk.org/ Tomorrow_s_Doctors_1214.pdf_48905759. pdf (accessed Dec 2015).

General Medical Council (GMC): Dornan T, Ashcroft D, Heathfield H *et al.* (2009b). *Final Report. An in Depth Investigation into Causes of Prescribing Errors by Foundation Trainees in Relation to their Medical Education. EQUIP Study.* Available at: http://www.gmc-uk.org/FINAL_ Report_prevalence_and_causes_of_prescribing_ errors.pdf_28935150.pdf (accessed Aug. 2012).

General Medical Council (GMC): Illing J, Morrow G, Kergon C *et al.* (2008) *How Prepared are Medical Graduates to Begin Practice? A Comparison of Three Diverse UK Medical Schools.* Available at: http://www.gmc-uk.org/FINAL_ How_prepared_are_medical_graduates_to_ begin_practice_September_08.pdf_29697834. pdf (accessed Aug. 2012).

Herbert M, Scott Brewster G, Lanctot-Herbert M (2000). Ten percent of patients who are allergic to penicillin will have serious reactions if exposed to cephalosporins. *West J Med* **172**: 341.

Kadowaki T, Hagura R, Kajinuma H *et al.* (1983). Chlorpropamide-induced hyponatremia: incidence and risk factors. *Diabetes Care* **6**: 468–71.

NHS National Patient Safety Agency (NPSA) (2007). *Safety in Doses Improving the Use of Medicines in the NHS. Learning from National Reporting.* National Reporting and Learning Service. Available at: www.nrls.npsa.nhs.uk/ resources/?entryid45=61625 (accessed Aug. 2012).

Nicholson TRJ (2012). *Pocket Prescriber*, 5th edn. Hodder Arnold, London.

Porter R, Kaplan J (2011). Hyponatraemia. In: *The Merck Manual for Health Care Professionals.* Merck Sharp & Dohme Corp: NJ, USA. Available at: http://www.merckmanuals.com/professional/ endocrine_and_metabolic_disorders/electrolyte_ disorders/hyponatremia.html (accessed Aug. 2012).

Sterns R (2011). *Diuretic-Induced Hyponatraemia.* Available at: http://www.uptodate.com/contents/ diuretic-induced-hyponatremia (accessed Aug. 2012).

Woodfield G, O'Sullivan M, Haddington N *et al.* (2014). Using simulation for prescribing; an evaluation. *Clinical Teacher* **11**: 24–8.

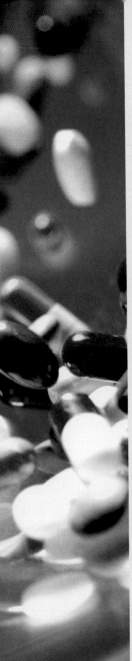

CHAPTER 2
Emergency Department

Victoria Taylor

Key topics:

NB. Other topics that would primarily be dealt with by emergency physicians or acute medicine physicians include: sepsis, acute arrhythmias, diabetic ketoacidosis and seizures. These are dealt with separately in the relevant specialty chapters.

Learning objectives

By the end of this chapter you should…

- …be able to recall the name, dose and route of administration for the key drugs used in anaphylaxis and cardiac arrest.

- …be able to describe the treatment of paracetamol overdose and acute alcohol withdrawal syndrome.

- …be aware of some of the difficulties of producing an evidence base for emergency scenarios.

Essential Practical Prescribing, First Edition. Georgia Woodfield, Benedict Lyle Phillips, Victoria Taylor, Amy Hawkins and Andrew Stanton. © 2016 by John Wiley & Sons, Ltd. Published 2016 by John Wiley & Sons, Ltd.

Cardiac arrest

> **Mr Thomas Lane**
>
> **Age: 62**
>
> **Hospital number: 123456**

🔍 Case study

Presenting complaint: *A 62-year-old man has been brought into the Emergency Department by ambulance with chest pains. The ambulance crew have already given him 300 mg aspirin.*

This is his ambulance sheet and rhythm strip (Figure 2.1):

Ambulance sheet:
A: *No known allergies*
M: *bisoprolol, ramipril, aspirin, omeprazole, tamsulosin*
P: *MI 5 years ago – two stents, HTN, borderline diabetes, prostate problem*
L: *2 hours ago*
E: *Chest pain started around 3 PM; tried taking Gaviscon but no improvement; some SoB; wife concerned so called 999. Smoker.*

Ambulance sheets

Ambulance sheets are often a great source of information. Paramedics sometimes record their information using the acronym AMPLE
A: Allergies
M: Medications
P: Past medical history
L: Last ate
E: Events

Before you manage to go and see him, an arrest call goes out.

Initial measures
Confirm cardiac arrest then ensure the call for help has gone out before immediately starting basic life support (BLS). Once further help is available, move to providing advanced life support (ALS) as per standard guidelines from the Resuscitation Council (see Further Reading).

Prescribing in cardiac arrest

Ideally, someone should be documenting the cardiac arrest as it happens; this includes keeping a record of medications that have been administered. There will not be time to prescribe each treatment before it is given and prescriptions may, in this exceptional circumstance, be written in retrospect.

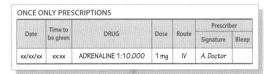

According to current ALS guidelines (Resuscitation Council (UK), 2015) adrenaline should be given every 3–5 minutes during cardiopulmonary resuscitation (CPR). It is important to state the *concentration* as well as the total *quantity* (dose) of

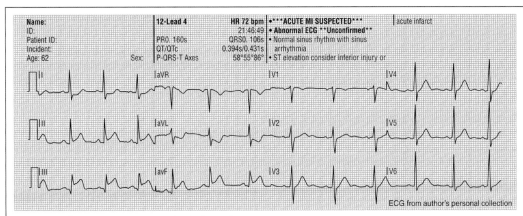

Figure 2.1 Cardiac arrest case study rhythm strip.

adrenaline being administered. You may know that adrenaline is also given in anaphylaxis but there are important differences in the prescriptions. In cardiac arrest the adrenaline is 10× as dilute (1:10 000 rather than 1:1000) **and** the route is different; it is intravenous (IV) as opposed to intramuscular (IM). Adrenaline given in anaphylaxis is concentrated so that 0.5 mL rather than 5 mL doses can be given IM.

Administering medications during resuscitation

Don't forget that without the usual pump action of the heart, there is no circulation of blood and, although chest compressions provide some degree of circulation, it is still much harder for the medications given to be distributed. It is therefore recommended that medications given intravenously during a cardiac arrest should be followed by a 20-mL flush to facilitate entry into the central circulation (Neumar *et al.*, 2010).

If intravenous access cannot be established, medication can be given via the intraosseous route. This has long been established as a means of gaining access in paediatric emergencies and can now also be recommended in adults. In the past, medications have been administered via the trachea but the absorption and doses are difficult to predict and alternative routes are preferred (Deakin *et al.*, 2010).

[TOP TIP] Adrenaline and other emergency medication often come pre-made-up in a special device, such as a 'mini-jet'. It's a good idea to learn how to use these before you need to use one in an emergency. You could ask your local Resus Officer or one of the emergency medicine physicians to show you.

Adrenaline in cardiac arrest: rationale and evidence

The theoretical benefit of adrenaline during cardiac arrest lies mainly in its ability to cause vasoconstriction of peripheral vasculature, thereby improving myocardial perfusion. However, there is little evidence to support its use and there is now some emerging evidence that it may be non-beneficial or even harmful (see Evidence). At the time of writing, the Resuscitation Council still favours its use during CPR,

although it is important to note that CPR should not be interrupted to administer this medication.

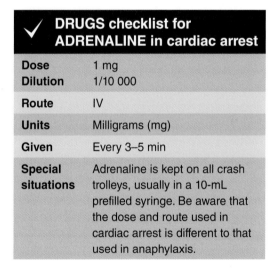

🔍 Evidence

Evidence is difficult to obtain in arrest situations but some studies have been carried out which suggest that adrenaline improves the chances of return of spontaneous circulation (ROSC). No study has determined the optimal dose or number of doses that should be used. There is no good evidence that the use of adrenaline during cardiac arrest improves the chances of survival to discharge and, worryingly, more recent reviews of the available evidence suggest that the use of adrenaline may be associated with poorer long-term outcomes (Callaway, 2013; Miller, 2013). Further studies are underway, including a randomised control trial (RCT).

✓ DRUGS checklist for ADRENALINE in cardiac arrest

Dose	1 mg
Dilution	1/10 000
Route	IV
Units	Milligrams (mg)
Given	Every 3–5 min
Special situations	Adrenaline is kept on all crash trolleys, usually in a 10-mL prefilled syringe. Be aware that the dose and route used in cardiac arrest is different to that used in anaphylaxis.

Adrenaline: essential pharmacology

Adrenaline (or epinephrine if you're American) is an adrenoceptor agonist and acts as a neurotransmitter in the sympathetic nervous system. Adrenoceptors are G-protein coupled receptors (GPCRs) which sit on the cell surface and, in response to an agonist (e.g. adrenaline), trigger specific intracellular events. Subtypes of adrenoceptor include $\alpha 1$, $\alpha 2$, $\beta 1$, $\beta 2$ and $\beta 3$ (Rang *et al.*, 2003). Some of the actions mediated by these receptors are listed below:

- $\alpha 1$-receptors mediate contraction of vascular smooth muscle, inducing peripheral vasoconstriction.

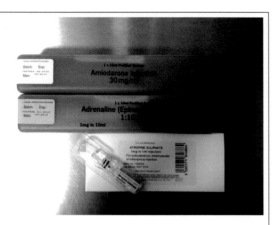

Figure 2.2 Medications from the cardiac arrest trolley.

- α2-receptors are responsible for negative feedback at nerve terminals and also decrease insulin secretion.
- β1-receptors mediate increases in the rate and force of myocardial contraction.
- β2-receptors mediate smooth muscle relaxation, inducing bronchodilation in the lungs, reduced motility of the GI tract and also relaxation of uterine muscle (tocolysis).
- β3-receptors promote lipolysis in adipose tissue.
  Be aware that beta-blockers and other adrenoceptor *antagonists* may blunt the effect of adrenaline in this situation.

Other medications used in cardiac arrest

Amiodarone: Expert consensus is that if ventricular fibrillation/ ventricular tachycardia (VF/VT) does not respond to three shocks, 300 mg IV amiodarone can be given as a bolus, followed by 900 mg IV amiodarone over the next 24 hours (Figure 2.2). If amiodarone is unavailable, lidocaine 1 mg/kg may be used.

Magnesium: This is only indicated if the arrest is due to polymorphic ventricular tachycardia (torsades de pointes).

Sodium bicarbonate: This is only indicated if the arrest is due to hyperkalaemia or tricyclic antidepressant overdose.

Case outcome

After one cycle of CPR, during which adrenaline was given, the rhythm was assessed and Mr Lane was found to be in VF: a shockable rhythm. He received a shock, and CPR was immediately resumed for 2 min. At the pulse check, he was found to have 'return of spontaneous circulation' (ROSC). He was stabilised and transferred to ITU. A coronary angiogram was subsequently performed which showed single-vessel disease. A drug-eluting coronary stent was used to open up the vessel and Mr Lane recovered in the Coronary Care Unit.

Although this case had a good outcome, less than 20% of patients who suffer an in-hospital cardiac arrest survive to discharge, despite the best care we can provide (Nolan *et al.*, 2014). The chances of surviving are higher if the patient develops a shockable rhythm.

Common pitfalls

- Be aware of the different concentrations of adrenaline available:
  - Adrenaline in cardiac arrest: 1 mg of **1:10 000** (10 mL)
  - Adrenaline in anaphylaxis: 500 micrograms of **1:1000** (0.5 mL).
- Note that atropine no longer appears in the ALS treatment algorithm (it previously appeared as part of the treatment of pulseless electrical activity (PEA)/ asystole arrests.

Every doctor should be familiar with the medications used in cardiac arrest, along with their doses and routes of administration. An ABC approach is warranted, as is early senior input, notably from an emergency physician or an anaesthetist.

SUMMARY

Key learning points

Cardiac arrest
- Currently recommended medication is: 1:10 000 adrenaline, 1 mg IV every 3–5 minutes.
- Adrenaline should be given as soon as possible in non-shockable cardiac arrest situations. Shocks should not be delayed to give adrenaline in shockable rhythms.

FURTHER READING

- The Resuscitation Council provides fantastic up-to-date guidelines for how to manage cardiac arrest and periarrest scenarios, available at: www.resus.org.uk/
- A good review of recent evidence with discussion of the potential benefits and harms of adrenaline in cardiac arrest is: Callaway CW (2013). Epinephrine for cardiac arrest. *Curr Opin Cardiol* 28: 36–42.

Anaphylaxis

Ms Carey Patterson

Age: 22

Hospital number: 123456

Case study

Presenting complaint: A 22-year-old woman was brought into the Emergency Department having suffered an allergic reaction of unknown cause. When the paramedics arrived she was short of breath with tongue swelling. She was treated for anaphylaxis and is being monitored in the Observation Unit. It is now 6 hours since she was first admitted and you are called to see her by one of the nurses as she is starting to feel short of breath.

PMH: Asthma (no previous ITU admissions)
DH: See prescription
Allergies: Oxytetracycline (causes a rash), aspirin (causes wheeze)
SH: Studying history at university; lives with 3 flatmates; non-smoker, alcohol: 15–30 units/week.
O/E: Ms Patterson is sitting upright and is clearly in distress. She is using her arms to fix her rib cage and support her breathing. She responds to questions by nodding/ shaking her head but cannot talk. There is a raised, red rash around her neck.

Airway: Unable to talk, mild stridor
Breathing: RR: 28; Sats: 96% OA
- *Air entry on both sides, mild wheeze*
Circulation: HR: 120; BP: 85/50
- *CRT <2 seconds; HS I+II+O*

PHARMACY STAMP	AGE 22	FORENAME, SURNAME Carey Patterson
	D.O.B. 12/02/1994	ADDRESS 2A, Southampton Street
		NHS NUMBER

SALBUTAMOL (100 micrograms per dose), inhaled.
Take 2 puffs as required.

BECLOMETASONE (100 micrograms per dose), inhaled.
Take 2 puffs twice a day.

MICROGYNON 30, oral.
Take as directed.

SIGNATURE OF PRESCRIBER	DATE

SP21000

Diagnosis

This patient has anaphylaxis (a severe allergic reaction) and has either been re-exposed to the allergen that triggered her initial episode or is experiencing the recurrence of symptoms, which is sometimes seen several hours after exposure, a so-called 'biphasic reaction'.

Initial measures

You should call for help. Assessment and treatment often occur concurrently in emergency situations such as this. An ABC approach should prompt you to assess and treat the most life-threatening symptoms before moving on to further assessment and treatment.

Prescribing for anaphylaxis

ONCE ONLY PRESCRIPTIONS						
Date	Time to be given	DRUG	Dose	Route	Prescriber Signature	Bleep
xx/xx/xx	xx:xx	OXYGEN	15L/minute	Inh	A. Doctor	
xx/xx/xx	xx:xx	ADRENALINE 1:1000	500 micrograms	IM	A. Doctor	
xx/xx/xx	xx:xx	CHLORPHENAMINE	10 mg	IV	A. Doctor	
xx/xx/xx	xx:xx	HYDROCORTISONE	200 mg	IV	A. Doctor	
xx/xx/xx	xx:xx	SALBUTAMOL	2.5 mg	Nebs	A. Doctor	

Concurrent assessment and treatment is required in anaphylaxis:

A: Tongue or lip swelling and stridor indicate there may also be pharyngeal or laryngeal oedema, both of which may obstruct the airway. **Adrenaline** is given to reverse these effects but an anaesthetist should be called in case there is a suboptimal response to medical therapy. **Oxygen** should be provided via a reservoir mask so that the gas that does get through is mainly oxygen.

B: You should check the S_pO_2 and listen for bilateral air entry as a silent chest suggests impending respiratory arrest. If the patient is deteriorating rapidly, it is appropriate to put out an arrest call. Bronchospasm can occur as part of an anaphylactic reaction, especially if the patient has underlying asthma. **Salbutamol** may be helpful to help relieve bronchospasm in these cases.

C: You should check the heart rate and blood pressure. If the patient doesn't already have IV access,

this would be the appropriate time to gain access, in order to give **hydrocortisone**, **chlorphenamine** and **IV fluids**. A fluid challenge (e.g. 500 mL of 0.9% saline) is appropriate to maintain a good circulating blood volume, as anaphylaxis may cause widespread vasodilation. Large volumes of fluid may be needed.

D: Always check the glucose and for evidence of neurological dysfunction.

E: Expose the patient for evidence of rashes or causes of the anaphylaxis and remove the trigger if you find one. This would include stopping any drug or colloid infusions or removing a bee sting etc.

The patient may also experience gastrointestinal disturbance and abdominal pain during an episode of anaphylaxis. Check the notes to ensure the history is consistent with anaphylaxis. Other causes of stridor include epiglottitis, which will not respond to the below medications and is likely to require surgical intervention.

It is important to note that not all healthcare staff may be aware that adrenaline given in anaphylaxis is an *intramuscular* medication. It is your responsibility to highlight this, to avoid it being accidentally given IV. Whilst intravenous adrenaline can be used in anaphylaxis, it should only be given by an experienced practitioner, such as an emergency physician or anaesthetist, at the appropriate dose and with appropriate cardiac monitoring (Brown, 1998).

Pathophysiology of anaphylaxis

Anaphylaxis is traditionally thought of as an IgE-mediated type 1 hypersensitivity reaction. However, other so-called anaphylactoid reactions have been noted to cause similar effects, with the same end result: degranulation of mast cells (and, to a lesser extent, basophils) releasing inflammatory mediators such as histamine, certain prostaglandins, leukotrienes, tryptase and platelet activating factor. These cause vasodilation and increased vascular permeability leading to decreased systemic vascular resistance, tissue oedema and shock (Kemp and Lockey, 2002). The smooth muscle contraction caused by the above substances can also lead to bronchospasm; those with pre-existing asthma are especially at risk of this.

The medications used in anaphylaxis aim to abate or reverse the above changes.

Adrenaline in anaphylaxis: rationale and evidence

Adrenaline is primarily used to reverse or prevent pharyngeal and laryngeal oedema via peripheral vasoconstriction. It also causes bronchodilation, which may help with any associated wheeze. There are also β-adrenergic receptors on mast cells and adrenaline should theoretically prevent further mast cell degranulation, which is perhaps why it is thought to be more effective the earlier it is used.

🔍 Evidence

There has been a Cochrane review of the use of adrenaline anaphylaxis but there were no studies of sufficient quality to satisfy their inclusion criteria (Sheik *et al.*, 2008). This highlights the ethical and methodological difficulties of performing trials in this unpredictable and life-threatening situation.

✓ DRUGS checklist for ADRENALINE in anaphylaxis

Dose **Dilution**	500 micrograms (or 0.5 mg) 1/1000
Route	IM (the best location is the thigh (Simons *et al.*, 2001), **never** into the hands or feet)
Units	Milligrams or micrograms
Given	'Stat'; may be repeated after 5 min if required
Special situations	Adrenaline is kept on all crash trolleys. Be aware that the dose and route used in anaphylaxis is different to that used in cardiac arrest. Adrenaline is more effective the earlier it is given.

Adrenaline: essential pharmacology

See Cardiac Arrest section for a review of adrenaline pharmacology.

Although adrenaline can cause side effects, including sweating, tremor, palpitations and nausea, it is relatively safe when given IM and its early use in anaphylaxis is potentially life-saving and unlikely to cause harm.

Chlorphenamine: rationale and evidence

The theoretical benefits of antihistamines in anaphylaxis (IgE-mediated) and anaphylactoid (non-IgE-mediated) reactions include helping counteract histamine-induced effects such as urticaria. However, histamine is only one of many inflammatory mediators released and antihistamines alone are insufficient to abate anaphylaxis (Brown, 1998). Although there is no good evidence for their benefit in this condition and some of their potential side effects (tachycardia and hypotension) could be harmful in this situation, they remain part of the recommended treatment in most current guidelines.

Although any antihistamine would have a similar effect, chlorphenamine is used as it is available as a parenteral preparation. Although it can be given IM, it is not required as a priority during initial treatment and can usually wait until IV access is established.

✓ DRUGS checklist for CHLORPHENAMINE

Dose	4–20 mg (24 mg is the maximum daily dose)
Route	PO/ slow IV injection/ IM
Units	Milligrams (mg)
Given	In anaphylaxis: 10–20 mg bolus For urticaria, hay fever, rhinitis: 4 mg up to 6 times per day
Special situations	Side effects are usually mild but include drowsiness, GI disturbances, blurred vision, dry mouth, urinary retention, tachyarrhythmias and hypotension.

Evidence

There has been a Cochrane review of the use of antihistamines in anaphylaxis but there were no studies of sufficient quality to satisfy the inclusion criteria (Sheik *et al.*, 2007).

Chlorphenamine: essential pharmacology

Chlorphenamine is an H1 antihistamine. Histamine receptors are G protein-couple receptors (GPCRs). There are several subtypes, the most clinically relevant of which are the H1 and H2 receptors. Each of these has specific or relatively specific antagonists and it is the H1 group of antihistamines that are employed in the treatment of anaphylaxis (Table 2.1). The H1 antihistamines work by binding to an allosteric site (i.e. not the histamine binding site) on the histamine receptor and are 'inverse agonists', that is they have the opposite effect to that of histamine (Church and Church, 2011). First-generation

Table 2.1 Comparison of H1 and H2 antihistamines.

	H1 antihistamines	H2 antihistamines
Examples	Chlorphenamine[a] Cetirizine[b] (no parenteral formulation) Loratadine[b] (no parenteral formulation)	Cimetidine Ranitidine
Therapeutic effects	Smooth muscle relaxation, vasoconstriction, decreased vascular permeability	Inhibition of gastric acid secretion, decreased myocardial rate and output
Side effects	Anti-α-adrenergic effects (hypotension), anticholinergic effects (dry mouth, blurred vision, urinary retention), sedation	

[a]First generation – crosses the blood–brain barrier.
[b]Second generation – limited penetration of the blood–brain barrier, thereby avoiding CNS effects.

H1 antihistamines such as chlorphenamine are not very selective for the histamine receptor and therefore have a number of side effects due to actions at other receptors. They have the ability to cross the blood–brain barrier interfering with histamine-mediated neurotransmission and causing central side effects such as drowsiness.

Hydrocortisone: rationale and evidence

Hydrocortisone is available as a parenteral preparation and is used for its anti-inflammatory and immunosuppressant actions. It has been suggested that glucocorticoid use may help avoid the prolonged or recurrent reactions (the so-called biphasic response) although the literature is far from conclusive in this regard (Lieberman, 2005).

Evidence

There has been a Cochrane review of the use of glucocorticoids in anaphylaxis but there were no studies of sufficient quality to satisfy the inclusion criteria (Choo *et al.*, 2012).

DRUGS checklist for HYDROCORTISONE

Dose	200 mg
Route	IV
Units	Milligrams (mg)
Given	As a one-off injection which may be followed up with a short course of oral steroid medication
Special situations	Typical steroid side effects occur with long-term use but should not be a problem with one-off use.

Hydrocortisone: essential pharmacology

Hydrocortisone is a type of steroid that has glucocorticoid actions including anti-inflammatory and immunosuppressive effects. It is about four times less potent than prednisolone and has about 27 times less potency than dexamethasone (BMA/RPS, 2015), that is 200 mg hydrocortisone = 50 mg prednisolone = 7.4 mg dexamethasone. The glucocorticoids are 90% bound to a steroid-binding globulin (SBG) in the circulation. Glucocorticoids act through several mechanisms. As well as being able to trigger intracellular signalling pathways via cell-surface receptors, they are also able to pass through the cell membrane (bound to SBG) to bind intracellular receptors. Inside the cell they can travel to the nucleus where they can have a direct effect on gene transcription or can alter gene transcription indirectly through interaction with transcription factors. In this way there is up-regulation and activation of anti-inflammatory proteins and inhibition and down-regulation of inflammatory proteins (Rhen and Cidlowski, 2005). As many of their effects manifest relatively slowly (i.e. through gene transcription), they are unlikely to act quickly enough to abate the initial symptoms of anaphylaxis, although they may prevent recurrence of symptoms. For a discussion of the side effects associated with long-term use of glucocorticoids, see Chapter 12 Rheumatology.

Further aspects of anaphylaxis management

The biphasic reaction

People presenting with anaphylaxis should be observed for a minimum of 6 hours following the initial reaction as a recurrence of symptoms can occur without re-exposure to the original allergen (Lieberman, 2005).

Mast cell tryptase

Tryptase is a major component of the mast cell granule and hence is released into the blood with mast cell degranulation. It is helpful, in cases of suspected anaphylaxis and once emergency treatment has been given, to take a blood sample for 'mast cell tryptase'. This should be repeated after 1–2 hours (plasma concentrations peak at 1–2 hours). A further sample for baseline tryptase levels can be taken at a later date or in clinic (NICE, 2011). This is particularly valuable in confirming the diagnosis of anaphylaxis in ambiguous cases.

Don't forget to look for a cause!

It is important to take a detailed history to look for the cause of the anaphylactic episode (see Common causes of anaphylaxis). If a drug reaction is suspected don't forget to cross off the medication on the drug chart and list the medication in the allergies section.

Patients should be referred to a specialist allergy service. When writing a referral, the following information should be included:

- A description of the event
- A list of treatments given
- Mast cell tryptase levels (if available at time of referral).

Common causes of anaphylaxis

- Nuts (especially peanuts)
- Seafood
- Bee or wasp stings
- Antibiotics
- Iodine (used in contrast medium and skin prep)
- Latex

Last but not least...

It is important to document in the notes and on the drug chart if a patient has a known allergy. If the reaction is to a medication, you should inform the MHRA via the **yellow card system**, which can be found online at: http://yellowcard.mhra.gov.uk/

 Guidelines

NICE provides the following guidance for post-acute management of suspected anaphylaxis (NICE, 2011):
Prior to discharge, all patients should
- Be observed for 6–12 hours
- Be offered an adrenaline autoinjector (these usually contain 300 micrograms of adrenaline) and be taught how to use it
- Be offered a referral to a specialist allergy clinic
- Be advised how to avoid the allergen, if known

- Be advised of the signs and symptoms of anaphylaxis, including the possibility of a biphasic reaction
- Be advised, in the event of further anaphylaxis, to use their adrenaline autoinjector and seek medical help

Case outcome and discharge medications

Ms Patterson recovered from her anaphylactic episode. Unfortunately the trigger could not be identified despite a detailed analysis of the hours preceding the anaphylactic reaction by the medical team. She was provided with an adrenaline autoinjector and shown how to use it and a referral was made to a specialist allergy clinic. She was warned of the symptoms and signs to look out for and advised to call 999 should another episode of anaphylaxis occur. She was given a short course of oral steroids and an antihistamine. She was advised that the antihistamine might make her drowsy and so not to drive whilst taking it.

New drugs have been prescribed in addition to her pre-existing inhalers and oral contraceptive pill.

DISCHARGE MEDICATION

Date	Medication	Dose	Route	Frequency	Supply	GP to continue?
xx/xx/xx	PREDNISOLONE	30 mg	PO	Once daily	5 days	N
xx/xx/xx	CHLORPHENAMINE	4 mg	PO	Three times daily	5 days	N
xx/xx/xx	EPIPEN™	300 micrograms	IM	As needed	One pen	Y
xx/xx/xx	SALBUTAMOL (100 micrograms per dose)	2 puffs	INH	As needed	14 days	Y
xx/xx/xx	BECLOMETHASONE (100 micrograms per dose)	2 puffs	INH	Twice daily	14 days	Y

Notes to patient/GP:
EpiPen provided (as well as appropriate training) in case of future episodes of anaphylaxis. No other changes to regular medications.

Common pitfalls

- Don't forget to highlight that the route of administration for adrenaline in anaphylaxis is **intramuscular**.
- Don't forget to look for the cause of anaphylaxis, cross off potentially causative drugs on the drug chart and document the potential allergy.

Anaphylaxis is a medical emergency and every doctor should know the medications, their doses and routes of administration by heart. An ABC approach is warranted, as is early senior input, notably from an emergency physician or an anaesthetist.

SUMMARY

🔑 Key learning points

Management of anaphylaxis:
- 1 : 1000 adrenaline, 500 micrograms, IM
- Oxygen: 15 L/min via a reservoir mask
- IV access: hydrocortisone, chlorphenamine and fluids
- Input from a clinician expert in airway management

(Continued)

⚷ Key learning points (*Continued*)

On discharge:
- Advice about anaphylaxis
- Adrenaline autoinjector
- Specialist allergy clinic referral
- Short course of steroids + antihistamines

FURTHER READING

- There is a good review of anaphylaxis treatment produced by the UK Resuscitation Council: Soar J, Pumphrey R, Cant A *et al*.; Working Group of the Resuscitation Council (UK) (2008). Emergency treatment of anaphylactic reactions–guidelines for healthcare providers. *Resuscitation* 77: 157–69.
- A good review article about anaphylaxis is: Simons FE, Sheik A (2013). Anaphylaxis: The acute episode and beyond. *BMJ* 346: f602.

Overdose

This section is primarily about the medications you might have to prescribe for a patient who has suffered an overdose. You are directed to other resources for full details of the management of drug overdoses.

Mr Robert Smith

Age: 32

Hospital number: 123456

⚲ Case study

Presenting complaint: *A 32-year-old man is brought into the department by his girlfriend who found him in his flat 1 hour ago. He was asleep and next to him were 2 empty packets of paracetamol (16 x 500 mg tablets) and a note. He was rousable and reported taking the overdose about 3 hours ago with 4 cans of strong cider.*

PMH: *Depression, appendicectomy*
DH: *See prescription*
Allergies: *None known*
SH: *Lives in a flat with his girlfriend, works as a software engineer*
He weighs 72 kg
O/E: *Feels sick but no vomiting*

A: *Intact: talking*
B: *RR 17, Sats 98% OA*
Equal expansion and air entry to both bases without added sounds
C: *Pulse 78 (regular); BP: 115/78; CRT <2 seconds; HS I + II + 0*
D: *Blood sugar 5.6; GCS 15*

Further examination:
Abdomen: No jaundice noted, soft and non-tender, bowel sounds present, no masses detected
Neurology: No focal abnormalities found

Diagnosis
Paracetamol overdose.
Features: Nausea and vomiting, abdominal pain. Look for evidence of hepatic injury such as jaundice, right subcostal pain, hepatic coma.

Initial measures
Poisoning is a medical emergency and warrants an ABC approach. You should look specifically at the GCS, respiratory rate and blood pressure, look for evidence of arrhythmias including examining the QT interval, be vigilant for seizure activity and don't forget to examine the pupils. Time of overdose is important to ascertain. Activated charcoal can be given orally within 1 hour of overdose in patients unlikely to develop a reduced level of consciousness.

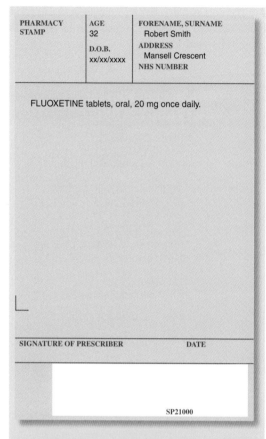

PHARMACY STAMP	AGE 32	FORENAME, SURNAME
		Robert Smith
	D.O.B.	ADDRESS
	xx/xx/xxxx	Mansell Crescent
		NHS NUMBER

FLUOXETINE tablets, oral, 20 mg once daily.

SIGNATURE OF PRESCRIBER   DATE

SP21000

After assessing the patient and taking a history if possible (you may need to call the patient's relative or friend), it is sensible to consult TOXBASE (National Poisons Information Service, 2015) to gain specific and up-to-date guidance on how to treat the overdose.

⊙ Guidelines

TOXBASE is a clinical toxicology resource (provided by the NPIS: National Poisons Information Service, which is itself commissioned by the government). The website provides up-to-date guidance about the diagnosis and management of poisoning with a wide range of substances. The website is password protected, with the password for a hospital usually held by its Emergency Department. It is available at: www.toxbase.org

Did you know?

Paracetamol is called **acetaminophen** in the USA.

Prescribing for paracetamol overdose

The antidote for paracetamol poisoning is **acetylcysteine** (also known as *N*-acetylcysteine or NAC). Trade names you may come across include Parvolex (don't get confused with Pabrinex; see Section Acute alcohol withdrawal).

When should acetylcysteine be used?

- When the 4-hour paracetamol level is above the treatment line (see Acetylcysteine: rationale and evidence)
- After a staggered overdose
- If the time of the overdose is unknown but a significant amount has been taken
- If the blood paracetamol levels will not be available within 8 hours of possible toxic overdose.

Acetylcysteine is given as three infusions of different concentrations over 21 hours: 150 mg/kg in 200 mL over the first 1 hour, then 50 mg/kg in 500 mL over 4 hours, then 100 mg/kg in 1000 mL over 16 hours. The dose of acetylcysteine will be different for each patient depending on their weight. Although a mg/kg dosing regimen is given, tables are also available that give the dose and infusion rate based on weight ranges (e.g. 70–79 kg) instead of individual weights. These are intended to reduce dosing errors and should be used wherever available, depending on local policy.

Calculation

In this case, the first infusion for this 72-kg man will contain 150 mg/kg of acetylcysteine:

$$150 \times 72 = 10800 \text{ mg}$$

FLUID CHART						
Date	Fluid	Additive	Rate	Time to be given	Signature	Print name
xx/xx/xx	5% GLUCOSE	ACETYLCYSTEINE 10800 mg	Over 1 hour	xx:xx	A. Doctor	A. Doctor
xx/xx/xx	5% GLUCOSE	ACETYLCYSTEINE 3600 mg	Over 4 hours	xx:xx	A. Doctor	A. Doctor
xx/xx/xx	5% GLUCOSE	ACETYLCYSTEINE 7200 mg	Over 16 hours	xx:xx	A. Doctor	A. Doctor

Acetylcysteine: rationale and evidence

Acetylcysteine is used with the aim of reducing the severity of liver damage caused by paracetamol overdose, although there are admittedly few high quality trials supporting interventions for paracetamol overdose. A Cochrane review (Brok *et al.,* 2008) concluded that whilst *N*-acetylcysteine 'seems preferable to placebo', there is a lack of evidence regarding how best to administer it and it remains unclear precisely which patient groups will benefit. It is not a risk-free medication and so the potential benefits must be weighed against the potential harms. In order to assess the risk posed to the patient by the overdose, you need to know:

- How many tablets were taken?
- When were they taken?

Calculation

In this case, a 72-kg man took 2 packets of 16 tablets each containing 500 mg of paracetamol, i.e. $2 \times 16 \times 500$ mg = 16 000 mg (or 16 g), approximately 4 hours ago

The mg/kg dose of paracetamol taken is therefore: 16 000 mg/72 kg = 222 mg/kg

---

The latest guidance is that all patients who have taken **more than 75 mg/kg** of paracetamol in a 24-hour period be medically assessed. Doses of <75 mg/kg are unlikely to cause serious harm and doses >150 mg/kg are likely to cause harm (TOXBASE).

Paracetamol levels: To further quantify the risk to the patient and decide whether they require treatment with acetylcysteine, paracetamol levels should be measured. Paracetamol takes 4 hours to be fully absorbed and so a **4-hour paracetamol level** is used to determine the risk to the patient. The level should be plotted on the nomogram (Figure 2.3; available on TOXBASE) and if the paracetamol level is above the treatment line, the patient should receive acetylcysteine.

Beware, there are **two different units** used to give paracetamol concentrations:

- mg/L
- mmol/L

Units are important! 151 mg/L = 1 mmol/L

The nomogram provides scales in both units but make sure you are using the correct units as there is a big difference!

✓	**DRUGS checklist for ACETYLECYSTEINE**
Dose	Total of 300 mg/kg
Route	IVI (mixed with 5% glucose)
Units	mg (comes in a 200 mg/mL concentration in a 10-mL vial)
Given	Over 21 hours as follows: 150 mg/kg in 200 mL over the first 1 hour then 50 mg/kg in 500 mL over 4 hours then 100 mg/kg in 1000 mL over 16 hours
Special situations	For patients weighing more than 110 kg, the dose is used as if they weighed 110 kg. For pregnant women, their prepregnancy weight is used. It should be noted that acetylcysteine comes in a solution containing sodium. Side effects include: may rarely cause an anaphylactoid reaction with nausea, vomiting, flushing, pruritis and dyspnoea. This is thought to be mediated by histamine release and can usually be treated by temporarily stopping the infusion and giving antihistamines. Those who have suffered previous anaphylactoid reactions can be given antihistamines prophylactically but should not be excluded from treatment with acetylcysteine. Most serious reactions have been due to administration errors.

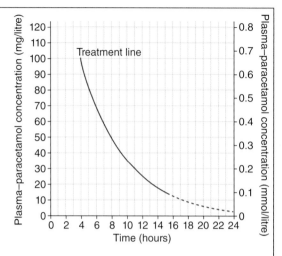

Figure 2.3 Paracetamol nomogram.

However, in paracetamol overdose more NAPQI is produced and glutathione stores are depleted until NAPQI can no longer be detoxified. NAPQI then binds to hepatocytes causing necrosis. Replacing the glutathione via use of acetylcysteine therefore prevents the hepatotoxic effects of paracetamol overdose (Heard, 2008).

There are some caveats to treatment with acetylcysteine in that while it is extremely effective in preventing liver damage when given in the first 8 hours after an overdose, its efficacy thereafter rapidly decreases. It may have some residual effect more than 24 hours after overdose, although the mechanism by which this occurs is not entirely clear (Smilkstein *et al.*, 1988).

Acetylcysteine can cause an anaphylactoid reaction, the severity of which correlates with plasma histamine concentrations (Pakravan *et al.*, 2008). The likelihood and severity of an anaphylactoid reaction has been found to be inversely proportional to the paracetamol level, with reactions rarely occurring in severe overdoses and much more serious reactions seen where the paracetamol dose was below the treatment line(Lynch and Robertson, 2004), which is why acetylcysteine is not recommended for all incidences of possible paracetamol poisoning.

Updated guidance: The first dose was previously given over 15 minutes but the duration of the initial infusion has recently been increased to 60 minutes. The MHRA released a 'drug safety update' (available at www.mhra.gov.org) in 2012 following a review carried out by the Commission on Human Medicines, which came to the conclusion that a slower infusion rate is less likely to cause a hypersensitivity reaction without compromising the efficacy of the treatment. In addition to this, the latest recommendations are that a previous hypersensitivity reaction to acetylcysteine is also no longer a contraindication to its subsequent use.

Acetylcysteine: essential pharmacology

Acetylcysteine works in early paracetamol overdose by replenishing stores of glutathione, a substance which protects the livers from the damage caused by reactive substances such as those produced in paracetamol overdose.

Paracetamol is metabolised by several pathways in the liver. One of these (involving CYP450 enzymes which usually only play a minor role in paracetamol metabolism) results in the production of a toxic metabolite called NAPQI (*N*-acetyl-*p*-benzo-quinoneimine). When therapeutic doses of paracetamol are taken, the smalls amounts of NAPQI produced are quickly detoxified by glutathione.

Further aspects of paracetamol poisoning

Accidental overdose

Due to low body weight: Toxicity can occur with doses only a little higher than the therapeutic dose and patients with low body weight are especially at risk. Many hospital guidelines recommend a lower total daily dose for patients with low body weight. The BNF advises that daily doses of paracetamol should not exceed 60 mg/kg when prescribed for adults weighing <50 kg (BMA/RPS, 2015). The maximum daily dose should be reduced to 3 g for adult patients with hepatocellular insufficiency, chronic alcoholism, chronic malnutrition or dehydration.

Due to co-administration of paracetamol-containing medications: Paracetamol is contained in many 'cold remedies' as well as combination medications such as co-codamol, which if taken together could potentially lead to overdose.

Hidden paracetamol overdose

Paracetamol levels should be taken in any cause of poisoning as mixed overdoses are common.

 Guidelines

NICE guidance suggests that paracetamol levels should also be checked in the following groups (NICE, 2004):
- Patients who present with a history of paracetamol overdose
- Patients who present with a history of opioid poisoning
- Patients who present unconscious where drug overdose is a possibility.

Case outcome and discharge

Mr Smith did not suffer any adverse physiological consequences as a result of his overdose. His liver function tests were normal. He was assessed by the psychiatry team the following day and referred to the community mental health services for further support and his fluoxetine was continued.

Discharge medication is shown on the prescription form.

DISCHARGE MEDICATION

Date	Medication	Dose	Route	Frequency	Supply	GP to continue?
xx/xx/xx	FLUOXETINE	20 mg	PO	Once daily	14 days	Y

Notes to patient/GP:
No changes to regular medications

Other medications seen in overdose

Opioid overdose and naloxone

Definition

Opioid: a substance that has similar effects to morphine and whose actions are blocked by naloxone.

Features of opioid overdose: CNS depression, respiratory depression, pinpoint pupils.

A note on the setting of opioid overdose: Although when we think of opioid overdose, it might conjure up images of people using illicit substances such as heroin, opioid overdose can also occur all too easily in the inpatient setting. This can occur because a patient receiving opioids such as morphine sulphate or even codeine has developed renal failure, because too high a dose has been prescribed, or because of a badly written prescription, for example where a prescription intended to say 2.5 mg has been misinterpreted as 25 mg. The duration of action of several opioids will be prolonged if the patient has renal impairment, as they or their metabolites are renally excreted, for example morphine sulphate, diamorphine and codeine.

If opiate toxicity is suspected, remember to examine patients thoroughly for opioids being given via patches.

Naloxone

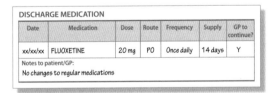

ONCE ONLY PRESCRIPTIONS

Date	Time to be given	DRUG	Dose	Route	Prescriber Signature	Bleep
xx/xx/xx	xx:xx	NALOXONE	400 micrograms	IV	A. Doctor	
xx/xx/xx	xx:xx	NALOXONE	800 micrograms	IV	A. Doctor	

Naloxone is the antidote to opioid poisoning. However, it usually has a shorter duration of effect than the medication it is being used to reverse, such that close monitoring is required for several hours after the initial dose of naloxone has been given.

There is a lack of evidence for the specific dose and route of administration of naloxone in opioid overdose. There are a number of reasons for this, including the difficulties of ascertaining exactly what was taken, the range of opioid preparations available and the difficulties of obtaining informed consent for participation in trials in patient presenting with a decreased GCS. Therefore, clinical judgment is needed as well as an awareness of the delicate balance between under-treatment and over-treatment. Under-treatment can result in ongoing respiratory depression whereas over-treatment can result in acute withdrawal (in chronic opioid users) and re-emergence of pain (in those using opioids for analgesia), neither of which are desirable.

It is recommended that the naloxone dose be titrated to reverse the respiratory depression (i.e. to a RR >10) rather than full recovery of GCS (Clarke *et al.*, 2005). There is no universally accepted initial dose but in the context of suspected acute overdose, TOXBASE recommends giving 400 micrograms IV in the first instance, followed by a further 800 microgram bolus, another 800 microgram bolus and then a 2 mg bolus at 1-minute intervals until the respiratory depression is reversed. Some sources suggest a smaller initial bolus (100 micrograms) (Clarke *et al.*, 2005, Datapharm, 2015). Once the patient has responded, TOXBASE recommends that they should then be monitored (RR and GCS) for a minimum of 6 hours (longer if the patient has taken a long-acting preparation). If repeated doses of naloxone are required to maintain a RR >10 after the initial recovery of respiratory rate, a naloxone infusion should be initiated. Patients requiring an infusion should be monitored in a high-dependency setting.

For full and up-to-date management guidelines, see TOXBASE.

Given	As a bolus or an infusion
	Infusion: 10 mg made up to 50 mL with 5% dextrose (i.e. 200 micrograms/mL). This should run at a rate of two-thirds of the initial dose required to achieve RR>10, per hour (Clarke *et al.*, 2005)
	For example: if a bolus of 800 micrograms achieved a RR>10, the infusion should run at 530 micrograms/hour or 2.7 mL/hour
Special situations	If there is no response after 10 mg naloxone, an alternative diagnosis should be considered.
	Be aware that reversal of opioid effect can precipitate acute withdrawal in chronic opioid users and can unmask pain where opioid is used as analgesia.
	Side effects: arrhythmias, nausea and vomiting, convulsions, pulmonary oedema.

DRUGS checklist for NALOXONE

Dose	100 micrograms to 2 mg initially, as IV boluses
Route	IV/ IM/ SC/ IVI
	NB. Slightly higher doses are required if administering naloxone IM or SC
Units	Micrograms or milligrams
	(Naloxone comes as 400 micrograms in 1 mL or 1 mg in 1 mL)

Benzodiazepine overdose and flumazenil

Features of benzodiazepine overdose: Drowsiness, ataxia, nystagmus, slurred speech, bradycardia, hypotension and respiratory depression.

Although there is an antidote to benzodiazepines (flumazenil), its utility is limited in the setting of drug overdose. It is not generally used in this setting unless there is coma or respiratory depression and the team are absolutely sure that no other medications were used in the overdose. It must not be used if there is suspicion of a mixed overdose as flumazenil may enhance the toxicity of other medications, notably the tricyclic antidepressants, leading to seizures and arrhythmias. It is also not recommended in those with a history of seizures or chronic benzodiazepine use. The main situation in which flumazenil can be safely used is by anaesthetists who have administered a benzodiazepine themselves and wish to reverse its sedative effects (Seger, 2004, Datapharm, 2015).

A note on charcoal: Activated charcoal can decrease the absorption of certain drugs, including aspirin. However, the evidence for its use is very limited and there are no good quality clinical trials demonstrating an improvement in *clinical* end points. Furthermore, its efficacy decreases sharply with time. It is therefore only recommended for use in patients who have ingested a potentially toxic dose of a substance known to be adsorbed to charcoal, within the first hour after ingestion. Where it is used, the adult dose is 50 g and it is administered orally or via nasogastric tube and only

in patients who can maintain their own airway (Chyka and Seger, 1997).

Common pitfalls

- Be aware that paracetamol concentration can be expressed using two different units – make sure you know which one you're using.
- Be careful when calculating the dose of acetylcysteine and use dosing tables wherever possible.
- Be aware when treating opioid overdose that naloxone is usually shorter acting than the opioid whose action it is reversing and therefore repeated doses or an infusion may be necessary.

SUMMARY

There are some general measures that apply when managing a patient who has taken an overdose and an ABC approach is sensible as many substances come with a risk of CNS depression in overdose, which can in turn compromise a patient's airway and breathing. Beyond this, the treatment is specific to the particular substance taken, as well as the amount taken and time since overdose. There is often a lack of a good evidence base when it comes to the treatment of emergencies such as overdose and clinicians should be aware of this when considering the risks and benefits of prescribing.

Key learning points

Paracetamol overdose:
- Acetylcysteine should be given if the paracetamol level measured at least 4 hours post-overdose is above the treatment line **or** straight away in the case of a staggered overdose.
- Mixed overdoses are common and paracetamol levels should be checked no matter what the reported overdose-medication is.

FURTHER READING

- TOXBASE contains up-to-date guidance on the diagnosis and management of overdose for a wide range of substances.
- A good review of the management of paracetamol overdose is: Ferner RE, Dear JW, Bateman DN (2011). Management of paracetamol poisoning. BMJ 342: d2218.

Acute alcohol withdrawal

> **Mr Bruce Stevenson**
>
> **Age: 72**
>
> **Hospital number: 123456**

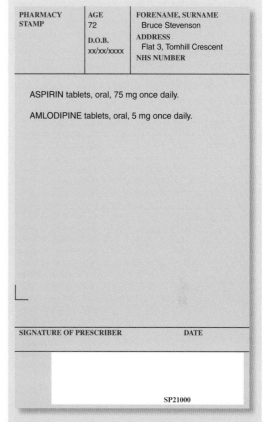 Case study

Presenting complaint: *Mr Stevenson was admitted via the Emergency Department yesterday having fallen at home. He has been seen by the orthopaedic team who confirmed a fractured pubis ramus, requiring a period of rehabilitation at a local community hospital. One of the nurses asks you to come and see him as he is starting to act strangely.*

PMH: *Hypertension, TIA*
DH: *See FP10*
Allergies: *Nil known*
SH: *Retired carpenter, lives alone, usually mobilises independently, ex-smoker; alcohol intake: 1 bottle of wine per night.*
O/E: *Mr Stevenson looks fidgety, agitated and sweaty. When you try to talk to him, he talks quickly and is dismissive of your questions. He looks thin.*
Airway: *Talking in sentences*
Breathing: *RR: 20; Sats: 98% OA*
Air entry on both sides
Circulation: *HR: 110; BP: 160/ 80*
CRT < 2 seconds; HS I+II+O
Abdomen: *Soft, non-tender*
Neurology: *Bilateral tremor, otherwise intact*
Blood sugar: *4.2*

You calculate his weekly alcohol intake at approximately 70 units per week.

Diagnosis

This patient is developing symptoms of acute alcohol withdrawal, due to an abrupt decrease in alcohol intake in someone who has developed alcohol dependence. Without treatment he may develop full-blown delirium tremens and potentially fatal seizures.

Initial measures

Treatment in the immediate setting is usually with a benzodiazepine, such as chlordiazepoxide or diazepam. Other agents in use include clomethiazole

PHARMACY STAMP	AGE 72	FORENAME, SURNAME Bruce Stevenson
	D.O.B. xx/xx/xxxx	ADDRESS Flat 3, Tomhill Crescent NHS NUMBER

ASPIRIN tablets, oral, 75 mg once daily.

AMLODIPINE tablets, oral, 5 mg once daily.

SIGNATURE OF PRESCRIBER	DATE

SP21000

and carbamazepine; however, only chlordiazepoxide and diazepam have UK marketing authorisation for the treatment of alcohol withdrawal. The aim of treatment is to maintain patient comfort during withdrawal and avoid complications such as delirium tremens or seizures. If seizures develop, you should treat these with IV/PR benzodiazepines. Phenytoin is not recommended for alcohol withdrawal seizures (NICE, 2010).

Prescribing for alcohol withdrawal

The drug charts below show examples of prescriptions for acute alcohol withdrawal.

Give pabrinex and a 'stat' dose of chlordiazepoxide straightaway.

ONCE ONLY PRESCRIPTIONS

Date	Time to be given	DRUG	Dose	Route	Prescriber Signature	Bleep
xx/xx/xx	xx:xx	PABRINEX	2 pairs	IV	A. Doctor	
xx/xx/xx	xx:xx	CHLORDIAZEPOXIDE	20 mg	PO	A. Doctor	

Regular IV pabrinex 1–2 pairs should be prescribed for 3 days then thiamine and vitamin B compound strong and don't forget to prescribe chlordiazepoxide 'as required' for breakthrough symptoms.

REGULAR PRESCRIPTIONS

DRUG PABRINEX					06				
Dose 2 pairs	Route IV	Freq BD	Start date xx/xx/xx		⑧				X
					12				
Signature A. Doctor		Bleep	Review		16				
Additional instructions					⑱				X
					22				

DRUG THIAMINE					06				
Dose 100 mg	Route PO	Freq OD	Start date xx/xx/xx		⑧	X	X	X	
					12				
Signature A. Doctor		Bleep	Review		16				
Additional instructions					18				
					22				

DRUG VIT B CO-STRONG					06				
Dose TT	Route PO	Freq OD	Start date xx/xx/xx		⑧	X	X	X	
					12				
Signature A. Doctor		Bleep	Review		16				
Additional instructions					18				
					22				

Circle/enter times below ↓ — Enter dates below: Day 1, Day 2, Day 3, Day 4

AS REQUIRED MEDICATION

DRUG CHLORDIAZEPOXIDE					Date	
					Time	
Dose 10 mg	Route PO	Max freq Hourly	Start date xx/xx/xx		Dose	
					Route	
Signature/Bleep A. Doctor		Max dose in 24 hrs	Review		Given	
Additional instructions					Check	

An example of a fixed-dose detox. regimen for a weekly intake of 70 units.

VARIABLE DOSE PRESCRIPTION

			Month & Year →				
						Date →	
			Start	Change	Change	Change	Change
DRUG CHLORDIAZEPOXIDE	Date →	Day 1	Day 2	Day 3	Day 4	Day 5	
	Time ↓	Dose	Dose	Dose	Dose	Dose	
Route	08.00	20 mg	10 mg	5 mg	5 mg	X	
	12.00	20 mg	10 mg	5 mg	X	X	
Surname DOCTOR	Signature A. Doctor	Bleep	18.00	20 mg	10 mg	5 mg	X	X
Additional instructions	22.00	20 mg	20 mg	10 mg	5 mg	5 mg	
Pharmacy							

Individual trusts are likely to have their own guidance and local protocols for medically assisted alcohol withdrawal. The regimen shown is only one example and is an example of a **fixed-dose reduction regimen**, where the doses given depend on the daily alcohol intake prior to admission and diminish day by day to wean the patient. The other main regimen you may come across is the **symptom-triggered regimen**. There are pros and cons to each regimen, discussed below. It is suggested that you follow local guidance where available.

In addition to chlordiazepoxide, B vitamins are given to prevent the development of Wernicke's encephalopathy and subsequent Korsakoff's psychosis.

Chlordiazepoxide in alcohol withdrawal: rationale and evidence

The neurobiology of alcohol is complex. Activation of opioid receptors with subsequent dopamine release is thought to contribute to its addictive qualities. However, it is the actions of alcohol on GABAergic and glutamatergic pathways in the brain that are thought to underlie its main effects of CNS depression as well as the tolerance seen with prolonged use.

Alcohol acts to enhance neuroinhibitory GABAergic pathways and depress neuroexcitatory glutamatergic pathways. With prolonged ethanol consumption, there is adaption. In response to the persistent stimulation of GABA receptors, they are down-regulated and in response to the ongoing inhibition of glutamate receptors, these are up-regulated. This adaptation means that when alcohol consumption abruptly ceases, there is hyperactivity within the brain, due to loss of the depressant effects of alcohol causing the symptoms of anxiety, autonomic overdrive and potentially seizures (Lees *et al.*, 2012; Nevo and Hamon, 1995). Medications such as benzodiazepines, which enhance GABA function, can compensate for the loss of inhibitory input from alcohol and can be used to engineer a controlled reduction in brain hyperactivity (see Evidence).

🔍 Evidence

There has been a systematic review (Amato *et al.*, 2010) looking at the use of agents in acute alcohol withdrawal. Although many of the studies were small and there was significant heterogeneity, there is evidence that benzodiazepines are more effective than placebo in preventing alcohol withdrawal seizures. However, the evidence did not show a benefit of any one agent as compared to another.

Fixed-dose reduction versus symptom-triggered regimen

As discussed above, there are several regimens for medically assisted alcohol withdrawal. Studies have favoured the symptom-triggered regimen (see Evidence) although this relies on the competent use of a symptom assessment tool such as 'CIWA-Ar' (the Clinical Institute Withdrawal Assessment of Alcohol scale, revised) and the availability of staff to perform assessments on a regular basis. As a compromise, some medical teams apply a symptom-triggered approach on day one and use the doses required to guide a subsequent fixed-dose regimen (Attard *et al.*, 2010). Generally, the more severe the dependence, the higher the initial/PRN doses of chlordiazepoxide given.

🔍 Evidence

Saitz *et al.* (1994) randomised 101 patients to receive either a fixed-dose or a symptom-triggered regimen to manage alcohol withdrawal. The patients receiving the symptom-triggered regimen required significantly less chlordiazepoxide (an average of 100 mg vs. 425 mg) and required a significantly shorter duration of treatment (an average of 9 hours vs. 68 hours) although there was no significant difference in the incidence of alcohol withdrawal seizures.

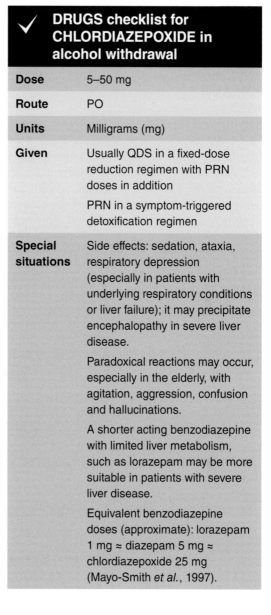

✓	DRUGS checklist for CHLORDIAZEPOXIDE in alcohol withdrawal	
Dose	5–50 mg	
Route	PO	
Units	Milligrams (mg)	
Given	Usually QDS in a fixed-dose reduction regimen with PRN doses in addition	
	PRN in a symptom-triggered detoxification regimen	
Special situations	Side effects: sedation, ataxia, respiratory depression (especially in patients with underlying respiratory conditions or liver failure); it may precipitate encephalopathy in severe liver disease.	
	Paradoxical reactions may occur, especially in the elderly, with agitation, aggression, confusion and hallucinations.	
	A shorter acting benzodiazepine with limited liver metabolism, such as lorazepam may be more suitable in patients with severe liver disease.	
	Equivalent benzodiazepine doses (approximate): lorazepam 1 mg ≈ diazepam 5 mg ≈ chlordiazepoxide 25 mg (Mayo-Smith *et al.*, 1997).	

Chlordiazepoxide: essential pharmacology

Chlordiazepoxide is a type of benzodiazepine. Benzodiazepines are thought to work by enhancing the action of the inhibitory neurotransmitter GABA (gamma aminobutyric acid) at the $GABA_A$-receptor. GABA-receptors, when activated, allow influx of chloride ions into a neuron, which hyperpolarises the neuron meaning the threshold for activation of that neuron is enhanced. The overall effect of GABA is therefore a 'damping-down' of activity in the brain. Benzodiazepines bind at an allosteric site on the GABA_A receptor and enhance the effects of GABA at the receptor (Rang *et al.*, 2003, Sandford *et al.*, 2000). This mimics the actions of alcohol on the brain, as described above, and allows controlled withdrawal of the effects of alcohol on the brain.

Chlordiazepoxide is mainly metabolised in the liver to active metabolites and is excreted via the kidneys. Specific characteristics of chlordiazepoxide (as opposed to other benzodiazepines) that make it suitable in this situation include a longer duration of action, which may help prevent breakthrough symptoms and a slower onset of action, which may lead to less abuse potential (Mayo-Smith *et al.*, 1997).

B vitamins in alcohol withdrawal: rationale and evidence

The rationale behind giving B vitamins in this situation is that patients who have a high alcohol intake often have poor nutritional status. Lack of thiamine (vitamin B_1) in particular can be detrimental, leading to a devastating neuropsychiatric condition, Wernicke–Korsakoff syndrome.

It can be difficult to distinguish the early symptoms of Wernicke–Korsakoff syndrome during acute alcohol withdrawal as both may present as an acute confusion state. In one study (Harper *et al.*, 1986), only 16% of cases of Wernicke–Korsakoff syndrome presented with the classic triad of ophthalmoplegia, ataxia and change in mental state. Therefore treatment is recommended for both at-risk and symptomatic patients, with a course of intravenous vitamins (Pabrinex), followed by

ongoing oral thiamine and vitamin B compound. The evidence base for this is scant (see Evidence) and the dose and duration of treatment remain non-evidence based. However, there are few risks to treatment and, when this is compared to the considerable risk of ongoing thiamine deficiency, most would agree that proving this treatment is an important consideration in managing alcohol withdrawal syndrome.

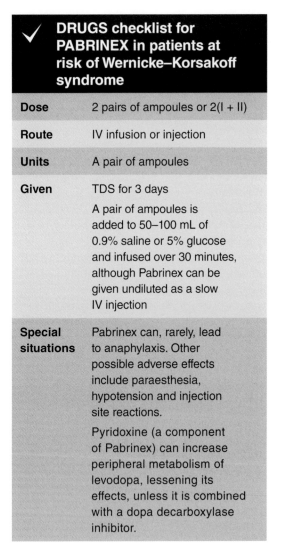

✓	DRUGS checklist for PABRINEX in patients at risk of Wernicke–Korsakoff syndrome	
Dose	2 pairs of ampoules or 2(I + II)	
Route	IV infusion or injection	
Units	A pair of ampoules	
Given	TDS for 3 days	
	A pair of ampoules is added to 50–100 mL of 0.9% saline or 5% glucose and infused over 30 minutes, although Pabrinex can be given undiluted as a slow IV injection	
Special situations	Pabrinex can, rarely, lead to anaphylaxis. Other possible adverse effects include paraesthesia, hypotension and injection site reactions.	
	Pyridoxine (a component of Pabrinex) can increase peripheral metabolism of levodopa, lessening its effects, unless it is combined with a dopa decarboxylase inhibitor.	

🔍 Evidence

A review of randomised controlled trials looking at the efficacy of thiamine in the prevention of Wernicke–Korsakoff syndrome (Day *et al.*, 2013) did not find any evidence of sufficiently high quality to draw conclusions about the dose, duration, frequency or efficacy of treatment.

Other uses for Pabrinex that you may come across include the treatment of patients at risk of refeeding syndrome.

✓ DRUGS checklist for THIAMINE

Dose	100–200 mg
Route	PO
Units	Milligrams (mg)
Given	As a once-daily dose
Special situations	Most people require 1.5 mg per day and body stores contain only 30–50 mg. Alcohol intake may impair thiamine absorption.
	No notable side effects; excess B vitamins are excreted.

✓ DRUGS checklist for VITAMIN B COMPOUND STRONG

Dose	2 tablets (TT)
Route	PO
Units	A tablet
Given	As a once-daily dose
Special situations	Contains pyridoxine, nicotinamide, riboflavin and thiamine.
	No notable side effects; excess B vitamins are excreted.

B vitamins: essential pharmacology

Pabrinex is an intravenous medication containing a range of vitamins (mainly B vitamins) which comes as two ampoules:

Ampoule 1: thiamine (vitamin B_1), riboflavin (vitamin B_2) and pyridoxine (vitamin B_6).

Ampoule 2: ascorbic acid (vitamin C), nicotinamide (vitamin B_3) and glucose.

B vitamins are essential for a range of bodily processes and form part of the co-enzymes involved in carbohydrate, protein and lipid metabolism (Eddleston *et al.*, 2008):

- Thiamine deficiency which occurs *gradually*, results in neuropathy, heart failure and peripheral oedema (as seen in beriberi), whereas the relatively *rapid* thiamine depletion seen in alcohol dependency tends to result in Werknicke–Korsakoff syndrome.
- Nicotinamide deficiency results in pellagra, which classically presents with a triad of dermatitis, diarrhoea and dementia.
- Pyridoxine deficiency can result in a peripheral neuropathy.
- Riboflavin deficiency is uncommon in isolation; it may precipitate anaemia and symptoms include stomatitis and atrophic glossitis.

Further aspects of alcohol withdrawal management

ⓘ Guidelines

NICE provides the following guidance (NICE, 2010):

- Patients suffering from or at high risk of acute alcohol withdrawal syndrome should be admitted to hospital.
- Patients who are alcohol dependent but who are not admitted to hospital should be advised not to stop drinking abruptly and should be given the details of local alcohol support services.

Biopsychosocial interactions

You need to consider whether there is there an underlying reason for alcohol use that you could help address. What support does the patient have at home? Are they in touch with any alcohol support services? Are there any safety issues surrounding the patient's alcohol use, either their own safety or that of others?

Look out for evidence of liver damage

Patients with prolonged high alcohol intake are at risk of liver damage, including fatty liver disease and cirrhosis. An admission with alcohol withdrawal is a good opportunity to look for evidence of liver damage and address strategies for preventing further damage and arrange follow-up appointments as needed. It is important that you address with the patient the adverse health consequences of continued high alcohol intake at an appropriate time.

You may also treat patients with established or decompensated liver cirrhosis who are undergoing alcohol withdrawal, either with withdrawal as their presenting complaint or during an admission for another reason. These patients are at higher risk from an episode of withdrawal and should ideally be managed by a clinician experienced in the management of liver disease.

Nutrition

It is often helpful to involve your local dietician if there is evidence of poor nutrition.

Case outcome and discharge medications

Mr Stevenson undergoes a standard detoxification regimen. After a few days, he is able to start his physiotherapy rehabilitation programme to regain his mobility. He admits to the team that he has been drinking at his current level for 5–6 years now, since his wife died. He is keen to make a change and is put in touch with the alcohol liaison specialist nurse who counsels him further and gives him the contact

details for local support groups. He is transferred to a local community hospital for ongoing rehabilitation for his pubic ramus fracture.

DISCHARGE MEDICATION

Date	Medication	Dose	Route	Frequency	Supply	GP to continue?
xx/xx/xx	VITAMIN B CO-STRONG	2 tablets	PO	Once daily	14 days	Y
xx/xx/xx	THIAMINE	100 mg	PO	Once daily	14 days	Y
xx/xx/xx	ASPIRIN	75 mg	PO	Once daily	14 days	Y
xx/xx/xx	AMLODIPINE	2.5 mg	PO	Once daily	14 days	Y

Notes to patient/GP:
Vitamin B co-strong and thiamine started in view of alcohol dependency

Common pitfalls

- Always obtain an accurate alcohol history and don't forget that alcohol misuse is often a hidden problem. Watch out for signs of withdrawal in patients with a high alcohol intake who are coming into hospital for other reasons and consider prescribing pre-emptive PRN chlordiazepoxide.
- Patients who are not actively withdrawing can be advised about how to decrease their alcohol intake gradually and should be put in touch with alcohol a support services but do not necessarily need to be admitted.
- Patients should not be discharged on chlordiazepoxide.

SUMMARY

Acute alcohol withdrawal is a medical emergency, which can easily go unrecognised and may mimic other conditions. Don't forget to take an accurate and detailed alcohol history when admitting patients for any reason.

Key learning points

Prescribing for acute alcohol withdrawal:
- Prescribe chlordiazepoxide or another benzodiazepine to alleviate symptoms and prevent alcohol withdrawal seizures.
- Prescribe B vitamins to prevent Wernicke–Korsakoff syndrome.
- Follow local guidelines where available.
- Manage seizures with benzodiazepines.
- On discharge, provide:
  - Education about the adverse consequences of high alcohol use
  - Contact details of alcohol advice services
  - Advice about the importance of adequate nutrition
  - Vitamin B supplements.

FURTHER READING

- A good review is available in the journal *Medicine*: Vale A (2006). The management of alcohol withdrawal. *Medicine* 34: 323–327.

Now visit **www.wileyessential.com/pharmacology** to test yourself on this chapter.

References

Amato L, Minozzi S, Vecchi S *et al.* (2010). Benzodiazepines for alcohol withdrawal. *Cochrane Database of Syst Rev* (3): CD005063.

Attard A, Torrens N, Holvey C (2010). Guy's and St Thomas' Foundation Trust Clinical Guideline: 1. The detection of alcohol misusers attending hospital 2. The management of alcohol withdrawal syndrome (AWS) 3. The management of Wernicke's Encephalopathy (WE). *Guy's and St Thomas' Foundation Trust*. Available at: www.guysandstthomas.nhs.uk/resources/our-services/acute-medicine-gi-surgery/elderly-care/alcohol-withdrawal-syndrome.pdf (accessed Sept. 2014).

British Medical Association and Royal Pharmaceutical Society of Great Britain (BMA/RPS) (2015). *British National Formulary 69*, 69th edn. BMJ group and Pharmaceutical Press, London.

Brok J, Buckley N, Gluud C (2008). Interventions for paracetamol (acetaminophen) overdose. *Cochrane Database Syst Rev* (2): CD003328.

Brown AF (1998). Therapeutic controversies in the management of acute anaphylaxis. *J Accid Emerg Med* 15: 89–95.

Callaway CW (2013). Epinephrine for cardiac arrest. *Curr Opin Cardiol* 28: 36–42.

Choo KJL, Simons FER, Sheikh A (2012). Glucocorticoids for the treatment of anaphylaxis. *Cochrane Database Syst Rev* (4): CD007596.

Church DS, Church MK (2011). Pharmacology of antihistamines. *World Allergy Organ J* 4: S22–S27.

Chyka PA, Seger DJ (1997). Position paper: single-dose activated charcoal. *Toxicol Clin Toxicol* 35: 721.

Clarke SFJ, Dargan PI, Jones AL (2005). Naloxone in opioid poisoning: walking the tightrope. *Emerg Med J* 22: 612–16.

Datapharm (2015). *Electronic Medicines Compendium (eMC) Summaries of Product Characteristics (SPC).* Available at: www.medicines.org.uk (accessed Dec. 2015).

Day E, Bentham PW, Callaghan R et al. (2013). Thiamine for prevention and treatment of Wernicke-Korsakoff Syndrome in people who abuse alcohol. *Cochrane Database Syst Rev* (7): CD004033.

Deakin CD, Nolan JP, Soar J et al. (2010). European resuscitation council guidelines for resuscitation 2010. Section 4. Adult advanced life support. *Resuscitation* 81: 1305–52.

Eddleston M, Davidson R, Brent A et al. (2008). *Oxford Handbook of Tropical Medicine*, 3rd edn, Oxford University Press: Oxford.

Harper CG, Giles M, Finlay-Jones R (1986). Clinical signs in the Wernicke-Korsakoff complex: a retrospective analysis of 131 cases diagnosed at necropsy. *J Neurol Neurosurg Psychiatr* 49: 341–5.

Heard K (2008). Acetylcysteine for acetaminophen poisoning. *N Engl J Med* 359: 285–92.

Kemp SF, Lockey RF (2002). Anaphylaxis: A review of causes and mechanisms. *J Allergy Clin Immunol* 100: 341–8.

Lees R, Lingford-Hughes A (2012). Neurobiology and principles of addiction and tolerance. *Medicine* 40: 633–6.

Lieberman P (2005). Biphasic anaphylactic reactions. *Ann Allergy Asthma Immunol* 95: 217–26.

Lynch RM, Robertson R (2004). Anaphylactoid reactions to intravenous N-acetylcysteine: a prospective case controlled study. *Accid Emerg Nurs* 12: 10–15.

Mayo-Smith MF, Cushman Jr P, Hill AJ et al. (1997). Pharmacological management of alcohol withdrawal: a meta-analysis and evidence-based practice guideline. *JAMA* 278: 144–51.

Medicines and Healthcare Products Regulatory Agency. Available at : www.gov.uk/government/organisations/medicines-and-healthcare-products-regulatory-agency (accessed Dec. 2015).

Miller C (2013). Towards evidence based emergency medicine: best BETs from the Manchester Royal Infirmary. BET 1: The use of adrenaline and long-term survival in cardiopulmonary resuscitation following cardiac arrest. *Emerg Med J* 30: 249–50.

Neumar, RW, Otto, CW, Link MS et al. (2010). Part 8: Adult advanced cardiovascular life support: 2010 American Heart Association guidelines for cardiopulmonary resuscitation and emergency cardiovascular care. *Circulation* 122: S729–67.

Nevo I, Hamon M (1995). Neurotransmitter and neuromodulatory mechanisms involved in alcohol abuse and alcoholism. *Neurochem Int* 26: 305–36.

NICE (2004). *Self-harm: the Short-term Physical and Psychological Management and Secondary Prevention of Self-harm in Primary and Secondary Care*, CG016. National Institute for Health and Care Excellence: London. Available at: http://guidance.nice.org.uk/CG016. (accessed March 2014).

NICE (2010). Alcohol-use Disorders: Diagnosis and Clinical Management of Alcohol-related Physical Complications, CG100. National Institute for Health and Care Excellence: London. Available at: https://www.nice.org.uk/guidance/cg100 (accessed Sept. 2014).

NICE (2011). *Anaphylaxis: Assessment to Confirm an Anaphylactic Episode and the Decision to Refer after Emergency Treatment for a Suspected Anaphylactic Episode*, CG134. National Institute for Health and Care Excellence: London. Available at: www.nice.org.uk/guidance/cg134 (accessed Nov. 2015).

Nolan JP, Soar J, Smith GB et al. (2014). National Cardiac Arrest Audit. Incidence and outcome of in-hospital cardiac arrest in the United Kingdom National Cardiac Arrest Audit. *Resuscitation* 85: 987–92.

Pakravan N, Waring S, Sharma S et al. (2008). Risk factors and mechanisms of anaphylactoid reactions to acetylcysteine in acetaminophen overdose. *Clin Toxicol* 46: 697–702.

Rang HP, Dale MM, Ritter JM et al. (2003). *Pharmacology*, 5th edn. Churchill Livingstone.

Resuscitation Council (UK) (2015). *Guidelines 2015. Adult Advanced Life Support.* Available at: www.resus.org.uk/pages/als.pdf (accessed Nov. 2015).

Rhen T, Cidlowski JA (2005). Antiinflammatory action of glucocorticoids — new mechanisms for old drugs. *N Engl J Med* 353: 1711–23.

Saitz R, Mayo-Smith MF, Roberts MS *et al.* (1994). Individualized treatment for alcohol withdrawal: randomized double-blind controlled trial. *JAMA* 272: 519–23.

Sandford JS, Argyropoulos SV, Nutt DJ (2000). The psychobiology of anxiolytic drugs: Part 1: Basic neurobiology. *Pharmacol Ther* 88: 197–212.

Seger DL. (2004). Flumazenil–treatment or toxin. *J Toxicol Clin Toxicol* 42: 209–16.

Sheikh A, Ten Broek V, Brown SG *et al.* (2007). H1-antihistamines for the treatment of anaphylaxis: Cochrane systematic review. *Allergy* 62: 830–7.

Sheikh A, Shehata YA, Brown SGA *et al.* (2008). Adrenaline (epinephrine) for the treatment of anaphylaxis with and without shock. *Cochrane Database Syst Rev* (4): CD006312.

Simons FE, Gu X, Simons KJ (2001). Epinephrine absorption in adults: intramuscular versus subcutaneous injection. *J Allergy Clin Immunol* 108: 871–3.

Smilkstein MJ, Knapp GL, Kulig KW *et al.* (1988). Efficacy of oral N-acetylcysteine in the treatment of acetaminophen overdose. *N Engl J Med* 319: 1557–62.

Soar J, Pumphrey R, Cant A *et al.*; Working Group of the Resuscitation Council (UK) (2008). Emergency treatment of anaphylactic reactions–guidelines for healthcare providers. *Resuscitation* 77: 157–69.

National Poisons Information Service (2015). *Toxbase*. Available at: www.toxbase.org (accessed July 2015).

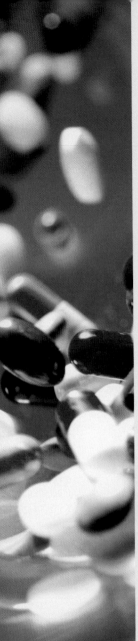

CHAPTER 3
Cardiology

Georgia Woodfield

Key topics:

Learning objectives

By the end of this chapter you should…

- …be able to write a prescription for patients with acute coronary syndrome, acute and chronic heart failure, a range of arrhythmias and hypertension, taking into account relevant contraindications, cautions and side effects.

- …be able to talk about the mechanisms of action of the key drugs used to treat these conditions.

- …be able to describe the pharmacological strategies employed in the long-term management of acute coronary syndrome, heart failure and hypertension.

- …be aware of some of the key trials that underpin the management of these conditions.

Essential Practical Prescribing, First Edition. Georgia Woodfield, Benedict Lyle Phillips, Victoria Taylor, Amy Hawkins and Andrew Stanton. © 2016 by John Wiley & Sons, Ltd. Published 2016 by John Wiley & Sons, Ltd.

Acute coronary syndrome

> **Mr Hamish Jenkins**
>
> **Age: 65**
>
> **Hospital number: 123456**

🔍 Case study

Presenting complaint: *A 65-year-old man presents to A&E with a 3-hour history of central crushing chest pain and breathlessness. The pain has almost resolved by the time of arrival at the ED.*

Background: *He lives with his wife in a house and mobilises with a stick. He is an ex-smoker (20 pack years) and drinks 5–6 units of alcohol per week.*

PMH: *Hypertension, type 2 diabetes*

Allergies: *codeine (causes nausea)*

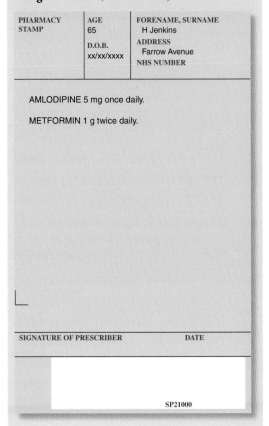

PHARMACY STAMP	AGE 65	FORENAME, SURNAME
		H Jenkins
	D.O.B.	ADDRESS
	xx/xx/xxxx	Farrow Avenue
		NHS NUMBER

AMLODIPINE 5 mg once daily.

METFORMIN 1 g twice daily.

SIGNATURE OF PRESCRIBER   DATE

SP21000

FH: *Father had an MI age 50*

Examination: *Pulse 80, BP 146/76, Sats 97% on air, RR 16, BM 10.2*

CVS: *Capillary refill time <2 seconds, pulse feels regular, JVP not seen, no pitting oedema, HS I + II + 0*

RS: *Equal expansion with air entry to both bases with no added sounds*

Abdo: *Soft, non-tender, no masses palpated, bowel sounds present*

Neuro: *Moving all four limbs, alert, mobilising*

ECG: *Sinus rhythm, 3 mm ST depression leads II, III and AVF, HR 80*

Bloods: *Hb 13.6, Plt 324, WCC 8.9, Na 136, K 4.3, Urea 6.5, Creat 136, INR 1.1*

Diagnosis

Acute coronary syndrome (ACS), possible non-ST-elevation ACS. This would be backed up by a supportive history and the presence of cardiac disease risk factors (hypertension, diabetes and being an ex smoker), as well as a raised troponin.

The spectrum of acute coronary syndrome pathology ranges from stable angina, to unstable angina to non-ST-elevation MI (NSTEMI) to ST-elevation MI (STEMI).

It is useful to be aware that the European Society of Cardiology has categorised ACS patients into two clinical categories (Roffi *et al.*, 2015):

- Patients with typical chest pain and persistent >20 minutes ST-segment elevation on the ECG. This is termed ST-elevation ACS (STE-ACS).
- Patients with acute chest pain but without persistent ST-segment elevation. They have transient or persistent ST-segment depression or T-wave inversion, flat T waves, pseudonormalisation of T waves or no ECG changes.

(Continued)

Case study (*Continued*)

ST-elevation ACS patients need to go directly to the cardiac catheterisation lab for coronary angiogram and consideration of primary percutaneous intervention (PCI), or be thrombolysed if primary PCI cannot be delivered within 120 minutes.

Patients with NSTE-ACS are suspected to be having an NSTEMI and may also warrant early coronary intervention, particularly in the setting of ongoing pain or dynamic ECG changes despite medical treatment.

Initial measures

This patient needs to be on a cardiac monitor as there is a risk of arrhythmias after MI. Blood pressure needs to be checked regularly in the event of acute left ventricular failure and cardiogenic shock post-MI. The patient needs to be reviewed by a cardiologist to determine the need for potential timing of cardiac catheterisation. Ideally, he should be managed on the coronary care unit.

Prescribing for suspected non-ST-elevation myocardial infarction

ONCE ONLY PRESCRIPTIONS

Date	Time to be given	DRUG	Dose	Route	Prescriber Signature	Bleep
xx/xx/xx	xx:xx	ASPIRIN	300 mg	PO	A. Doctor	
xx/xx/xx	xx:xx	MORPHINE	2.5–10 mg	IV	A. Doctor	
		Titrate to pain.				
xx/xx/xx	xx:xx	GLYCERYL TRINITRATE	2 sprays	SL	A. Doctor	
xx/xx/xx	xx:xx	OXYGEN	Aim sats 94–98%	INH	A. Doctor	
xx/xx/xx	xx:xx	CLOPIDOGREL	300 mg	PO	A. Doctor	
xx/xx/xx	xx:xx	FONDAPARINUX	2.5 mg	SC	A. Doctor	
xx/xx/xx	xx:xx	METOCLOPRAMIDE	10 mg	PO/IV	A. Doctor	

The management of suspected acute coronary syndrome depends on the extent of ECG changes. If there is significant ST elevation on the ECG, transfer to the cardiac catheterisation lab is needed urgently for primary PCI, or where this is not available, thrombolysis.

Where there are ischaemic ECG changes that do not fit criteria for PCI/thrombolysis, aggressive antiplatelet/ anticoagulation treatment is essential.

Often there are no initial ECG changes in patients ultimately found to have ACS, and often you may not know the troponin result when you see the patient. In such circumstances patients are treated as presumed ACS until diagnosis is confirmed or disproved, although an aggressive anticoagulation strategy (such as the one shown here) in patients with a normal ECG at presentation is unnecessary. In such situations treatment with aspirin and prophylactic dose low molecular weight heparin (LMWH) is not unreasonable – many units have specific protocols to use in the different situations – make sure you check.

Guidelines

- The National Institute for Health and Care Excellence (NICE) has complete guidelines on the managements of unstable angina and NSTEMI: *Unstable Angina and NSTEMI: Early Management*, CG94, 2010. Available at: www.nice.org.uk/guidance/cg94/resources (accessed Dec. 2015).
- The European Society of Cardiology (ESC) has guidelines on management of acute MI in patients presenting without ST segment elevation:
  - *Acute Coronary Syndromes (ACS) in Patients Presenting without ST-Segment Elevation (Management of)*, 2015. Available at: www.escardio.org/Guidelines-&-Education/Clinical-Practice-Guidelines/Acute-Coronary-Syndromes-ACS-in-patients-presenting-without-persistent-ST-segm (accessed Dec. 2015).
  - *Stable Coronary Artery Disease (Management of)* (European Society of Cardiology, 2013). Available at: www.escardio.org/Guidelines-&-Education/Clinical-Practice-Guidelines/Stable-Coronary-Artery-Disease-Management-of (accessed Dec. 2015).

Aspirin: rationale and evidence

Three drugs are given for management of thrombus in the coronary arteries. Aspirin 300 mg is given providing there are no contraindications.

This can be given per rectum or via an enteral feeding tube. For patients intolerant of aspirin (see below), it is withheld. If the patient is at high risk of gastrointestinal bleeding, a proton pump inhibitor (e.g. omeprazole) should be given as well. Aspirin is given initially as a one-off stat dose. After this the patient should continue on a daily 75-mg maintenance dose.

Evidence

Aspirin in MI

Aspirin has been shown to decrease mortality and reduce reinfarction in acute myocardial infarction. It should be administered routinely to all patients with evolving acute MI unless contraindicated.

Summary of ISIS-2 trial

In the Second International Study of Infarct Survival (ISIS-2), more than 17 000 men and women, within 24 hours of onset of symptoms of suspected MI, were randomly assigned to 162 mg of aspirin or placebo daily for 30 days (ISIS-2, 1988). After 5 weeks patients allocated to receive aspirin had statistically significant reductions in risk of vascular mortality (23%), non-fatal reinfarction (49%), and non-fatal stroke (46%). There was no increase in haemorrhagic stroke or gastrointestinal bleeding in the treated group and only a small increase in minor bleeding.

Thus, aspirin has perhaps the best benefit-to-risk ratio of any proven therapy for acute MI.

DRUGS checklist for ASPIRIN

Dose	300 mg once only in acute MI 75 mg in primary/ secondary prevention of thrombus formation and thromboembolic disease
Route	PO or PR; can also be given via nasogastric tube
Units	mg
Given	Once daily
Special situations	May predispose to GI bleeding. Can cause a hypersensitivity reaction with bronchospasm, rhinorrhoea, urticaria and angioedema.

Aspirin: essential pharmacology

How does it work?

Aspirin has three main clinical effects: at low doses it inhibits platelet aggregation, at medium doses it has an analgesic effect, and at higher doses it has anti-inflammatory properties (it has been classed as an NSAID). In current clinical practice, it is used mainly as an antiplatelet agent in the prevention and treatment of arterial thromboses, for example MI and stroke. Aspirin works by irreversibly inhibiting the cyclo-oxygenase (COX) enzyme, which is present in nearly all tissues. This leads to decreased production of inflammatory mediators called 'prostanoids'. Its antiplatelet effect can be explained by its actions on a particular prostanoid called thromboxane A_2 (TXA_2). This is usually synthesised in platelets in response to endothelial damage and promotes platelet aggregation. This in turn initiates haemostasis, clot formation and endothelial repair (but also thrombosis). By irreversibly inhibiting COX in platelets, aspirin reduces TXA_2 levels and therefore reduces platelet aggregation. MIs occur when thrombus blocks one or more of the coronary arteries, hence inhibition of thrombus formation is key to relieving the obstructed coronary arteries.

Interestingly, although low-dose aspirin has a short half-life (minutes to hours), it only needs to be given once a day. This is because platelets lack nuclei and therefore cannot synthesise new proteins, including COX. Therefore the antiplatelet effect of aspirin persists until more platelets are produced (the lifespan of a platelet is 8–10 days).

Unwanted effects

The side effects of aspirin are also related to its ability to deplete prostanoids. Certain prostanoids, namely prostacyclin and prostaglandin E2, inhibit gastric acid production and promote gastric mucus production, both of which protect the mucosa from erosions and ulcers. Therefore the depletion of these prostanoids, caused by the inhibition of COX by aspirin, leads to an increased risk of gastric erosions and ulcers. Because of aspirin's antiplatelet activity, the risk of bleeding from these ulcers and erosions is also increased.

Aspirin hypersensitivity is caused by an imbalance between prostanoids and leukotrienes. These are both inflammatory mediators produced from the same precursor, arachidonic acid. When aspirin inhibits COX, more arachidonic acid is available for conversion into leukotrienes by the enzyme lipoxygenase (LOX). The imbalance between the prostanoids and the leukotrienes leads to leukotriene-mediated inflammation in the airways and upper respiratory tract. In some people, this leads to symptoms of rhinitis, angioedema, bronchospasm and urticaria, especially if they already have asthma. This also explains why leukotriene *antagonists* such as 'montelukast' are used to treat asthma.

For details of aspirin overdose, see Chapter 2.

Clopidogrel: rationale and evidence

Clopidogrel 300 mg is given in addition to aspirin, providing there are no contraindications. It has been shown to reduce the risk of subsequent cardiovascular events such as stent thrombosis or recurrent ACS.

This can be given per rectum or via an enteral feeding tube. For patients intolerant of clopidogrel, it is withheld. If the patient is already on warfarin with a therapeutic INR, aspirin and clopidogrel are usually still given without the third agent. This is because the risk of bleeding is generally outweighed by the benefit that these agents will have on the coronary circulation. However, this varies in some centres. If the patient has an INR above 3 this may also influence the decision to withhold clopidogrel, due to high bleeding risk. If you are unsure, discuss with a senior.

Note from NICE guidelines Unstable angina and NSTEMI: early management, CG94 (NICE, 2010a)

There is emerging evidence about the use of a 600-mg loading dose of clopidogrel for patients undergoing PCI within 24 hours of admission. Clopidogrel does not have UK marketing authorisation for use at doses above 300 mg. The guideline development group was not able to formally review all the evidence for a 600-mg loading dose and was therefore not able to recommend this at the time of publication (March 2010). However, subsequently, the ARMYDA-2 trial showed a reduction in cardiovascular events in patients

undergoing PCI who received 600 mg loading as opposed to 300 mg clopidogrel up to 8 hours preprocedure (Patti *et al.*, 2005).

 Guidelines

NICE has complete guidelines on the management of acute coronary syndromes: *Clopidogrel in the Treatment of non-ST-Segment-Elevation Acute Coronary Syndrome*, TA80, 2004. Available at: www.nice.org.uk/guidance/ta80 (accessed Dec. 2015).

 Evidence

Clopidogrel in MI
The CURE trial showed that 300 mg clopidogrel followed by daily 75 mg clopidogrel (in addition to aspirin) for NSTEMI resulted in a significant reduction in major adverse cardiac events, i.e. recurrent ischaemia and infarction, as well as deaths from cardiovascular causes, non-fatal myocardial infarction and stroke (11.4–9.3% P <0.0001) (Yusuf *et al.*, 2001).

The COMMIT trial showed that the addition of clopidogrel 75 mg to aspirin within the first 24 hours of acute NSTEMI reduced mortality and major vascular events in the first 2 weeks (note 93% of these patients had STEMI) (Chen *et al.*, 2005).

Note regarding clopidogrel alternatives

Alternates to clopidogrel include prasugrel and ticagrelor. Prasugrel is recommended only for patients on an invasive strategy because existing data comes from patients treated by percutaneous interventions (Wiviott *et al.*, 2007). Ticagrelor is a new direct-acting reversible inhibitor of the adenosine diphosphate receptor P2Y12. The PLATO study (Wallentin *et al.*, 2009) showed significant reduction in major adverse cardiac events at 12 months compared to clopidogrel. Some centres have therefore adopted ticagrelor over clopidogrel as standard.

✓	**DRUGS checklist for CLOPIDOGREL**
Dose	300 mg stat (in acute MI) then 75 mg daily in primary/secondary prevention of thrombus formation
Route	PO, can also be given via nasogastric tube
Units	mg
Given	Once daily
Special situations	Increases bleeding risk.

Clopidogrel: essential pharmacology

Clopidogrel is a $P2Y_{12}$ adenosine diphosphate (ADP) receptor blocker. The $P2Y_{12}$ protein is found mainly on the surface of platelets, and is an important regulator in blood clotting (Dorsam and Kunapuli, 2004). Clopidogrel prevents coagulation by inhibiting the binding of ADP to $P2Y_{12}$ platelet receptors. It is specifically the low affinity receptors that are affected, as the high-affinity binding sites are unaffected by clopidogrel. Clopidogrel inhibits ADP by inhibiting adenylyl cyclase down-regulation, protein tyrosine phosphorylation, activation of the GPIIb-IIIa complex and fibrinogen binding, as well as inhibition of aggregation and release (Savi *et al.*, 1998).

Occasionally, patients are resistant to clopidogrel, that is they receive no antiplatelet benefit from it. In these situations the $P2Y_{12}$ level can be checked to confirm this.

Low molecular weight heparin and fondaparinux: rationale and evidence

Fondaparinux is a synthetic pentasaccharide and is given in addition to aspirin and clopidogrel, providing there are no contraindications. It is increasingly used as an alternative to other LMWHs. Other LMWHs licensed for NSTEMI are enoxaparin and dalteparin. These are all subcutaneous injections.

For patients intolerant of heparins, it is withheld. If the patient is already on warfarin with a therapeutic INR, this third agent is generally not given due to increased risk of bleeding.

Fondaparinux is a one-off stat dose and is usually given for up to 5 days in total once ACS/NSTEMI is confirmed, depending on local protocol. However, it is possible to receive it once daily for up to 10 days. After this the patient should continue 75 mg aspirin and/or clopidogrel maintenance dose.

🔍	**Evidence**

Fondaparinux in MI

Fondaparinux was shown to be similar to enoxaparin in reducing the risk of ischemic events at 9 days, but it substantially reduced major bleeding and improved long-term mortality and morbidity. It is therefore recommended for patients with non-ST-elevation ACS (Yusuf *et al.*, 2006).

!	**Guidelines**

NICE guidelines 2010 recommend:
- Offer fondaparinux to patients who do not have a high bleeding risk, unless coronary angiography is planned within 24 hours of admission.
- Offer unfractionated heparin as an alternative to fondaparinux to patients who are likely to undergo coronary angiography within 24 hours of admission.

✓	**DRUGS checklist for FONDAPARINUX**
Dose	2.5 mg in acute MI once daily for up to 5 days
Route	SC
Units	mg
Given	Once daily
Special situations	Increased bleeding risk. Do not use in severe renal failure (eGFR <30 mL/min).

Fondaparinux: essential pharmacology

Fondaparinux is a synthetic pentasaccharide factor Xa inhibitor. It is derived from the minimal antithrombin binding region of heparin. It acts as an anticoagulant by binding with high affinity to antithrombin. This causes a conformational change in antithrombin that significantly increases its ability to inactivate factor Xa (a prothrombotic clotting factor). In contrast to heparin, fondaparinux does not inhibit thrombin (factor IIa).

Advantages of fondaparinux over LMWH or unfractionated heparin are:

1. Lower risk for heparin-induced thrombocytopenia (HIT). This is because fondaparinux does not interact with platelets or platelet factor 4, and thus, unlike heparin, is not expected to induce thrombocytopenia. Furthermore, there have been case reports of fondaparinux being used to anticoagulate patients with established HIT as it has no affinity to platelet factor 4.
2. Fondaparinux is 100% bioavailable after subcutaneous injection.
3. The half-life of fondaparinux is much longer (mean 17 hours) than that of heparin and LMWHs, allowing it to be given once daily.

The disadvantage is that it is renally excreted therefore cannot be used in patient with severe renal dysfunction.

Licensed LMWHs that can be used instead of fondaparinux are shown in Table 3.1.

Table 3.1 Licensed low molecular weight heparins (LMWHs) that can be used instead of fondaparinux.

LMWH	Dose	Frequency
Enoxaparin	1 mg/kg	OD until stable (usually 5–8 days)
Dalteparin	120 IU/kg (maximum 10000 IU)	12 hourly until stable (usually 5–8 days)

Other medications used in acute coronary syndrome

The following drugs are given to relieve symptoms of chest pain and breathlessness but do not necessarily prolong survival.

Oxygen

Oxygen therapy is indicated if the patient is hypoxic (i.e. if the oxygen saturations are outside the target range of 94–98%). There is conflicting evidence about routine use of oxygen in all patients, but it is recommended in acutely unwell patients (BTS oxygen guidelines: O'Driscoll *et al.*, 2008) and ultimately most patients do receive oxygen (Cabello *et al.*, 2013).

Morphine sulphate

Morphine acts as a potent analgesic. It is given IV as this is fast acting with good effect. Opiates cause respiratory depression and sedation so the dose must be titrated according to response. If any signs of decreasing respiratory rate or decreasing consciousness occur, then stop morphine. In the event of overdose, naloxone can be used. Please see information on analgesia in Chapter 7.

Evidence

Enoxaparin versus unfractionated heparin in MI

Subcutaneous enoxaparin and aspirin was shown to be more effective than continuous IV unfractionated heparin and aspirin at reducing ischaemic events in those with NSTEMI (Cohen *et al.*, 1997).

Similarly, Fragmin (dalteparin) showed benefit in the FRISC study (FRISC Study Group, 1996).

Guidelines

NICE guidelines state: 'Offer pain relief as soon as possible. This may be achieved with GTN (sublingual or buccal), but offer intravenous opioids such as morphine, particularly if an acute myocardial infarction (MI) is suspected.'

NICE. *Chest Pain of Recent Onset: Assessment and Diagnosis*, CG95, 2010. Available at: www.nice.org.uk/guidance/cg95 (accessed Dec. 2015).

✓ DRUGS checklist for MORPHINE SULPHATE

Dose	2.5–10 mg for chest pain
Route	IV; different formulations of morphine can be given via different routes (see Chapter 7)
Units	mg
Given	No maximum; dose is titrated according to response, and presence of any signs of opiate toxicity such as respiratory depression and decreasing consciousness
Special situations	Regular opiate users may have very high requirements, whereas opiate naïve patients may find 2.5 mg sufficient.

Metoclopramide

Patients having an MI often experience nausea and vomiting. Morphine is well known to cause nausea and vomiting also. Vomiting could be potentially harmful to the patient if it inhibits absorption of other important medications. Metoclopramide is therefore given with morphine as symptomatic relief. If not tolerated, the other antiemetics can be used, for example ondansetron (which is often used by ambulance crews).

Please see Chapter 7 for details of antiemetics.

✓ DRUGS checklist for METOCLOPRAMIDE

Dose	10 mg
Route	PO or IV
Units	mg
Given	Up to three times in 24 hours
Special situations	Metoclopramide can cause an oculogyric crisis due to its effect on dopamine receptors (see Chapter 7). This occurs particularly in young women, although is rare. Procyclidine reverses this unwanted symptom.

Glyceryl trinitrate

Glyceryl trinitrate (GTN) can be given as a sublingual spray or as an infusion. It relieves chest pain by dilating the coronary vessels thereby allowing greater oxygenated blood flow to the heart. GTN spray is used in the community as a treatment for angina pain, as it is easy for a patient to carry with them. In the setting of an MI it is used as a spray initially. However, for ACS/NSTEMI if the patient is getting ongoing chest pain it can be set up as an infusion. Ongoing chest pain must be assumed to be representing ongoing myocardial ischaemia, therefore cardiac circulation must be optimised. Dynamic ECG changes may also ensue. Ideally, aim for the maximum dose, or a dose that will adequately control pain. However, this is often limited by a drop in blood pressure secondary to vasodilation, thereby potentially decreasing cardiac perfusion. For this reason GTN infusions must be slowly titrated up whilst closely monitoring blood pressure, aiming for a systolic above 90 mmHg.

ⓘ Guidelines

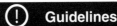

NICE guidelines state: 'Offer pain relief as soon as possible. This may be achieved with GTN (sublingual or buccal), but offer intravenous opioids such as morphine, particularly if an acute myocardial infarction (MI) is suspected.'

NICE. *Chest Pain of Recent Onset: Assessment and Diagnosis*, CG95, 2010. Available at: www.nice.org.uk/guidance/cg95 (accessed Dec. 2015).

✓ DRUGS checklist for GLYCERYL TRINITRATE (GTN) SPRAY

Dose	2 sprays (each spray is 0.3 mg)
Route	Sublingual
Units	Sprays
Given	0.3–1 mg at a time, repeat as required
Special situations	Causes headache due to vasodilation of vessels in the head (as well as the desired coronary vessels). This can limit use.

✓ DRUGS checklist for GLYCERYL TRINITRATE (GTN) INFUSION

Dose	1–10 mg per hour
Route	IV
Units	mg
Given	As an infusion over 24 hours
Special situations	Titrate to blood pressure, as it will invariably drop blood pressure due to vasodilation. Ideally aim for the maximum dose, or dose that will adequately control pain without dropping BP to less than 90 systolic. Again, it can cause headache.

FLUID CHART

Date	Fluid	Additive	Rate	Time to be given	Signature	Print name
xx/xx/xx	GTN 50 mg	Diluted in 50 ml NaCl 0.9%	1–10 mg/hour	xx:xx	A. Doctor	A. Doctor

GTN is a prodrug. The active metabolite is nitric oxide (NO). GTN must therefore first be denitrated in order to produce NO and to have any clinical effect. The mechanism by which nitrates produce NO is widely disputed. It has been suggested that nitrates produce NO by reacting with sulphhydryl groups. Other suggestions involve enzymatic bioactivation of GTN, with enzymes such as glutathione S-transferases, cytochrome P450 (CYP) and xanthine oxidoreductase.

The main clinical effect of vasodilation is caused by NO. NO is a potent activator of guanylyl cyclase. This activation results in cGMP formation from cyclic guanosine triphosphate (cGTP). Thus, NO increases the level of cGMP within the cell. Increased cGMP causes increased smooth muscle relaxation by decreasing intracellular calcium levels.

Ticagrelor

This is a relatively new antiplatelet agent used instead of clopidogrel for STEMIs or NSTEMIs. Like clopidogrel it is given with aspirin for 12 months post-MI. It is an oral, reversible direct $P2Y_{12}$ ADP receptor inhibitor, which is active in its native form; therefore it has rapid onset of action and more pronounced platelet inhibition. The PLATO study showed significant reduction in major adverse cardiac events at 12 months compared to clopidogrel (Wallentin *et al.*, 2009).

 Guidelines

NICE guidelines: *Ticagrelor for the Treatment of Acute Coronary Syndromes*, TA236, 2011. Available at: www.nice.org.uk/guidance/ta236 (accessed Dec. 2015).

Further aspects of ACS management

Glycoprotein IIa/IIIb antagonists

Glycoprotein IIa/IIIb antagonists such as tirofiban or eptifibatide are considered for those patients with NSTEMI with high risk of recurrent events. These are given in addition to aspirin, clopidogrel and fondaparinux. This is a senior decision to prescribe, as some of the trials were done before clopidogrel and LMWH were routinely used for NSTEMI. It is therefore uncertain what the role of glycoprotein IIa/IIIb antagonists is, when used in addition to these agents. In general they are reserved for situations where there is evidence of ongoing myocardial ischaemia despite treatment with standard treatment, especially where urgent percutaneous intervention is not available.

GP IIb/IIIa inhibitors are not routinely given in acute STEMI or in NSTEMI where a primary PCI is planned.

For elective PCI, abciximab (also a glycoprotein IIa/IIIb antagonist) can be considered as an adjunct to PCI for patients with diabetes, and those undergoing complex procedures (e.g. multivessel PCI , multiple stents).

They are also not currently licensed in the UK for use as an adjunct to thrombolytic therapy.

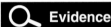

Evidence

Glycoprotein IIa/IIIb antagonists in NTEMI
Treatment with eptifibatimide was shown to reduce the risk of death or MI in patients with NSTEMI, particularly among those at risk of recurrent events (PURSUIT Trial Investigators, 1998).

Aspirin as secondary prevention

Long-term aspirin 75 mg therapy is recommended post-MI, to be continued indefinitely. It has been shown to reduce risk of subsequent MI, stroke, and vascular death among patients with a wide range of prior manifestations of cardiovascular disease.

If a patient has aspirin hypersensitivity then clopidogrel monotherapy should be given as an alternative.

Evidence

Aspirin as secondary prevention
The 1994 Antiplatelet Trialists' Collaboration overview analysed results of randomised trials of antiplatelet therapy among more than 54 000 high-risk patients with prior evidence of cardiovascular disease. These trials included patients with prior MI, stroke, transient ischemic attacks (TIAs), unstable angina, stable angina, revascularisation surgery, angioplasty, atrial fibrillation, valvular disease and peripheral vascular disease. Aspirin therapy reduced risk of subsequent vascular events by about one- quarter in these patients

(non-fatal MI plus non-fatal stroke plus vascular death); 75 mg was the most widely tested regimen in the secondary prevention trials (Antiplatelet Trialists Collaboration, 1994).

Clopidogrel as secondary prevention

Clopidogrel should be continued for 12 months after the most recent acute episode of non-ST-segment-elevation acute coronary syndrome (NSTEMI), in addition to aspirin (Yusuf *et al.*, 2001). After this, aspirin should be given alone unless there are other indications to continue dual antiplatelet therapy.

If a patient has aspirin hypersensitivity then clopidogrel monotherapy should be given as an alternative.

After an ST-segment-elevation MI (STEMI), patients treated with a combination of aspirin and clopidogrel during the first 24 hours after the MI should continue this treatment for at least 4 weeks. After this, aspirin should be given alone unless there are other indications to continue dual antiplatelet therapy. However, after PCI/angioplasty/stent insertion dual antiplatelet therapy is also continued for 12 months.

Evidence

Clopidogrel versus aspirin as secondary prevention
Clopidogrel (75 mg/day) was compared with aspirin (325 mg/day) in a randomised trial of 19 185 patients with recent ischemic stroke, MI or peripheral arterial disease as part of the CAPRIE trial (CAPRIE Steering Committee, 1996). Annual rates of the composite outcome of ischemic stroke, MI and vascular death showed no major differences reported in the safety of the two regimens.

Beta-blockers as secondary prevention

Beta-blockers should be started once a patient has been haemodynamically stabilised post-MI, with the aim of prevention of reinfarction, arrhythmias and reducing mortality.

The choice of beta-blocker may depend on any other co-morbidities; carvedilol is generally preferred for heart failure patients, whereas propranolol/metoprolol may be favoured for diabetic patients. Other commonly used beta-blockers post-MI include bisoprolol or atenolol.

Evidence

Beta-blockers as secondary prevention
- COMMIT trial: early metoprolol decreases the risk of reinfarction and ventricular fibrillation, but increases the risk of cardiogenic shock post-MI (Chen *et al.*, 2005).
- BHAT trial: propranolol decreases mortality post-MI (BHAT Research Group, 1982).
- Norwegian Multicenter Study Group: timolol decrease mortality and reinfarction post-MI (Norwegian Multicenter Study Group, 1981).
- CAPRICORN trial: carvedilol reduces mortality and reinfarction post-MI in patients with heart failure (LV ejection fraction <40%) (CAPRICORN Investigators, 2001).
- ISIS-1: Atenolol given within the first 24 hours improved mortality post-MI. (ISIS-1 Collaborative Group, 1986).

ACE inhibitors and ARBs as secondary prevention

Angiotensin converting enzyme inhibitors (ACEIs) should be started early after an acute MI, and continued long term regardless of left ventricular function. ACE inhibitor therapy should be initiated at the appropriate dose and titrated upwards at short intervals (for example every 1–2 weeks) until the maximum tolerated or target dose is reached. Where ACEIs are not tolerated, angiotensin receptor blockers (ARBs) should be substituted. This is recommended in the NICE guidelines.

The benefit of ACEIs may be due to their beneficial effect on LV remodelling, as remodelling occurs after any significant MI to varying degrees. LV remodelling post-MI causes slow dilation of the ventricles, leading to a decrease in left ventricular ejection fraction. ACEIs slow this process and discourage dilation.

Evidence

ACEIs as secondary prevention
- ISIS-4 trial: early ACE inhibitors have a significant survival benefit. In fact, one-third of the survival benefit evident at 35 days was apparent in the first 24 hours following intervention (ISIS-4 Collaborative Group, 1995).
- Survival and Ventricular Enlargement Trial and Acute Infarction Ramipril Efficacy (AIRE) Study: ACE inhibitors improve survival in patients with reduced LV systolic function or heart failure after MI (Acute Infarction Ramipril Efficacy (AIRE) Study Investigators, 1993).

Statins as secondary prevention

Statins are recommended for all patients post-MI. Statins have been shown to significantly reduce risk of all-cause mortality, CVD mortality, CHD mortality, fatal MI, non-fatal MI, unstable angina, hospitalisation for unstable angina, non-fatal stroke, new or worsening intermittent claudication and coronary revascularisation (Mills *et al.*, 2011; Pedersen *et al.*, 1994). Statins are also recommended for treatment of hypercholesterolaemia as primary prevention for vascular events (including MI and stroke) (Brugts *et al.*, 2009). Statins inhibit 3-hydroxy-3-methylglutaryl coenzyme A (HMG CoA) reductase, an enzyme involved in cholesterol synthesis. Inhibition of HMG CoA reductase lowers LDL levels by slowing down the production of cholesterol in the liver and increasing the liver's ability to remove the LDL already in the blood. Five statins currently have a UK marketing authorisation: atorvastatin, fluvastatin, pravastatin, rosuvastatin and simvastatin.

Guidelines

NICE has complete guidelines on statins as primary and secondary prevention: *Cardiovascular Disease: Risk Assessment and Reduction, including Lipid Modification,* CG181, 2014. Available at: http://www.nice.org.uk/guidance/cg181 (accessed Dec. 2015).

Antihypertensives as secondary prevention

Hypertension is a risk factor for coronary artery disease. Control of blood pressure is therefore important as secondary prevention post-MI. In light of the additional benefits of beta-blockers and ACEIs/ARBs (as explained in Sections Beta Blockers as Secondary Prevention and ACE Inhibitors and ARBs as Secondary Prevention), these are the first choice antihypertensive agents. This may be different to general antihypertensive guidelines for age-matched equivalent patients who have not had MIs. See Section Hypertension.

 Guidelines

NICE has complete guidelines on secondary prevention post- MI: *MI – Secondary Prevention: Secondary Prevention in Primary and Secondary Care for Patients Following a Myocardial Infarction*, CG48, 2007. Available at: www.nice.org.uk/guidance/cg48 (accessed Dec. 2015).

Other considerations

Thromboprophylaxis: MI patients may be less mobile than usual during their stay in hospital, and may well have other VTE risk factors. However, as they are likely to be already on two antiplatelet agents and a pentasaccharide/LMWH, additional prophylaxis is not required. DVT prevention stockings are, however, perfectly reasonable.

Diabetes: A fasting blood glucose level should be checked to ensure that the patient is not diabetic. Sliding scales should be used when blood glucose levels are above 11 mmol/L, but otherwise the patient's usual diabetic medication is often as effective. The DIGAMI2 trial showed that a generally applied aggressive insulin regimen post-MI did not significantly improve survival.

ECG/ 24-hour ECG recording: If atrial fibrillation (AF) is diagnosed, it should be treated as for AF in any other situation (see Section Atrial Fibrillation).

Heart failure: Patients may well develop a degree of left ventricular/right ventricular failure depending on the area of infarction of the heart. Echocardiograms are routinely done post-MI for this reason. Heart failure is treated as described in Section Chronic Heart Failure.

Case outcome and discharge

Mr Jenkins will be discharged when his chest pain has resolved and he is haemodynamically stable. He needs to be aware of his new medication regimen of aspirin, clopidogrel, beta-blocker, ACEI and statin. The GP can up titrate doses in the community.

Mr Jenkins's new prescription is shown on the prescription form. Note amlodipine has been replaced with antihypertensives that have prognostic benefit post-MI.

DISCHARGE MEDICATION

Date	Medication	Dose	Route	Frequency	Supply	GP to continue?
xx/xx/xx	ASPIRIN	75 mg	PO	Once daily	14 days	Y
xx/xx/xx	CLOPIDOGREL	75 mg	PO	Once daily	14 days	Y
xx/xx/xx	BISOPROLOL	2.5 mg	PO	Once daily	14 days	Y
xx/xx/xx	RAMIPRIL	2.5 mg	PO	Once daily	14 days	Y
xx/xx/xx	SIMVASTATIN	40 mg	PO	Once at night	14 days	Y
xx/xx/xx	METFORMIN	1 g	PO	Twice daily	14 days	Y

Notes to patient/GP:
These medications are to continue lifelong as secondary prevention of acute coronary syndrome. Amlodipine was stopped and ramipril started instead.

If not already done, investigations in the short term will be an echocardiogram, cholesterol and glucose blood levels check, and often an angiogram. These may be done as an outpatient.

Patients should be advised not to drive for 4 weeks post-MI, or 1 week if they have been successfully treated with coronary angioplasty. HGV drivers cannot drive for 6 weeks, and must meet functional test requirements. Occasionally, patients require CABG for revascularisation. These patients must not drive for 4 weeks, and there are more stringent requirements for HGV drivers, who cannot drive for 3 months and need a satisfactory echocardiogram and functional test result before relicensing.

Patients should be advised about the importance of healthy diet, moderation of alcohol, regular exercise and smoking cessation.

Common pitfalls

1. Renal function: ACEIs and ARBs cause an increase in creatinine and drop in eGFR. Urea and Electrolytes need to be checked 1–2 weeks after commencing therapy.
2. Maximising doses: Often patients are started on the correct medications prior to discharge, but these are not always titrated up to the maximum tolerated dose. ACEIs doses can be titrated upwards at short intervals (for example, every 12–24 hours). Beta-blockers may need longer titrations. However, if maximum doses are not reached, make it clear in the discharge summary to the GP that is the intention. NICE guidelines state that maximum titration should be completed within 4–6 weeks of hospital discharge (NICE, 2013).
3. Blood pressure: Hypotension may limit optimal therapy with beta-blockers, ACEIs and ARBS.
4. Avoid Ca^{2+} channel blockers post-MI unless they are needed for hypertension control. Beta-blockers, ACEIs and ARBs are prognostically beneficial post-MI, and also control blood pressure, therefore are the better choices.
5. If beta-blockers are contraindicated or need to be discontinued, diltiazem or verapamil may be considered for secondary prevention in patients without pulmonary congestion or left ventricular systolic dysfunction.
6. If a patient has chronic heart failure, amlodipine is the only Ca^{2+} channel blocker that is safe to use. Avoid verapamil and diltiazem.
7. Avoid flecainide in any patient with coronary vessel disease, as it can be arrhythmogenic in these patients.

SUMMARY

There are a number of pharmacological interventions that can improve the outcome and prognosis in myocardial infarction. As with all medical interventions there are risks as well as benefits and the decision to administer a potentially harmful treatment should be supported by good evidence where possible. Suspected ACS is treated as unstable angina/NSTEMI whilst the troponin is awaited. If the troponin comes back negative and the ECGs show no change, alternate investigations or alternative diagnoses need to be considered. In these cases the ongoing management detailed in this chapter does not apply. It is important to recognise that pharmacological intervention represents only one facet of treatment in MI, particularly in secondary prevention. Lifestyle modifications such as smoking cessation, exercise and healthy diet are crucial.

🔑 Key learning points

Acute coronary syndrome

- Any ST elevation on the ECG indicates a STEMI. The patient needs urgent transfer to the cardiac catheterisation laboratory for primary PCI. These patients can have aspirin and clopidogrel but not the other ACS medications (risk of bleeding during procedure).
- Suspected unstable angina or NSTEMI is treated in the same way.
- Give 300 mg aspirin, 300 mg clopidogrel and 2.5 mg fondaparinux as a one-off dose.
- Oxygen is recommended only if the patient is hypoxic.

Secondary prevention

- Consider continuation of antiplatelet agents. Addition of cardioselective beta blocker and ACEi/ARB, as this is shown to have prognostic benefit post-MI.
- Consider other antihypertensive medications, cholesterol-lowering drugs, as well as considering the treatment of related conditions such as diabetes, AF and heart failure.

FURTHER READING

- A comprehensive review of recent ACS trials can be found in the British Medical Journal (Carville *et al.*, 2013).

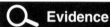 **Evidence**

Primary PCI in MI

'The benefit of prompt, expertly performed primary percutaneous coronary intervention over thrombolytic therapy for acute ST elevation myocardial infarction is now well established' (Keeley *et al.*, 2003).

- Grines *et al.*, 1993.
- The Global Use of Strategies to Open Occluded Coronary Arteries in Acute Coronary Syndromes (GUSTO IIb) Angioplasty Substudy Investigators, 1997.

Thrombolysis in MI

Thrombolytic therapy is indicated for the treatment of STEMI if the drug can be administered within 12 hours of the onset of symptoms, the patient is eligible based on exclusion criteria and primary PCI is not immediately available. The effectiveness is highest in the first 2 hours (Antman *et al.*, 2004; Morrison *et al.*, 2000).

ⓘ **Guidelines**

NICE has complete guidelines on the management of:

- Chest pain of recent onset: assessment and diagnosis, CG 95, 2010. Available at: www.nice.org.uk/guidance/cg95 (accessed Dec. 2015).

- Guidance on the use of drugs for early thrombolysis in the treatment of acute myocardial infarction, TA52, 2002. Available at: www.nice.org.uk/guidance/ta52 (accessed Dec. 2015).
- Myocardial infarction with ST-segment elevation: acute management, CG167, 2013. Available at: www.nice.org.uk/guidance/cg167 (accessed Dec. 2015).
- A useful summary of these guidelines has been published (Carville *et al.*, 2013).

Evidence

Rescue angioplasty in STEMI

'In patients with ECG evidence of failed reperfusion after fibrinolytic treatment for acute MI, rescue angioplasty is associated with lower adverse event rates than conservative care or repeat fibrinolysis' (Gershlick *et al.*, 2005).

Early angioplasty in NSTEMI

Early PCI for patients with NSTEMI was shown to reduce angina, reduce death and reduce recurrent non-fatal MI in comparison to a conservative strategy.

Early PCI (optimal timing remains uncertain) is recommended for patients who have had an NSTEMI and who have refractory angina, haemodynamic instability or high risk of future cardiac events (Fox *et al.*, 2002).

Acute left ventricular failure

> **Mrs Jenny Clive**
>
> **Age: 70**
>
> **Hospital number: 123456**

🔍 Case study

PC: *A 70-year-old woman is brought in to A&E by ambulance. She is acutely breathless. She had acute onset palpitations this morning whilst reading. These have now resolved. There was no chest pain.*

PMH: *Hypertension, high cholesterol, paroxysmal AF, angina*

Allergies: *None*

Examination:
HR 120 reg, RR 24, BP 160/70, Sats 92% on air, afebrile, BM 6.5, Looks breathless.

PHARMACY STAMP	AGE 70	FORENAME, SURNAME Jenny Clive
	D.O.B. xx/xx/xxxx	ADDRESS Newlands Road NHS NUMBER

BISOPROLOL 2.5 mg once daily.

FUROSEMIDE 20 mg once daily.

SIMVASTATIN 40 mg once daily.

WARFARIN 2 mg daily as per INR.

GTN SPRAY 2 puffs as required.

SIGNATURE OF PRESCRIBER   DATE

SP21000

CVS: *Capillary refill time <2 seconds, pulse feels regular, JVP raised +6 cm*
Bilateral pitting leg oedema up to knees, HS I + II + 0

RS: *Bilateral fine inspiratory crepitations up to midzones bilaterally with quiet polyphonic wheeze*

Abdo: *Soft, non-tender, no masses palpated, bowel sounds present*

Chest X-ray *shows pulmonary oedema*

ECG *shows sinus tachycardia*

Bloods: *Hb 13.6, Plt 324, WCC 8.9, Na 136, K 4.3, Urea 6.5, Creat 136, INR 1.1*

Diagnosis
Acute pulmonary oedema due to acute left ventricular failure. Likely precipitants include an acute arrhythmia, as she has known paroxysmal atrial fibrillation. She may have gone into fast AF causing acute LVF, and has now reverted back to sinus rhythm. In light of her history of angina, there needs to be a high index of suspicion for acute coronary syndrome as a precipitant.

Initial measures
ABC measures are a priority. The airway should be checked and high-flow oxygen given. The pulse, BP and respiratory function should be assessed. It is important to secure IV access, check glucose levels and get senior help. An ECG is important, as myocardial infarction and arrhythmias are well known triggers for acute LVF. These need to be treated alongside the pulmonary oedema, if present, as they will drive it further.

Prescribing for acute left ventricular failure

ONCE ONLY PRESCRIPTIONS					Prescriber	
Date	Time to be given	DRUG	Dose	Route	Signature	Bleep
xx/xx/xx	xx:xx	OXYGEN	15 L/min	INH	A. Doctor	
xx/xx/xx	xx:xx	FUROSEMIDE	40 mg	IV	A. Doctor	
xx/xx/xx	xx:xx	GTN	2 puffs	SL	A. Doctor	
xx/xx/xx	xx:xx	MORPHINE	1–2.5 mg	IV	A. Doctor	
xx/xx/xx	xx:xx	GTN	1–10 mg/hour	IV infusion	A. Doctor	

This patient is hypoxic and needs high-flow oxygen. The priority here is breathing, hence the lungs need to be offloaded of fluid. GTN causes vasodilation, including in coronary arteries. However, for this reason it also causes hypotension. GTN infusion is therefore only started if breathlessness and/or chest pain is not resolving and systolic BP is greater then 90 mmHg. BP must be regularly monitored whilst on the infusion.

⊘ Guidelines

- Complete guidelines are available online from the American Heart Association (Williams *et al.*, 1995).
- Complete guidelines are available online from the European Society of Cardiology: *Acute and Chronic Heart Failure*, 2012. Available at: www.escardio.org/Guidelines-&-Education/Clinical-Practice-Guidelines/Acute-and-Chronic-Heart-Failure (accessed Dec. 2015).

Furosemide: rationale and evidence

Furosemide is a loop diuretic, which acts on the loop of Henle in the kidney to cause fluid loss. It is fast acting and therefore good for an acute situation like this. Fluid is lost from the circulation into the urine, which reduces afterload on the heart. This allows fluid to be more easily offloaded from the lungs and re-enter the circulation. This decrease in pulmonary congestion allows more effective breathing and oxygenation.

🔍 Evidence

Furosemide in acute LVF
Loop diuretics improve dyspnoea in patients with acute heart failure. This observation has been confirmed in the placebo groups of the Value of Endothelin Receptor Inhibition with Tezosentan in Acute Heart Failure Studies and the Efficacy of Vasopressin Antagonism in Heart Failure Outcome Study with Tolvaptan (McMurray *et al.*, 2007; Gheorghiade *et al.*, 2007).

✓ DRUGS checklist for FUROSEMIDE

Dose	40 mg as a starting point
Route	IV; can be given PO but will take longer to work
Units	mg
Given	As required
Special situations	If patient is already on high doses of furosemide, 40 mg may not be enough. Consider doubling patient's usual maintenance.

Furosemide: essential pharmacology

Furosemide is a loop diuretic, which acts of the loop of Henle in the kidney. It causes sodium ions not to be reabsorbed, which means water follows the sodium ions out into the urine. This therefore causes water to be lost from the circulation into the urine. In light of this mechanism of action, sodium is lost and also potassium. These electrolytes therefore need to be monitored. Furosemide helps symptoms of pulmonary oedema by reducing volume, and therefore afterload of the heart. This decreases pulmonary congestion and allows clearance of the fluid into the circulation.

Glyceryl trinitrate: rationale and evidence

This can be given as a sublingual spray or as an infusion. It relieves pulmonary oedema by dilating the pulmonary vessels, therefore decreasing pressure and encouraging fluid to seep out of the lung interstitium back into the circulation. General vasodilation also causes a decrease in afterload and therefore decreased back pressure on the pulmonary circulation, and more effective ventricular filling. Unlike in myocardial infarction, two sprays of GTN is rarely enough and often an infusion has to be prescribed. Ideally, aim for the maximum dose as this will optimise fluid offload. However, the dosing is often limited by a drop in blood pressure secondary to vasodilation, thereby potentially decreasing cardiac perfusion. For this reason GTN infusions must be slowly titrated up whilst closely monitoring blood pressure, aiming for a systolic blood pressure above 90 mmHg.

🔍 Evidence

GTN in acute LVF

Buccal, oral or intravenous GTN has been shown to reduce filling pressures in patients with acute decompensated heart failure, although no randomised trial has demonstrated superiority of GTN in reduction of dyspnoea, or determined optimal dose (Verma *et al.*, 1989). Some studies have shown that an aggressive vasodilator regimen was superior to diuretics in short-term outcomes, with a trend toward reduced myocardial infarction and in-hospital mortality rates (Sharon *et al.*, 2000; Cotter, 1998).

✓ DRUGS checklist for GLYCERYL TRINITRATE (GTN) SPRAY

Dose	2 sprays (each spray is 0.3 mg)
Route	Sublingual
Units	Sprays
Given	0.3–1 mg at a time, repeat as required
Special situations	Causes headache due to vasodilation of vessels in the head (as well as the desired coronary vessels). This can limit use.

✓ DRUGS checklist for GLYCERYL TRINITRATE (GTN) INFUSION

Dose	1–10 mg per hour
Route	IV
Units	mg
Given	As an infusion over 24 hours
Special situations	Titrate to blood pressure, as it will invariably drop blood pressure due to vasodilation. Ideally aim for the maximum dose, or dose that will adequately control pain without dropping BP to less than 90 mmHg systolic. Again can cause headache.

Glyceryl trinitrate : essential pharmacology

Please see Section Glyceryl Trinitrate in the Acute Coronary Syndrome section of this chapter.

Morphine sulphate: rationale and evidence

Morphine not only acts as an analgesic but also has vasodilator properties. It has been considered a central drug in the treatment of pulmonary oedema for many years. It causes venodilatation, peripheral venous pooling and reduces pulmonary congestion by decreasing afterload. It also affects the central nervous system to slow breathing and act as an anxiolytic. This is very helpful as it may help the fear element that exacerbates any cause of dyspnoea. Lower doses are needed when given for this intention. Despite its frequent use there are no large studies showing increase in survival or long-term benefit. In fact, some studies have shown an increase in adverse events and mortality with morphine for acute heart failure patients (Peacock *et al.*, 2008).

Morphine for acute LVF is given IV as this is fast acting and with good effect. Opiates cause respiratory depression and sedation so the dose must be titrated according to response. If any signs of rapidly decreasing respiratory rate or decreasing consciousness occur, then stop morphine. Respiratory depression could be fatal in someone who already has respiratory distress and is relying on a fast respiratory rate to maintain adequate oxygenation.

In the event of overdose naloxone can be used (see Chapter 1).

✓ DRUGS checklist for MORPHINE SULPHATE	
Dose	2.5–5 mg for pulmonary oedema
Route	IV; different formulations of morphine can be given via different routes (see Chapter 7)
Units	mg
Given	No maximum however this is being given for vasodilation and calming effect, therefore high doses are not required. Dose is titrated according to response, and consciousness levels
Special situations	Monitor carefully for respiratory depression or decreasing consciousness as this is very detrimental to a patient already in respiratory distress.

Morphine sulphate: essential pharmacology

Please see Chapter 7.

Other medications used in acute heart failure

Metoclopramide

Metoclopramide is an antiemetic commonly used with morphine. Patients with acute heart failure may have diminished circulation to the gut, causing nausea, as the body prioritises brain and chest circulation. Morphine is well known to cause nausea and vomiting also. Vomiting could be potentially harmful to the patient if it inhibits absorption of other important medications. Metoclopramide

is therefore given with morphine as symptomatic relief. If not tolerated, other antiemetics can be used.

✓ DRUGS checklist for METOCLOPRAMIDE	
Dose	10 mg
Route	PO or IV
Units	mg
Given	Up to three times in 24 hours
Special situations	Metoclopramide can cause an oculogyric crisis due to its effect on dopamine receptors (see Chapter 7). This occurs particularly in young women, although is rare. Procyclidine reverses this unwanted symptom.

For pharmacology please see Chapter 7.

Further aspects of acute left ventricular failure management

Acute LVF should not be thought of as a diagnosis in itself, as there is usually a cause of acute decompensation. Common causes are non-compliance with medications, disease progression, excess fluid intake, ischaemia, arrhythmias, new pulmonary embolus (PE), new anaemia, thyrotoxicosis, pregnancy, vitamin deficiency states (e.g. beri beri) and also drugs that cause decompensation (e.g. NSAIDs) and renal failure.

Oxygen: High-flow oxygen should be given to any patient in respiratory distress. This can be decreased as pulmonary oedema is corrected, and would be guided by the blood gas and saturation readings.

Arrhythmias: These are common precipitants for acute LVF and must be treated alongside (see Atrial Fibrillation and Arrhythmia Sections). In the setting of concurrent arrhythmia and LVF, caution must be taken with beta-blockers for rate control as these can precipitate acute heart failure. See the Common Pitfalls sections of the Arrhythmia section for advice about this. For example, if our patient had fast AF as well as acute LVF, we could consider digoxin rather than beta-blocker to control heart rate.

Acute coronary syndrome: MIs are common precipitants of acute LVF. Previous MIs also cause chronic LVF, which predisposes to episodes of acute LVF. Acute MI needs to be treated alongside acute LVF, as if left untreated it will continue to drive the problem (see Acute Coronary Syndrome Section for management).

Cardiogenic shock: In acute left ventricular with an ongoing underlying cause, cardiogenic shock may ensue. In our patient, the precipitating arrhythmia is no longer acutely present therefore shock is less likely. However, in ischaemic causes, ongoing arrhythmias or in underlying chronic left ventricular dysfunction, this is more likely. Cardiogenic shock will not respond to fluids in the same was as many other causes of shock. In fact, fluids would further overload a failing left ventricle and worsen pulmonary oedema. Any patient with cardiogenic shock needs to be discussed with a senior and considered for transfer to ITU for inotropes, and potentially for an intra-aortic balloon pump.

Thromboprophylaxis: Heart failure is a VTE risk factor therefore inpatients should be given prophylactic LMWH (see Chapter 7).

Fluid balance: Fluid balance will be critical in the few days after acute LVF. Any excess fluid intake can precipitate further pulmonary oedema. Patients may be put on fluid and salt restriction by the cardiology team to prevent this, particularly if there is chronic left ventricular failure (see Chronic Heart Failure Section). On top of any fluid restriction, patients will also have been heavily diuresed and therefore may be at risk of dehydration and acute kidney injury. This creates a difficult fluid balance situation. For this reason, urinary catheterisation is essential management of acute left ventricular failure with accurate fluid input and output balance recorded.

Chronic left ventricular failure: Patients with acute left ventricular failure may already have a degree of chronic left ventricular failure, or will go on to develop it. There are therefore other more chronic prescribing considerations (see Chronic Heart Failure Section). Investigations such as 24-hour ECGs and echocardiograms are likely to be part of the future investigation of any patient presenting with acute left ventricular failure.

Mechanical support: Devices are available to augment and support a failing left ventricle, both in the acute and chronic setting. Intra-aortic balloon pumps aim to temporarily improve coronary blood flow, and left ventricular assist devices (LVAD) can be inserted by specialist centres as a bridge to heart transplant. This is beyond the scope of this book. Specific prescribing considerations for these devices are surrounding anticoagulation, as foreign material in the circulation is extremely thrombogenic.

Ventilatory support: In patients with ongoing hypoxia (Po_2 <8 kPa) despite optimum oxygen delivery and other measures above, use of continuous positive airways pressure (CPAP) delivered non-invasively can be of benefit. For patients who have significantly decompensated ventilatory failure with a respiratory acidosis, non-invasive ventilation may be inadequate and invasive ventilation may be required where appropriate (Gray *et al.*, 2009).

 Guidelines

ESC heart failure guidelines recommend the following investigations in 'all' suspected heart failure: 12-lead ECG, echocardiogram, blood chemistry (urea and electrolytes, thyroid function tests, liver enzymes) and full blood count (McMurray *et al.*, 2012).

Case outcome and discharge

Mrs Clive responded well to diuretics and nitrates, and her breathlessness resolved. She was referred to a cardiologist to address control of her underlying arrhythmia, as it is likely to be an episode of fast AF that precipitated this episode. Prior to this appointment, an echocardiogram and 24-hour ECG were arranged to better assess the chronic function of the heart and assess frequency of arrhythmias. The echocardiogram showed good left ventricular systolic function with no valvular abnormalities. The only change to her medication in the short term was an increase in her dose of loop diuretic to a more conventional maintenance dose. On seeing the cardiologist after recovery, her bisoprolol dose was also increased to help prevent further episodes of fast AF.

DISCHARGE MEDICATION

Date	Medication	Dose	Route	Frequency	Supply	GP to continue?
xx/xx/xx	BISOPROLOL	5 mg	PO	Once daily	14 days	Y
xx/xx/xx	FUROSEMIDE	40 mg	PO	Once daily	14 days	Y
xx/xx/xx	SIMVASTATIN	40 mg	PO	Once daily	14 days	Y
xx/xx/xx	WARFARIN	2 mg	PO	Once daily as per INR	14 days	Y
xx/xx/xx	GTN SPRAY	2 puffs	PO	As required	14 days	Y

Notes to patient/GP:
These medications are to continue lifelong. Furosemide and bisoprolol doses were doubled during admission for control of heart failure.

Common pitfalls

- If a patient is already on a long-term cardioselective beta-blocker when they present with acute LVF, this is likely not to be the cause, and can usually be continued (unless patient is bradycardic or hypotensive).
- Furosemide can paradoxically increase blood pressure in the context of fluid overload, as a decrease in the afterload allows more effective left ventricular filling and a stronger systole, leading to a better systolic blood pressure. Therefore, if a patient is hypotensive, this does not automatically rule out furosemide as a therapy. Discuss with your senior.

What not to give

> **What not to give in acute LVF**
> - Beta-blockers
> - Calcium channel blockers
> - Antihypertensives

Beta-blockers: Despite the proven long-term benefits of beta-blockers in chronic heart failure (see Section Chronic Heart Failure), initial commencement or increase in beta-blocker dose can precipitate acute heart failure in the short term. This is due to the negatively inotropic effects of beta-blockers, as they decrease heart rate and contractility. This causes an acute drop in LV ejection fraction (Hall *et al.*, 1995). This increases fluid retention and reduces efficacy of ventricular emptying, which can worsen pulmonary oedema acutely. Usually, this can be treated by increasing diuretics doses, but sometimes beta-blocker dose has to be reduced or the drug stopped despite known improvement in survival. If a patient is already on a cardioselective beta-blocker when they develop acute heart failure, it is generally continued unless low blood pressure or bradycardia make this impossible. Generally, beta-blockers are not started or uptitrated until the patient is euvolaemic.

Ca^{2+} channel blockers: If a patient has chronic heart failure, and Ca^{2+} channel blockers are required for control of hypertension, amlodipine is the safest to use. Avoid verapamil and diltiazem (NICE, 2010b). Calcium channel blockers block the calcium channels in the cell membrane of cells, preventing calcium uptake. More specifically, they block L-type calcium channels, which are responsible for allowing influx of calcium for excitation of skeletal, smooth and cardiac muscle cells. By blocking excitation of vascular smooth muscle, they cause arterial dilation (there is no effect on venous smooth muscle). This decreases afterload and reduces blood pressure, hence their use for hypertension. However, in heart failure this benefit is outweighed by the dampening effect on myocardial cells, causing a lowering in heart rate and reduced force of contraction. This negatively inotropic effect can cause an acute deterioration on left ventricular function and worsening of heart failure symptoms.

Antihypertensives: Antihypertensives cause a drop in blood pressure. In the setting of an acutely failing left ventricle, systolic blood pressure is already likely to drop. Additional antihypertensives can therefore cause dangerously low blood pressure, which may lead to syncope and end organ damage, and also confuse the picture with cardiogenic shock.

SUMMARY

Acute LVF is a medical emergency and every doctor should be aware of the initial steps in its management. An ABC approach is warranted, as is early senior input. Junior doctors would be expected to initiate treatment for this, and should have an awareness of the treatments available, along with their side effects and interactions. All junior doctors will encounter these medications at some point in their career and it is important to be aware of the large base of evidence behind this management.

FURTHER READING

- McMurray JJ, Adamopoulos S, Anker SD, *et al.* (2012). ESC guidelines for the diagnosis and treatment of acute and chronic heart failure 2012. *Eur Heart J* 33: 1787–847.
- American College of Cardiology/ American Heart Association (1995). Guidelines for the Evaluation and Management of Heart Failure Report of the American College of Cardiology/ American Heart Association Task Force on Practice Guidelines (Committee on Evaluation and Management of Heart Failure). *Circulation* 92: 2764–84.

🔑 Key learning points

Acute left ventricular failure
- Start with ABCDE approach.
- Oxygen is recommended if the patient is hypoxic or in respiratory distress.
- Give 40 mg IV furosemide, GTN spray and morphine initially.
- Add GTN infusion if continued dyspnoea.
- Portable CXR can be done quickly and will aid diagnosis.
- Dropping BP can signal impending cardiogenic shock; call the cardiologist and alert intensive care department.
- Stop any aggravating medications.
- Treat any causal factors.
- Acute LVF should not be thought of as a diagnosis in itself – look for the cause of decompensation.

Chronic heart failure

> **Mrs Vera Roads**
>
> **Age: 75**
>
> **Hospital number: 123456**

Case study

Presenting complaint: *A 75-year-old woman presents to A&E with gradual worsening of shortness of breath. She has been unable to take her medication due to inability to mobilise to the GP surgery due to leg swelling.*

Background: *She lives with her husband in a house and mobilises with a frame. She is an ex smoker (20 pack years) and drinks 5–6 units of alcohol per week.*

PMH: *Hypertension, myocardial infarction (7 years ago), osteoarthritis and a right knee replacement (3 years ago).*

Allergies: *Oxytetracycline (causes a rash)*

Examination:
HR 120 reg, RR 24, BP 116/70, Sats 97% on air, afebrile, BM 6.5,

CVS: *Capillary refill time <2 seconds, pulse feels regular, JVP raised +6 cm*
Bilateral pitting leg oedema up to knees, HS I + II + soft pansystolic murmur

RS: *Bibasal fine inspiratory crepitations, no wheeze*

Abdo: *Soft, non-tender, 1 cm pulsatile liver edge palpable, bowel sounds present*

Chest X-ray *shows clear lung fields but some upper lobe blood diversion*

ECG *shows sinus tachycardia with tall QRS complexes in chest leads*

Bloods: *Hb 13.6, Plt 324, WCC 8.9, Na 136, K 4.3, Urea 6.5, Creat 136, INR 1.1*

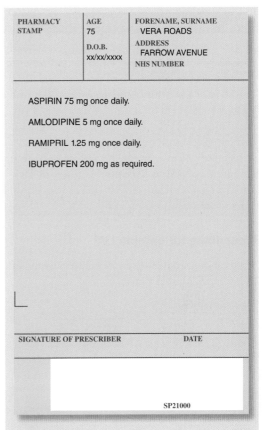

PHARMACY STAMP	AGE 75	FORENAME, SURNAME VERA ROADS
	D.O.B. xx/xx/xxxx	ADDRESS FARROW AVENUE
		NHS NUMBER

ASPIRIN 75 mg once daily.

AMLODIPINE 5 mg once daily.

RAMIPRIL 1.25 mg once daily.

IBUPROFEN 200 mg as required.

SIGNATURE OF PRESCRIBER   DATE

SP21000

Diagnosis

This patient has symptomatic congestive cardiac failure.

Signs of right-sided heart failure are raised JVP, peripheral oedema and hepatomegaly. Signs of left-sided heart failure are bibasal crepitations with upper lobe blood diversion on CXR. This could have been initially caused by ischaemic heart disease in light of her history. It may have been made worse by the fact she has not been taking her diuretic lately. Coronary artery disease is the most common cause of chronic heart failure in the western world.

Initial measures

Chronic heart failure is not reversible; however, measures can be taken to improve symptoms, reduce hospital admissions, prevent deterioration in heart function and improve prognosis and quality of life.

(Continued)

🔍 Case study (*Continued*)

Treatment for heart failure is therefore centred not only around pharmacological interventions, but also patient education, compliance and identification of any contributory co-morbidities such as hypertension, coronary artery disease, arrhythmias and anaemia.

Pharmacological treatments are split in to two categories: disease-modifying treatments and symptom-control treatments. Disease modifying-treatments include ACEIs, ARBS, beta-blockers and aldosterone antagonists.

Prescribing for chronic LVF

A typical drug chart for a heart failure patient with an ischaemic cause is shown.

REGULAR PRESCRIPTIONS				Circle/enter times below ↓	Enter dates below ↘			
					Day 1	Day 2	Day 3	Day 4
DRUG RAMIPRIL				06				
				08				
Dose 5 mg	Route PO	Freq BD	Start date xx/xx/xx	12				
Signature A. Doctor		Bleep	Review	16				
				18				
Additional instructions				22				
DRUG CARVEDILOL				06				
				08				
Dose 25 mg	Route PO	Freq BD	Start date xx/xx/xx	12				
Signature A. Doctor		Bleep	Review	16				
				18				
Additional instructions				22				
DRUG SPIRONOLACTONE				06				
				08				
Dose 25 mg	Route PO	Freq OD	Start date xx/xx/xx	12				
Signature A. Doctor		Bleep	Review	16				
				18				
Additional instructions				22				
DRUG FRUSEMIDE				06				
				08				
Dose 20 mg	Route PO	Freq BD	Start date xx/xx/xx	12				
Signature A. Doctor		Bleep	Review	16				
				18				
Additional instructions				22				
DRUG ASPIRIN				06				
				08				
Dose 75 mg	Route PO	Freq OD	Start date xx/xx/xx	12				
Signature A. Doctor		Bleep	Review	16				
				18				
Additional instructions				22				
DRUG SIMVASTATIN				06				
				08				
Dose 40 mg	Route PO	Freq OD	Start date xx/xx/xx	12				
Signature A. Doctor		Bleep	Review	16				
				18				
Additional instructions				22				

Target doses of key drugs in heart failure are given in Table 3.2. Doses may be limited by low heart rate, low blood pressure or development of side effects/intolerances.

ACE inhibitors: rationale and evidence

In heart failure with reduced ejection fraction, preload is already elevated. Increasing the preload further will not necessarily increase stroke volume and could in fact exacerbate pulmonary oedema. Emphasis is therefore on decreasing afterload to increase overall cardiac output. ACEIs cause vasodilation, which decreases afterload and significantly enhances ventricular stroke volume and decreases preload, thereby improving ejection fraction (Dr Jubin Joseph, Oxford University, personal communication).

ACEIs also have a beneficial effect on ventricular remodelling and arterial pressure. ACEIs are first-line treatment in all patients with heart failure and have been shown to reduce hospitalisations and improve survival (see Evidence).

✓ DRUGS checklist for ENALAPRIL

Dose	2.5 mg aiming for 10–20 mg
Route	PO
Units	mg
Given	Start at 2.5 mg BD, aiming for 10–20 mg BD
Special situations	ACEIs will cause a degree of renal impairment. Allow a <50% deterioration in baseline creatinine; however, renal function that is poor may limit dosing.

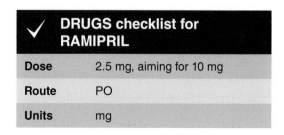

✓ DRUGS checklist for RAMIPRIL

Dose	2.5 mg, aiming for 10 mg
Route	PO
Units	mg

Given	Start at 2.5 mg OD, aiming for 10 mg OD
Special situations	ACEIs will cause a degree of renal impairment. Allow a <50% deterioration in baseline creatinine; however, renal function that is poor may limit dosing.

✓ DRUGS checklist for LISINOPRIL

Dose	2.5 mg aiming for 20–35 mg
Route	PO
Units	mg
Given	Start at 2.5 mg OD, aiming for 20–35 mg OD
Special situations	ACEIs will cause a degree of renal impairment. Allow a <50% deterioration in baseline creatinine; however, renal function that is poor may limit dosing.

🔍 Evidence

CONSENSUS (Cooperative North Scandinavian Enalapril Survival Study) trial of 253 patients with severe congestive heart failure (NYHA IV) with increased heart size. All were on digoxin and diuretics. Enalapril resulted in:

- Reduced all-cause mortality
- Reduced death due to progression of heart failure.

SOLVD-T (Studies of Left Ventricular Dysfunction Treatment) trial of 2569 patients with clinically stable chronic heart failure (mostly NYHA II and III) and decreased ejection fraction (<0.35). Long-term enalapril resulted in:

- Reduced death due to all causes
- Reduced death or hospitalisation due to heart failure
- Greatest effect in reducing death due to progressive heart failure
- Greater benefit in patients with lower ejection fraction.

Table 3.2 Target doses of key drugs in heart failure.

Drug category	Drug	Starting dose (mg)	Target dose (mg)
ACEI	Ramipril	2.5 OD	10 OD
	Enalapril	2.5 BD	10–20 BD
	Lisinopril	2.5–5.0 OD	20–35 OD
ARB	Candesartan	4 or 8 OD	32 OD
	Valsartan	40 BD	160 BD
Aldosterone antagonist	Eplerenone	25 OD	50 OD
	Spironolactone	25 OD	25–50 OD
Beta-blocker	Bisoprolol	1.25 OD	10 OD
	Carvedilol	3.125 BD	25–50 BD
	Metoprolol	50 OD	200 OD

Contraindications for ACEIs

- History of angioedema
- Bilateral renal artery stenosis
- Severe aortic stenosis
- Pregnancy.

Common problems (see BNF (BMA/RPS, 2015)):

- Worsening renal function/hyperkalaemia – a small increase in creatinine, urea and K$^+$ is expected, but if creatinine is deteriorating (>50% baseline or >200 mol/L) or hyperkalaemia (K >5.5 mmol/L) consider stopping or reducing doses of other nephrotoxic drugs, non-essential vasodilators, potassium supplements or potassium-retaining agents and diuretics (if not fluid overloaded).
- Symptomatic hypotension – if symptoms of dizziness, confusion or collapse consider stopping other non-essential vasodilators and, if not overloaded, diuretics.
- Cough – typically dry, irritating cough, triggered by bradykinin release. If this occurs, consider swapping for an ARB. Cough can develop even after years on an ACEI and can take some weeks to resolve after cessation. However, ensure that this symptom is not due to pulmonary oedema before altering the ACEI.

Alternatives to ACEI: ARBs (see Section Other Medications Used in Chronic Heart Failure).

ACE inhibitors: essential pharmacology

ACEIs reduce the conversion of angiotensin I to angiotensin II, disrupting the body's main mechanism for vasoconstriction and fluid retention, the renin-angiotensin-aldosterone system. Angiotensin II is found in the pulmonary circulation and in the endothelium of many blood vessels, and is a potent vasoconstrictor. By inhibiting production of this, ACEIs cause arterial and venous dilatation, increase cardiac stroke volume and increased excretion of sodium in the urine. Angiotensin converting enzyme inactivates bradykinin, hence ACEIs cause an increase in bradykinins (Dr Jubin Joseph, Oxford University, personal communication).

ACEIs also have a beneficial effect on ventricular remodelling. This is because ACE stimulates a number of pro-oncogenes, which cause fibrogenesis and apoptosis, contributing to ventricular remodelling and ventricular hypertrophy. ACEIs prevent this (Khatter, 2003).

Beta-blockers: rationale and evidence

Cardioselective beta-blockers are first-line therapy in all patients with heart failure, and include bisoprolol, carvedilol and metoprolol. They have been shown to improve left ventricular ejection fraction, improve survival, reduce deaths from cardiovascular causes and reduce hospitalisations. They should be started at low dose then titrated up to the desired dose, providing excessively low heart rate or excessive drop in blood pressure don't prevent this dose increase.

Despite the proven long-term benefits of beta-blockers, initial commencement or increase in dose can cause acute heart failure in the short term. This is due to the increased fluid retention that peripheral vasodilation may cause, which can worsen pulmonary oedema acutely. Usually this can be treated by increasing diuretic doses, but sometimes beta-blocker dose has to be reduced or the drug stopped despite known improvement in long-term survival.

✓ DRUGS checklist for BISOPROLOL	
Dose	1.25 mg starting, aiming for 10 mg
Route	PO
Units	mg
Given	OD, aiming for 10 mg OD
Special situations	None

✓ DRUGS checklist for CARVEDILOL	
Dose	3.125 mg BD starting dose
Route	PO
Units	mg
Given	BD, aiming for 25–50 mg BD
Special situations	None

✓ DRUGS checklist for METOPROLOL

Dose	50 mg starting, aiming for 200 mg
Route	PO, can also be given IV but not for chronic LVF
Units	mg
Given	OD, aiming for 200 mg OD
Special situations	None

Contraindications for beta-blockers (BNF (BMA/RPS, 2015)):
- Reversible airways disease
- Severe asthma
- Second or third-degree atrioventricular block
- Hypotension.

Cautions for beta-blockers:
- Severe (New York Heart Association [NYHA] class IV) heart failure
- Recent exacerbation of heart failure
- Heart block
- Sick sinus syndrome
- Heart rate <60 bpm
- Severe peripheral vascular disease.

🔍 Evidence

MERIT-HF (Metoprolol Randomized Intervention Trial in congestive Heart Failure Study Group) 3991 patients with LVEF <0.40 and NYHA class II-IV heart failure, stabilised by optimum standard therapy (any combination of diuretics + ACE inhibitor) randomised to either metoprolol or placebo. Study was halted early because all-cause mortality was significantly lower in the metoprolol group (34% risk reduction) and there were significantly fewer cardiovascular deaths, sudden deaths and death from heart failure (Hjalmarson *et al.*, 1999).

CIBIS II (Cardiac Insufficiency Bisoprolol Study II) 2647 patients with LVEF <35% and NYHA class III/IV receiving standard therapy (diuretic plus ACE inhibitor/other vasodilator) were randomised to bisoprolol or placebo. Study was halted early because all-cause mortality was significantly less in the bisoprolol group than in the placebo group and there was a significant reduction in sudden deaths, all cardiovascular deaths and all-cause hospitalisation. Treatment effects were independent of severity or cause of heart failure (Klein *et al.*, 1999).

COPERNICUS (Carvedilol Prospective Randomized Cumulative Survival Trial) 2289 patients with NYHA III/IV and LVEF <25%, receiving standard therapy (diuretic plus ACEI/ARB) randomised to carvedilol or placebo. The study halted early because there was a significant reduction in all-cause mortality in the carvedilol group (35% relative risk reduction) and a significant reduction in combined endpoint of death or hospitalisation (Eichhorn *et al.,* 2001).

Beta-blockers: essential pharmacology

Beta-blockers block beta-2-adrenoceptors, which are key in potentiating the sympathetic response. The sympathetic response consists of tachycardia, increased blood pressure, anxiety, sweating and pupillary dilation. Beta-blockers prevent excess sympathetic stimulation, therefore cause slowing of the heart rate and decreasing of the blood pressure (Arcangelo and Peterson, 2006). Reduction in heart rate causes prolongation of diastolic filling time therefore improved ejection fraction. Beta-blockers may also improve ventricular relaxation. Despite the fact that beta-blockers are negatively inotropic, they can actually improve left ventricular ejection fraction in heart failure patients by allowing increased diastolic filling time. This also has beneficial effects on cardiac remodelling (Khattar, 2003). These beneficial effects are widely accepted but the exact mechanism by which beta-blockers confer their benefit is still being researched.

Aldosterone receptor antagonists: rationale and evidence

Mineralocorticoid/aldosterone receptor antagonists such as spironolactone and eplerenone have been shown to improve symptoms, reduce hospital admissions and increase survival when added to standard therapy in patients with a reduced left ventricular ejection fraction (LVEF) and symptomatic heart failure (see Evidence). Spironolactone is used in routine practice and eplerenone is used following myocardial infarction. This is because eplerenone is shown to have beneficial effects on cardiac remodelling in this group (Pitt *et al.*, 2003).

An aldosterone antagonist should be considered in patients who remain in severe heart failure (NYHA class III or IV) despite treatment with a diuretic, ACEI (or ARB) and beta-blocker. They should be initiated early in patients with post infarction-related severe heart failure.

As with ACEIs, treatment with an aldosterone antagonist should be initiated at a low dose with careful monitoring of serum electrolytes and renal function.

✓ DRUGS checklist for SPIRONOLACTONE

Dose	25 mg starting dose, aiming for 50 mg
Route	PO
Units	mg
Given	OD
Special situations	Note that this chronic heart failure dose is different to the higher dose used in chronic liver disease and other situations requiring more significant diuresis.

✓ DRUGS checklist for EPLERENONE

Dose	25 mg starting dose, aiming for 50 mg
Route	PO
Units	mg
Given	OD
Special situations	Eplerenone is used in preference to spironolactone post-MI.

Common problems (BNF (BMA/RPS, 2015)):

- Hyperkalaemia and uraemia are the adverse effects of greatest concern (as with ACEIs and ARBs).

🔍 Evidence

RALES (Randomized Aldactone Evaluation Study) 1663 patients in NYHA class III/IV with LVEF <35% and receiving an ACEI, loop diuretic and (most patients) digoxin were randomised to placebo or 25 mg spironolactone. Trial stopped early because all-cause mortality significantly reduced in spironolactone group (30% relative risk reduction). The effect was mostly due to reduction in sudden death and death due to heart failure progression. Benefit was independent of age, ejection fraction, cause of heart failure and concurrent therapy (Pitt *et al.*, 1999).

EMPHASIS-HF (Eplerenone in Mild Patients Hospitalization and Survival Study in Heart Failure) 2737 patients less than 55 years with NHYA II symptoms and LVEF less than 33% receiving ACEI, ARB, or both, beta-blocker and either hospitalisation with heart failure (HF) in last 6 months or elevated BNP. Treatment with eplerenone (50 mg) led to 37% relative risk reduction in cardiovascular death or HF hospitalisation over average 21 months treatment (Zannad *et al.*, 2010)

EPHESUS (Eplenerone Post Acute Myocardial Infarction Heart Failure Efficacy and Survival) 6632 patients enrolled 3–14 days after acute MI with ejection fraction 40% and HF or diabetes. Eplenerone (25–50 mg) plus ACEI/ARB and beta-blocker. Treatment with eplenerone led to relative risk reduction of 15% in death over 16 months (Pitt *et al.*, 2001).

Aldosterone receptor antagonists: essential pharmacology

Spironolactone and eplerenone are aldosterone antagonists and act as potassium-sparing diuretics. This means that they block the mineralocorticoid receptor so that aldosterone cannot bind. This prevents resorption of sodium in the collecting duct of the kidney and therefore prevents the fluid retention that would follow. In preventing resorption of sodium, these drugs also prevent excretion of potassium by disruption of the sodium/potassium ion exchange process (Rossi, 2006). On the one hand this is good because it means that these drugs don't cause hypokalaemia (potassium sparing); however, it also means that they increase risk of hyperkalaemia.

Spironolactone acts at mineralocorticoid receptors and therefore is also an antagonist of androgen receptors. This means it acts as an antiandrogen, inhibiting androgen production. This makes it useful for conditions associated with androgen excess such as acne and polycystic ovarian syndrome. However, it also means that it causes gynaecomastia and testicular atrophy as an unwanted effect in heart failure patients (Loriaux et al., 1976).

Diuretics: rationale and evidence

Diuretics are a symptom-modifying treatment in chronic heart failure. They have not been shown to improve survival or modify the course of the disease; however, almost all patients will require them for symptom relief.

The main two classes of diuretics used for chronic heart failure are loop diuretics (i.e. furosemide), which results in a rapid onset of an intense but short-lived diuresis (especially in patients with concomitant renal dysfunction) and thiazide diuretics (i.e. bendroflumethiazide), which has a longer lasting but gentler effect (used in patients with milder symptoms) (Dr Jubin Joseph, Oxford University, personal communication). Bendroflumethiazide is also useful in severe heart failure, where the effects of long-term administration of a loop diuretic may be diminished by increased sodium reabsorption at the distal tubule. Thiazides overcome this problem as they blocks sodium reabsorption in the distal tubule.

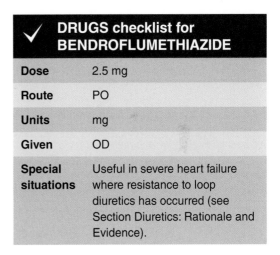

DRUGS checklist for FUROSEMIDE

Dose	20–120 mg (max dose daily, discuss with senior)
Route	PO
Units	mg
Given	OD or BD
Special situations	Titrate dose to tolerance, blood pressure and electrolyte control. Heart failure patients will be on other medications that are beneficial to survival, hence furosemide dose must fit around the optimum doses of these medications as first priority.

DRUGS checklist for BENDROFLUMETHIAZIDE

Dose	2.5 mg
Route	PO
Units	mg
Given	OD
Special situations	Useful in severe heart failure where resistance to loop diuretics has occurred (see Section Diuretics: Rationale and Evidence).

Common problems (Dr Jubin Joseph, Oxford University, personal communication): Patients may develop resistance to oral diuretics for unknown reasons (possibly due to gut oedema, hypotension or reduced renal blood flow) and in this situation either a bolus or an infusion of intravenous loop diuretic may be required. Loop and thiazide diuretics work by blocking sodium reabsorption. They therefore can cause hyponatraemia and hypokalaemia, which if severe may require potassium replacement and/or limit these as treatment options.

Diuretics: essential pharmacology

Furosemide is a loop diuretic, bendroflumethiazide is a thiazide diuretic. They act by blocking sodium reabsorption at specific sites in the renal tubule, thereby enhancing urinary excretion of sodium and water, which results in rapid and effective reduction in symptoms and signs of fluid overload.

Other medications used in chronic heart failure

Angiotensin receptor blockers

ARBs are a good alternative to ACEIs in cases where ACEIs are contraindicated due to allergy or cough. ARBs block the binding of angiotensin II to the angiotensin receptor. This is different to ACEIs, as these inhibit the production of angiotensin II.

Unlike ACEIs, ARBS do not inhibit the breakdown of bradykinin, which is the main mechanism for cough (Abdi *et al.*, 2002). It is therefore a good alternative for these patients. ARBS have been shown to produce similar benefits to ACEIs, so are good alternative.

As second-line therapy, an ARB used in addition to an ACEI and beta-blocker improves LVEF and symptoms whilst reducing hospital admissions and the risk of cardiovascular death (see Evidence). However, adding an aldosterone antagonist to an ACEI is of benefit to these patients but the safety of an ACEI, beta-blocker, ARB and aldosterone antagonist combination is uncertain and therefore not recommended. Therefore, in symptomatic patients already on ACEI and beta-blocker, an ARB or aldosterone antagonist can be added, but not both.

✓	**DRUGS checklist for VALSARTAN**
Dose	40 mg aiming for 160 mg BD
Route	PO
Units	mg
Given	Start at 40 mg BD, aiming for 160 mg BD

Special situations	ARBs (like ACEIs) will cause a degree of renal impairment. Allow a <50% deterioration in baseline creatinine; however, renal function that is poor may limit dosing.

Contraindications:

- Bilateral renal artery stenosis
- Severe aortic stenosis

Common problems (same as with ACEIs):

- Hypotension
- Renal dysfunction
- Hyperkalaemia

These adverse effects are encountered as frequently as with an ACEI.

🔍 Evidence

Val-HeFT (Valsartan Heart Failure Trial, 2000) 5010 patients with NYHA class II–IV (mostly II–III) on standard therapy (ACEI, diuretics and digoxin) were randomised to placebo or to valsartan. At 2-year follow-up, valsartan did not significantly affect all-cause mortality but did significantly reduce the combined endpoint of mortality and morbidity. This effect largely mediated through a reduction in HF hospitalisations (Cohn, 2001).

Ivabradine

Ivabradine is used in patients who have heart failure of NYHA class II–IV who are in sinus rhythm with a heart rate of greater than 70 bpm (Dr Jubin Joseph, Oxford University, personal communication). It is given in combination with standard therapy, including beta-blocker therapy or when beta-blocker therapy is contraindicated/not tolerated.

When added to standard heart failure medication, ivabradine decreases cardiovascular death rate and risk of hospitalisation (see Evidence).

Ivabradine acts on the If ion current, which is a mixed Na$^+$–K$^+$ inward current (f is for funny). This current is highly expressed in the sinus node and is modulated by the autonomic nervous system.

Blocking this channel reduces sinus node activity, therefore reducing heart rate. It is a good alternative when beta-blockers are not tolerated, as it has much less of an effect on blood pressure than beta-blockers yet still controls heart rate effectively.

Contraindications: sick sinus syndrome.

Common problems: luminous phenomena (sensation of enhances brightness) – usually mild.

Evidence

SHIFT (Systolic Heart failure treatment with the IF inhibitor ivabradine Trial) 6558 patients in sinus rhythm with a resting heart rate of >70 bpm, chronic heart failure for >4 weeks with an admission for worsening heart failure during the previous 12 months and LVEF of <35% on optimum management were randomised to ivabradine or placebo. Ivabradine reduced admissions due to worsening heart failure. Patients with heart rates higher than the median were at increased risk of an event and experienced a greater reduction in events with ivabradine than those with lower heart rates (Swedberg, 2010).

Digoxin

Digoxin is most commonly used as rate control for patients in atrial fibrillation (see Section Atrial Fibrillation). However, it has been shown to reduce hospital admissions in patients with heart failure when used in addition to ACEIs and diuretics (even where patients are in sinus rhythm) (Digitalis Investigation Group, 1997). Digoxin is therefore used as an additional therapy in heart failure patients in sinus rhythm who remain symptomatic despite ACEIs, beta-blockers and ARB/mineralocorticoids . Where patients are in atrial fibrillation, it may be used at an earlier stage if betablockade fails to control the ventricular rate, as it has an additional rate-controlling action.

Digoxin increases myocardial contractility by inhibiting cell membrane Na^+/K^+ ATP pumps, and therefore increasing intracellular calcium. It also enhances parasympathetic activity, thereby slowing heart rate.

✓ DRUGS checklist for DIGOXIN

Dose	250 micrograms
Route	PO
Units	micrograms
Given	OD
Special situations	Note this dose differs from the higher doses that may be used for rate control of atrial fibrillation. Digoxin levels must be monitored as it has a narrow therapeutic window (see Digoxin Toxicity). Levels are best taken 7–10 days after starting treatment.

Contraindications (BNF (BMA/RPS, 2015)): second-degree or third-degree atrioventricular block and pre-excitation syndromes.

Cautions: sick sinus syndrome.

Common problems:

- Hypokalaemia: digoxin causes this, but also increases susceptibility to the adverse effects of hypokalaemia. Potassium must therefore be checked and corrected
- Poor renal function: reduce dose to 125 micrograms or 62.5 micrograms and check levels.
- Digoxin toxicity: anorexia, nausea, sinoatrial and atrioventricular block, arrhythmias, confusion and visual disturbances. Withhold drug, or if levels >10 ng/mL or life-threatening arrhythmia then treat with digoxin-specific antibody fragments (Digibind).

Evidence

DIG (Digitalis Investigation Group, 1997) 6800 patients with an EF <45% with heart failure category NYHA II–IV receiving standard therapy (ACE-inhibitor and diuretic) were randomised to placebo or digoxin. At 3-year follow-up treatment with digoxin did not alter all-cause mortality, but decreased hospital admissions for worsening HF.

Hydralazine and isosorbide dinitrate

Hydralazine is a powerful direct-acting arterial vasodilator with an unknown mechanism of action. Nitrates dilate both veins and arteries, reducing preload and afterload.

Neither of these drugs has shown a significant benefit in heart failure outcomes, except for in African Americans.

Hydralazine and isosorbide dinitrate (ISDN) should therefore be given as an additional treatment in African American patients, and considered for other patients who remain symptomatic on other proven therapies. These medications can also be used as substitute in patients with intolerance to an ACEI and an ARB (Dr Jubin Joseph, Oxford University, personal communication).

Evidence

V-HeFT (Vasodilator–Heart Failure Trial) 642 men were randomized to placebo, prazosin or hydralazine and isosorbide dinitrate (H-ISDN) added to a diuretic and digoxin. At 2-year follow-up patients in the H-ISDN group showed a trend to a reduction in all cause mortality (RRR 22%) increased exercise capacity and LVEF (Cohn, 1986).

A-HeFT (African-American Heart Failure Trial) 1050 African-American men and women in NYHA III/IV on standard therapy (diuretic, ACE-inhibitor, beta blocker) were randomised to placebo or H-ISDN. The trial was discontinued prematurely after a median follow-up of 10 months, as patients receiving H-ISDN had a significant reduction in mortality (RRR 43%), a reduction in the risk of HF hospitalisation (RRR 33%) and improved quality of life (Franciosa, 2002).

Inotropes and phosphodiesterase inhibitors

Inotropic drugs increase stroke volume, increase ejection fraction and reduce preload. Examples are sympathomimetics, such as adrenaline, and phosphodiesterase inhibitors, such as milrinone. These effects are ideal for encouraging optimal cardiac output.

However, these are IV infusions and require a patient to be in hospital. They are also very good for short-term treatment of heart failure, but prolonged use has been shown to worsen the outcome and increase mortality in some patients.

These drugs may be used in end-stage heart failure during a time of acute illness, or as a bridge to cardiac transplant/VAD placement.

Further aspects of chronic heart failure management

Implantable cardiac defibrillators

Patients with chronic heart failure are at increased risk of ventricular and other arrhythmias and therefore have increased risk of sudden cardiac death. Implantable cardiac defibrillators (ICDs) have been shown to improve survival in patients with NYHA class II–III heart failure due to systolic dysfunction (see Evidence). They are also used in selected patients post-MI.

As a result, all patients with NYHA class II and III heart failure with LVEF <35% and an expected survival of greater than 1 year should be considered for an ICD as a primary prevention device. In addition, patients who have survived cardiac arrest or who have symptomatic ventricular arrhythmias should be considered for device therapy as secondary prevention.

Evidence

SCD-HeFT (Sudden Cardiac Death in Heart Failure Trial) 2521 patients with non-ischaemic dilated cardiomyopathy or ischaemic HF, no prior symptomatic ventricular arrhythmia and an EF <35% with NYHA II/III. These patients were randomised to placebo, amiodarone or an ICD, in addition to conventional treatment (ACE-inhibitor/ARB and a beta blocker). At 4-year follow-up ICD treatment led to a reduction in mortality (23%). Amiodarone had no effect on survival (Bardy *et al.*, 2005).

MADIT-II (Multicenter Automatic Defibrillator Implantation Trial II) 1232 patients with a prior myocardial infarction (not within previous 4 weeks) and an EF <30% were randomised to conventional treatment or conventional treatment plus an ICD. Use of an ICD led to a reduction in mortality (31% RRR), largely driven through a reduction in sudden cardiac death (Moss *et al.*, 2002).

Cardiac resynchronisation therapy

Widening of the QRS complex in cardiac failure is a sign of abnormal electrical activation between the ventricles, causing dys-synchronous contraction and less efficient ventricular emptying. Cardiac resynchronisation therapy (CRT) is a biventricular pacemaker which optimises atrioventricular timing, ventricular synchrony and improves effectiveness of cardiac contraction. CRT can therefore be considered for patients with a wide QRS complex (>120 ms) who remain symptomatic (NYHA II–IV) despite maximal medical therapy and a reduced LVEF (<35%). In these patients, CRT has been show to improve pump function, relieve symptoms, prolong exercise capacity and reduce the composite of death or hospital admission. CRT devices can also have a defibrillator capacity.

🔍 Evidence

COMPANION (Comparison of Medical Therapy, Pacing, and Defibrillation in Heart Failure) 600 patients with NYHA III/IV with QRS >120 ms and P–R interval >150 ms with a HF hospitalisation or equivalent in the preceding year were randomised to conventional therapy, conventional therapy plus CRT or conventional therapy plus CRT

with an ICD. Patient with a CRT had a reduced risk of death from any cause and hospital admission for worsening HF (24% RRR with CRT-P [pacing] and of 36% RRR with CRT-D [defibrillating]) (Bristow *et al.*, 2000).

CARE-HF (Cardiac Resynchronization in Heart Failure Study) 813 patients with NYHA III/IV despite conventional treatment, an LVEF <35%, and QRS duration >120 ms were randomised to conventional treatment or conventional treatment plus a CRT device. (Patients with a QRS duration <150 ms were also required to have echocardiographic confirmation of ventricular dys-synchrony). At 2-year follow-up, patients in the CRT group had a lower mortality (36% RRR) and hospital admission with HF (52% RRR) (Cleland *et al.*, 2005).

MADIT-CRT (Multicenter Automatic Defibrillator Implantation Trial with Cardiac Resynchronisation Therapy) 1820 patients with NYHA I/II and LVEF <30% and QRS duration >130 ms with conventional medical therapy were randomised to receive CRT-D or ICD. At follow-up averaging 2.4 years, patients with CRT-D had a lower combined mortality and non-fatal HF event, largely driven by a reduction in HF events (41% RRR) (Moss *et al.*, 2009).

MIRACLE-ICD (Multicentre InSync ICD Randomized Clinical Evaluation) evaluated 369 patients with NYHA III/IV heart failure and CRT-D devices where 182 had the CRT function switched off. The CRT group had greater improvement in quality of life score and functional class compared to controls. There was no difference in survival, LV size or function, overall heart failure status and rates of hospitalization. (Young *et al.*, 2003).

Cardiac transplantation

Cardiac transplantation is an option in selected patients with end-stage heart failure with severe symptoms, a poor prognosis and no further treatment options. Many patients may not be candidates for this given the need for major surgery with a long general anaesthetic, ITU stay, intensive postoperative rehabilitation and need for lifelong immunosuppression. Co-morbidities are important deciding factors, as well as the fact that organs are in short supply and may not be available in time for severely unwell patients.

Left ventricular assist devices

Left ventricular assist devices (LVAD) are mechanical pumps implanted in the ventricle that augment cardiac output. At present, mechanical circulatory support with an LVAD is seen as a 'bridge to transplantation' and therefore not a long-term solution. Wider use is limited by the high cost of implantation and of the device itself, as well frequent complications such as bleeding, thromboembolism, infection and device failure.

Case outcome and discharge

This patient was initially treated with IV furosemide and fluid restriction to decrease pulmonary congestion, then was commenced on long-term cardiac failure medications. Amlodipine was substituted for a beta-blocker, in light of known prognostic benefits. Ramipril was doubled to 2.5 mg. Ibuprofen was stopped as NSAIDs can worsen symptoms of heart failure due to increasing fluid retention (Bleumink *et al.*, 2003).

In the GP summary it should be made clear that beta-blocker and ACEI doses should be slowly increased until the target dose is reached (if tolerated).

Contact was also established during the admission with the hospital cardiac failure nurse. Such specialist nurses are a valuable resource, giving ongoing advice and liaison for patients and health professionals in the community as well assisting in up-titration of heart failure medications.

As chronic heart failure is a deteriorating chronic condition with a high mortality, palliative care specialists can be invaluable in helping symptoms and improving quality of life.

NB: When initiating ACEIs, renal function needs to be checked 2 weeks afterwards. An increase in creatinine is to be expected, but large increases may limit doses.

DISCHARGE MEDICATION						
Date	Medication	Dose	Route	Frequency	Supply	GP to continue?
xx/xx/xx	ASPIRIN	75 mg	PO	Once daily	14 days	Y
xx/xx/xx	BISOPROLOL	2.5 mg	PO	Once daily	14 days	Y
xx/xx/xx	RAMIPRIL	2.5 mg	PO	Once daily	14 days	Y
xx/xx/xx	FUROSEMIDE	40 mg	PO	Twice daily	14 days	Y
xx/xx/xx	SPIRONOLACTONE	25 mg	PO	Once daily	14 days	Y
xx/xx/xx	PARACETAMOL	1 g	PO	Up to four times daily, as required	7 days	N

Notes to patient/GP:

Paracetamol prescribed to replace Ibuprofen. Amlodipine was stopped, Ramipril dose was doubled. Medications are to continue lifelong for control of chronic heart failure.

Common pitfalls

- Avoid calcium channel blockers in chronic heart failure. This is because calcium channel blockers reduce myocardial contractility and have negatively ionotropic effects. Dihydropyridines such as nifedipine are worse than amlodipine, which can be used if necessary for blood pressure control.
- Particularly avoid rate-controlling calcium channel blockers such as verapamil and diltiazem, as these have highly negatively ionotropic effects in heart failure patients.
- Antiarrhythmics can have unpredictable effects in heart failure. Amiodarone is considered the safest for arrhythmias in heart failure.
- Avoid NSAIDs in heart failure as they have been associated with symptoms of heart failure in several case reports and studies due to effects on fluid retention. They have also been shown to increase the risk of MI and stroke (this does not include aspirin).
- Renal and hepatic dysfunction often coexist in patients with heart failure, so any drug excreted predominantly by the kidneys or metabolised by the liver may accumulate.
- Patients may develop resistance to oral diuretics for unknown reasons (possibly due to gut oedema, hypotension or reduced renal blood flow). In this

situation either a bolus or an infusion of intravenous loop diuretic may be required.

■ Anaemia and iron deficiency, depression, gout and renal dysfunction are very common in patients with heart failure. These should be recognised and treated or monitored where present.

SUMMARY

The management of chronic heart failure is a multidisciplinary task fundamentally based on use of medications, patient education and ongoing support. Education and support are key in improving compliance with medication and recognising signs of deterioration. Many areas provide specialised heart failure teams with community nurses to facilitate this.

Treatments for systolic heart failure include disease-modifying treatments as well as symptomatic treatments, with emerging uses for implantable devices, surgical assist devices and transplantation.

No treatment has yet been shown to convincingly reduce morbidity and mortality in patients with diastolic heart failure. However, symptomatic management, patient education and the treatment of co-morbidities remains the same in both groups.

FURTHER READING

■ The European Society of Cardiology has up to date guidelines on many aspects of cardiology and is an excellent learning resource. Available at: www.escardio.org (accessed Dec. 2015).

■ The American Heart Association has a website useful for both professionals and patients. Available at: www.heart.org/HEARTORG/ (accessed Dec. 2015).

Atrial fibrillation

> **Mrs Mavis Hilton**
>
> **Age: 67**
>
> **Hospital number: 123456**

🔍 Case study

PC: *A 67-year-old woman self presents to A&E by ambulance. She had been aware of intermittent palpitations for a few weeks and feels they have worsened throughout the day. She now feels uncomfortable and is more breathless than usual. There is no chest pain.*

PMH: *Diabetes type 2, previous MI*

Allergies: *Penicillin*

Examination:
HR 100–140 irregularly irregular, RR 24, BP 170/100, Sats 99% on air, afebrile, BM 9.5
Looks anxious; tongue moist

CVS: *Capillary refill time <2 seconds, JVP not raised, no oedema*
HS I + II + 0

RS: *Clear lung fields*

Abdo: *Soft, non-tender, no masses palpated, bowel sounds present*

Chest X-ray *clear lung fields*

ECG *shows fast atrial fibrillation rate 110–140*

(Continued)

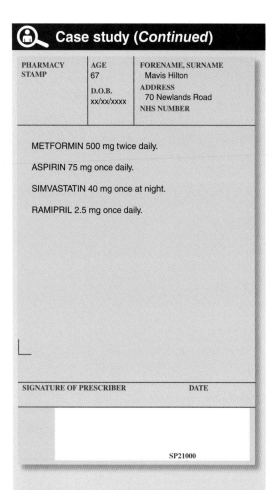

Case study (*Continued*)

PHARMACY STAMP	AGE 67	FORENAME, SURNAME
		Mavis Hilton
	D.O.B. xx/xx/xxxx	ADDRESS
		70 Newlands Road
		NHS NUMBER

METFORMIN 500 mg twice daily.

ASPIRIN 75 mg once daily.

SIMVASTATIN 40 mg once at night.

RAMIPRIL 2.5 mg once daily.

SIGNATURE OF PRESCRIBER   DATE

SP21000

Diagnosis

This patient has fast AF on a background of likely paroxysmal AF, given the history of intermittent palpitations. There may be a trigger such as sepsis/PE/hypovolaemia/thyroid disorders, but this is at present unknown.

Signs of instability with AF are:

- chest pain
- pulmonary oedema
- systolic BP <90 mmHg
- reduced conscious level or syncope.

Signs of cardiac instability should prompt consideration for direct current (DC) cardioversion and/or amiodarone to restore to sinus rhythm. This is not done for stable patients in the acute setting due to risk of emboli from atrial/ventricular thrombi that may have formed during the arrhythmia (if not fully anticoagulated).

This patient has no signs of cardiac instability, despite feeling uncomfortable. The priority is therefore rate control rather than urgent cardioversion (rhythm control).

Guidelines

Resuscitation Council (UK) tachycardia management algorithm available at www.resus.org.uk/pages/tachalgo.pdf (accessed Dec. 2015).

Initial measures

ABC. Airway is clear, give oxygen if hypoxic. Check BP and HR and get IV access. ECG is required to confirm diagnosis, and look for additional problems (such as ischaemia, as an MI may have provoked AF). Tachycardia itself can cause a degree of ischaemic change on the ECG ('rate-related ischaemia') so this must be correlated with history and risk factors. Check glucose and send bloods particularly for electrolytes (low/high Mg, K, Ca can precipitate arrhythmias), thyroid function and CRP (sepsis can drive AF). Anaemia also contributes to tachycardias of all types. Examine patent for signs of LVF and do a CXR for pulmonary oedema, as this is a sign of cardiac instability and requires a different treatment approach. Look also for other clinical signs that may point towards a cause of AF (hypovolaemia, fever, signs of infection, signs of Graves' disease, previous cardiac operations).

The patient needs to be on a cardiac monitor in case the rate or rhythm changes.

Prescribing for atrial fibrillation

Rhythm control

DC cardioversion and/or chemical cardioversion with amiodarone (or sometimes flecainide) are considered in patients who are unstable or who have new-onset AF within the past 24–48 hours. This is because an

LV/LA thrombus is less likely to have formed within 48 hours; also because new-onset arrhythmias are much more likely to respond to cardioversion than established arrhythmias. The aim of these treatments is to restore sinus rhythm. Our patient Mrs Hilton has paroxysmal AF and has had palpitations on previous days, so we cannot be sure as to the exact time of fast AF onset. She is also haemodynamically stable, therefore urgent cardioversion is not indicated and may well be unsuccessful anyway due to the recurrence of this arrhythmia on previous occasions.

Rate control

Where patients are stable but remain in fast AF, the focus is on rate control. Rate-controlled AF is unlikely to cause symptoms to the patient. Triggers for the fast AF need also to be identified and treated. If the driving factor is treated, this may in fact obviate the need for rate-control medication

The main aim for this case is rate control, where first-line treatments are beta-blockers.

ONCE ONLY PRESCRIPTIONS						
Date	Time to be given	DRUG	Dose	Route	Prescriber	
					Signature	Bleep
xx/xx/xx	STAT	BISOPROLOL	5 mg	PO	A. Doctor	
xx/xx/xx	xx:xx	MAGNESIUM SULPHATE	2 g	IV over 2 hours	A. Doctor	

If a faster onset of action is required, for example in a very anxious/uncomfortable patient, then metoprolol can be given IV or orally as it is faster acting.

Another option for patients who can't have beta-blockers or who are elderly and less mobile is digoxin. This is effective for rate control at rest but less so on exertion, which is why beta-blockers are the first-line treatment.

ONCE ONLY PRESCRIPTIONS						
Date	Time to be given	DRUG	Dose	Route	Prescriber	
					Signature	Bleep
1/1/15	14:00	DIGOXIN	500 micrograms	IV	A. Doctor	
1/1/15	20:00 (6 hours later)	DIGOXIN	250 micrograms	PO	A. Doctor	

This is a digoxin loading regime. This may then be followed by a regular oral regime of daily digoxin, where dosing ranges usually from 62.5 micrograms to 250 micrograms daily titrated to response.

REGULAR PRESCRIPTIONS					Circle/enter times below ↓	↘ Enter dates below		
						Day 1	Day 2	Day 3
DRUG DIGOXIN					06			
					(08)			
Dose 125 micrograms	Route PO	Freq OD	Start date 2/1/15		12			
Signature A. Doctor		Bleep	Review		16			
Additional instructions					18			
					22			

Further prescribing of beta-blockers and/or digoxin very much depends on response, and both of these medications may be required. IV magnesium is often given as replacement, even if the serum magnesium level is not yet back.

Beta-blockers: rationale and evidence

Beta-blockers block beta-2-adrenoceptors, which are key in potentiating the sympathetic response. The sympathetic response consists of tachycardia, increased blood pressure, anxiety, sweating and pupillary dilation. Beta-blockers prevent excess sympathetic stimulation, therefore cause slowing of the heart rate and decreasing of the blood pressure (Arcangelo and Peterson, 2006). In the situation of acute AF, beta-blockers are required solely for their rate-limiting properties, rather than for any long-term or prognostic benefits.

Metoprolol acts quickly, within 5–10 minutes if given IV. Oral dosing is used if a patient is asymptomatic, but if they are uncomfortable then IV is often used instead.

Long-term maintenance dosing after the initial acute treatment will generally consist of a longer-acting beta-blocker (such as bisoprolol) purely for the convenience of once-daily dosing. Metoprolol maintenance would require three times daily dosing if it were continued long term.

✓ DRUGS checklist for BISOPROLOL

Dose	2.5 mg (up to maximum of 10 mg)
Route	PO
Units	mg
Given	OD
Special situations	Do not use in asthma/COPD, uncontrolled heart failure, sick sinus syndrome, heart block, hypotension or severe peripheral vascular disease.

✓ DRUGS checklist for ORAL METOPROLOL

Dose	50 mg
Route	PO
Units	mg
Given	TDS; can give up to 300 mg daily in divided doses
Special situations	Do not use first line in asthma/COPD, uncontrolled heart failure, sick sinus syndrome, heart block, hypotension or severe peripheral vascular disease.

✓ DRUGS checklist for IV METOPROLOL

Dose	1–5 mg, give in 1 mg aliquots max total dose is 15 mg
Route	IV
Units	mg
Given	Give, then wait 5–10 minutes, repeat if no response 5 mg is a common dose, but it is less risky to give smaller doses and repeat rather than give the full 5 mg at the start

Special situations	Do not use first line in asthma/COPD, uncontrolled heart failure, sick sinus syndrome, heart block, hypotension or severe peripheral vascular disease.

Beta-blockers: essential pharmacology

Please see Section Chronic Heart Failure.

Digoxin: rationale and evidence

Digoxin is used for rate control in AF, particularly where beta-blockers are contraindicated or in the elderly or immobile where there may be concern about the potential hypotension that may accompany beta-blocker therapy. Digoxin is effective for controlling resting heart rate, but has limited rate control effect on exertion, hence its use in less mobile patients. It also can be used first line in AF with chronic cardiac failure, as digoxin has additional benefits in heart failure. It has been shown to reduce hospital admissions for chronic cardiac failure when used in combination with ACEIs and diuretics (Digitalis Investigation Group, 1997).

✓ DRUGS checklist for DIGOXIN

Dose	500 microgram loading dose ×2 (separated by 6 hours)
Route	PO or IV
Units	micrograms
Given	Give second dose after 4–6 hours then continue daily oral maintenance dose of 62.5–250 micrograms once daily
Special situations	May be used first line for AF in the elderly, immobile or where beta-blockers are contraindicated. Check digoxin levels after 24–48 hours as maintenance dose may need adjustment. Typically, digoxin levels should be 1.0–2.0 ng/mL.

Special situations (*Cont.*)	Do not use in heart block, Wolff–Parkinson–White syndrome, ventricular tachycardias (VT) as it may potentiate the use of the abnormal conduction pathways by slowing the atrioventricular (AV) node (normal) conduction.

Digoxin is usually given orally, but can also be given by slow IV injection in urgent situations (heart rhythm should be monitored). Both IV and oral digoxin have a very long distribution half-life into the cardiac tissue. This delays its onset of action. In patients with normal renal function the half-life is about 36 hours. This is prolonged in patients with decreased renal function, therefore the maintenance dose should be reduced (guided by digoxin levels).

Evidence

Digoxin in AF
The *European Heart Journal* has published conflicting studies about mortality with digoxin in AF, questioning its appropriateness. In conclusion, evidence is lacking regarding the hypothesis that digoxin increases mortality as a treatment for atrial fibrillation. It is therefore still used as a mainstay of treatment in the UK (Gheorghiade *et al.*, 2013).

For continuous AF in chronic heart failure, there is evidence that a combination of digoxin and beta-blockers may be more effective and may allow lower doses to be used (see Evidence Combination therapy for long term AF in heart failure).

Evidence

Combination therapy for long-term AF in heart failure
A combination of digoxin and beta blockers more effective for reducing symptoms, improving ventricular function and leads to better rate control than either agent used alone. A combination of digoxin and beta blockers may allow lower doses to be used, thereby improving tolerability and decreasing the risk of toxicity (Khand *et al.*, 2003; Veloso and de Paola, 2005; Gheorghiade *et al.*, 2004).

Digoxin: essential pharmacology

Digoxin is a cardiac glycoside that is similar to digitoxin extracted from the foxglove plant, *Digitalis lanata* (Hollman, 1996). Digoxin slows the heart rate and increases myocardial contractility by binding to the cell membrane Na^+/K^+ ATPase pump on the myocyte, thereby inhibiting it. This leads to an increase in the amount of sodium in the myocyte. Increased sodium concentrations disrupt the sodium/calcium exchanger on the cell membrane (as this relies on an inward sodium gradient in order to pump calcium out of the cell). This leads to an increase in intracellular calcium. Increased intracellular calcium causes increased contractility of the cell and a decreased heart rate (Gheorghiade *et al.*, 2004).

Digoxin also slows heart rate by enhancing parasympathetic activity, which slows depolarisation of the pacemaker cells in the AV node, and therefore slowing conduction rate (Gheorghiade *et al.*, 2004). This in turn allows an increased stroke volume, and therefore an increased blood pressure and better tissue perfusion.

Interactions (BNF (BMA/RPS, 2015)): Digoxin elimination relies on P-glycoprotein. This means that is has significant clinical interactions with other drugs commonly used in patients with heart problems, including spironolactone, verapamil and amiodarone. Quinidine also interacts. This is because these drugs all inhibit P-glycoprotein, and hence reduce digoxin clearance. This can increase the risk of digoxin toxicity if the digoxin dosing is not carefully monitored.

Adverse effects: Digoxin has a narrow therapeutic index, meaning that there is a only a small dosing range within which it is effective without causing toxicity. This narrow margin makes the likelihood of toxicity and side effects greater. Digoxin toxicity is rare when the plasma concentration is <0.8 micrograms/L, and is more common in patients with hypokalaemia (Rossi, 2006). This is because digoxin competes with K⁺ ions for the same binding site on the Na⁺/K⁺ ATPase pump. Less potassium therefore allows increased digoxin cell binding. It is therefore important to replace potassium in patients on digoxin, and consider this where toxicity is suspected.

Signs of digoxin toxicity

- Nausea and vomiting
- Confusion
- Headache
- Hypotension
- ECG changes: bradycardia, prolonged PR interval, bidirectional ventricular tachycardia, 'reverse tick' sign)
- Disturbed colour vision (yellow/green)
- Hypokalaemia

Treatment for digoxin toxicity: Digoxin immune Fab ('digibind'), made up of antidigoxin immunoglobulin fragments (Flanagan and Jones, 2004). This is available in A&E or the hospital pharmacy.

Other medications used in AF: rate control

Rate-controlling calcium channel blockers

Diltiazem or verapamil are recommended as an alternative to beta-blockers for rate control of AF, both by NICE guidelines and by the UK resuscitation council. They are both class 4 antiarrhythmics:

- Diltiazem is a non-dihydropyridine (non-DHP) calcium channel blocker
- Verapamil is a phenylalkylamine calcium channel blocker.

These can be used in the treatment of hypertension, angina pectoris and some types of arrhythmia, including fast atrial fibrillation.

These medications blocks voltage-dependent calcium channels, which are particularly abundant in the sinoatrial (SA) and atrioventricular (AV) node. Blocking the calcium channels decreases conduction through these nodes, thereby slowing the heart rate. They are also potent vasodilators, as calcium channels are also present in smooth muscle. This, however, means that they can precipitate hypotension.

Rate-limiting calcium channel blockers are negatively ionotropic; they decrease cardiac output, slow the heart rate and may impair atrioventricular conduction. This decrease in heart muscle contractility leads to reduced myocardial oxygen consumption, hence they are also useful for angina. However, these affects meant that they may therefore precipitate heart failure and hypotension, and should not be used with beta-blockers (although diltiazem is less negatively ionotropic than verapamil, hence beta-blockers may be used with caution).

✓	**DRUGS checklist for DILTIAZEM**
Dose	60 mg
Route	PO or IV
Units	mg
Given	TDS
Special situations	Do not give in heart failure, hypotension, sick sinus syndrome, bradycardia, 2nd or 3rd degree heart block (without pacemaker), AF with WPW, VT, pregnancy and breast feeding. Caution with beta-blockers – risk of bradycardia, AV block and arrhythmias. NB: there are numerous longer-acting maintenance formulations where brand name must be specified, e.g. Adizem-SR and Tildiem LA. Seek advice from senior/ cardiologist if you are unfamiliar with this drug.

✓ DRUGS checklist for VERAPAMIL

Dose	40 mg oral or 5 mg IV
Route	PO or IV
Units	mg
Given	TDS
Special situations	Do not give in heart failure, hypotension, sick sinus syndrome, bradycardia, 2nd or 3rd degree heart block (without pacemaker), AF with WPW, VT, pregnancy and breast feeding. Do not give with beta-blockers – risk of bradycardia, AV block and arrhythmias. Seek advice from senior/ cardiologist if you are unfamiliar with this drug.

Other medications used in AF: rhythm control

Amiodarone

Amiodarone is a rhythm-control agent, and is used for chemical cardioversion of tachyarrhythmias in an emergency. It is an alternative to emergency DC cardioversion, which would require presence of an anaesthetist for sedation and airway management (please see Tachycardia Section).

In the situation of atrial fibrillation it is used where the patient is tachycardic and cardiovascularly unstable. It would therefore not be used in Mrs Hilton's case of stable fast AF, assuming that she responded to beta-blockers or digoxin.

Had she not responded, amiodarone can also be used in a non-emergency setting where beta-blockers and/or digoxin have failed. Chemical cardioversion can be done with relatively low risk of thromboembolic stroke where the arrhythmia commenced less than 48 hours ago, or where the patient has been anticoagulated with a consistently therapeutic INR (between 2 and 3) for at least 3 weeks (NICE, 2006). In practice it may be difficult to confirm these factors, hence a transoesophageal echocardiogram may need to be performed to confirm absence of atrial or ventricular thrombus prior to cardioversion. Elective (planned) DC cardioversion may be a preferable option in these circumstances, as it avoids the side effects of long-term amiodarone and may be more effective. Post-DC cardioversion, patients may need a rate-control medication to maintain sinus rhythm. The first line maintenance is beta-blockers.

Amiodarone may also been given as a long-term daily medication in patients with AF to prevent them from having tachycardic episodes. This is generally managed by cardiologists.

If a patient has heart failure and fast AF then digoxin or amiodarone may be used as alternatives to beta-blockers for rate control, as beta-blockers can precipitate acute pulmonary oedema (see Tachycardia Section).

Flecainide

Flecainide is an option for management of episodes of paroxysmal AF and may be taken by patients as a 'pill in the pocket' strategy for managing tachycardic episodes (see Tachycardia Section).

It is generally the treatment of choice for chemical cardioversion in patients with clearly defined recent-onset AF who do not have, or who are at very low risk of, underlying coronary artery or structural heart disease (e.g. patients <50 years of age with no cardiac risk factors).

Flecainide cannot be used in patients with any structural heart disease or ischaemic heart disease because of the risk of precipitating ventricular fibrillation. The decision to use this should be taken by a registrar or above.

ⓘ Guidelines

- NICE has complete guidelines on the management of atrial fibrillation: *Atrial Fibrillation: The Management of Atrial Fibrillation*, CG36, 2006. Available at: nice.org.uk/guidance/CG36 (accessed Dec. 2015).
- The European Society of Cardiology has complete guidelines on the management of atrial fibrillation (Camm *et al.*, 2012). Available at: www.escardio.org/guidelines-surveys/esc-guidelines/Pages/atrial-fibrillation.aspx (accessed Dec. 2015).

Further aspects of AF management

Management decisions regarding persistent AF are based on of the same principles of rate and/or rhythm control as new AF. Options include use of beta-blockers, digoxin, rate-controlling calcium channel blockers or amiodarone. Fast AF episodes are managed as above, mostly in hospital.

Other considerations in the setting of persistent AF as an outpatient are:

- Referral for AF ablation. This requires mapping of the aberrant pathways by an electrophysiologist at a specialist cardiology centre, then ablation of the area. This may require subsequent pacemaker insertion should the ablation result in heart block post procedure. Ablation is more likely to be considered in young patients, those with troublesome symptoms and where there is no other correctable cause for AF. It can be 6 months before ablation success is confirmed by way of a continuous rhythm strip, as arrhythmias can happen immediately post procedure, which may not correlate with long-term resolution.
- Referral for elective DC cardioversion. This requires careful anticoagulation in the weeks leading up to the procedure and may also require exclusion of an atrial or ventricular thrombus via a transoesophageal echocardiogram. Post-DC cardioversion, patients may need a rate control medication to maintain sinus rhythm. The first-line maintenance is beta-blockers.
- Anticoagulation. Patients with AF are at increased risk of thromboembolic stroke and need to be risk stratified using the CHA2DS-VASc score and HASBLED score to determine their need for anticoagulation versus risk of bleeding. Anticoagulation could be with warfarin or one of the new oral anticoagulant drugs. This is discussed in detail in Chapter 16.
- AV node ablation and permanent pacemaker implantation. Where adequate rate or symptom control is not possible with drugs, or their side effects are not tolerated, this is an option for troublesome AF. Complete heart block is induced with AV node ablation, and the patient becomes completely dependent on a permanent pacemaker. This brings dramatic symptom improvement in those with no previous treatment efficacy. The life expectancy of patients with normal hearts is unchanged.

Evidence

- The European Heart Association recommends the CHADS2-VASc score for guiding anticoagulation decisions in patients with AF (Camm et al., 2010).
- The HAS-BLED score original article is Pisters et al., 2010.
- Rate Control versus Electrical Cardioversion for Persistent Atrial Fibrillation Trial (522 patients). The trial indicated that that rate control was not inferior to rhythm control for preventing death and morbidity from cardiovascular causes in patients with recurrent AF after DC cardioversion (Van Gelder et al., 2002).

Case outcome and discharge

Mrs Hilton received a number of investigations to look for underlying driving factors to precipitate fast AF. Her electrolytes including magnesium were normal, as were her thyroid function tests. She had no evidence of sepsis as shown by her history, lack of signs of sepsis, with normal CXR and negative urine dip. However, she had had a recent viral infection with a few episodes of diarrhoea and vomiting.

She was therefore diagnosed with paroxysmal AF, with an episode of fast AF probably precipitated by a recent viral illness.

She remained on a cardiac monitor whilst an inpatient and had an echocardiogram to look for structural causes of AF, particularly in light of her MI history. This came back showing a normal LV ejection fraction with resolution of AF at the time of the study.

She was successfully rate controlled and discharged with a regular beta-blocker for maintenance of rate control. She was no longer in AF on discharge, but is highly likely to have recurrent episodes.

Anticoagulation needs to be considered in paroxysmal AF, as she is at increased risk of stroke, as shown by her CHA2DS2-VASc score of 3 (age, diabetes, female). She was therefore counselled about taking warfarin and started on it whilst in hospital with referral to the anticoagulation clinic on discharge for INR monitoring and dosing adjustment (see Chapter 16). She was advised of the need to keep her INR within a therapeutic range for stroke prevention.

She was referred back to her GP but with a low threshold for cardiology referral should episodes reoccur or AF become persistent, as she could be a candidate for DC cardioversion or ablation in future.

She was advised against heavy caffeine, alcohol or recreational drug consumption, as these are known precipitants for atrial fibrillation.

Mrs Hilton's new prescription is shown.

Common pitfalls

- Mrs Hilton has been discharged on a beta-blocker, yet she has diabetes. Beta-blockers can blunt the effect of hypoglycaemia so that patients are unaware that they need to ingest glucose to prevent coma. This is less of an issue with type 2 diabetics as hyperglycaemia tends to be their main problem rather than hypoglycaemia. Metformin itself doesn't cause hypoglycaemia as it increase the body's sensitivity to its own insulin, rather than affecting amount of insulin. She should, however, be counselled about good glycaemic control and its health benefits in preventing cardiovascular disease.

DISCHARGE MEDICATION

Date	Medication	Dose	Route	Frequency	Supply	GP to continue?
xx/xx/xx	BISOPROLOL	5 mg	PO	Once daily	14 days	Y
xx/xx/xx	WARFARIN	2 mg	PO	Once daily (as per INR, aiming for INR 2-3)	14 days	Y
xx/xx/xx	METFORMIN	500 mg	PO	Twice daily	14 days	Y
xx/xx/xx	SIMVASTATIN	40 mg	PO	Once per night	14 days	Y
xx/xx/xx	RAMIPRIL	2.5 mg	PO	Once daily	14 days	Y

Notes to patient/GP:
These medications are to continue lifelong. Aspirin was stopped in favour of warfarin for new atrial fibrillation.

SUMMARY

The management of AF is different according to whether the patient is haemodynamically stable or unstable. Within these categories it is also broken down into rate control and rhythm control, where emergency treatments for unstable AF will generally address both areas (DC cardioversion or amiodarone).

Many patients are asymptomatic with AF as long as it is adequately rate controlled. Those who are young or who have troublesome palpitations or frequent admissions despite antiarrhythmic drugs should be prioritised for more definitive management, with ablation or elective DC cardioversion. These treatments would aim for return to sinus rhythm rather than rate control of AF.

Key learning points

Fast atrial fibrillation
- If the patient is unstable, consider DC cardioversion and/or chemical cardioversion with amiodarone.
- If patient is haemodynamically stable, the focus is first on rate control, unless onset of AF is known to be within 24-48 hours. Here consideration should be given to chemical/electrical cardioversion.

(Continued)

Key learning points (Continued)

- Treat any precipitating factors first, e.g. sepsis, hyperthyroidism.
- If no obvious driver for AF is found, give a beta blocker, e.g. bisoprolol, or digoxin if beta blockers are contraindicated.
- If not effective involve senior early.
- In the event of ECG changes, discuss with senior. There could be concurrent ischaemic heart disease requiring treatment, or simply rate-related ischaemia that will resolve with rate control.
- When the rate is controlled, prescribe maintenance longer-acting rate control.
- All patients require cardiac monitoring, a CXR and an echo.

Rate-controlled persistent AF
- Assess risk of thromboembolic stroke with CHA2DS2-VASc score to guide anticoagulation decisions.
- May warrant referral to cardiologists for consideration of definitive therapies such as ablation or elective DC cardioversion.

(!) **Guidelines**

- NICE has complete guidelines on the managements of atrial fibrillation: *Atrial Fibrillation: The Management of Atrial Fibrillation*, CG36, 2006. Available at: nice .org.uk/guidance/CG36 (accessed Dec. 2015).
- The Resuscitation Council has guidelines on how to manage emergency tachyarrhythmias including AF. Available at: www.resus.org.uk/ (accessed Dec. 2015).

Tachycardia

Miss Mignon Korn

Age: 37

Hospital number: 123456

 Case study

PC: A 37-year-old woman self presents to A&E. She has had palpitations for the past hour making her feel uncomfortable and breathless. There is no chest pain but she feels dizzy on exertion. This has happened once before but self-terminated.

PMH: nil

Allergies: nil

Examination:
HR 180 regular, RR 24, BP 170/100, Sats 99% on air, afebrile, BM 9.5
Looks uncomfortable; tongue moist

CVS: Capillary refill time <2 seconds, JVP not raised, no oedema
HS I + II + 0

RS: Clear lung fields

Abdo: Soft, non-tender, no masses palpated, bowel sounds present

Chest X-ray clear lung fields

ECG shows a regular narrow complex tachycardia, difficult to define p waves

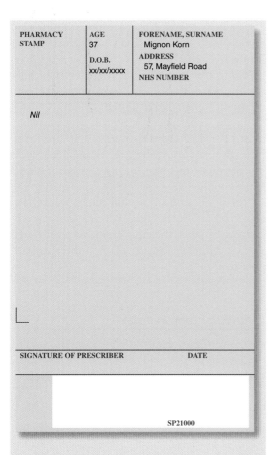

PHARMACY STAMP	AGE 37	FORENAME, SURNAME
		Mignon Korn
	D.O.B.	ADDRESS
	xx/xx/xxxx	57, Mayfield Road
		NHS NUMBER

Nil

SIGNATURE OF PRESCRIBER   DATE

SP21000

Diagnosis

This patient has a supraventricular tachycardia. Other differentials could include fast atrial flutter, but it is difficult to tell at this heart rate, particularly if there is no previous diagnosis. There may be a trigger such as sepsis/ PE/ hypovolaemia/ thyroid disorders, but this is at present unknown. Caution should be exercised with diagnosing the type of tachycardia if you are not confident with ECGs, as sinus tachycardia is a possibility. Sinus tachycardia is a physiological response to illness, hence it is the underlying cause that needs treatment rather than the tachycardia per se.

Signs of instability with tachycardias are:

- Chest pain
- Pulmonary oedema
- Systolic BP <90 mmHg
- Reduced conscious level or syncope.

Signs of cardiac instability should prompt consideration for DC cardioversion and/or amiodarone to restore to sinus rhythm. This is not done for stable patients in the acute setting due to risk of emboli of ventricular thrombi that may have formed during the arrhythmia (if not fully anticoagulated).

This patient has no signs of cardiac instability, despite feeling uncomfortable and breathless. The priority is therefore rate control rather than urgent cardioversion (rhythm control). Rate control is also diagnostically useful with SVT, as the underlying rhythm may be clarified once the rate is slower.

 Guidelines

Resuscitation Council (UK) tachycardia management algorithm. Available at: www .resus.org.uk/pages/tachalgo.pdf (accessed Dec. 2015).

Initial measures

Follow the ABC sequence. The airway of the patient is clear, give oxygen if hypoxic. Check BP and HR and get IV access. An ECG is required to confirm presence of SVT and look for additional problems (such as ischaemia, as an MI may have provoked SVT). Tachycardia itself can cause a degree of ischaemic change on the ECG ('rate-related ischaemia') so this must be correlated with history and risk factors. Check glucose and send bloods, particularly for electrolytes (low/high Mg, K, Ca can precipitate arrhythmias), thyroid function and CRP (sepsis can drive SVT). Anaemia also contributes to tachycardias of all types. Examine the patient for signs of LVF and do a CXR for pulmonary oedema, as this is a sign of cardiac instability and requires a different treatment approach. Look also for other clinical signs that may point towards a cause of SVT (hypovolaemia, fever, signs of infection, signs of Graves' disease, previous cardiac operations).

The patient needs to be on a cardiac monitor.

(Continued)

🔍 Case study (*Continued*)

If the diagnosis is SVT (as above), attempts can be made at slowing SVT by first using vagal manoeuvres. These increase vagal tone, thereby activating the parasympathetic nervous system and encouraging relative bradycardia.

Vagal manoeuvres include carotid sinus massage, where the carotid sinus on one side of the neck is firmly massaged, whilst watching the cardiac monitor. This should not be attempted if the patient has carotid stenosis (often this is unknown).

Valsalva manoeuvres can also be attempted to increase vagal tone. These include blowing into a syringe or exhaling against a closed mouth and nose. If effective, the monitor should show a pause, then return of sinus rhythm (Ramrakha and Hill, 2006). If these are ineffective, give IV adenosine.

For an ECG showing SVT cardioverting to sinus rhythm with administration of adenosine, see Figure 3.1.

Sometimes, the SVT does not revert to sinus rhythm but instead slows down enough to reveal the flutter waves of atrial flutter.

In the situation of atrial flutter, the patient must be treated as if this were fast atrial fibrillation. This would involve prescribing beta-blockers or digoxin first line (see Section Atrial Fibrillation).

Atrial flutter can be difficult to treat, and ablation may be the best way to terminate it. The patient will therefore probably need referral to a cardiologist, particularly if the rhythm is persistent.

Ventricular tachycardias

Ventricular tachycardia (VT) can be a life-threatening rhythm and is associated with cardiac arrest. However, non-sustained VT with a pulse is relatively common, particularly in patients with heart failure or dilated cardiomyopathies. These patients may already have ICDs in situ. Treatment includes rate control and rhythm control with beta-blockers or amiodarone, and addressing any suspected causes or triggers (Figure 3.2). Management is generally guided by a cardiologist, as these

Prescribing for tachyarrhythmias

| | | | | | Prescriber | |
Date	Time to be given	DRUG	Dose	Route	Signature	Bleep
xx/xx/xx	xx:xx	ADENOSINE	6 mg	IV	A. Doctor	
		If unsuccessful				
xx/xx/xx	xx:xx	ADENOSINE	12 mg	IV	A. Doctor	

ONCE ONLY PRESCRIPTIONS

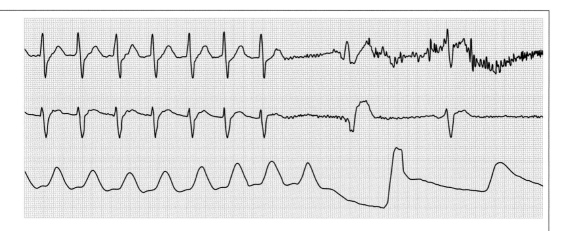

Figure 3.1 SVT cardioverting to sinus rhythm with administration of adenosine.

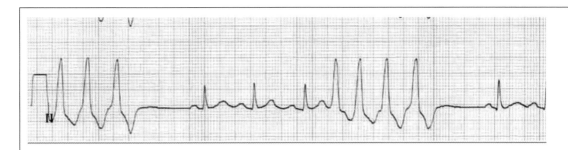

Figure 3.2 Rhythm strip showing non-sustained ventricular tachycardia.

patient are at high risk of cardiac arrest and may already have pacemakers with/without an ICD function.

For beta-blocker prescription, see Section Atrial Fibrillation. Patients may be loaded on amiodarone to try and terminate the rhythm and control the heart rate.

ONCE ONLY PRESCRIPTIONS						
Date	Time to be given	DRUG	Dose	Route	Prescriber	
					Signature	Bleep
xx/xx/xx	xx:xx	AMIODARONE	300 mg loading	IV via a central line over 1 hour	A. Doctor	
		Followed by				
xx/xx/xx	xx:xx	AMIODARONE	900 mg	IV via a central line over 23 hours	A. Doctor	

Adenosine: rationale and evidence

Adenosine is a class V antiarrhythmic agent and causes transient atrioventricular node blockade. This means that any re-entrant supraventricular tachycardia involving the AV node is abruptly halted. Re-entry supraventricular tachycardias include AV re-entry tachycardia (AVRT) or AV nodal re-entry tachycardia (AVNRT). Clinically, transient AV node blockade shows as a period of ventricular asystole on the cardiac monitor. This can be a frightening and sometimes uncomfortable experience for a patient. Patients should be warned that they may experience transient chest pain and that they may 'feel like they are going to die'. This is exactly how many patients describe it afterwards, and is also a scary few seconds for any junior doctor giving adenosine for the first time. Adenosine has a short half-life of 10–30 seconds.

Tachyarrhythmias that are confined to the atria (e.g. atrial fibrillation, atrial flutter) or ventricles (e.g. monomorphic ventricular tachycardia) do not involve the AV node as part of the re-entrant circuit. These rhythms are therefore not halted by adenosine. However, the ventricular response rate is temporarily slowed with adenosine in such cases, as the AV block reduces the number of conducted beats. Adenosine also has an indirect effect on atrial tissue causing a shortened refractory period. This means that adenosine can have the role of 'revealing' the underlying rhythm and therefore clarifying the cause for tachycardia. Where underlying atrial flutter or fibrillation is seen, adenosine will be ineffective in terminating the rhythm, but may show this as the diagnosis.

Evidence

Adenosine in SVT

'Adenosine may be used safely and effectively to terminate acute episodes of supraventricular tachycardia that involve the AV node in the reentry pathway' (DiMarco *et al.*, 1983).

Adenosine was subsequently approved by the FDA for the treatment of supraventricular tachycardia in 1990.

✓	**DRUGS checklist for ADENOSINE**
Dose	6 mg
Route	IV
Units	mg
Given	Stat. If ineffective, repeat with 9 mg, then 12 mg if required
Special situations	Must be given via large-bore cannula in antecubital fossa and flushed immediately with 5–10 mL normal saline otherwise it will not be effective. Do not use in Wolff–Parkinson–White syndrome or where there is a known aberrant pathway. Adenosine will block the AV node and therefore potentiate conduction through the abnormal pathway in these situations. Adenosine can precipitate AF due to its effect of atrial tissue. Where there is an aberrant pathway present, this can precipitate VT or VF due to conduction of AF down the aberrant pathway. Contraindications: asthma or bronchospasm from other causes.

Adenosine: essential pharmacology

Adenosine is a purine nucleoside present in every cell of the human body. When administered IV, adenosine causes transient AV node blockade. It does this by inhibiting adenylyl cyclase at the A_1 receptor, which has the effect of reducing cAMP. This leads to cell hyperpolarisation by causing increased outward flux of potassium ions.

Adenosine also affects endothelial cells inside coronary artery walls, causing smooth muscle relaxation and arterial dilation. The dilation only occurs where endothelium is in contact with the tunica media of the artery, that is not separated from the tunica media by an atherosclerotic plaque. This feature allows cardiologists to determine presence of atherosclerotic disease inside arteries at the time of coronary angiogram, as dilation is exaggerated in the normal segments and decreased in the diseased segments of artery (DiMarco et al., 1983; Conti, 1991; Pijls and De Bruyne, 2000).

Amiodarone: rationale and evidence

Amiodarone can be used for the treatment of most types of arrhythmia, particularly when other drugs are contraindicated or ineffective. It can be used for paroxysmal supraventricular tachycardias including atrial flutter and fibrillation, as well as nodal and ventricular tachycardias. It can also be used in Wolff–Parkinson–White syndrome and during cardiac arrests due to ventricular tachycardia or ventricular fibrillation. Due to its extensive interactions, cautions and adverse effects, it should only be initiated under specialist supervision, ideally in hospital. It can be given IV or orally, and has the advantage of causing minimal cardiac depression (Wyse et al., 2002; Roy et al., 2000).

✓	**DRUGS checklist for AMIODARONE first dose**
Dose	300 mg loading dose
Route	IV via a central line (or at very least through large bore cannula in antecubital fossa – check with local guidance)
Units	mg
Given	Over 1 hour
Special situations	Irritant to blood vessels, hence preferable to give IV amiodarone via a central line. If it is given via a peripheral cannula and then extravasates, it causes painful inflammation to skin. Can cause hypokalaemia and hypotension when given IV. Can cause severe hepatocellular toxicity, even acutely. Can cause arrhythmias due to the fact it can prolong the QT interval, hence use in extreme caution with other drugs that cause prolonged QT.

Contraindications: sinus bradycardia, sinoatrial heart block (unless pacemaker fitted), iodine sensitivity.

Main things to remember are:
- Arrhythmogenic
- Check thyroid and liver function tests every 6 months
- Can cause hypokalaemia
- Check colour vision.

✓ DRUGS checklist for AMIODARONE second dose

Dose	900 mg prolonged loading dose, given after the first 300 mg loading dose has run through
Route	IV via a central line
Units	mg
Given	Over 23 hours
Special situations	As above. Maximum dose is 1.2 g in 24 hours.

After the initial loading dose amiodarone is given as a maintenance drug every day.

✓ DRUGS checklist for maintenance AMIODARONE

Dose	200 mg maintenance dose
Route	oral
Units	mg
Given	Three times daily for 1 week then twice daily for 1 week then once daily
Special situations	Different cardiologists may alter this typical regimen of oral dosing, also practices in different trusts vary. Amiodarone has many long-term side effects, many of which are irreversible. It is a toxic and unpleasant drug. See Section Amiodarone: Essential Pharmacology for numerous side effects and cautions.

🔍 Evidence

Amiodarone for secondary prevention of VT
Whilst amiodarone is effective for secondary prevention of VT, meta-analysis of three large studies showed clear superiority of implantable cardiac defibrillators over amiodarone, particularly where ejection fraction was <35%.

Patients with a history of VT with normal left ventricular function had similar outcomes whether they were randomised to an implantable cardiac defibrillator or amiodarone (Connolly *et al.*, 2000).

🔍 Evidence

Amiodarone for AF/atrial flutter
Amiodarone is more effective than sotalol or propafenone for the prevention of recurrences of atrial fibrillation (Roy *et al.*, 2000).

However: 'Management of atrial fibrillation with the rhythm-control strategy offers no survival advantage over the rate-control strategy, and there are potential advantages, such as a lower risk of adverse drug effects, with the rate-control strategy. Anticoagulation should be continued in this group of high-risk patients' (Wyse *et al.*, 2002).

Amiodarone is therefore a useful drug for treatment of difficult AF; however, if the rate can be controlled by drugs that are better tolerated with fewer side effects (such as beta blockers), then this is a preferable management strategy.

Amiodarone: essential pharmacology

Amiodarone is a benzofuran derivative class III antiarrhythmic agent. However, despite its class III classification, it exhibits all four of the classic Vaughan Williams mechanisms of action, namely sodium and potassium channel blockade, a mild antisympathetic action and some calcium channel blockade. It prolongs the refractory period in all cardiac tissues. It also has coronary and peripheral artery dilation properties (Campbell, 2005) (Table 3.3).

One mechanism of action is by prolongation of phase 3 of the cardiac action potential. This is the repolarisation phase where there is normally decreased calcium permeability and increased potassium permeability. Amiodarone affects potassium channels, causing increased duration of the action potential and prolonging the refractory period.

Amiodarone also affects sodium channels, causing generalised slowing of intracardiac conduction. Amiodarone also has beta-blocker-like and potassium channel blocker-like actions by increasing the refractory periods of the SA and AV nodes and thereby slowing conduction.

Amiodarone chemically resembles thyroxine and binds to the nuclear thyroid receptor. This may contribute to some of its pharmacological and toxic actions.

Amiodarone takes a long time to build up to therapeutic levels in the blood stream, hence the necessity of a loading regimen. It has a very long half-life of up to several weeks, and may take weeks or months to reach a steady concentration in the bloodstream. This is important because drug interactions and side effects can therefore occur months after initiation of treatment. Because of its long half-life, amiodarone needs only to be taken once daily. However, it is very likely to cause nausea at doses greater than 100 mg at a time, therefore initial maintenance doses are split throughout the day. Amiodarone is metabolised by the liver.

Amiodarone has numerous drug interactions, including with other antiarrhythmics, HMG CoA reductase inhibitors (statins), drugs metabolised by cytochrome P450, warfarin and any drugs that prolong the QT interval. Consult the *BNF* (BMA/RPS, 2015) and seek specialist advice.

Non-cardiac effects

- Most patients taking amiodarone develop corneal microdeposits. These are visible on fundoscopy and rarely interfere with vision. However, they may cause dazzling from headlights when driving at night. They are usually reversed on withdrawal of treatment. However, amiodarone can rarely cause optic neuritis or neuropathy and must be stopped to prevent blindness in these situations. These patients should be referred to an ophthalmologist.
- Amiodarone contains iodine and can cause both hypothyroidism and hyperthyroidism. Thyroid function tests should be done pretreatment and every 6 months. If thyroid dysfunction occurs, amiodarone is usually withdrawn. However, if amiodarone is necessary for arrhythmia control, hyperthyroidism can be treated with carbimazole or hypothyroidism with thyroxine replacement without altering the amiodarone regimen. Thyroid disorders may be transient or permanent, even after stopping therapy.
- Amiodarone causes increased skin photosensitivity. Sunscreen is therefore advised, including for 3 months after stopping therapy. It can also cause persistent slate-grey skin discoloration.
- Amiodarone is associated with development interstitial pneumonitis and pulmonary fibrosis. This may be irreversible.
- Amiodarone can cause peripheral neuropathy.
- Amiodarone is associated with hepatotoxicity and should be discontinued if liver function becomes deranged.

Table 3.3 Vaughan Williams classification of antiarrhythmic drugs.

Class	Mechanisms of action
I	Sodium channel blockade
II	Beta-blockade
III	Potassium channel blockade
IV	Calcium channel blockade

Other medications used for tachycardias

Verapamil

This is a rate-controlling calcium channel antagonist (see Section Atrial Fibrillation). It can be used for SVT, but usually adenosine is first choice. Verapamil may be used instead of adenosine in asthmatics. It can be given initially IV, then as an oral maintenance dose. It should not be used in tachycardias using an accessory pathway (e.g. Wolff–Parkinson–White syndrome). It must not be given with beta-blockers.

Flecainide

Flecainide is a class 1c antiarrhythmic drug. It works by regulating the flow of sodium ions in cardiac muscle, causing prolongation of the cardiac action potential and therefore slowing tachycardias. It is an option for management of episodes of recurrent SVT and may be taken by patients as a 'pill in the pocket' strategy for managing tachycardic episodes. It also may be used for symptomatic ventricular arrhythmias, junctional re-entry tachycardias and paroxysmal atrial fibrillation.

Flecainide cannot be used in patients with any structural heart disease or ischaemic heart disease due to risk of serious arrhythmias. In cases where this is not clear, an echocardiogram at least may be required.

Propafenone

Propafenone has a complex mechanism of action. It slows influx of sodium ions like a class I antiarrhythmic, yet also has weak beta-blocking activity. It can be used for the prophylaxis and treatment of ventricular arrhythmias and also for some supraventricular arrhythmias. It is only really started under specialist guidance.

Magnesium sulphate

ONCE ONLY PRESCRIPTIONS						
Date	Time to be given	DRUG	Dose	Route	Prescriber Signature	Bleep
xx/xx/xx	xx:xx	MAGNESIUM SULPHATE	2 g	IV over 2 hours	A. Doctor	

Low plasma magnesium levels may lower the threshold for arrhythmias. Magnesium increases sinus node refractoriness and prolongs conduction in the AV node (Stühlinger *et al.*, 2000). It is therefore worth replacing this electrolyte in patients with even borderline low levels. Regardless of magnesium levels, intravenous magnesium is a treatment in its own right for tachycardias secondary to Torsade de pointes, digitalis toxicity and multifocal atrial tachycardias (Wills, 1986). In addition, patients with ventricular arrhythmias secondary to neuroleptics or tricyclic antidepressants may benefit.

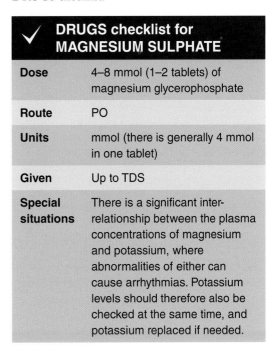

✓	**DRUGS checklist for MAGNESIUM SULPHATE**
Dose	2 g
Route	IV
Units	grams
Given	over 2 hours
Special situations	This dose is for rapid replacement of Mg rather than everyday prescribing.

For daily maintenance of chronically low magnesium levels, treatment is shown in a separate DRUGS checklist.

✓	**DRUGS checklist for MAGNESIUM SULPHATE**
Dose	4–8 mmol (1–2 tablets) of magnesium glycerophosphate
Route	PO
Units	mmol (there is generally 4 mmol in one tablet)
Given	Up to TDS
Special situations	There is a significant inter-relationship between the plasma concentrations of magnesium and potassium, where abnormalities of either can cause arrhythmias. Potassium levels should therefore also be checked at the same time, and potassium replaced if needed.

Potassium chloride

Low potassium levels (or high levels) can predispose patients to have arrhythmias (both tachycardias and bradycardias). This is because one of the functions of potassium is to maintain the excitability of nerve and muscle tissue. Alterations therefore affect membrane excitability by alterations in the resting membrane potential (Wills, 1986).

Replacement is generally given where the potassium is less than 3 mmol/L, but if a patient is particularly vulnerable to arrhythmias, potassium is replaced when levels are less than 3.5 mmol/L (lower end of normal range).

✓	DRUGS checklist for POTASSIUM CHLORIDE
Dose	20–40 mmol of KCl in 1 L of 0.9% saline
Route	IV
Units	mmol
Given	No faster than 10 mmol KCl per hour (max rate)
Special situations	KCl given neat would cause fatal arrhythmias, hence it is always diluted in saline 0.9% or dextrose 5% in a premixed fluid bag and given slowly. Nurses no longer make up the fluid bags on the ward for fear of concentration errors. This situation may be different in intensive care settings, but even in ITU the pharmacy tends to mix the fluid for non-standard potassium prescriptions. There is a significant inter-relationship between the plasma concentrations of magnesium and potassium, where abnormalities of either can cause arrhythmias. Magnesium levels should therefore also be checked at the same time, and Mg replaced if needed.

Further aspects of tachycardia management

Tachycardias may be triggered or driven by an underlying cause. It is important to consider these, as the tachycardia may be resolved by treatment of the underlying cause.

Precipitating factors for tachycardia

- **Underlying cardiac conditions:**
  - Ischaemic heart disease
  - Recent MI
  - Angina
  - Mitral valve disease
  - LV aneurysm
  - Congenital heart disease
  - Baseline ECG abnormalities (short PR showing pre-excitation or long QT syndrome)
- **Drugs:**
  - Antiarrhythmics
  - Beta agonists
  - Cocaine
  - Antidepressants, particularly tricyclic antidepressants
  - Aminophylline
  - Caffeine
  - Alcohol
- **Metabolic abnormalities:**
  - High or low potassium
  - High or low calcium
  - High or low magnesium
  - Hypoxia
  - Hypercarbia
  - Acidosis
- **Endocrine abnormalities:**
  - Thyrotoxicosis
  - Phaeochromocytoma
- **Miscellaneous:**
  - Febrile illness
  - Emotional stress
  - Smoking
  - Fatigue

The management of arrhythmias secondary to re-entry pathways such as Wolff–Parkinson–White has not been discussed here. This needs specialist advice as some antiarrhythmics may worsen the situation by potentiating the conduction down the abnormal pathway.

Other non-pharmacological considerations for patients with persistent tachycardias are similar to those discussed in Section Atrial Fibrillation:

- Referral for SVT or VT ablation. This require mapping of the aberrant pathways via a specialist electrophysiologist at a tertiary cardiology centre, then ablation of the area. This may require subsequent pacemaker insertion should the ablation result in heart block post procedure. Ablation is more likely to be considered in young patients, those with troublesome symptoms, and where there is no other correctable cause for SVT or VT. It can be 6 months before ablation success is confirmed by way of a continuous rhythm strip, as arrhythmias can happen immediately post-procedure, which do not correlate with long-term resolution.
- Referral for elective DC cardioversion. This requires careful anticoagulation in the weeks leading up the procedure and may also require exclusion of an atrial or ventricular thrombus via a transoesophageal echocardiogram. Post-DC cardioversion, patients may need a rate control medication to maintain a controlled heart rate. The first-line maintenance is generally beta-blockers unless there are contraindications.
- Insertion of internal cardiac defibrillators. Patients who have VT may qualify for an ICD. Particularly if they have a low ejection fraction (MADIT Executive Committee, 1991).
- Cardiac resynchronisation therapy (CRT). This is a treatment for patients with a low ejection fraction and a prolonged QRS complex designed to optimise systolic function, not treat arrhythmias. However, in the setting of someone with recurrent VT caused by heart failure, a CRT may help prevent VT by optimising cardiac function. Please see Section Chronic Heart Failure. Many CRT devices are also ICDs, and in reality patients with heart failure and VT would probably be upgraded from a CRT-P (pacing) device to a CRT-D (defibrillating) device.
- If a patient's VT is due to hypertrophic cardiomyopathy (HOCM), this may require

additional surgical myectomy or alcohol septal ablation, both under highly specialist cardiology guidance.

- Anticoagulation. Patients with paroxysmal AF are at increased risk of thromboembolic stroke and need to be risk stratified using the CHA2DS-VASc score and HASBLED score to determine their need for anticoagulation versus risk of bleeding. Anticoagulation could be with aspirin, warfarin, or one of the new oral anticoagulant drugs. This is discussed in detail in Chapter 16. SVT does not generally need anticoagulation as the atria still contract, hence thromboembolic risk is low.

Evidence

ICDs reduce mortality in those with high risk of sudden cardiac death

The Multicentre Automatic Defibrillator Implantation Trial (MADIT) randomised 300 patients with a history of ventricular tachycardia or Q wave MI (>1 month previously) and LVEF <35% to receive either ICD or drug therapy (most commonly amiodarone). There was a 54% reduction in all-cause mortality in ICD group compared to non-device group (MADIT Executive Committee, 1991).

The Multicenter UnSustained Tachycardia Trial (MUSTT) also showed a reduced risk of arrhythmic death, cardiac arrest, and overall mortality in selected patients who were given ICDs (Buxton *et al.*,1999).

Case outcome and discharge

Miss Korn had SVT diagnosed by successful termination of the rhythm with adenosine, after failed vagal manoeuvres.

She received a number of investigations to look for underlying driving factors to precipitate SVT. Her electrolytes including magnesium were normal, as were her thyroid function tests. She had no evidence of sepsis as shown by her history, lack of signs of sepsis, with normal CXR and negative urine dip. She was booked for an outpatient echocardiogram to look for any underlying structural heart abnormalities.

She had returned to sinus rhythm on discharge; however, it is possible that this could happen again. She was therefore referred back to her GP but with a low threshold for cardiology referral should SVT episodes recur, as she could be a candidate for SVT ablation in future.

Unlike atrial fibrillation, there is not a significant increased risk of stroke with SVT. This is because it is a regular tachycardia and there is no protracted period of atrial standstill.

She was advised against heavy caffeine, alcohol or recreational drug consumption, as these are known precipitants for SVT.

She was given a daily beta-blocker to act as a preventative for future episodes, although this was stopped prior to the 24-hour tape, as it may reduce the chance of detecting underlying frequently occurring arrhythmias.

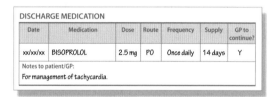

DISCHARGE MEDICATION						
Date	Medication	Dose	Route	Frequency	Supply	GP to continue?
xx/xx/xx	BISOPROLOL	2.5 mg	PO	Once daily	14 days	Y
Notes to patient/GP:						
For management of tachycardia.						

Common pitfalls

- Diagnosing SVT can be difficult particularly if the rate is so fast that AF can't be excluded. This should not be a problem as administration of adenosine should reveal the underlying rhythm by transiently slowing the conduction rate. If it is SVT, then adenosine itself is the treatment and the rhythm may cardiovert back to sinus rhythm.

- A big clue to underlying atrial flutter is when the rate is exactly 150 bpm – look for subtle 'saw-toothing' on the ECG. Adenosine is still appropriate to help in the diagnosis of this if it is unclear from the ECG.

- When used, amiodarone should be given via a central line. However, the loading dose of 300 mg can be given via a large peripheral line where the rate needs to be controlled quickly. In these situations, if the patient reverts to sinus rhythm then the 900-mg dose can be omitted and the patient put straight on to oral amiodarone. This negates the need for central access, which can be difficult to organise on a non-specialist ward.

- All tachycardic patients should be put on a cardiac monitor as rhythms may change, or the patient may stop tolerating the tachycardia and start developing ischaemia. This also provides a record of the rhythm, which can be printed at a later date.

- If adenosine is reported to have no effect on a tachycardia, check how the drug was given. If it was given slowly through a small line then it may have zero effect as the half life is so short. Also consider aberrant pathways and ventricular rhythms in this scenario.

SUMMARY

Tachycardia management differs according to whether the patient is haemodynamically stable or unstable. It also depends on whether the arrhythmia originates from the atria (supraventricular) or ventricles (ventricular). Within these groups there are subdivisions of arrhythmia, which guide management. ECG interpretation is therefore the underpinning essential skill for this area of cardiology.

🔑 Key learning points

Supraventricular tachycardia
- If the patient is unstable, consider DC cardioversion and/or chemical cardioversion with amiodarone.
- If the patient is haemodynamically stable, the focus is first on rate control.
- Treat any precipitating factors first, e.g. sepsis, hyperthyroidism.
- If no obvious driver for SVT, try vagal manoeuvres and/or carotid sinus massage in the first instance, watching the cardiac monitor.
- If not effective, give adenosine 6 mg to terminate rhythm.
- This can be repeated at up to 12 mg if ineffective.
- If the SVT is actually fast atrial flutter, giving adenosine will slow the rate enough to reveal the flutter waves; this will therefore direct further management.
- When the rate is controlled, referral to cardiology may be required for consideration of future DC cardioversion (if persistent prolonged episodes) or SVT ablation, particularly if it is a recurrent problem or very disabling.

Ventricular tachycardias
- Sustained VT leads to cardiac arrest and needs electrical. cardioversion urgently, as per the cardiac arrest ALS algorithm.
- Non-sustained VT with a stable patient still requires urgent treatment. VT may be controlled with beta blockers or amiodarone, but always under cardiology guidance. These patients are at risk of cardiac arrest in future.
- There is often an underlying structural cause for persistent VT episodes, such as heart failure or HOCM (due to dilated or hypertrophied ventricles).
- Treatment with VT ablation or DC cardioversion, or prevention of cardiac arrest with ICD implantation must be considered.

⃝ Guidelines

The European Society of Cardiology has complete guidelines on:
- *Supraventricular Arrhythmias (ACC/AHA/ESC Guidelines for the Management of Patients with)*, 2003. Available at: www.escardio.org/guidelines-surveys/esc-guidelines/Pages/supraventricular-arrhythmias.aspx (accessed Dec. 2015).
- *Ventricular Arrhythmias and the Prevention of Sudden Cardiac Death,* 2015. Available at: www.escardio.org/Guidelines-&-Education/Clinical-Practice-Guidelines/Ventricular-Arrhythmias-and-the-Prevention-of-Sudden-Cardiac-Death (accessed Dec. 2015).

Bradycardia

Mr Andrew Raymond

Age: 75

Hospital number: 123456

Case study

PC: *A 75-year-old man is brought in by ambulance after a collapse in a shop. He is conscious but confused and unable to sit up. History from the family reveals that he has had three falls in the past 2 months with a number of dizzy episodes.*

(Continued)

Case study (Continued)

PMH: *Previous MI, diabetes type 2, hypertension, hypercholesterolaemia*

Allergies: *Nil known*

Examination:
HR 35 regular, RR 24, BP 95/55, Sats 99% on air, afebrile, BM 9.5

CVS: *Capillary refill time <2 seconds, JVP not raised, no oedema*
HS I + II + 0

RS: *Clear lung fields*

Abdo: *Soft, non-tender, no masses palpated, bowel sounds present*

Chest X-ray *clear lung fields*

ECG *shows sinus bradycardia with no signs of ischaemia*

PHARMACY STAMP	AGE 75	FORENAME, SURNAME
		Andrew Raymond
	D.O.B.	ADDRESS
	xx/xx/xxxx	85, Elmfield Way
		NHS NUMBER

SIMVASTATIN 40 mg once at night.

ASPIRIN 75 mg once daily.

RAMIPRIL 10 mg once daily.

ATENOLOL 25 mg once daily.

SIGNATURE OF PRESCRIBER	DATE

SP21000

Diagnosis

This patient has symptomatic sinus bradycardia precipitated by beta-blocker treatment. Other potential driving causes of sinus bradycardia include sick sinus syndrome, endocrine disease (hypothyroidism, Addison's disease), hypothermia or physiological bradycardia in athletes. Careful consideration needs to be given to more serious bradyarrhythmias such as second-degree or third-degree heart block, but the resting ECG should (unless intermittent) reveal these. There may be a trigger such as sepsis/PE/hypovolaemia/thyroid disorders, but this is at present unknown.

Signs of instability with bradycardia are:
- Chest pain or signs of myocardial ischaemia
- Heart failure
- Systolic BP <90
- Reduced conscious level or syncope.

Indications for risk of asystole are:
- Recent asystole
- Mobitz II AV block
- Complete heart block with broad QRS
- Ventricular pause >3 seconds.

Signs of cardiac instability or a patient at risk of asystole should prompt consideration for emergency external pacing in ED. This is done with the pads from the defibrillation machine. This is not done for stable patients in the acute setting, as it requires an anaesthetist for sedation and can be very uncomfortable for the patient. It is also only a temporary solution until a temporary pacing wire is fitted, and/or a permanent pacemaker implanted (Resuscitation Council UK, 2015).

This patient has signs of cardiac instability as he is confused, which could be secondary to his bradycardia, and his blood pressure is a potential concern but there is likely to be time to try atropine first before pacing.

 Guidelines

Resuscitation Council (UK) bradycardia management algorithm available at:
www.resus.org.uk/resuscitation-guidelines/

Initial measures

ABC. Airway is clear, give oxygen if hypoxic. Check BP and HR and get IV access. ECG is required to confirm diagnosis, and look for additional problems (such as ischaemia, as an MI may have caused new complete heart block). Bradycardia itself can cause a degree of ischaemic change on the ECG, as the heart is a muscle like any other, which reacts poorly to decreased perfusion. Check glucose and send bloods, particularly for electrolytes, thyroid function, cortisol and troponin if MI is suspected. Examine the patient for signs of LVF and do a CXR for pulmonary oedema. Look also for other clinical signs that may point towards a cause of bradycardia (signs of hypothyroidism or Addison's disease, recent cardiac operations and look at the drug chart).

The patient needs to be on a cardiac monitor.

Prescribing for bradycardia

ONCE ONLY PRESCRIPTIONS					Prescriber	
Date	Time to be given	DRUG	Dose	Route	Signature	Bleep
xx/xx/xx	xx:xx	ATROPINE	500 micrograms	IV	A. Doctor	

If this dose of atropine is not effective, repeat up to a dose of 3 mg. If atropine has none or limited effect (in terms of maintaining conscious level/ reasonable blood pressure), given the likely precipitant has been a beta-blocker, IM glucagon 1 mg could be considered. Otherwise, if the clinical situation remains unstable, the patient may require urgent pacing. Given the likelihood of the beta-blocker being responsible, if there is response to atropine and the situation settles, no further cardiological investigations would be needed.

Atropine: rationale and evidence

Atropine blocks the effect of the vagal nerve on the sinoatrial (SA) and atrioventricular (AV) node, thereby increasing sinus automaticity and facilitating AV node conduction to increase heart rate (Rang *et al.*, 2015).

DRUGS checklist for ATROPINE

Dose	0.5 mg
Route	IV
Units	mg
Given	Stat
	Give up to 3 mg if ineffective at first
Special situations	May be ineffective in third-degree heart block.
	If an overdose is given, the antidote is physostigmine or pilocarpine.
	Side effects are dose related: blurred vision, dry mouth, urinary retention.
	Can cause confusion in the elderly.

For prevention of recurrent symptomatic bradycardia episodes, a pacemaker may be required.

Atropine: essential pharmacology

Atropine is a naturally occurring tropane alkaloid extracted from plants from the Solanceae family. This family includes deadly nightshade (*Atropa belladonna*), Jimson weed (*Datura stramonium*) and mandrake (*Mandragora officinarum*). Atropine is a competitive antagonist of the muscarinic acetylcholine receptors (Rang *et al.*, 2015). These are the main receptors used by the parasympathetic nervous system, most importantly the vagus nerve (which is the parasympathetic nervous supply to sinoatrial node). Atropine opposes parasympathetic effects, causing increased heart rate, pupil dilation and reduced salivation. Atropine may have no effect at all on complete heart block or Mobitz type 2 heart block, particularly if there is a ventricular escape rhythm or a rhythm originating low in the Purkinje fibres. There may be some effect if the bradycardia is caused by third-degree heart block with an AV nodal escape rhythm, or where the rhythm is originating from high in the Purkinje fibres.

Other medications used in bradycardia

Isoprenaline: Isoprenaline can be given IV at 5 micrograms per minute for bradycardia under cardiology or intensive care team guidance. It is a beta-adrenergic agonist and induces positive chronotropic, dromotropic and inotropic effects. It is structurally similar to adrenaline (Porter and Kaplan, 2011).

Adrenaline: Adrenaline can be given via infusion at 2–10 micrograms per minute IV.

Glucagon: Glucagon is given for bradycardia caused by beta-blockers or calcium channel blocker overdose.

Dopamine: Dopamine is the precursor of the naturally occurring catecholamines adrenaline or noradrenaline. It is a positive ionotrope, which is dose dependent. It can be given under cardiology or intensive care guidance as an infusion in bradycardia.

Further aspects of bradycardia management

It is important to note that different people tolerate different degrees of bradycardia. Even if a patient has a persistent bradycardia of 40 bpm, if they are well and completely asymptomatic, this may be observed under a cardiology clinic and never treated. Symptoms are the main drive for treatment.

However, persistent symptomatic bradycardic episodes may require pacemaker implantation. However a pacemaker-induced systole can never perfectly imitate a physiological heart beat, and over time there may be pacemaker complications. This can include fibrosis around the pacing wires leading to a decreased ejection fraction as well as other complications.

For this reason, most pacemakers for bradycardia are on-demand pacemakers, therefore they only pace when they detect that there has been no p wave, or no subsequent QRS complex. In this way, the majority of the heart beats will ideally be physiological and only a minority will be paced beats. The number of paced beats also depends on the pacemaker setting, as some people function very well with a heart rate of 50 bpm, yet others need a heart rate of 70 bpm.

All patients with a pacemaker have 6-monthly checks at the pacing clinic, where the rate is adjusted and the percentage of pacing time required is analysed by interrogation of the device.

 Guidelines

Pacemakers for bradycardia
NICE has complete guidelines: *Dual-Chamber Pacemakers for Symptomatic Bradycardia due to Sick Sinus Syndrome and/or Atrioventricular Block*, TA88, 2005. Available at: www.nice.org.uk/guidance/ta88 (accessed Dec. 2015).

Case outcome and discharge

Mr Raymond responded to atropine whilst in the emergency department and his heart rate returned to normal. He remained on a cardiac monitor overnight and his rate remained above 50 bpm. His beta-blocker was stopped and his GP was advised to refer to cardiology in the event of further episodes. Other medications were kept the same.

DISCHARGE MEDICATION

Date	Medication	Dose	Route	Frequency	Supply	GP to continue?
xx/xx/xx	SIMVASTATIN	40 mg	PO	Once per night	14 days	Y
xx/xx/xx	ASPIRIN	75 mg	PO	Once daily	14 days	Y
xx/xx/xx	RAMIPRIL	10 mg	PO	Once daily	14 days	Y

Notes to patient/GP:
Atenolol stopped due to bradycardia.

Common pitfalls

■ Atropine used to be recommended for asystole/pulseless electrical activity (PEA) as part of the cardiac arrest algorithm. However, atropine is no longer routinely recommended for this, as asystole during cardiac arrest is usually caused by a primary myocardial pathology rather than excessive vagal tone. There was therefore insufficient evidence to keep it as a mandatory cardiac arrest drug (Field *et al.*, 2010).

■ Beware of diagnosing syncope secondary to bradycardia, as bradycardia can be secondary to other causes of syncope such as vasovagal syncope. A vasovagal episode occurs due to over-effect of the parasympathetic nervous system in response to a number of factors. One of these effects is bradycardia. The link between the bradycardia and syncopal episode must therefore be investigated by a thorough history and symptom diary.

■ Third-degree heart block can occur transiently after inferior myocardial infarction.

This usually resolves after 10 days, therefore permanent pacing is not usually necessary. In this situation, the patient would only require emergency pacing if they had signs of instability or new escape ventricular rhythms were developing. If third-degree heart block occurs after an anterior MI, this is a different situation and the patient requires a temporary pacing wire.

■ Atropine can be detrimental for some types of bradycardia, particularly where the QRS is wide. Bradycardia with wide QRS must be discussed with a cardiologist. This is because a wide QRS indicates that the rhythm may be originating from low down in the conduction system/ Purkinje fibres. Giving atropine disrupts the innate escape rhythm provided by the Purkinje fibres, and may cause asystole.

Bradycardia may be asymptomatic, but symptomatic bradycardia requires treatment. Emergency treatment consists of transcutaneous pacing or transvenous pacing (temporary pacing wire). However, even in unstable patients, pharmacological measures are usually tried first as they are rapid acting.

SUMMARY

🔑 Key learning points

Bradycardia

- In patients who are unstable or at risk of asystole, consider transcutaneous pacing. This requires an anaesthetist to administer sedation (unless life-threatening) or insertion of a transvenous pacing wire.
- In the meantime give atropine 500 micrograms IV, repeated up to 3 mg.
- Treat any precipitating factors, e.g. stop beta blockers/rate-controlling calcium channel blockers.
- All patients require cardiac monitoring throughout.
- Referral to cardiology may be required for consideration of a permanent pacemaker, if bradycardia episodes are recurrent and symptomatic.

FURTHER READING

- Neumar RW, Otto CW, Link MS, *et al.* (2010) Part 8: adult advanced cardiovascular life support: 2010 American Heart Association Guidelines for Cardiopulmonary Resuscitation and Emergency Cardiovascular Care. *Circulation* 122 (18 Suppl. 3): S729–67.
- Porter RS, Kaplan JL (2011). Arrhythmias and conduction disorders. In: *Merck Manuals: Online Medical Library,* 19th edn. Merck Sharp and Dohme Corp.

Hypertension

Mrs Jane Goodings

Age: 59

Hospital number: 123456

🔍 Case study

PC: *A 59-year-old woman is found to have persistent hypertension by her GP. She is asymptomatic.*

PMH: *Hypercholesterolaemia*

Allergies: *Nil*

Examination:
HR 80 regular, RR 18, BP 150/120, Sats 99% on air, afebrile, BM 9.5
Looks uncomfortable
No rash or meningism

CVS: *Capillary refill time <2 seconds, JVP not raised, no oedema*
HS I + II + 0

RS: *Clear lung fields*

Abdo: *Soft, non-tender, no masses palpated, bowel sounds present*

Neuro: *No focal neurology, on fundoscopy no papilloedema is seen*

Bloods: *FBC and U&Es normal, CRP 1*

Chest X-ray *clear lung fields*

ECG *shows regular sinus rhythm*

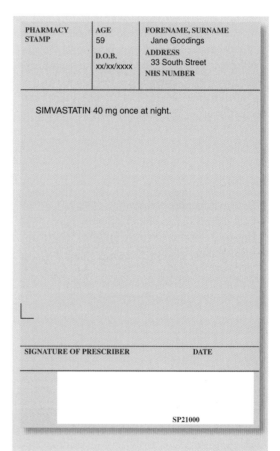

| PHARMACY STAMP | AGE 59 | FORENAME, SURNAME Jane Goodings |
| | D.O.B. xx/xx/xxxx | ADDRESS 33 South Street NHS NUMBER |

SIMVASTATIN 40 mg once at night.

SIGNATURE OF PRESCRIBER   DATE

SP21000

Diagnosis

This patient is hypertensive. This is classified as a blood pressure persistently over 140/90. The majority of hypertension has unknown aetiology and is therefore classed as essential or primary hypertension. The patient should be checked for signs of secondary organ damage, mainly kidney dysfunction and hypertensive retinopathy. Causes of secondary hypertension should also be considered, such as endocrine pathology (Cushing's syndrome, Conn's syndrome, hyperthyroidism, phaeochromocytoma), sepsis, renal artery stenosis and nephritic syndrome. These can be investigated for according to clinical suspicion.

Hypertension should be treated not only because it can cause secondary organ dysfunction, but also because it is a major risk factor for MI, stroke, vascular disease and coronary artery disease. The risk of morbidity increases as blood pressure rises, as each 2 mmHg rise in systolic blood pressure is associated with a 7% increased risk of mortality from ischaemic heart disease and a 10% increased risk of mortality from stroke (NICE, 2011).

Initial measures

This patient is stable in the outpatient setting. Neurology examination is important to look for papilloedema and signs of raised intracranial pressure. ECG may show signs of longstanding hypertension, and there may be LVH. Send bloods for renal function, thyroid function, cortisol and CRP (sepsis can worsen hypertension). Urine dip and microscopy for casts may reveal renal pathology. A renal ultrasound or CT angiogram may be required in due course if nephritic syndrome or renal artery stenosis are suspected.

Prescribing for chronic hypertension

There are clear guidelines, which are mainly based on age, co-morbidities, race and patient choice.

> ### ⓘ Guidelines
>
> The NICE guidelines on hypertension is an essential read. This includes a clear flow chart of management for patients of different demographics, available at: http://pathways.nice.org.uk/pathways/hypertension (accessed Dec. 2015).
>
> The full guideline is *Hypertension in Adults: Diagnosis and Management*, CG127, 2011. Available at: www.nice.org.uk/guidance/cg127 (accessed Dec. 2015).

Essentially, those below the age of 55 should commence an ACEI as treatment for primary hypertension, or ARB if not tolerated (abbreviations are explained in Table 3.4).

The exceptions to this rule, however, are patients who are diabetic, have had an MI or have known coronary or vascular disease. These patients have other prognostically significant reasons for being on an ACEI (see Section Acute Coronary Syndrome). These individuals should have therefore already been started on an ACEI regardless of blood pressure, so this should also be their first-line antihypertensive agent regardless of age.

Those above the age of 55 or who are black with African or Caribbean family origin should be offered calcium channel blockers or thiazide-like diuretics as first-line for primary hypertension.

If this is ineffective, add either an ACEI or calcium channel blocker, whichever one they are not already taking.

If this is not effective, add a thiazide-like diuretic in addition.

Table 3.4 Treatment for primary hypertension.

Abbreviation	Definition	Example
ACEI	Angiotensin converting enzyme inhibitor	Ramipril, lisinopril, enalapril
ARB	Angiotensin receptor blocker	Losartan, candesartan, irbesartan, valsartan
CCB	Calcium channel blocker	Amlodipine, nifedipine, felodipine (dihydropropine class), verapamil and diltiazem (phenylalkylamine class)

If three agents are ineffective this is resistant hypertension. Consider adding a beta-blocker, alpha-blocker and further diuretic, and consider expert advice.

Mrs Goodings is a 59-year-old British female without diabetes or coronary artery disease, where secondary hypertension has been excluded.

First line is amlodipine.

REGULAR PRESCRIPTIONS				Circle/enter times below ↓	Enter dates below		
					Day 1	Day 2	Day 3
DRUG AMLODIPINE				06			
				⑧			
Dose 5 mg	Route PO	Freq OD	Start date xx/xx/xx	12			
Signature A. Doctor		Bleep	Review	16			
Additional instructions				18			
				22			

If amlodipine 5 mg is ineffective after 1 week, the dose should be up-titrated to 10 mg. If this is ineffective after 4 weeks, ramipril can be added.

REGULAR PRESCRIPTIONS				Circle/enter times below ↓	Enter dates below		
					Day 1	Day 2	Day 3
DRUG RAMIPRIL				06			
				⑧			
Dose 2.5 mg	Route PO	Freq OD	Start date xx/xx/xx	12			
Signature A. Doctor		Bleep	Review	16			
Additional instructions				18			
				22			

Ramipril can be up-titrated to 10 mg. If this is ineffective after 4 weeks, bendroflumethiazide can be added.

REGULAR PRESCRIPTIONS				Circle/enter times below ↓	Enter dates below		
					Day 1	Day 2	Day 3
DRUG BENDROFLUMETHIAZIDE				06			
				⑧			
Dose 2.5 mg	Route PO	Freq OD	Start date xx/xx/xx	12			
Signature A. Doctor		Bleep	Review	16			
Additional instructions				18			
				22			

Other essential treatments are lifestyle modifications, healthy low-salt diet, maintenance of healthy BMI and smoking cessation. These discussions must be a part of every patient visit (Chobanian et al., 2003).

ACE inhibitors: rationale and evidence

ACEIs are first-line treatment for essential hypertension in those aged under 55 years. However, if a patient is over 55 but has diabetes, a history of MI or cardiovascular disease, heart failure or stroke, then it should be used as first line. Choice of ACEI agent is dependent on local practice, cost and tolerability.

🔍 Evidence

ACEIs for primary hypertension
ACEIs are effective for reducing blood pressure, and reduce BP measured 1 to 12 hours after the dose by about 11/6 mm Hg on average. There are no clinically meaningful BP lowering differences between different ACE inhibitors (Heran et al., 2008).

✓ DRUGS checklist for RAMPRIL

Dose	2.5–10 mg
Route	PO
Units	mg
Given	OD
Special situations	ACEIs will cause a degree of renal impairment. Allow a <50% deterioration in baseline creatinine; however, renal function that is poor may limit dosing. Contraindicated in renal artery stenosis, due to substantial reduction on glomerular filtration rate, leading to severe and progressive renal failure.

✓ DRUGS checklist for ENALAPRIL

Dose	2.5–20 mg
Route	PO
Units	mg
Given	OD
Special situations	ACEIs will cause a degree of renal impairment. Allow a <50% deterioration in baseline creatinine; however, renal function that is poor may limit dosing.

Contraindicated in renal artery stenosis, due to substantial reduction on glomerular filtration rate, leading to severe and progressive renal failure. |

✓ DRUGS checklist for LISINOPRIL

Dose	2.5–35 mg
Route	PO
Units	mg
Given	OD
Special situations	ACEIs will cause a degree of renal impairment. Allow a <50% deterioration in baseline creatinine; however, renal function that is poor may limit dosing.

Contraindicated in renal artery stenosis, due to substantial reduction on glomerular filtration rate, leading to severe and progressive renal failure. |

ACE inhibitors: essential pharmacology

One mechanism by which blood pressure is maintained is by the renin–angiotensin–aldosterone system. Renin is released from the kidney in response to low blood pressure, dehydration, low sodium or low plasma volume. This catalyses the conversion of angiotensinogen to angiotensin I. Angiotensin I is then converted to angiotensin II by ACE. Angiotensin II is found in the circulation and in blood vessel endothelium, and causes vasoconstriction in order to increase blood pressure. The release of angiotensin also signals the adrenal gland to produce the hormone aldosterone. Aldosterone is a potent vasoconstrictor and causes sodium retention. Angiotensin II also stimulates the posterior pituitary to produce antidiuretic hormone, which causes increased water reabsorption by the kidney (Solomon and Anavekar, 2005).

ACEIs inhibit angiotensin converting enzyme, the enzyme responsible for catalysing the conversion of angiotensin I to angiotensin II. They therefore lower arteriole resistance, cause venous dilation and lower blood pressure.

Common adverse drug reactions include hypotension, cough and hyperkalaemia. The cough is caused by an increase in bradykinin levels produced by ACEIs. If this symptom is troublesome, the patient may need to be switched to an angiotensin II receptor antagonists (see Section Angiotensin Receptor Blockers). Increased bradykinin levels can also cause angioedema in some patients (Rossi, 2006).

Renal dysfunction is caused by ACEIs, and creatinine can be expected to rise a small amount in every patient. This is because angiotensin II vasoconstricts the efferent arterioles of the glomeruli of the kidney, thereby increasing glomerular filtration rate (GFR). ACEIs reverse this by inhibiting production of angiotensin II. ACEIs therefore cannot be used in those with poor glomerular filtration rates or in those with renal artery stenosis (Sidorenkov and Navis, 2014). Renal dysfunction will be increased if ACEIs are used in combination with NSAID and a diuretic, therefore this combination should be avoided where possible, or at least closely monitored.

Angiotensin receptor blockers: rationale and evidence

Angiotensin receptor antagonists are used where ACEIs are not tolerated. They treat hypertension and reduce stroke risk in hypertensive patients with left ventricular hypertrophy.

✓ DRUGS checklist for LOSARTAN

Dose	50 mg
Route	PO
Units	mg
Given	OD
Special situations	Note this is a higher dose than when used for chronic heart failure (12.5 mg). Dose can be up-titrated to 100 mg OD.
	Use with caution in renal artery stenosis.
	Use with caution in chronic renal impairment; contraindicated where eGFR <60 mL/min/1.73 m².

✓ DRUGS checklist for CANDESARTAN

Dose	8 mg
Route	Oral
Units	mg
Given	OD
Special situations	Max dose is 32 mg. Dose for heart failure is usually lower (4 mg starting dose).
	See DRUGS checklist for losartan for cautions.

🔍 Evidence

ARBs

The data do not suggest that any one ARB is better or worse at lowering BP. ARBs reduced BP measured 1–12 hours after the dose by about 12/7 mmHg (Heran *et al.*, 2008).

ARBs versus ACE inhibitors for primary hypertension

A 2014 Cochrane review of nine studies and 11 007 patients found no evidence of a difference in total mortality or cardiovascular outcomes for ARBs as compared with ACEIs. However, ARBs have not been directly studied in placebo-controlled trials for hypertension. ARBs caused slightly fewer withdrawals due to adverse events than ACE inhibitors (Li *et al.*, 2014).

ARBs: essential pharmacology

ARBs have properties similar to those of ACEIs. However, one difference is that they do not inhibit the breakdown of bradykinin and are therefore less likely to cause a dry cough (Abdi *et al.*, 2002). They are therefore a useful alternative for patients who develop this troublesome symptom on ACEIs. They are used for hypertension and chronic heart failure as second line instead of ACEIs (first line).

ARBs block the activation of angiotensin II receptors thereby inhibiting the renin–angiotensin–aldosterone system as explained above. This leads to vasodilation, reduced secretion of ADH and reduced aldosterone levels. All of these lead to a reduction in blood pressure.

ARBs are usually well tolerated. Common adverse drug reactions include dizziness, headache and hyperkalaemia.

Beta-blockers: rationale and evidence

Beta-blockers are not recommended as first-line treatment for hypertension due to their modest effect on reduction of stroke and no significant reduction in mortality or coronary heart disease (see Evidence). This makes them inferior to other antihypertensive drugs when used for hypertension treatment. They are also not recommended for routine treatment of hypertension in diabetic patients, as beta-blockers can reduce awareness of hypoglycaemia.

🔍 Evidence

Beta-blockers for hypertension
A Cochrane review of 13 randomised controlled trials showed that patients initiating beta blockers for treatment of hypertension had modest reductions in cardiovascular disease and no significant difference in mortality compared to placebo. The effects of beta-blockers were inferior to those of other antihypertensive drugs (calcium channel blockers, ACEIs and ARBs) (Wiysonge *et al.*, 2012).

✓ DRUGS checklist for ATENOLOL

Dose	25–50 mg
Route	PO
Units	mg
Given	OD
Special situations	This is a lower dose than for arrhythmias and angina (up to 100 mg daily). Contraindicated in asthma and COPD with bronchoconstriction.

✓ DRUGS checklist for BISOPROLOL

Dose	5–20 mg
Route	PO
Units	mg
Given	OD
Special situations	Used as an adjunct in heart failure, usually at 1.25–10 mg, Contraindicated in asthma and COPD with bronchoconstriction.

Beta-blockers: essential pharmacology

Beta-blockers (beta-adrenergic receptor antagonists) are a class of drugs that target the beta-receptor. The beta-receptor is found in tissues involved in the sympathetic nervous system, including cardiac muscle cells, smooth muscle, arteries and the kidneys. Beta-blockers interfere with the binding of adrenaline and noradrenaline to the beta-receptor (Arcangelo and Peterson, 2006). This prevents the sympathetic stress response of tachycardia, vasoconstriction and hypertension and therefore has the reverse effects. β_1 receptors are located mainly in the heart and in the kidneys whereas β_2-adrenergic receptors are mainly in the lungs, gastrointestinal tract, liver, uterus, vascular smooth muscle and skeletal muscle. This explains the adverse drug reaction of bronchospasm with beta-blockers, and explains why they are contraindicated in those with asthma or COPD with bronchospasm.

Calcium channel blockers: rationale and evidence

Calcium channel blockers are recommended for treatment of hypertension in patients over the age of 55 or patents who are of black or Caribbean origin. They have been shown to be effective for primary hypertension.

🔍 Evidence

CCBs versus diuretics for primary hypertension
In a Cochrane review of 18 randomised controlled trials, diuretics were found to be better at reducing total cardiovascular events than CCBs, and CCBs were found to be better at reducing total cardiovascular events than beta-blockers (Chen *et al.*, 2010).

✓ DRUGS checklist for AMLODIPINE

Dose	5–10 mg
Route	PO
Units	mg
Given	OD
Special situations	Common side effect is peripheral oedema.

✓ DRUGS checklist for FELODIPINE

Dose	5–10 mg
Route	PO
Units	mg
Given	OD
Special situations	Common side effect is peripheral oedema.

Nifedipine is not usually recommended for hypertension, and neither are the phenylalkylamine class of calcium channel blockers (verapamil, diltiazem) as they are relatively selective for myocardium. They are therefore more often used for angina rather than hypertension.

Calcium channel blockers: essential pharmacology

Calcium channels are embedded in cell membranes, allowing calcium to enter into the cell when signalled. This causes cell excitation. CCBs mostly act on the L-type voltage-gated calcium channel, which is responsible for excitation and contraction of skeletal, smooth and cardiac muscle cells, and for hormone secretion (Yousef *et al.*, 2005). CCBs cause reduced contraction of vascular muscle and therefore a drop in arterial blood pressure. In the myocardium they also slow the conduction and decrease force of contraction of the heart; CCBs are therefore negatively ionotropic. This negatively ionotropic effect is useful for angina and symptoms of ischaemic heart disease; however, it is not good for heart failure or cardiomyopathy. Dihydropyridines (amlodipine, felodipine) mainly affect arterial vascular smooth muscle and lower blood pressure by causing vasodilation. The phenylalkylamine group (diltiazem, verapamil) mainly affect the cells of the heart and have negative inotropic and negative chronotropic effects. The benzothiazepine class of CCBs combine effects of the other two classes.

Thiazide diuretics: rationale and evidence

It is established that low-dose thiazides reduce mortality as well as cardiovascular morbidity in patients with hypertension.

🔍 Evidence

Thiazide diuretics for primary hypertension

A Cochrane review of 60 trails showed that thiazides reduced average blood pressure compared to placebo by 9 mmHg/4 mmHg. Different thiazide drugs have similar effects in lowering blood pressure (Musini *et al.*, 2014).

Thiazides reduce the risk of death, stroke, MI and heart failure due to hypertension (Wright and Musini, 2009).

✓ DRUGS checklist for INDAPAMIDE

Dose	2.5 mg
Route	PO
Units	mg
Given	OD
Special situations	Commonly causes hyponatraemia.

✓ DRUGS checklist for BENDROFLUMETHIAZIDE

Dose	2.5–10 mg
Route	PO
Units	mg
Given	OD
Special situations	

✓	**DRUGS checklist for METOLAZONE**
Dose	5 mg
Route	PO
Units	mg
Given	OD on alternate days
Special situations	Metolazone is a potent diuretic and can cause profound prerenal renal dysfunction. For this reason low doses are given for hypertension treatment, often on alternate days.
	For resistant oedema higher doses of 80 mg (maximum) can be given, but this is a very high dose.

Thiazide diuretics: essential pharmacology

Thiazides cause diuresis, a fall in plasma volume and thereby lower blood pressure. They do this by inhibiting reabsorption of sodium and chloride ions from the distal convoluted tubules of the kidney, as a result of blocking the thiazide-sensitive Na^+-Cl^- symporter (Mastroianni *et al.*, 1996). They also increase calcium reabsorption at the distal tubule. After chronic use thiazides also cause a reduction in blood pressure by lowering peripheral resistance (by vasodilation). The mechanism of this is not fully understood (Duarte and Cooper-DeHoff, 2010).

Other medications used for hypertension

Alpha-blockers

Alpha-blockers (or α-adrenergic antagonists) act as receptor antagonists of α-adrenergic receptors. Alpha-blockers may be used in addition to standard agents where blood pressure is difficult to control, mainly doxazosin and terazosin. Tamsulosin is another selective alpha-blocker but this is used mainly in benign prostatic hyperplasia to ease the passage of urine.

Hydralazine

Hydralazine is a direct-acting vasodilator, which has been used for hypertension treatment for over 60 years. Because of its propensity to cause side effects, it has largely been replaced by newer antihypertensive drugs. However, it is still used widely in developing countries due to its lower cost. Side effects include reflex tachycardia, haemolytic anaemia, vasculitis, glomerulonephritis and a lupus-like syndrome.

There were no randomised controlled trials found by a 2011 Cochrane review that compared hydralazine to placebo for primary hypertension (Kandler *et al.*, 2011), and it is not in UK guidelines for primary care initiated treatment. It is, however, used in resistant hypertension under specialist guidance.

Further aspects of hypertension management

Low-salt diet

A reduction in dietary salt has long been advised for those with hypertension and/or hypercholesterolaemia. This is an effective life-style modification for lowering blood pressure by around 1–3.5%. However, this is often an inadequate reduction for many.

🔍 Evidence

Low-salt diet for primary hypertension
A Cochrane review of 167 studies showed that sodium reduction resulted in a 1% decrease in blood pressure in normotensives, a 3.5% decrease in hypertensives, a significant increase in plasma renin, plasma aldosterone, plasma adrenaline and plasma noradrenaline, a 2.5% increase in cholesterol, and a 7% increase in triglyceride. In general, these effects were stable in studies lasting for 2 weeks or more (Graudal *et al.*, 2011).

Management in a GP or outpatient setting

Blood pressure cannot be assessed on one reading, and is influenced greatly by the situation, time of day and anxiety levels. Blood pressure is therefore better monitored by the GP in the community, to prevent over treatment in hospitals. Ambulatory blood pressure monitoring is being encouraged by GPs and is now part of the 2011 NICE guidance to aid diagnosis and monitoring of treatment.

Hypertensive emergencies

Hypertensive emergencies (also called hypertensive crises) are classified as hypertension with a systolic blood pressure greater than 179 mmHg or a diastolic blood pressure that is greater than 109 mmHg combined with evidence of end-organ damage (Varon and Malik, 2003). This could include hypertensive encephalopathy, dissecting aortic aneurysm, acute left ventricular failure with pulmonary oedema, acute myocardial ischemia, eclampsia, acute renal failure or symptomatic microangiopathic haemolytic anaemia.

The term 'hypertensive urgency' is used for patients with severely elevated blood pressure (as above) but without evidence of end-organ damage. This is the case in the majority of patients with severely elevated blood pressure. The term malignant hypertension is no longer used (Varon and Marik, 2003).

Treatment of hypertensive emergencies/crises may require sodium nitroprusside, particularly if there is acute pulmonary oedema and/or severe left ventricular dysfunction or in patients with aortic dissection (Brewster and Sutters, 2006; Varon and Marik, 2003). Labetalol is used in other situations (Pearce and Wallin, 1994). Nifedipine is no longer used as it drops blood pressure too quickly (Komsuoglu *et al.*, 1992; Varon and Marik, 2003).

For hypertensive urgency, oral agents should be used aiming to bring blood pressure down gradually over 24–48 hours. Rapid reduction of blood pressure can lead to significant morbidity (Bertel *et al.*, 1987; Reed and Anderson, 1986).

Case outcome and discharge

Mrs Goodings was commenced on amlodipine by her GP and she decided to buy a home blood pressure monitor. This showed that amlodipine had a moderate effect, but after 2 months her blood pressure was still often over the target range of 140/90. She was therefore commenced on ramipril in addition. These two drugs in combination controlled her blood pressure effectively. She was given advice regarding a low-salt diet to prevent the need for increasing her medication doses, and was also advised on the benefit of exercise, smoking cessation and maintenance of a healthy weight in preventing cardiovascular disease. This is particularly relevant for Mrs Goodings as she has high cholesterol as well as hypertension.

| PHARMACY STAMP | AGE 59 | FORENAME, SURNAME Jane Goodings |
| | D.O.B. xx/xx/xxxx | ADDRESS 33 South Street NHS NUMBER |

AMLODIPINE 10 mg once daily.

RAMIPRIL 5 mg once daily.

SIMVASTATIN 40 mg once at night.

| SIGNATURE OF PRESCRIBER | DATE |

SP21000

Common pitfalls

- Amlodipine and other calcium channel blockers cause oedema, a common side effect which may limit tolerance.
- ACEIs cause cough in 8% of patients, requiring a switch to ARBs.

- ACEIs are contraindicated in renal artery stenosis, due to substantial reduction in glomerular filtration rate, leading to severe and progressive renal failure.
- Do not give beta-blockers in combination with rate-controlling calcium channel blockers (verapamil, diltiazem) due to the risk of bradycardia.
- In patients with renal disease, management is altered by the fact that ACEIs and ARBs may cause an unacceptable rise in creatinine.

Hypertension is very common and there is increased prevalence as age increases. The most common is essential hypertension; however, all patients should be considered for secondary causes depending on their presentation and risk factors.

   Management is clearly set out according to a step-wise algorithm described in the NICE guidelines, related to age, ethnicity and co-morbidities.

SUMMARY

 Key learning points

Essential hypertension
- Treat any precipitating factors first, e.g. sepsis, hyperthyroidism, renal dysfunction.
- A diagnosis of primary hypertension is based on an average blood pressure greater than 140/90. With ambulatory BP measuring, this is assessed on at least two measurements per hour during the person's usual waking hours. With home BP measuring, this is assessed on twice-daily BP measurements over 4–7 days
- In patient under 55 years, first-line treatment is either with an ACEI or ARB.
- In those over 55 years of age or of African or Caribbean origin, first-line treatment is with a CCB or thiazide-like diuretic.
- Co-morbidities affect choice of agent, e.g. all patients with diabetes, previous MI, heart failure or stroke should be on an ACEI regardless of BP, and patients with ischaemic heart disease or heart failure should be an a beta blocker.
- If a second agent is required, an ACEI or CCB/thiazide should be added (depending on what they are already taking)
- Beta blockers are no longer used first-line for hypertension but are a useful addition in combination with other agents where BP control is insufficient.
- Resistant hypertension needs referral for specialist guidance.

 Guidelines

NICE has complete guidelines on the clinical management of primary hypertension in adults. Hypertension in adults: diagnosis and management, CG127, 2011. Available at: www.nice.org.uk/guidance/cg127 (accessed Dec. 2015).

Now visit **www.wileyessential.com/pharmacology**
to test yourself on this chapter.

References

Abdi R, Dong V, Lee C *et al.* (2002). Angiotensin II receptor blocker-associated angioedema: on the heels of ace inhibitor angioedema *Pharmacotherapy* 22: 1173–5.

Acute Infarction Ramipril Efficacy (AIRE) Study Investigators (1993). Effect of ramipril on mortality and morbidity of survivors of acute myocardial infarction with clinical evidence of heart failure. *Lancet* 342: 821–8.

Antiplatelet Trialists Collaboration (1994). Collaborative overview of randomised trials of antiplatelet treatment, for prevention of vascular death, MI and stroke in high risk patients. *Br Med J* 308: 235–46.

Antman EM, Anbe DT, Armstrong PW *et al.* (2004). ACC/AHA guidelines for the management of patients with ST-elevation myocardial infarction: a report of the American College of Cardiology/American Heart Association Task Force on Practice Guidelines (Committee to Revise the 1999 Guidelines for the Management of Patients With Acute Myocardial Infarction). *J Am Coll Cardiol* 44: 671–719.

Arcangelo VP, Peterson AM (2006). *Pharmacotherapeutics for Advanced Practice: a Practical Approach*, 2nd edn. Lippincott Williams & Wilkins: Philadelphia: 205.

Bardy GH, Lee KL, Mark DB *et al.* (2005). Amiodarone or an implantable cardioverter-defibrillator for congestive heart failure. *N Engl J Med* 352: 225–37.

Bertel O, Marx BE, Conen D (1987). Effects of antihypertensive treatment on cerebral perfusion. *Am J Med* 82: 29–36.

Beta-Blocker Heart Attack Trial Research Group (BHAT Research Group) (1982). A randomized trial of propranolol in patients with acute myocardial infarction: I. Mortality results. *JAMA* 247: 1707–14.

Bleumink G, Feenstra J, Sturkenboom M *et al.* (2003). Nonsteroidal anti-inflammatory drugs and heart failure. *Drugs* 63: 525–34.

Brewster LM, Sutters M (2006). *Hypertensive Urgencies and Emergencies.* Available at: www .health.am/hypertension/hypertensive-urgencies-emergencies/ (accessed May 2015).

Bristow M, Feldman A, Saxon L (2000). Heart failure management using implantable devices for ventricular resynchronization: Comparison of medical therapy, pacing, and defibrillation in chronic heart failure (COMPANION) trial. *J Card Fail* 6: 276–85.

British Medical Association and Royal Pharmaceutical Society of Great Britain (BMA/RPS) (2015). *British National Formulary 69*, 69th edn. BMJ group and Pharmaceutical Press, London. Available at: www.bnf.org (accessed Dec. 2015).

Brugts JJ, Yetgin T, Hoeks SE *et al.* (2009). The benefits of statins in people without established cardiovascular disease but with cardiovascular risk factors: meta-analysis of randomised controlled trials. *BMJ* 338: b2376.

Buxton AE, Lee KL, Fisher JD *et al.* (1999). A randomized study of the prevention of sudden death in patients with coronary artery disease. Multicenter UnSustained Tachycardia Trial Investigators. *N Engl J Med* 341: 1882–90.

Cabello JB, Burls A, Emparanza JI *et al.* (2013). Oxygen therapy for acute myocardial infarction. *Cochrane Database Syst Rev* (8): CD007160.

Camm AJ, Kirchhof P, Lip GY *et al.*; European Heart Rhythm Association; European Association for Cardio-Thoracic Surgery (2010). Guidelines for the management of atrial fibrillation: the Task Force for the Management of Atrial Fibrillation of the European Society of Cardiology (ESC). *Eur Heart J* 31: 2369–429.

Camm AJ, Lip GY, De Caterina R *et al.* (2012) Atrial Fibrillation (management of) 2010 and focused update (2012). An update of the 2010 European Society of Cardiology guidelines for the management of atrial fibrillation. *Eur Heart J* 33: 2719–47.

Campbell T (2005). Amiodarone. *Australian Prescriber* 28: 150–4.

CAPRICORN Investigators (2001). Effect of carvedilol on outcome after myocardial infarction in patients with left-ventricular dysfunction: the CAPRICORN randomised trial. *Lancet* 357: 1385.

CAPRIE Steering Committee (1996). A randomised, blinded trial of clopidogrel versus aspirin in patients at risk of ischaemic events (CAPRIE). *Lancet* 348: 1329–39.

Carville S, Harker M, Henderson R *et al.* (2013). Acute management of myocardial infarction with ST-segment elevation: summary of NICE guidance. *BMJ* 347: f4006.

Chen N, Zhou M, Yang M *et al.*; Editorial Group: Cochrane Hypertension Group (2010). Calcium channel blockers versus other classes of drugs for hypertension. *Cochrane Database Syst Rev* (8): CD003654.

Chen ZM, Jiang LX, Chen YP *et al.* COMMIT (Clopidogrel and Metoprolol in Myocardial Infarction Trial) Collaborative Group (2005). Addition of clopidogrel to aspirin in 45,852 patients with acute myocardial infarction: randomised placebo-controlled trial. *Lancet* 366: 1607–21.

Chobanian, Bakris GL, Black HR, *et al.* (2003). The Seventh Report of the Joint National Committee on Prevention, Detection, Evaluation, and Treatment of High Blood Pressure: The JNC 7 Report. *JAMA* 289: 2560–71.

Cleland JG, Daubert JC, Erddman E *et al.*: for the Cardiac Resynchronization-Heart Failure (CARE-HF) Study Investigators (2005). The effect of cardiac resynchronization on morbidity and mortality in heart failure. *N Engl J Med* 352: 1539–49.

Cohen M, Demers C, Gurfinkel E *et al.* (1997). ESSENCE Study (Efficacy and Safety of Subcutaneous Enoxaparin in Non-Q-wave Coronary Events). A comparison of low-molecular-weight heparin with unfractionated heparin for unstable coronary artery disease. *N Engl J Med* 337: 447–52.

Cohn J, Archibald J, Ziesche S (1986). Effect of vasodilator therapy mortality in chronic congestive heart failure (V-HeFT). *N Engl J Med* 3124: 1547–52.

Cohn J, Tognoni G (2001). A randomized trial of the angiotensin-receptor blocker valsartan in chronic heart failure (Val-HeFT). *N Engl J Med* 345: 1667–75.

Connolly SJ, Hallstrom AP, Cappato R *et al.* (2000). Meta-analysis of the implantable cardioverter defibrillator secondary prevention trials. *Eur Heart J* 21: 2071–8.

Conti C (1991). Adenosine: Clinical pharmacology and applications. *Clin Cardiol* 14: 91–3.

Cotter G, Metzkor E, Kaluski E *et al.* (1998). Randomised trial of high-dose isosorbide dinitrate plus low-dose furosemide versus high-dose furosemide plus low-dose isosorbide dinitrate in severe pulmonary oedema. *Lancet* 351: 389–93.

Digitalis Investigation Group (1997). The effect of digoxin on mortality and morbidity in patients with heart failure. *N Engl J Med* 336: 525–33.

DiMarco J, Sellers T, Berne R *et al.* (1983). Adenosine: electrophysiologic effects and therapeutic use for terminating paroxysmal supraventricular tachycardia. *Circulation* 68: 1254–63.

Dorsam RT, Kunapuli SP (2004). Central role of the P2Y12 receptor in platelet activation. *J Clin Invest* 113: 340–5.

Duarte JD, Cooper-DeHoff RM (2010). Mechanisms for blood pressure lowering and metabolic effects of thiazide and thiazide-like diuretics. *Expert Rev Cardiovasc Ther* 8: 793–802.

Eichhorn E, Bristow M (2001). carvedilol prospective randomized cumulative survival trial (COPERNICUS). *Curr Control Trials Cardiovasc Med* 2: 20–3.

European Society of Cardiology (2013). Management of stable coronary artery disease. *Eur Heart J* 34: 2949–3003.

Field JM, Hazinski MF, Sayre MR *et al.* (2010). Part 1: executive summary: 2010 American Heart Association guidelines for cardiopulmonary resuscitation and emergency cardiovascular care. *Circulation* 122 (Suppl.): S640–56.

Flanagan RJ, Jones AL (2004). Fab antibody fragments: some applications in clinical toxicology. *Drug Safety* 27: 1115–33.

Fox KA, Poole-Wilson PA, Henderson RA *et al.*; Randomized Intervention Trial of unstable Angina Investigators. RITA 3 trial (British Heart Foundation Intervention Trial of unstable Angina) (2002). Interventional versus conservative treatment for patients with unstable angina or non-ST-elevation myocardial infarction. *Lancet* 360: 743–51.

Franciosa J, Taylor A, Cohn J *et al.* (2002). A-HeFT (African-American Heart Failure Trial. *J Card Fail* 8: 128–35.

FRISC Study Group (1996). Low-molecular-weight heparin during instability in coronary artery disease, fragmin during instability in coronary artery disease. *Lancet* 347: 561–8.

Gershlick AH, Stephens-Lloyd A, Hughes S *et al.* (2005). REACT trial (Rescue Angioplasty vs Conservative treatment or repeat Thrombolysis). Rescue angioplasty after failed thrombolytic therapy for acute myocardial infarction. *N Engl J Med* 353: 2758–68.

Gheorghiade M, Adams KF Jr, Colucci WS (2004). Digoxin in the management of cardiovascular disorders. *Circulation* 109: 2959–64.

Gheorghiade M, Fonarow G, van Veldhuisen D *et al.* (2013). Lack of evidence of increased mortality among patients with atrial fibrillation taking digoxin: findings from post hoc propensity-matched analysis of the AFFIRM trial. *Eur Heart J* 34: 1489–97.

Gheorghiade M, Konstam MA, Burnett JC Jr, *et al.* for the Efficacy of Vasopressin Antagonism in Heart Failure Outcome Study With Tolvaptan I (2007). Short-term clinical effects of tolvaptan, an oral vasopressin antagonist, in patients hospitalized for heart failure: the EVEREST Clinical Status Trials. *JAMA* 297: 1332.

Graudal NA, Hubeck-Graudal T, Jurgens G; Editorial Group: Cochrane Hypertension Group (2011). Effects of low sodium diet versus high sodium diet on blood pressure, renin, aldosterone, catecholamines, cholesterol, and triglyceride. *Cochrane Database Syst Rev* (11): CD004022.

Gray AJ, Goodacre S, Newby DE *et al.*; 3CPO Study Investigators (2009). A multicentre randomised controlled trial of the use of continuous positive airway pressure and non-invasive positive pressure ventilation in the early treatment of patients presenting to the emergency department with severe acute cardiogenic pulmonary oedema: the 3CPO trial. *Health Technol Assess* 13: 1–106.

Grines CL, Browne KF, Marco J *et al.* (1993). A comparison of immediate angioplasty with thrombolytic therapy for acute myocardial infarction. The Primary Angioplasty in Myocardial Infarction Study Group. *N Engl J Med* 328: 673–9.

Hall SA, Cigarroa CG, Marcoux L *et al.* (1995). Time course of improvement in left ventricular function, mass and geometry in patients with congestive heart failure treated with beta-adrenergic blockade. *J Am Coll Cardiol* 25: 1154–61.

Heran B, Wong M, Heran I, Wright J; Editorial Group for Cochrane Hypertension Group (2008). Blood pressure lowering efficacy of angiotensin converting enzyme (ACE) inhibitors for primary hypertension. *Cochrane Database Syst Revi* (4): CD003823.

Hjalmarson A, Goldstein S, Fagerberg B *et al.* Metoprolol Randomized Intervention Trial in congestive Heart Failure Study Group (1999). Effect of metoprolol CR/XL in chronic heart failure: Metoprolol CR/XL Randomised Intervention Trial in Congestive Heart Failure (MERIT-HF). *Lancet* 353: 2001–7.

Hollman A (1996). Digoxin comes from Digitalis lanata. *BMJ* 312: 912.

ISIS-1 (First International Study of Infarct Survival) Collaborative Group (1986). Randomised trial of intravenous atenolol among 16 027 cases of suspected acute myocardial infarction: ISIS1. *Lancet* 12: 57–66.

ISIS-2 (Second International Study of Infarct Survival) Collaborative Group (1988). Randomised trial of intravenous streptokinase, oral aspirin, both, or neither among 17,187 cases of suspected acute myocardial infarction: ISIS-2. *Lancet* 2: 349.

ISIS-4 (Fourth International Study of Infarct Survival) Collaborative Group (1995). A randomised factorial trial assessing early oral captopril, oral mononitrate, and intravenous magnesium sulphate in 58 050 patients with suspected acute myocardial infarction. ISIS-4 Collaborative Group. *Lancet* 345: 669–82.

Kandler M, Mah G, Tejani A, *et al.*; Editorial Group: Cochrane Hypertension Group (2011).

Hydralazine for essential hypertension. *Cochrane Database Syst Rev* (9): CD004934.

Keeley EC, Boura JA, Grines CL (2003). Primary angioplasty versus intravenous thrombolytic therapy for acute myocardial infarction: a quantitative review of 23 randomised trials. *Lancet* 361: 13–20.

Khand AU, Rankin AC, Martin W *et al.* (2003). Carvedilol alone or in combination with digoxin for the management of atrial fibrillation in patients with heart failure? *J Am Coll Cardiol* 42: 1944–51.

Khattar RS (2003). Effects of ACE-inhibitors and beta-blockers on left ventricular remodeling in chronic heart failure. *Minerva Cardioangiol* 51:143–54.

Klein W, Brunhuber R,Hofmann P *et al.* (1999) The Cardiac Insufficiency Bisoprolol Study II (CIBIS-II): a randomised trial *Lancet* 353: 9–13.

Komsuoglu SS, Komsuoglu B, Ozmenoglu M *et al.* (1992). Oral nifedipine in the treatment of hypertensive crises in patients with hypertensive encephalopathy. *Int J Cardiol* 34: 277–82.

Li E, Heran B, Wright J; Editorial Group: Cochrane Hypertension Group (2014). Angiotensin converting enzyme (ACE) inhibitors versus angiotensin receptor blockers for primary hypertension. *Cochrane Database Syst Rev* (22): CD009096.

Loriaux L, Menard R, Taylor A *et al.* (1976). Spironolactone and endocrine dysfunction. *Ann Intern Med* 85: 630–6.

MADIT Executive Committee (1991). Multicenter automatic defibrillator implantation trial. *Pacing Clin Electrophysiol* 14: 920–7.

Mastroianni N, De Fusco M, Zollo M *et al.* (1996). Molecular cloning, expression pattern, and chromosomal localization of the human Na-Cl thiazide-sensitive cotransporter (SLC12A3). *Genomics* 35: 486–93.

McMurray J, Adamopoulos S, Anker S *et al.*; The Task Force for the Diagnosis and Treatment of Acute and Chronic Heart Failure 2012 of the European Society of Cardiology (2012). ESC Guidelines for the diagnosis and treatment of acute and chronic heart failure 2012, developed in collaboration with the Heart Failure Association (HFA) of the ESC. *Eur Heart J* 33: 1787–847.

McMurray JJ, Teerlink JR, Cotter G *et al.* (2007). Effects of tezosentan on symptoms and clinical outcomes in patients with acute heart failure: the VERITAS randomized controlled trials. *JAMA* 298: 2009–19.

Mills EJ, WU P, Chong G *et al.* (2011). Efficacy and safety of statin treatment for cardiovascular disease: a network meta-analysis of 170,255 patients from 76 randomized trials. *QJM* 104: 109–24.

Morrison LJ, Verbeek PR, McDonald AC *et al.* (2000). Mortality and prehospital thrombolysis for acute myocardial infarction: A meta-analysis. *JAMA* 283: 2686–92.

Moss AJ, Hall WJ, Cannom DS, Klein H *et al.*, for the MADIT-CRT Trial Investigators (2009). Cardiac-resynchronization therapy for the prevention of heart-failure events. *N Engl J Med* 361: 1329–38.

Moss A, Zareba W, Hall W *et al.*, for the Multicenter Automatic Defibrillator Implantation Trial II Investigators (2002). Prophylactic implantation of a defibrillator in patients with myocardial infarction and reduced ejection fraction. *N Engl J Med* 346: 877–83.

Musini V, Nazer M, Bassett K, Wright J; Editorial Group: Cochrane Hypertension Group (2014). Blood pressure-lowering efficacy of monotherapy with thiazide diuretics for primary hypertension. *Cochrane Database Syst Rev* (29): CD003824.

National Institute for Health and Care Excellence (NICE) (2006) *Atrial Fibrillation: The Management of Atrial Fibrillation*, CG36, Available at: nice.org.uk/guidance/CG36 (accessed Dec. 2015).

National Institute for Health and Care Excellence (NICE) (2007). *MI – Secondary Prevention: Secondary Prevention in Primary and Secondary Care for Patients Following a Myocardial Infarction*, CG48. Available at: www.nice.org.uk/guidance/cg48 (accessed Dec. 2015).

National Institute for Health and Care Excellence (NICE) (2010a). *Unstable Angina and NSTEMI: Early Management*, CG94. Available at: www.nice.org.uk/guidance/cg94 (accessed Dec. 2015).

National Institute for Health and Care Excellence (NICE) (2010b). *Chronic Heart failure in Adults: Management*, CG108. Available at: www.nice.org.uk/guidance/cg108/ (accessed Dec. 2015).

National Institute for Health and Care Excellence (NICE) (2011). *Hypertension in Adults: Diagnosis and Management*, CG127. Available at: www.nice.org.uk/guidance/cg127 (accessed Dec. 2015).

National Institute for Health and Care Excellence (NICE) (2013). *Myocardial Infarction: Cardiac Rehabilitation and Prevention of Further MI*, CG172. Available at: www.nice.org.uk/guidance/cg172 (accessed Dec. 2015).

Norwegian Multicenter Study Group (1981). Timolol-induced reduction in mortality and reinfarction in patients surviving acute myocardial infarction. *N Engl J Med* 304: 801–7.

O'Driscoll BR, Howard LS, Davison AG, British Thoracic Society (2008). BTS guideline for emergency oxygen use in adult patients. *Thorax* 63 (Suppl. 6): vi1–68.

Patti G, Colonna G, Pasceri V *et al.* (2005). Randomized trial of high loading dose of clopidogrel for reduction of periprocedural myocardial infarction in patients undergoing coronary intervention: results from the ARMYDA-2 (Antiplatelet therapy for Reduction of MYocardial Damage during Angioplasty) Study. *Circulation* 111: 2099–106.

Peacock W, Hollander J, Diercks D *et al.* (2008). Morphine and outcomes in acute decompensated heart failure: an ADHERE analysis. *Emerg Med J* 25: 205–9.

Pearce CJ, Wallin JD (1994). Labetalol and other agents that block both alpha- and beta-adrenergic receptors. *Cleve Clin J Med* 61: 59–69.

Pedersen TR, Kjekshus J, Berg K, (1994). Randomized trial of cholesterol lowering in 4444 patients with coronary heart disease: the Scandinavian Simvastatin Survival Study (4S). *Lancet* 344: 1383–9.

Pijls NHJ, De Bruyne B (2000). *Coronary Pressure*, 2nd edn. Springer: Dordrecht.

Pisters R, Lane DA, Nieuwlaat R *et al.* (2010). A novel user-friendly score (HAS-BLED) to assess 1-year risk of major bleeding in patients with atrial fibrillation: the Euro Heart Survey. *Chest* 138: 1093–100.

Pitt B, Remme W, Zannad F, *et al.*: Eplerenone Post–Acute Myocardial Infarction Heart Failure Efficacy and Survival Study Investigators (2003). Eplerenone, a selective aldosterone blocker, in patients with left ventricular dysfunction after myocardial infarction. *N Engl J Med* 348: 1309–21.

Pitt B, Williams G (2001). EPHESUS (Eplenerone in patients with heart failure due to systolic dysfunction complicating acute myocardial infarction. *Cardiovas Drugs Therapy* 15: 79–87.

Pitt B, Zannad F, Remme WJ, *et al.* (1999). The effect of spironolactone on morbidity and mortality in patients with severe heart failure: Randomized Aldactone Evaluation Study Investigators. *N Engl J Med* 341: 709–17.

Porter RS, Kaplan JL (2011). *Merck Manual*, 19th edn. MerckSharp and DohmeCorp.: West Point, PA.

PURSUIT Trial Investigators (1998). PURSUIT trial (Platelet Glycoprotein IIb/IIIa in Unstable Angina: Receptor Suppression Using Integrilin Therapy). Inhibition of platelet glycoprotein IIb/IIIa with eptifibatide in patients with acute coronary syndromes. *N Engl J Med* 339: 436–43.

Ramrakha P, Hill J (2006). Arrhythmias. In: *Oxford Handbook of Cardiology*. Oxford University Press: Oxford: 357–409.

Rang HR, Dale MM, Ritter JM *et al.* (2015). *Pharmacology*, 8th edn. Elsevier, Churchill Livingstone.

Reed WG, Anderson RJ (1986). Effects of rapid blood pressure reduction on cerebral blood flow. *Am Heart J* 111: 226–8.

Resuscitation Council (2015). *Advanced Life Support*, 7th edn. Resuscitation Council, UK. Available at: www.resus.org.uk/resuscitation-guidelines/ (accessed Dec. 2015).

Roffi R, Patrono C, Collet J-P; European Society of Cardiology (2015). *2015 ESC Guidelines for the management of acute MI in patients presenting without ST segment elevation*. *Eur Heart J* in press: doi/10.1093/eurheartj/ehv320.

Rossi S (2006). *Australian Medicines Handbook*. Australian Medicines Handbook Pty Ltd.: Adelaide.

Roy D, Talajic M, Dorian P *et al.* (2000). Amiodarone to prevent recurrence of atrial fibrillation. *N Engl J Med* 342: 913–20.

Savi P, Nurden P, Nurden A *et al.* (1998). Clopidogrel: a review of its mechanism of action. *Informa Healthcare* 9: 251–5.

Sharon A, Shpirer I, Kaluski E *et al.* (2000). High-dose intravenous isosorbide-dinitrate is safer and better than Bi-PAP ventilation combined with conventional treatment for severe pulmonary edema. *J Am Coll Cardiol* 36: 832–7.

Sidorenkov G, Navis G (2014). Safety of ACE inhibitor therapies in patients with chronic kidney disease. *Expert Opini Drug Safety* 13: 1383–95.

Solomon S, Anavekar N (2005). A brief overview of inhibition of the renin-angiotensin system: emphasis on blockade of the angiotensin ii type-1 receptor. *Medscape Cardiology* 9 (1).

Stühlinger HG, Kiss K, Smetana R (2000). Significance of magnesium in cardiac arrhythmias. *Wien Med Wochenschr* 150: 330–4.

Swedberg K, Komajda M, Böhm M (2010). SHIFT (systolic heart failure treatment with the IF inhibitor ivabradine trial). *Eur J Heart Fail* 12: 75–81.

The Global Use of Strategies to Open Occluded Coronary Arteries in Acute Coronary Syndromes (GUSTO IIb) Angioplasty Substudy Investigators (1997). A clinical trial comparing primary coronary angioplasty with tissue plasminogen activator for acute myocardial infarction. *N Engl J Med* 336: 1621–8.

Van Gelder IC, Hagens VE, Bosker HA *et al.*; Rate Control versus Electrical Cardioversion for Persistent Atrial Fibrillation Study Group (2002). A comparison of rate control and rhythm control in patients with recurrent persistent atrial fibrillation. *N Engl J Med* 347: 1834–40.

Varon J, Marik P (2003). Clinical review: The management of hypertensive crises. *Critical Care* 7: 374–84.

Veloso HH, de Paola AA (2005). Beta-blockers versus digoxin to control ventricular rate during atrial fibrillation. *J Am Coll Cardiol* 45: 1905–6.

Verma SP, Silke B, Reynolds GW *et al.* (1989). Nitrate therapy for left ventricular failure complicating acute myocardial infarction: a haemodynamic comparison of intravenous, buccal, and transdermal delivery systems. *J Cardiovasc Pharmacol* 14: 756–62.

Wallentin L, Becker R, Budaj A *et al.* (2009). Ticagrelor versus clopidogrel in patients with acute coronary syndromes for the PLATO investigators. *N Engl J Med* 361: 1045–57.

Williams J, Bristow M, Fowler M *et al.* (Committee on Evaluation and Management of Heart Failure) (1995). Guidelines for the evaluation and management of heart failure. Report of the American College of Cardiology/ American Heart Association Task Force on Practice Guidelines. *Circulation* 92: 2764–84.

Wills MR (1986). Magnesium and potassium. Inter-relationships in cardiac disorders. *Drugs* 31 (Suppl. 4): 121–31.

Wiviott S, Braunwald E, McCabe C *et al.* for the TRITON–TIMI 38 Investigators (2007). Prasugrel versus clopidogrel in patients with acute coronary syndromes. *N Engl J Med* 357: 2001–15.

Wiysonge C, Bradley H, Volmink J *et al.*; Editorial Group: Cochrane Hypertension Group (2012). Beta-blockers for hypertension. *Cochrane Database Syst Rev* (14): CD002003.

Wright JM, Musini VM (2009). First-line drugs for hypertension. *Cochrane Database Syst Rev* (8): CD001841.

Wyse DG, Waldo AL, DiMarco JP *et al.*, Atrial Fibrillation Follow-up Investigation of Rhythm Management (AFFIRM) Investigators (2002). A comparison of rate control and rhythm control in patients with atrial fibrillation. *N Engl J Med* 347: 1825–33.

Young JB, Abraham WT, Smith AL *et al.* for The Multicenter InSync ICD Randomized Clinical Evaluation (MIRACLE ICD) Trial Investigators (2003). Combined cardiac resynchronization and implantable cardioversion defibrillation in advanced chronic heart failure : the MIRACLE ICD trial. *JAMA* 289: 2685–94.

Yousef W, Omar A, Morsy M *et al.* (2005). The mechanism of action of calcium channel blockers in the treatment of diabetic nephropathy. *Int J Diabetes Metabolism* 13: 76–82.

Yusuf S, Mehta SR, Chrolavicius S *et al.*: Fifth Organization to Assess Strategies in Acute Ischemic Syndromes Investigators (2006). Comparison of fondaparinux and enoxaparin in acute coronary syndromes. *N Engl J Med* 354: 1464–76.

Yusuf S, Zhao F, Mehta SR *et al.*; Clopidogrel in Unstable Angina to Prevent Recurrent Events Trial Investigators (2001). Effects of clopidogrel in addition to aspirin in patients with acute coronary syndromes without ST-segment elevation. *N Engl J Med* 345: 494–502.

Zannad F, McMurray J (2010). Eplerenone in mild patients hospitalization and survival study in heart failure (EMPHASIS-HF). *Eur J Heart Fail* 12: 617–22.

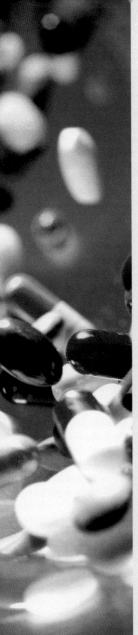

CHAPTER 4
Respiratory
Andrew Stanton

Key topics:

Learning objectives

By the end of this chapter you should…

- …be able to write a prescription for patients with common acute presentations of respiratory disease.

- …be able to recall the mechanisms of action of the key drugs used to treat these conditions.

- …be able to describe the principles of the pharmacological strategies employed in the long-term management of asthma and COPD.

- …be aware of some of the key evidence that underpins the management of these conditions.

Essential Practical Prescribing, First Edition. Georgia Woodfield, Benedict Lyle Phillips, Victoria Taylor, Amy Hawkins and Andrew Stanton. © 2016 by John Wiley & Sons, Ltd. Published 2016 by John Wiley & Sons, Ltd.

Acute asthma

> ### Jane Dalton
> ### Age: 35
> ### Hospital Number: 123456

🔍 Case study

Presenting complaint: *A 35-year-old woman is admitted with 5 days progressive breathlessness, wheeze and dry cough. Her symptoms have not been helped with multiple doses of her reliever inhaler. In the last month she has been waking most nights coughing and with a little wheeze, needing to use her reliever inhaler.*

Background: *She lives with her husband and two children and works as a sales representative.*

PMH: *Asthma, eczema*

Allergies: *nil*

Examination:
Pulse 95, BP 132/76, Sats 93% on air, RR 26, BM 5.2. Struggling to complete sentences in one breath
Peak flow: 200 L/min (predicted 480 L/min)

CVS: *Capillary refill time <2 seconds, pulse regular, JVP not seen, no pitting oedema, HS I + II + 0*

RS: *Equal expansion with generalised wheeze throughout both lung fields*

Abdo: *Soft, non-tender, no masses palpated, bowel sounds present*

Neuro: *Nil focal*

ECG: *Normal sinus rhythm*

Bloods: *Hb 13.2, Plt 416, WCC 7.9, Na 137, K 4.2, Urea 5.5, Creat 86, CRP 6.3*

CXR: *No focal consolidation/ pneumothorax*

Diagnosis
Acute asthma.

| PHARMACY STAMP | AGE 35 | FORENAME, SURNAME J Dalton |
| | D.O.B. xx/xx/xxxx | ADDRESS Ball Lane NHS NUMBER |

CLENIL INHALER 200 2 puffs twice daily.

SALBUTAMOL INHALER 100 mcg 2 puffs as required.

SIGNATURE OF PRESCRIBER   DATE

SP21000

Initial measures
Severity of asthma exacerbation needs to be determined. She is struggling to complete sentences, has a respiratory rate of >25 breaths/minute along with her peak flow below 50% predicted (but above 33%), indicating this is severe acute asthma. Immediate attention to ABC required, in particular starting high-flow oxygen with continuous saturation monitoring. ABG is **not** required given her saturations are above 92% and she has no features of life-threatening asthma.

Prescribing for acute asthma

The initial pharmacological management of acute asthma is guided by severity assessment and central to this is measurement of peak expiratory flow rate

ONCE ONLY PRESCRIPTIONS

Date	Time to be given	DRUG	Dose	Route	Prescriber Signature	Bleep
xx/xx/xx	STAT	SALBUTAMOL	5 mg	NEB	A. Doctor	
xx/xx/xx	STAT	ATROVENT	0.5 mg	NEB	A. Doctor	
xx/xx/xx	STAT	PREDNISOLONE	40 mg	PO	A. Doctor	

REGULAR PRESCRIPTIONS

			Circle/enter times below ↓	Day 1	Day 2	Day 3	Day 4
DRUG SALBUTAMOL			(06)				
Dose 5 mg	Route NEB	Freq 6 hourly	Start date xx/xx/xx	08 (12)			
Signature A. Doctor	Bleep	Review	16				
Additional instructions			(18) (22)				
DRUG ATROVENT			(06)				
Dose 0.5 mg	Route NEB	Freq 6 hourly	Start date xx/xx/xx	08 (12)			
Signature A. Doctor	Bleep	Review	16				
Additional instructions			(18) (22)				
DRUG PREDNISOLONE			06				
Dose 40 mg	Route PO	Freq OD	Start date xx/xx/xx	(08) 12			
Signature A. Doctor	Bleep	Review	16				
Additional instructions			18 22				
DRUG CLENIL 200			06				
Dose 2 puffs	Route INH	Freq BD	Start date xx/xx/xx	(08) 12			
Signature A. Doctor	Bleep	Review	16				
Additional instructions			(20) 22				

Table 4.1 Clinical features to guide assessment of acute asthma.

Near fatal asthma	Raised $Paco_2$ and/or requiring mechanical ventilation with raised inflation pressures
Life-threatening asthma	Any one of the following in a patient with severe asthma: Clinical signs/measurements Altered conscious level Exhaustion Spo_2 <92% Arrhythmia Pao_2 <8 kPa Hypotension Inappropriately 'normal' $Paco_2$ (4.6–6.0 kPa) Cyanosis Silent chest Poor respiratory effort
Severe acute asthma PEFR 33–50% best or predicted	Any one of: PEF 33–50% best or predicted Respiratory rate ≥25/min Heart rate ≥110/min Inability to complete sentences in one breath
Moderate asthma exacerbation PEFR 50–75% best or predicted	Increasing symptoms PEF >50–75% best or predicted No features of acute severe asthma

PEFR, peak expiratory flow rate.

(PEFR) as a percentage of best, or if not known, predicted (for age, sex and height). Numerous easily accessible on-line calculators for this are available to calculate predicted PEFR.

Table 4.1 gives more detail on other clinical features to guide assessment.

Acute management priorities are:

- Oxygenation
  - Oxygen should be prescribed aiming for target saturations of 94–98%.

    Depending on initial saturations, a delivery device giving between 35% and 60% would be appropriate.

Measurement of arterial blood gases is only indicated in patients with saturations below 92% or features of life-threatening asthma, as otherwise the risk of hypercapnia is very low (BTS SIGN, 2014).

- Bronchodilation
  - Salbutamol is the initial drug of choice, with doses repeated depending on clinical response.

Ipratropium is recommended as initial therapy in severe or life-threatening asthma only.

- Anti-inflammatory treatment
  - Patients with acute asthma need corticosteroid treatment and this should be given as soon as possible. Guidelines advise this should be achieved within 1 hour for severe or life-threatening asthma.

> ## (!) Guidelines
>
> - British Thoracic Society (BTS) guideline for emergency oxygen use in adults (O'Driscoll *et al.*, 2008).
> - British guideline on the management of asthma (BTS SIGN, 2014).
> - National Institute for Health and Care Excellence (NICE) *Asthma NICE Quality Standard*, QS25, 2013. Available at: www.nice.org.uk/guidance/qs25 (accessed Dec. 2015).

Salbutamol: rationale and evidence

Salbutamol is a fast-acting bronchodilator, which will provide clinical benefit in the overwhelming majority of patients with acute severe asthma. It is delivered by an oxygen-driven nebuliser, which ensures maximum delivery to the airways while minimising risk of desaturation and hypoxaemia. Unless repeated doses are given, side effects are rare but with more frequent dosing (sometimes with 4-hourly, often with more frequent dosing), tremor and tachycardia can occur, so lower doses in these circumstances (2.5 mg) may well suffice. Nebulised salbutamol has had a place in the management of acute asthma for decades (McFadden, 1986).

> ## ✓ DRUGS checklist for SALBUTAMOL (in acute asthma)
>
> | | |
> |---|---|
> | **Dose** | 5 mg in acute asthma |
> | **Route** | Nebulised (driven by oxygen **not** air) |
> | **Units** | mg |
> | **Given** | 4–6 hourly |
> | **Special situations** | In acute severe asthma not responding to initial treatment or in life-threatening asthma, can be given up to every 15–30 minutes. Once clinical stability/improvement obtained, 2.5 mg may be adequate (especially if side effects predominate). Repeated dosing, especially if more than 4–6 hourly, is associated with risk of lactic acidosis. |

Salbutamol: essential pharmacology

Salbutamol acts directly on β_2 adenoreceptors to cause relaxation by increasing intracellular cAMP, activation of protein kinase, in turn inactivating myosin light chain kinase, therefore inhibiting contraction. Although relatively selective for β_2 receptors, found in bronchial and uterine smooth muscle (hence its use in premature labour; see Chapter 14), there will be some effects mediated through β_2 receptors in skeletal muscle (tremor) and some β_1 receptors in the heart (tachycardia). The mechanism by which salbutamol can cause a lactic acidosis (more often seen with very high frequency dosing), in the absence of poor tissue perfusion, is not entirely clear but may relate to excess glycogenolysis within skeletal muscle, mediated through higher intracellular cAMP (Tomar, 2012).

Atrovent (ipratropium bromide): rationale and evidence

By providing bronchodilation through a different mechanism to beta agonists, it is rational to expect ipratropium to provide benefit over and above that of salbutamol. Meta-analyses of randomised controlled trials (RCTs) of ipratropium in acute asthma have found that in combination with salbutamol, ipratropium produces improvements in lung function and speeds clinical recovery (Stoodley *et al.*, 1999; Rodrigo *et al.*, 1999). These meta-analyses have also found that patients with more severe airflow obstruction have more to gain from this combination approach, hence its recommendation only in severe or life-threatening acute asthma.

✓	**DRUGS checklist for ATROVENT (ipratropium bromide)**
Dose	0.5 mg
Route	Nebulised (driven by oxygen **not** air)
Units	mg
Given	4–6 hourly
Special situations	Unlike salbutamol additional clinical benefit is not seen with more frequent dosing. Not indicated in moderate acute asthma.

Atrovent (ipratropium bromide): essential pharmacology

Ipratropium is a non-selective muscarinic receptor antagonist that exerts a bronchodilatory effect through antagonism of the M_3 receptors found in bronchial smooth muscle and so blocking any acetylcholine-mediated bronchospasm. Its effectiveness is limited by its blockade of M_2 autoreceptors on cholinergic nerves, hence increasing acetylcholine release. It has minimal systemic absorption and so systemic side effects are uncommon but can cause dry mouth because of its direct effect on secretions. Its effect will last for 3–5 hours, hence there is no need to dose more frequently than 6-hourly in acute asthma.

Prednisolone: rationale and evidence

Airway inflammation is the underlying pathology in asthma and in the context of an asthma exacerbation this is very intense and requires systemic anti-inflammatory treatment in addition to topical treatment from inhaled steroids. Although there is often debate about were the line is drawn between simply increasing asthma symptoms (necessitating increase in maintenance therapy) and an exacerbation, it is unlikely a patient presenting to secondary care with asthma is doing so because of the former, and so systemic steroids are indicated in all patients. The oral route should be the default method for administration unless the patient is unable to swallow or has life-threatening asthma.

Steroid treatment in acute asthma reduces mortality, relapses and subsequent hospital admissions, and requirement for β_2 agonist therapy (BTS guidelines). Reviews of published evidence suggest that that the earlier they are given, the better the outcome in asthma (Rowe *et al.*, 2001b).

🔍	**Evidence**

One Cochrane review of early administration of corticosteroids found that the administration of early steroid, within 1 hour, significantly reduced the admission rate (pooled odds ration 0.4) with an estimated number needed to treat (NNT) of 8 (Rowe *et al.*, 2001a).

✓	**DRUGS checklist for PREDNISOLONE in asthma**
Dose	40–50 mg
Route	PO
Units	mg
Given	Stat, then once daily for at least 5 days. 'Tailing off' steroid dosage is not necessary unless the patient is on regular maintenance oral steroid or if the patient has been on high-dose steroid for 3 or more weeks (very rare)
Special situations	In life-threatening asthma, or if oral route not possible, give 100 mg hydrocortisone IV as equivalent.

Prednisolone: essential pharmacology

See Chapter 12.

Other medications used in acute asthma

Magnesium

Magnesium causes bronchodilation, possibly through depletion of intracellular calcium and inhibition of calcium's interaction with myosin in smooth muscle, thereby causing muscle relaxation. In addition, it may inhibit mast cell degranulation and stimulate nitric oxide and prostacyclin synthesis, thereby reducing asthma severity.

Current guidelines recommend its use only in life-threatening asthma or in severe asthma not responding to initial therapy with nebulised bronchodilators and steroids (see Evidence).

✓ DRUGS checklist for MAGNESIUM in asthma

Dose	1.2–2 g
Route	IV
Units	g
Given	Once only as IV infusion over 20 minutes in 100 mL 5% dextrose or normal saline
Special situations	Only give in life-threatening asthma, or in severe acute asthma not responding to initial therapy. No evidence of benefit of repeated administration. Reason for varying dose relates to fact different doses have been used in different studies (see Evidence).

Aminophylline

Methylxanthines such as theophylline block the α_1 (adenosine) receptor on mast cells, reducing release of mediators that cause mucous secretion and bronchoconstriction. In addition, they may promote bronchodilation through phosphodiesterase inhibition and increase of cAMP. Despite the lack of benefit of IV aminophylline seen in RCTs (Parameswaran et al., 2000) there may be some patients with near-fatal or life-threatening asthma who derive benefit. Its role in severe acute asthma is not really supported by good evidence but most units will use this in patients with severe acute asthma who have ongoing bronchospasm and respiratory distress despite adequate treatment with bronchodilators, steroids and magnesium.

✓ DRUGS checklist for AMINOPHYLLINE in acute asthma

Dose	5 mg/kg loading dose then 0.5 mg/kg/h infusion
Route	IV
Units	mg
Given	As loading dose over 20 minutes then continuous IV infusion
Special situations	Loading dose must not be given if the patient is on maintenance theophylline preparation – take blood level then commence maintenance infusion.

Antibiotics

There is no evidence to justify routine use of antibiotics in asthma exacerbations as most are likely to be viral in nature. There is ongoing investigation into the use of azithromycin in exacerbations of asthma (AZALEA trial).

Leukotriene antagonists

Although drugs such as montelukast or zafirlukast have a role in the management of some asthma patients with chronic asthma, there is no evidence of efficacy in acute asthma.

🔍 Evidence

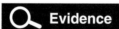

Magnesium
A Cochrane review (Powell et al., 2014) of 16 clinical trials of nebulised magnesium in acute asthma found no evidence of improved lung function or advantage in terms of hospital admissions with nebulised magnesium in addition to beta agonist and/or ipratropium.

Goodacre et al. (2013) found no evidence of benefit of 2 g IV magnesium in patients with severe (but not life-threatening) asthma in terms of symptoms or need for hospital admissions.

An earlier pooled analysis of seven trials of IV magnesium (using 1.2–2 g IV magnesium) in acute asthma found no overall evidence of benefit but improved lung function parameters in patients with severe acute asthma (Rowe *et al.*, 2000). A more recent review (Kew *et al.*, 2014) found that in patients who had not responded to first-line treatment, IV magnesium (again doses varying in trials 1.2–2 g) reduced hospital admissions (seven fewer for every 100 treated) and improves lung function.

Aminophylline

Although some individual trials in adults have suggested that aminophylline in addition to standard therapy is of benefit, a review (Nair *et al.*, 2012) found no evidence that aminophylline an addition to standard therapy is of consistent proven benefit.

Other aspects of asthma exacerbation management

All patients admitted to hospital with an exacerbation of asthma should have an assessment of their background level of control to determine whether their regular maintenance treatment should be modified. The detailed aspects of regular maintenance treatment of asthma and stepwise management of asthma are out with the scope of this book but further details of various inhaled therapies for asthma are detailed in Section Long-acting beta agonists – LABAs.

Unless there is clear evidence of good background control and a definite acute precipitant (e.g. recent infection), patients admitted with an exacerbation are likely to require an escalation of their background maintenance inhaled therapy. An exception to this rule would be that any patient with an asthma exacerbation who was not on any maintenance inhaled steroid, would need to be commenced on such treatment immediately.

Assessment of asthma control should be done by a number of means such as:

- The Royal College of Physicians three questions
  - How many days in the last fortnight/ month have you:
    1. Had symptoms from your asthma?
    2. Had activities limited by your asthma?
    3. Been disturbed at night by your asthma?
- Asthma control test (ACT)
- Mini-AQLQ (Mini Asthma Quality Of Life Questionnaire).

Prior to discharge all patients with asthma should:

- Be stable on usual inhaled therapy for at least 12 hours (often 24 hours) to ensure they are stable off nebulised therapy
- Have had their inhaler technique reviewed
- Have been given a Personal Asthma Action Plan (PAAP)
- Have GP follow-up arranged within 2 working days
- Have respiratory clinic follow-up arranged within 4 weeks.

Case outcome and discharge

Over the next 48 hours, Mrs Dalton improved with significant reduction in cough, wheeze and breathlessness. Her PEFR gradually came up to 430 L/min 2 days after admission. Her nebulisers were stopped and she was assessed by the respiratory nurse specialist. Given she described symptoms of poor asthma control in the month leading up to admission, her inhaled therapy was escalated (as per BTS guidelines) to include a long-acting bronchodilator (budesonide/ eformoterol 200/6 2 puffs BD). This new inhaler was in a different device than her previous one (dry powder Turbohaler as opposed to the metered dose inhaler she had been used to) and so required instruction on appropriate technique. She was given a PAAP with instructions to monitor her PEFR daily until review in the respiratory clinic in 4 weeks time.

Mrs Dalton's new prescription is shown.

DISCHARGE MEDICATION						
Date	Medication	Dose	Route	Frequency	Supply	GP to continue?
xx/xx/xx	SYMBICORT INHALER 200/6	2 puffs	INH	Twice daily	28 days	Y
xx/xx/xx	SALBUTAMOL INHALER 100 micrograms	2 puffs	INH	As required	28 days	Y
xx/xx/xx	PREDNISOLONE	40 mg	PO	Once daily	5 days (to complete 7 days)	N
Notes to patient/GP:						

Common pitfalls

- There is often a knee-jerk measurement of blood gases in all patients with asthma exacerbations and this is unnecessary in the majority of cases. BTS/SIGN guidelines advise this only in patients with saturations below 92% irrespective of whether they are on oxygen or not. The principle reason for doing an ABG is to make sure CO_2 is not abnormal and this is exceptionally unlikely in the non-hypoxic patient.
- Failure to continue to monitor PEFR regularly (e.g. QDS) following admission, making assessment of progress harder.

- Remember to prescribe usual inhaled steroid during admission in addition to oral steroid
- IV steroid is only indicated if life-threatening asthma or oral route is not available.
- Instructing patients to 'tail off' steroid dose unnecessarily.
- In planning discharge make sure the patient has been reviewed by one of the respiratory team and is stable on usual inhaled medication for at least 12 hours prior to discharge.

SUMMARY

Acute asthma is a common medical emergency, with the key priorities in management being maintaining adequate oxygenation, bronchodilation and steroid treatment. All patients require a background level of control measures and a determination made of the appropriate level of discharge medication, and clear plans for follow-up and monitoring made.

Key learning points

- All patients with acute asthma need to have severity of their exacerbation assessed.
- Priorities in management are oxygenation, nebulised salbutamol (+/– atrovent depending on severity) and oral prednisolone.
- Additional IV therapies (magnesium/ aminophylline) are indicated only in life-threatening exacerbations or severe acute asthma not responding to initial therapy.
- Make sure all patients have a structured respiratory review before discharge and appropriate follow-up arranged.

FURTHER READING

- SIGN and NICE guidelines give excellent guidance about the treatment of asthma and are regularly updated.

Chronic asthma

Prescribing in chronic asthma

There are a huge number of potential specific inhaled therapies for asthma and detailed description of them all is out with the scope of this book. Furthermore, the majority of any changes in asthma treatment are performed by GPs, or by respiratory teams during admissions for acute exacerbations or in the outpatient clinic.

There are a number of principles that are worth bearing in mind, however, when patients arrive in hospital, both for and with asthma, in terms of prescribing their inhaled therapies.

As a general rule, prescribing generically is less important as it will generally be the case that the patient's existing inhaler should be prescribed. It is easy to be confused by the plethora of different therapies on the market, especially when trade names sound similar to the names of component drugs.

When writing the prescription make sure you write in the drug name, the inhaled product and the dose. Historically, the number on the inhaler describes the dose (in micrograms) of the drug intended to be delivered by each actuation or puff. Recent changes in pharmaceutical regulations, however, stipulate that the number must refer to the amount of drug that is delivered at the mouth, rather than that contained within the medication blisters in the inhaler device. This explains why newer devices will have numbers that seem a bit 'less round'. In the dose section of the chart, write the number of puffs to be taken, for example two puffs.

There are four main classes of drugs licensed for the use in asthma, some just as reliever medications (R), some as purely maintenance therapies (M) and some for both maintenance and relief of symptoms, with increasing variety of some of these classes in combination (Table 4.2).

The following sections outline the key drugs and products used in asthma that may be encountered on the wards. Many drugs are available in both metered dose inhalers (MDIs), breath actuated aerosol inhalers and dry powder inhalers.

Table 4.2 Classes of drugs licensed for use in asthma.

Drugs	Class
Short-acting beta agonists (SABAs)	R therapy only
Long-acting beta agonists (LABAs)	Largely M, one drug R
Inhaled corticosteroids (ICS)	All M therapies
ICS/LABA combinations	Generally M, some M+R
Long-acting muscarinic antagonist (LAMA)	M only (one)

M, maintenance therapy; R, reliever medications.

Short-acting beta agonists

Short-acting beta agonists (SABAs) are licensed only for reliever therapy for asthma and are appropriate as monotherapy only in patients with very mild intermittent asthma who have minimal and rare need for reliever medication.

AS REQUIRED MEDICATION			
DRUG SALBUTAMOL	TRADE NAME VENTOLIN		Date
			Time
Dose per actuation 100 micrograms	Prescribed dose 2 puffs PRN	Start date xx/xx/xx	Dose
			Route
Signature/Bleep A. Doctor		Review	Given
			Check
Additional instructions Acts within 5 minutes, effects can last 4–6 hours			

AS REQUIRED MEDICATION			
DRUG TERBUTALINE	TRADE NAME BRICANYL		Date
			Time
Dose per actuation 500 micrograms	Prescribed dose 1 puff PRN	Start date xx/xx/xx	Dose
			Route
Signature/Bleep A. Doctor		Review	Given
			Check
Additional instructions Onset of action up to 30 minutes, lasts approx. 4 hours			

Long-acting beta agonists

There are two long-acting beta agonists (LABAs) currently licensed for asthma as single agents – salmeterol and eformoterol. Both must only be prescribed alongside an inhaled corticosteroids (ICS) as their use as maintenance therapy without ICS in poorly controlled asthma is associated with a risk of asthma death. The key differences between them are that salmeterol exhibits a logarithmic dose–response curve, and so is only effective at one dose, while eformoterol has a linear dose response curve and so escalating doses can provide additional bronchodilation. Eformoterol also has an onset of action similar to salbutamol (within 5 minutes) and so is also licensed for reliever therapy as well as maintenance therapy. Vilanterol is a new once-daily LABA but is not licensed or available other than in combination with fluticasone furoate (see Section Combined ICS/LABA therapies).

The use of LABAs in a single inhaler is now unusual, with the common use of combined ICS/LABA products.

✓ DRUGS checklist for LABAs in asthma

	Salmeterol	Eformoterol
Dose	50 micrograms	6–12 micrograms
Route	Inhaled	Inhaled
Units	micrograms	micrograms
Given	BD	1–2 puffs BD/ PRN
Special situations	Available in Accuhaler DPI (dry powder inhaler) (50 micrograms/puff), 1 puff BD and MDI (metered dose inhaler) (25 micrograms/puff, 2 puffs BD). Non-generic name: Serevent.	Available in Turbohaler DPI. Maximum recommended total dose 96 micrograms/day. Non-generic names: Oxis, Atimos, Foradil.

Inhaled corticosteroids

Any patient with asthma who has more than very intermittent asthma symptoms requires treatment with an inhaled steroid. Studies of patients dying or suffering near-fatal attacks of asthma have identified lack of regular ICS use as an associated factor, emphasising their importance as the cornerstone of asthma therapy.

There are numerous different ICS products that are licensed for asthma in various dosages. The most frequently used ICS are beclomethasone, budesonide and fluticasone. In prescribing ICS it is important to realise that fluticasone is twice as potent as beclomethasone and budesonide (the latter two are largely equivalent) so this must be borne in mind if one is substituted one for another. Furthermore, beclomethasone is also available in a preparation with 'extrafine' particles (QVAR), which allow delivery of the drug to smaller airways and is effectively twice as potent as 'standard' beclomethasone.

You may see some ICS preparation doses described as 'BDP equivalent (beclomethasone dipropionate equivalent)' reflecting that particular ICS equivalence to beclomethasone.

✓ DRUGS checklist for ICSs in asthma

	Beclomethasone	Budesonide	Fluticasone propionate	Extrafine beclomethasone
Dose	100–400 micrograms	100–400 micrograms	100–500 micrograms	50–200 micrograms
Route	Inhaled	Inhaled	Inhaled	Inhaled

Units	micrograms	micrograms	micrograms	micrograms
Given	BD	BD	BD	BD
Special situations	Maximum daily licensed dose is 800 micrograms BD. Non-generic names: Becotide, Becloforte, Asmabec, Clenil.	Maximum daily licensed dose is 800 micrograms BD. Non-generic name: Pulmicort	Maximum daily licensed dose is 1000 micrograms BD. Non-generic name: Flixotide	Non-generic name: Qvar.

In addition, you may come across patients taking ciclesonide (trade name Alvesco), which is a longer-acting ICS and is associated with a lower risk of oropharyngeal side effects than other ICS.

Combined ICS/LABA therapies

Patients with asthma who require both ICS and LABA therapy to control their asthma are rarely prescribed separate inhaler devices for each drug, and so most will be prescribed these drugs in combination. There is no evidence that any combination gives greater efficacy than the two products taken separately, but it is likely that patient compliance is improved with this strategy and also it minimises the risk (discussed in Section Long-Acting Beta Agonists) of patients taking LABAs without an ICS.

There are currently four different combination products available and licensed for asthma.

Two generic products have also been launched in 2015, reflecting expiry of patents for Symbicort and Seretide:

- Spiromax DuoResp (budesonide/eformoterol combination)
- Sirdupla (fluticasone propionate/salmeterol combination).

The cornerstone for the license for all of these products is the use of fixed doses as maintenance therapy. Due to the fast onset of eformoterol, products containing this are licensed for reliever therapy in addition (e.g. Symbicort/Fostair maintenance and reliever therapy [SMART/FMART] regimens). When using the inhaler in this way, generally, a lower dose of maintenance therapy (e.g. Symbicort 200/6 1 puff) is used, with the same strength used as reliever therapy. There is evidence that this strategy can improve asthma outcomes (e.g. levels of control and exacerbations).

✓ DRUGS checklist for ICS/LABAs in asthma

Product	Symbicort	Seretide	Fostair	Relvar Ellipta	Flutiform
Individual components	Budesonide + eformoterol	Fluticasone (propionate) + salmeterol	Beclomethasone (extra-fine particle) + formoterol	Fluticasone (furoate) + vilanterol	Fluticasone (propionate) + formoterol
Dose (ICS/LABA)	100/6 or 200/6	See below	100/6	92/22 or 184/22	50/5 125/5 250/10
Route	Inhaled	Inhaled	Inhaled	Inhaled	Inhaled

(Continued)

✓ DRUGS checklist for ICS/LABAs in asthma (*Continued*)				
Units	micrograms	micrograms	micrograms	micrograms	micrograms
Given	1–2 puffs BD +/- PRN	1–2 puffs BD depending on device Not licensed for reliever therapy	1–2 puffs BD	1 puff OD	2 puffs BD
Special situations	Turbohaler device. Also licensed for maintenance and reliever therapy (SMART Symbicort maintenance and reliever therapy). Generally with this 1 puff is taken BD with 1 puff for relief as needed (max. dose is 8 puffs of 200/6 strength/day).	3 different licensed doses each for the Accuhaler dry powder device (100, 250, 500 micrograms fluticasone, each containing the full 50 micrograms of salmeterol per actuation) and the Evohaler MDI (50, 125, 250 micrograms fluticasone, containing 25 micrograms salmeterol per actuation. Accuhaler devices are therefore 1 puff BD and Evohaler devices 2 puffs BD.	Available in MDI and newer dry powder (NEXThaler) device. Also licensed for maintenance and reliever therapy (Fostair maintenance and reliever therapy, FMART) as 1 puff BD + 1 puff PRN, max. 4 puffs/day.	Fluticasone furoate is a different molecule with much higher affinity for glucocorticoid receptor, hence lower dose required. It is a long-acting once-daily ICS.	Not licensed as reliever therapy.

Long-acting muscarinic antagonists

There is currently only one long-acting muscarinic antagonists (LAMA) licensed for use in asthma – tiotropium via the Respimat device (see Section Long-Acting Bronchodilators –

Rationale and Evidence for DRUGS list). It is licensed for patients poorly controlled and experiencing ≥1 severe exacerbation per year despite moderate-dose ICS (800 micrograms/day BDP or equivalent).

Acute exacerbation of COPD

> **James Carterton**
> **Age: 69**
> **Hospital Number: 123456**

🔍 Case study

Presenting complaint: A 69-year-old man is admitted with progressive worsening of shortness of breath, wheeze and cough productive of purulent sputum.

Background: He has had a diagnosis of chronic obstructive pulmonary disease (COPD) for 10 years, tends to get episodes of 'bronchitis' in the winter months and usually needs two courses of prednisolone each year from his GP. He gets breathless on about 200 metres but is usually independent in undertaking normal daily activities. He stopped smoking 5 years ago.

PMH: Hypertension, AF

Allergies: Nil

Examination:
Pulse 102, BP 146/85, Sats 87% on air, RR 26, BM 5.2, Temp 37.8. Struggling to complete sentences in one breath

CVS: Capillary refill time <2 seconds, pulse irregular, JVP not seen, no pitting oedema, HS I + II + 0

RS: Reduced expansion with generalised wheeze throughout both lung fields

Abdo: Soft, non-tender, no masses palpated, bowel sounds present

Neuro: Intact

ECG: AF, rate 105, no acute changes

Bloods: Hb 14.2, Plt 530, WCC 15.4, neut 12.4, Na 142, K 3.9, urea 6.5, creat 42, INR 2.4, CRP 54

CXR: No focal consolidation/ pneumothorax.

| PHARMACY STAMP | AGE 69 | FORENAME, SURNAME J Carterton |
| | D.O.B. xx/xx/xxxx | ADDRESS White Road NHS NUMBER |

SYMBICORT INHALER 400/12 1 puff twice daily.

TIOTROPIUM INHALER 18 mcg once daily.

SALBUTAMOL INHALER 100 mcg 2 puffs as required.

BISOPROLOL 5 mg oral once daily.

BENDROFLUAZIDE 2.5 mg oral once daily.

WARFARIN as per INR oral once daily (usual dose 6 mg).

SIGNATURE OF PRESCRIBER   DATE

SP21000

Diagnosis
Infectious exacerbation of COPD.

Initial measures
Controlled oxygen needs to be started, aiming for saturations of 88–92%, alongside measurement of ABG to clarify whether there is evidence of ventilatory failure, as indicated by a raised CO_2, and whether there is any evidence of acute or chronic respiratory acidosis. The patient needs to be sat up so that any airway secretions can be cleared, often urgent physiotherapy is needed for this. He has evidence of SIRS (systemic inflammatory response syndrome) as evident by his pulse >90, resp. rate over 20 and WCC >12, but does not have sepsis (no evidence of pneumonia on CXR, no focal signs of parenchymal infection) (see Chapter 11). Despite this, taking of blood cultures and commencement of IV fluids to support circulation would be perfectly reasonable.

Prescribing for acute exacerbation of COPD

ONCE ONLY PRESCRIPTIONS

Date	Time to be given	DRUG	Dose	Route	Prescriber Signature	Bleep
xx/xx/xx	STAT	SALBUTAMOL	5 mg	NEB	A. Doctor	
xx/xx/xx	STAT	ATROVENT	0.5 mg	NEB	A. Doctor	
xx/xx/xx	STAT	PREDNISOLONE	30 mg	PO	A. Doctor	
xx/xx/xx	STAT	AMOXICILLIN	500 mg	PO	A. Doctor	

REGULAR PRESCRIPTIONS

	Circle/enter times below ↓	Day 1	Day 2	Day 3	Day 4
DRUG SALBUTAMOL	06				
Dose 5 mg / Route NEB / Freq 6 hourly / Start date xx/xx/xx	08 / 12				
Signature A. Doctor / Bleep / Review	16 / 18				
Additional instructions	22				
DRUG ATROVENT	06				
Dose 0.5 mg / Route NEB / Freq 6 hourly / Start date xx/xx/xx	08 / 12				
Signature A. Doctor / Bleep / Review	16 / 18				
Additional instructions	22				
DRUG PREDNISOLONE	06				
Dose 30 mg / Route PO / Freq OD / Start date xx/xx/xx	08 / 12				
Signature A. Doctor / Bleep / Review	16 / 18				
Additional instructions	22				
DRUG AMOXICILLIN	06				
Dose 500 mg / Route PO / Freq TDS / Start date xx/xx/xx	08 / 12				
Signature A. Doctor / Bleep / Review	14 / 18				
Additional instructions	22				
DRUG SYMBICORT 400/12	06				
Dose 1 puff / Route BD / Freq INH / Start date xx/xx/xx	08 / 12				
Signature A. Doctor / Bleep / Review	16 / 20				
Additional instructions	22				
DRUG BISOPROLOL	06				
Dose 5 mg / Route PO / Freq OD / Start date xx/xx/xx	08 / 12				
Signature A. Doctor / Bleep / Review	16 / 18				
Additional instructions	22				
DRUG BENDROFLUAZIDE	06				
Dose 2.5 mg / Route PO / Freq OD / Start date xx/xx/xx	08 / 12				
Signature A. Doctor / Bleep / Review	16 / 18				
Additional instructions	22				
DRUG WARFARIN	06				
Dose As per INR / Route PO / Freq OD / Start date xx/xx/xx	08 / 12				
Signature A. Doctor / Bleep / Review	16 / 18				
Additional instructions	22				

Oxygen: rationale and evidence

Oxygen must be given in a controlled manner aiming to maintain saturations between 88% and 92%. This will allow delivery of adequately oxygenated haemoglobin to body tissues, but without risking suppressing respiratory drive in a chronically hypoxic patient. We don't really know whether our patient has chronic ventilatory failure yet as we don't have the ABG, but he is at risk of this given his background and so current guidelines would advise aiming for this initial target saturation.

Delivering 'controlled' oxygen requires using devices that give a specific inspired oxygen concentration irrespective of the patient's inspiratory flow rate – 'venturi devices'. The patient breathes a mixture of room air (21% oxygen) and oxygen from a gas supply (100% oxygen). By varying the flow rate of the 100% oxygen from the gas supply and the amount of room air that is entrained in (through the design of the apertures in the coloured nozzle), these masks are able to give fixed inspired oxygen concentrations of (most commonly) 24%, 28%, 31%, 35%, 40% and 60% (Figure 4.1). To give the required inspired oxygen concentrations the oxygen flow rate needs to be set at a fixed rate for the relevant mask (as detailed on the nozzle).

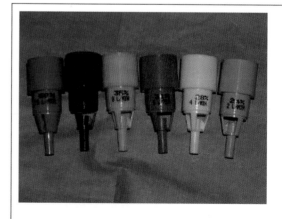

Figure 4.1 Venturi masks; note also the different size apertures in 60% mask compared with 24%.

By contrast, using nasal cannulae would deliver a highly variable inspired oxygen concentration that would purely depend on the patients inspiratory flow rate. In patients with high inspiratory flow rates (e.g. tachypnoeic patients), supplementation of breathing room air at 21% by the 100% oxygen through nasal cannulae at, for example, 2 L/min would result in a much lower inspired oxygen concentration than if the same patient had a much lower inspiratory flow rate (because here there would be less dilution of the 100% oxygen by the room air).

In our patient, it would be appropriate to start with a 28% mask and monitor saturations. Assuming they remained in the 88–92% range and that there was no evidence of a respiratory acidosis on the ABG further, routine measurement of the ABG would not be required unless the clinical situation changed.

 Guidelines

BTS oxygen guidelines (Hardinge *et al.*, 2015).

Salbutamol in COPD: rationale and evidence

As discussed in Section Acute Asthma, salbutamol is a fast-acting bronchodilator that should provide rapid relief of breathlessness in acute exacerbations of COPD. There are no RCTs confirming benefit but its use is well established and not questioned. In contrast to patients with asthma, salbutamol should be delivered by air driven nebuliser rather than oxygen.

✓ DRUGS checklist for OXYGEN

Dose	Most units ask you to prescribe according to target saturations, either 88–92% or 94–98% depending on whether the patient has, or is at risk of, ventilatory failure
	Often you will be required to select an initial delivery device only, e.g. Venturi 24%
Route	Inhaled
Units	Specify device (e.g. venture mask/ non-rebreathe) and oxygen flow rate
Given	Continuously
Special situations	See text. Be very careful of using nasal cannulae in patients with low respiratory rates who are at risk of ventilatory failure – can result in unexpectedly high inspired oxygen concentrations.

✓ DRUGS checklist for SALBUTAMOL (in COPD)

Dose	5 mg
Route	Nebulised (driven by air **not** oxygen)
Units	mg
Given	4–6 hourly
Special situations	As with asthma dosage can be repeated within 15–30 minutes if poor clinical response.
	If significant desaturation occurs while using air-driven nebuliser, supplement with oxygen via nasal cannulae (but exercise care as per Section Long-acting Beta Agonists).

Atrovent (ipratropium bromide) in COPD: rationale, evidence and essential pharmacology

Again as in asthma, in theory, supplementing salbutamol with Atrovent will provide additional bronchodilation and clinical benefit. There is lack of confirmed benefit of this strategy however. A Cochrane review of four trials comparing salbutamol with ipratropium found that neither were superior, and that there was no evidence of improvement by using the two together (McCrory and Brown, 2002). These studies concentrated on lung function parameters

(FEV_1), with the impact on level of symptoms, hospital stay or need for escalation of therapy not clear. Despite the absence of evidence of benefit, the strategy of combining both bronchodilators is recommended and usually well tolerated.

In patients with COPD exacerbations who are already on long-acting antimuscarinics (e.g. tiotropium), these must be stopped while patients are being given nebulised Atrovent. Neither tiotropium nor ipratropium discriminate between muscarinic receptors, with both drugs mediating bronchodilation through direct action on M_3 receptors in airway smooth muscle. In using ipratropium there is the risk that by action on M_2 receptors, there is greater release of acetyl choline and therefore any action on M_3 receptors is impeded, but also anticholinergic side effects could be more pronounced. Studies have found that in clinical use there is evidence of increased bronchodilator effect with the two drugs used together but that the risk of anticholinergic effects, especially urinary retention, is significantly increased (Cole et al., 2012). Current advice is that the two drugs should not be administered concomitantly.

DRUGS checklist for ATROVENT (ipratropium bromide) in COPD

Dose	0.5 mg
Route	Nebulised (driven by air **not** oxygen)
Units	mg
Given	4–6 hourly
Special situations	Unlike salbutamol, additional clinical benefit is not seen with more frequent dosing. Stop any LAMA (e.g. tiotropium) while on nebulised Atrovent.

Prednisolone in COPD: rationale and evidence

Inflammation plays a key role in COPD exacerbations and so use of systemic corticosteroids plays a key role in management. As the airway inflammation present in a COPD exacerbation is different to that in an asthma exacerbation (largely neutrophilic rather than eosinophilic), the degree to which the inflammation quickly responds to steroid is less in COPD than asthma and so there is not the same degree of urgency in the need for administration of steroids in COPD. Two key RCTs of oral steroid use demonstrated primarily reduced hospital stay alongside some improvements in measurement of lung function by using 2 weeks of either 30 mg prednisolone (Davies et al., 1999) or combinations of methylprednisolone and tapering prednisolone doses over both 2 and 8 weeks (Niewoehner et al., 1999). Current NICE guidelines recommend a dose of 30 mg prednisolone for 7–14 days, but there is evidence that 40 mg prednisolone over 5 days is not inferior to the same dose over 14 days (Leuppi et al., 2013).

 Guidelines

NICE guidelines *Chronic Obstructive Pulmonary Disease in over 16s: Diagnosis and Management*, CG101, 2010. Available at: www.nice.org.uk/guidance/cg101 (accessed Dec. 2015).

DRUGS checklist for PREDNISOLONE in COPD

Dose	30 mg
Route	PO
Units	mg
Given	Stat, then once daily for 7–14 days (although 5 days 40 mg probably adequate)
	'Tailing off' steroid dosage is not necessary unless patient is on regular maintenance oral steroid (a strategy not favoured in COPD) or if patient has been on high-dose steroid for 3 or more weeks
Special situations	Use of the IV route is rarely justified.

Antibiotics in COPD: rationale and evidence

Bacteria that are most commonly associated with exacerbations of COPD are *Streptococcus pneumoniae*, *Haemophilus influenzae* and *Moraxella cattarrhalis*, with Gram-negative bacilli and *Pseudomonas* increasingly recognised in patients with more severe underlying COPD (Monso *et al.*, 1995; Soler *et al.*, 1998). Exacerbations of COPD can be caused by viruses, and there is often little way to identify the likely precipitant on clinical grounds. There is evidence to suggest, however, that patients who have increased sputum purulence alongside either increased sputum volume or dyspnoea may benefit from antibiotics (Stockley *et al.*, 2000). Current NICE guidelines advise using antibiotics in such patients. The choice of agent should be guided by sputum culture but initial empirical therapy should be with only one antibiotic, with amoxicillin, clarithromycin or doxycycline the recommended first-line agents. In patients who have not responded to one antibiotic, it is not unreasonable to either add in another or switch to co-amoxiclav. The use of the IV route is rarely justified and increases the risk of antibiotic-related complications (e.g. *Clostridium difficile* diarrhoea).

In patients who do not have increased sputum purulence but have evidence of a marked inflammatory response (e.g. fever, high CRP), there is no evidence base to justify antibiotic treatment but often there may be clinical anxiety about not using antibiotics. If antibiotics are used, sensible antibiotic stewardship should be exercised, that is restrict to monotherapy, oral route and short duration of treatment.

Other medications used in acute exacerbations of COPD

Aminophylline

Studies looking at IV aminophylline in acute exacerbations of COPD have found that the effect on objective parameters such as lung function, hospital stay and symptoms is marginal (Barbera *et al.*, 1992; Duffy *et al.*, 2005) but it is recommended by NICE guidelines as an adjunct if there is an inadequate response to nebulised bronchodilators. It should not delay the use of non-invasive ventilation (NIV) in patients with a respiratory acidosis.

Magnesium

In contrast to asthma, the bronchodilatory effect of magnesium does not appear to translate into clinical benefit in COPD. In three RCTs of IV magnesium, some improvement in lung function parameters have been variably reported, but with no translation into improved symptoms, hospital stay or treatment escalation (Shivanthan and Rajapakse, 2014). Nebulised magnesium has also not been found to be of benefit either (Edwards *et al.*, 2013). Accordingly, the use of magnesium is not recommended in COPD exacerbations.

Other aspects of COPD exacerbation management

The main non-pharmacological treatment that may be of benefit in COPD exacerbations is non-invasive ventilation, which should be considered in the context of a respiratory acidosis (pH < 7.35) that does not respond to initial medical therapy (i.e. controlled oxygen therapy and nebulised bronchodilators). It has been recognised for some time (Lightowler *et al.*, 2003) that NIV improves mortality, the need for intubation and treatment failure compared with standard therapy. It is worth bearing in mind that most patients in these studies did not have severe acidosis (pH< 7.25) and so care must be exercised in initiating NIV in such patients who perhaps are less likely to derive the same amount of benefit and have higher risk of death. It is imperative to decide early on the ceiling of care for all patients admitted with acute exacerbations of COPD, and so in deciding to use NIV it must be clear whether treatment should be escalated to intubation and ventilation if NIV fails. This decision must be made by a senior member of medical staff (registrar and/or consultant) and must be made on the balance of all available information, in particular background functional status and likely physiological reserve. There is no one single parameter which completely contraindicates intubation and ventilation.

Otherwise care must be taken to ensure adequate hydration and nutrition, alongside venous thromboembolism prophylaxis.

Patients with COPD often have associated cardiovascular morbidity and may have good reasons to be on cardioselective beta blockers (e.g. post myocardial infarction/ atrial fibrillation). There is no evidence that such treatment causes risk to patients with COPD (in contrast to asthma where beta blockers are contraindicated), and, if anything, there is a suggestion that they may be of benefit, which seems to be a consistent finding in retrospective studies (Short *et al.*, 2011; Etminan *et al.*, 2012), although prospective evidence is not available. Whether this is because of confounding from improved outcomes for other pathology rather than an effect on COPD per se remains debated.

As with asthma, patients with COPD need to have their inhaler technique checked prior to discharge. Ongoing support in the community is important, either through hospital at home schemes, where patients may be managed at home for much of their exacerbation, or with community matron support. Principle indications for secondary care follow-up would include the need for long-term oxygen assessment, where there is diagnostic uncertainty or clarification on need for specific treatment requirements. All patients with COPD who are breathless should be referred for pulmonary rehabilitation.

Case outcome and discharge

Mr Carterton ABG showed no evidence of a respiratory acidosis and so he did not require NIV. He gradually improved over 48 hours. At that point his oxygen saturations had improved to 91% on air, was much less wheezy, his temperature had settled and his CRP was falling. His nebulisers were stopped and he was put back on his usual inhaled medication. His inhaler technique was

adequate and he was referred for pulmonary rehabilitation in the community. Because his saturations were still low, arrangements were made for him to attend for repeat saturation measurement with/without ABG in 6 weeks time to make sure he did not need further assessment for the need for long-term oxygen.

His discharge medications are shown.

DISCHARGE MEDICATION							
Date	Medication	Dose	Route	Frequency	Supply	GP to continue?
xx/xx/xx	SYMBICORT INHALER 400/12	1 puff	INH	Twice daily	28 days	Y
xx/xx/xx	TIOTROPIUM INHALER 18 micrograms	1 puff	INH	Once daily	28 days	Y
xx/xx/xx	SALBUTAMOL INHALER 100 micrograms	2 puffs	INH	As required	28 days	Y
xx/xx/xx	AMOXICILLIN	500 mg	PO	Three times daily	4 days then stop (to complete 7 days)	N
xx/xx/xx	PREDNISOLONE	30 mg	PO	Once daily	4 days then stop (to complete 7 days)	N
xx/xx/xx	BISOPROLOL	5 mg	PO	Once daily	28 days	Y
xx/xx/xx	BENDROFLUAZIDE	2.5 mg	PO	Once daily	28 days	Y
xx/xx/xx	WARFARIN	3 mg	PO	Once daily	28 days	Y
Notes to patient/GP:						

Common pitfalls

- Not giving initial therapy (controlled oxygen/ nebulisers) time to improve a relatively mild respiratory acidosis before commencing NIV.
- Not attending to adherence to controlled oxygen delivery and prescription.
- Unnecessary use of IV route for both steroids and broad spectrum-antibiotics when oral route and narrow spectrum are perfectly adequate.
- Assuming prednisolone courses need slow tapering.
- Worrying that oxygen saturations are not quite normal despite clinical improvement – it can take some weeks for this to be fully realised.

COPD exacerbations are a common medical emergency with prompt attention needed to airway and breathing through controlled oxygen and nebulised bronchodilators. Steroids are important in the management but probably more in speeding recovery over subsequent days and preventing relapse rather than any more immediate improvement in outcome. Patients with a respiratory acidosis need consideration for NIV and the ceiling of care should be decided early and documented. Narrow-spectrum oral antibiotics are indicated in selected patients felt likely to have bacterial infection as the precipitant to their exacerbation.

SUMMARY

🔑 Key learning points

- Patient with COPD exacerbation should have oxygen delivered in a controlled manner via venture masks to target saturations between 88 and 92%.
- Nebulised bronchodilators salbutamol and atrovent should be given regularly and driven by air.
- Steroid treatment consists of short-course oral prednisolone.
- Give an oral antibiotic only to those with purulent sputum with increased sputum volume or dyspnoea unless good clinical reason to consider otherwise.
- Don't forget about the role of NIV.

COPD – long-term management

Principles of prescribing in chronic COPD

In contrast to asthma, where everyone with an asthma exacerbation requires careful evaluation prior to discharge about the level of specific therapy required to control symptoms, it is less common to alter COPD treatment following exacerbations unless there is a clear need for adding in more therapy to reduce the likelihood of exacerbations. One of the key determinants of the appropriate level of therapy for COPD is FEV_1 which falls during an exacerbation and measurement at the time will not give a clear indication of the true level of severity of disease.

The key features that determine the level of inhaled treatment patients with COPD require for maintenance therapy are:

- Breathlessness and/or exercise limitation
- Whether or not they are prone to exacerbations (defined as two or more courses of steroids per year)
- Whether they have severe COPD, as defined by FEV_1 <50% predicted.

The strategy for the pharmacological management of chronic COPD is summarised within NICE guidance in the flow chart shown in Figure 4.2.

The classes of drugs used in the treatment for COPD are:

- Short-acting bronchodilators – short-acting beta agonist (SABA), short-acting muscarinic antagonist (SAMA)
- Long-acting beta agonists (LABA)
- Long-acting muscarinic antagonists (LAMA)
- Combined inhaled steroid (ICS)/LABA

ICS as separate inhaled therapy are not licensed in COPD.

Although medication regimes are not commonly altered during hospital admissions, it is important to be familiar with the sort of medications patients with COPD can be on in the community as they will require prescribing whenever patients with COPD are admitted to hospital, whether it is for COPD or not. Confusion often arises, in particular, in relation to the combined ICS/LABA products as only certain ones are licensed in COPD. The situation is only likely to get more confusing as several new LABA/LAMA combinations, and even

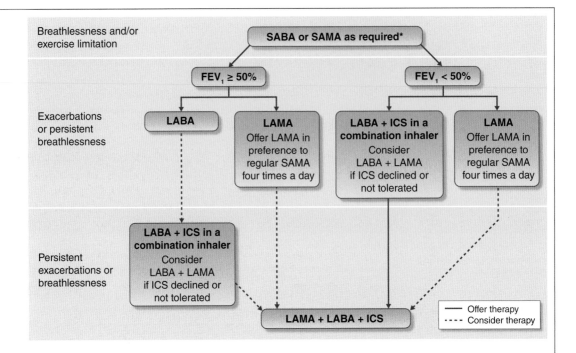

Figure 4.2 Strategy for the pharmacological management of chronic COPD. SABA, short-acting beta agonist; SAMA, short-acting muscarinic antagonist; LABA, long-acting beta agonist; LAMA, long-acting muscarinic antagonist; ICS, inhaled corticosteroid. * SABA (as required) may continue at all stages. Source: National Institute for Health and Care Excellence (2010) CG101. Chronic obstructive pulmonary disease. London: NICE. Available at: www.nice.org.uk/guidance/CG101. Reproduced with permission.

ICS/LABA/LAMA combinations, are being introduced to the market.

As discussed in Section Combined ICS/LABA Therapies, the only situation where maintenance therapy should not be prescribed as usual is if the patient is being prescribed nebulised Atrovent, in which case any LAMA should be withheld.

Long-acting bronchodilators – rationale and evidence

Any patient who requires any more than episodic reliever inhaled medication with either a SABA or SAMA and who has exertional breathlessness from COPD should be on a long-acting bronchodilator of some description. Both between different LABAs and LABAs versus LAMAs show similar efficacy in comparison with each other, but there is a suggestion that tiotropium is more effective than the LABAs in reducing likelihood of exacerbations. For patients on individual LAMAs (less severe COPD, tend not to exacerbate), preference tends to be towards products that can be taken just once daily for patient convenience and compliance. Differential cost also drives availability of different long-acting bronchodilators.

✓	DRUGS checklist for LABAs in COPD			
	Salmeterol	**Eformoterol**	**Indacaterol**	**Olodaterol**
Dose	50 micrograms	12 micrograms	150 micrograms	2.5 micrograms
Route	Inhaled	Inhaled	Inhaled	Inhaled

Units	micrograms	micrograms	micrograms	micrograms
Given	BD	1 puff BD	1 puff OD	2 puffs OD
Special situations	Available in Accuhaler (DPI, 50 micrograms/puff), 1 puff BD and MDI (25 micrograms/puff), 2 puffs BD.	Available in Turbohaler DPI.	Administered via Breezhaler, fast onset of action similar to eformoterol.	Administered via Respimat device.

In addition, there are other once-daily LABAs at the time of writing not yet licensed as monotherapies but likely to be available in the near future, for example vilanterol (available in combination, see DRUGS checklist for ICS/LABAs in COPD) and carmoterol.

✓ DRUGS checklist for LAMAs in COPD

	Tiotropium (Handihaler device)	Tiotropium (Respimat device)	Aclidinium	Glyco-pyrronium	Umeclidinium
Dose	18 micrograms/puff	2.5 micrograms/puff	400 micrograms	44 micrograms	55 micrograms
Route	Inhaled	Inhaled	Inhaled	Inhaled	Inhaled
Units	micrograms	micrograms	micrograms	micrograms	micrograms
Given	OD	2 puffs OD	1 puff BD	1 puff OD	1 puff OD
Special situations			Administered via Genuair device.	Administered via Breezhaler.	Administered via Ellipta device.

Combined inhaled steroid/ LABA in COPD – rationale and evidence

Numerous studies have shown that patients with severe COPD (FEV_1 <50% predicted) who are prone to exacerbations and who are symptomatic despite use of LABA alone, derive benefit from using combined ICS/LABA. There are currently four products licensed for COPD in this situation. The principle benefit from these products is reduction in exacerbation frequency over and above the benefit from the LABA component, which primarily improves breathlessness and exercise tolerance. Some products are licensed for use in milder disease but the cost effectiveness of using them routinely in such patients is not clear and is not supported by current NICE/SMC (Scottish Medicines Consortium) guidance. Patients with COPD who do not meet these criteria should not be prescribed inhaled steroid as part of their maintenance regime. All inhaled steroids are associated with an increased risk of pneumonia when used in patients with COPD.

✓ DRUGS checklist for ICS/LABAs in COPD

Product	Symbicort	Seretide	Fostair	Relvar Ellipta
Individual components	Budesonide + Eformoterol	Fluticasone (propionate) + salmeterol	Beclomethasone (extra fine particle) + formoterol	Fluticasone (furoate) + vilanterol
Dose (ICS/LABA)	400/12 1 puff BD or 200/6 2 puffs	500/50	100/6	92/22
Route	Inhaled			
Units	micrograms	micrograms	micrograms	micrograms
Given	BD	1 puff BD	2 puffs BD	1 puff OD
Special situations	Turbohaler device.	Other seretide formulations are not licensed in COPD and should not be used.		Fluticasone is a different molecule with much higher affinity for glucocorticoid receptor, hence lower dose.

Note that the newer products tend to have less 'round' numbers for doses of their individual components. This is due to a recent change in the drug marketing regulations whereby products have to detail the amount of drug that is expelled from the inhaler device at the mouth (e.g. 92 micrograms fluticasone furoate in Relvar Ellipta) rather than the amount of drug that is included in each actuation within the inhaler (e.g. 200 micrograms budesonide in Symbicort).

As discussed in Section Combined ICS/LABA Therapies, given the expiry of patents on Symbicort and Seretide, there are equivalent generic products available which are also licensed for COPD – Spiromax DuoResp (budesonide/ eformoterol) and Sirdupla Diskus dry powder inhaler (fluticasone propionate/salmeterol).

Finally, look out for newer combination inhalers with LAMA/LABA components, which may be initiated in outpatient or primary care setting. These are primarily indicated for increasingly breathless (but non-exacerbating) patients with moderate COPD not responding to initial single-agent bronchodilator therapy. Currently there are four products available in the UK:

- Ultibro – Indacaterol / glycopyrronium (once daily administration)
- Anoro Ellipta – Vilanterol / umeclidinium (once daily)
- Duaklir – Eformoterol / aclidinium (twice daily)
- Spiolto – Oldaterol / tiotropium (once daily).

Community-acquired pneumonia

Stuart Jenkins

Age: 54

Hospital Number: 123456

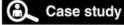 **Case study**

Presenting complaint: A 54-year-old man is admitted with 3 days' shortness of breath, cough *productive of purulent sputum, fever and left sided pleuritic chest pain.*

Background: *Usually fit and well, smoker of 20 cigarettes per day for 30 years*

PMH: *Type II diabetes*

Allergies: *Nil*

Examination:
Pulse 115, BP 96/54, Sats 84% on air, RR 33, BM 5.2, Temp 38.5. Struggling to complete short sentences

CVS: *Capillary refill time 3 seconds, pulse regular, JVP not seen, no pitting oedema, HS I + II + 0*

RS: *Reduced expansion on left side with dullness to percussion and bronchial breathing over left lower zone.*

Abdo: *Soft, non-tender, no masses palpated, bowel sounds present*

Neuro: *Intact, AMT 10/10*

ECG: *Sinus tachycardia, no acute changes*

Bloods: *Hb 13.6, Plt 587, WCC 19.5, Neut 16.4, Na 137, K 3.7, Urea 9.4, Creat 96, CRP 364*

CXR: *Left lower lobe consolidation.*

Diagnosis
Severe community-acquired pneumonia (CAP).

Initial measures
Support of his breathing through high-flow oxygen and circulation through good IV access with fluid bolus would be key. He meets the criteria for sepsis (SIRS + signs of new infection). He needs measurement of blood gases to check no evidence of hypoventilation and whether acidosis (either metabolic, including lactate, part of sepsis 6) or respiratory. Blood cultures must be taken. He has 'severe' pneumonia on account of his urea >7.0, respiratory rate >30, and diastolic BP <60. A senior member of the team needs to be made aware of his situation to consider liaising with HDU.

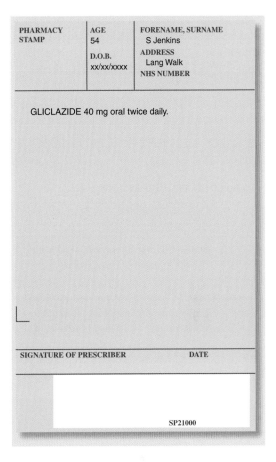

GLICLAZIDE 40 mg oral twice daily.

Prescribing for community-acquired pneumonia

The initial prescription depends on the severity of pneumonia. The CURB-65 is a robustly validated tool to estimate a patient's risk of death from pneumonia and to guide initial treatment. It was developed prospectively in over 1000 patients (Lim *et al.*, 2003) and has been subsequently studied on over 12 000 patients. Risk of death progressively rises as components of the CURB-65 score are accumulated (Table 4.3).

In addition to these core features of pneumonia severity, there are further features that are independently predictive for risk of death in pneumonia and can, alongside one or another of the core features, sway one towards thinking about managing more as severe, rather than moderate pneumonia.

Table 4.3 CURB-65 score.

CURB-65 score	Pneumonia severity	Risk of death
0	Mild	0.7%
1	Mild	2.1%
2	Moderate	9–12%
3–5	Severe	15–40%

Components of CURB-65 score

C	Confusion, defined as a score of <8 on the AMT
U	Urea >7.0 (unless known to be raised, difficult in patients on diuretics)
R	Respiratory rate >30
B	Blood pressure less than 90 mmHg (systolic) and/or 60 mmHg (diastolic)
65	Age >65.

ONCE ONLY PRESCRIPTIONS

Date	Time to be given	DRUG	Dose	Route	Prescriber Signature	Bleep
xx/xx/xx	STAT	NORMAL SALINE 0.9%	500 ml	IV	A. Doctor	
xx/xx/xx	STAT	CO-AMOXICLAV	1.2 g	IV	A. Doctor	
xx/xx/xx	STAT	CLARITHROMYCIN	500 mg	PO	A. Doctor	

REGULAR PRESCRIPTIONS

DRUG CO-AMOXICLAV				times	Day 1	Day 2	Day 3	Day 4
Dose 1.2 g	Route IV	Freq TDS	Start date xx/xx/xx	06 ⑧ 12 ⑭ 18 ㉒				
Signature A. Doctor	Bleep	Review						
Additional instructions								

DRUG CLARITHROMYCIN								
Dose 500 mg	Route PO	Freq BD	Start date xx/xx/xx	06 ⑧ 12 16 18 ⑳				
Signature A. Doctor	Bleep	Review						
Additional instructions								

DRUG GLICLAZIDE								
Dose 40 mg	Route PO	Freq BD	Start date xx/xx/xx	06 ⑧ 12 16 18 ⑳				
Signature A. Doctor	Bleep	Review						
Additional instructions								

These include significant hypoxaemia, multilobar involvement on CXR, presence of co-existing illness, positive blood cultures and WCC <4 or >20.

The principles of prescribing in CAP are:

1. Fluid resuscitation (where appropriate), e.g. initial fluid bolus, further prescription depending on response, urine output etc.
2. Antibiotics, including the principles of antibiotic stewardship:
   (a) narrow any initial broad-spectrum antibiotics once any causative organism is identified
   (b) IV to oral switch as soon as clinically appropriate (no hard and fast rules but in general consider definite clinical improvement and afebrile in prior 24 hours).
3. Review prescription and consider withholding potential nephrotoxic/ hypotensive drugs (especially diuretics, ACEI).
4. Watch for interactions, e.g. using macrolide in patients on warfarin as this may increase INR.

Antibiotics in community-acquired pneumonia – rationale and evidence

There are no placebo-controlled RCTs of antibiotics in the treatment of CAP but it is clear that untreated CAP with pneumococcal bacteraemia carries a high mortality of over 80% (Austrian and Gold, 1964). The initial choice of antibiotics regimen depends on the severity of pneumonia, local antibiotic guidelines and any concern regarding likely causative organism. The term 'atypical pneumonia' is not recommended because there are no clinical features that can consistently and reliably be used to predict likely causative organism, other than, for example, when there is known high community incidence of legionella. The term 'atypical pathogen' is therefore preferred in reference to less frequently causative organisms (e.g. legionella pneumonia, mycoplasma pneumonia). The organism most frequently responsible for CAP is *Streptococcus pneumoniae* (approx 40% in hospital studies) so any initial antibiotic regimen must cover this. Atypical pathogens are rarely responsible for CAP managed in the community (<2%) but more so in patients managed in hospital (*Mycoplasma pneumoniae* approx 10%, *Chlamydophila pneumoniae* 13%). There is a low incidence of β-lactam resistance by *S. pneumoniae* within the UK (not so in areas of continental Europe, e.g. Spain), therefore in mild CAP (CURB-65 0 or 1), monotherapy with amoxicillin is the treatment of choice. Alternatives (e.g. in allergy) would be doxycycline or clarithromycin. As the severity of pneumonia increases, one should be more cautious about covering a wider spectrum of pathogens, as they are more likely to be causative; therefore dual therapy with (e.g. β-lactam and macrolide) becomes more appropriate.

Table 4.4 shows one example of an initial antibiotic strategy according to CURB-65 score. In general, the oral route is sufficient for mild and moderate CAP whereas the IV route is recommended for severe CAP.

In many units, IV benzylpenicillin will be recommended (1.2 g QDS) rather than co-amoxiclav

Table 4.4 Example of an initial antibiotic strategy according to the CURB-65 score.

CURB score	First line
0	Amoxicillin 500 mg TDS
1	Amoxicillin 500 mg TDS
2	Amoxicillin 500 mg TDS + clarithromycin 500 mg BD
3–5	Co-amoxiclav 1.2 g TDS + clarithromycin 500 mg BD

in severe CAP. This often relates to local anxieties about the risk of broad-spectrum antibiotics (in particular *Clostridium difficile* rates). Co-amoxiclav will give broader cover than benzylpenicillin, in particular for Gram-negative bacilli and *Staphylococcus aureus,* which are uncommon causes of CAP but are associated with high mortality. Other alternative IV agents in severe CAP include cefuroxime 1.5 g TDS, cefotaxime 1 g TDS or ceftriaxone 2 g OD.

For essential pharmacology see Chapter 11.

✓ **DRUGS checklist for CAP**	Amoxicillin/ ampicillin	Co-amoxiclav	Clarithromycin
Dose	500 mg	1.2 g (IV) 625 mg (PO)	500 mg
Route	PO (amoxicillin) IV (ampicillin)	IV	PO
Units	mg	mg	mg
Given	TDS	TDS	BD
Special situations		Some units use IV benzylpenicillin 1 g QDS instead in severe CAP.	Although can be given IV there is minimal difference in bioavailability and oral route should be used unless patient unable to swallow. IV also carries risk of local thrombophlebitis.

⊙ Guidelines

BTS CAP guidelines (see Further reading).

Further aspects of CAP management

Careful attention to IV fluid resuscitation (and ongoing hydration) and oxygenation is key in all patients. Most patients admitted with moderate/ severe CAP will benefit from physiotherapy to aid expectoration of secretions. In patients with severe CAP or clinical deterioration, a low threshold should exist for discussion with ITU/ critical care. Patients with persisting hypoxaemia despite optimum oxygen delivery may need intubation. The development of a respiratory acidosis is a poor prognostic sign and should prompt consideration of intubation and ventilation. Non-invasive ventilation is unlikely to help in this situation and is not recommended.

Testing extensively for atypical pathogens is rarely helpful in the acute setting as many tests rely on the identification of differential acute and convalescent serology (e.g. in diagnosis of *Mycoplasma pneumoniae* infection). Atypical pathogens are rarely cultured from sputum or blood. In severe CAP (or in presence of confirmed local outbreak), however, it is recommended that urine is sent for legionalla antigen testing, results of which are usually available within 24 hours, and is of high sensitivity (>95%) and specificity (approximately 80%) (Birtles *et al.*, 1990). Similarly, testing for pneumococcal antigen in the urine is much more sensitive than blood or sputum culture in diagnosis of pneumococcal disease and should be performed in patients with moderate and severe CAP (Smith *et al.*, 2003).

Assuming correct guidelines have been followed, poor response to antibiotic therapy usually reflects severity of pneumonia rather than inappropriate antibiotics. In this situation, consideration must always be given to either an alternative or additional diagnosis (most commonly development of pleural infection, e.g. where fever/ inflammatory response persists).

Case outcome and discharge

Two days after admission, blood culture grew *S. pneumoniae*, in addition to pneumococcal antigen in the urine being positive. The organism was sensitive to amoxicillin. By that point his temperature had settled, he was haemodynamically stable and able to be switched to oral antibiotics. Given this, his antibiotic regimen was narrowed accordingly. He was discharged with plans for him to attend the chest clinic for a repeat CXR in 6 weeks time to ensure resolution of the consolidation on CXR.

His discharge drugs are shown.

DISCHARGE MEDICATION						
Date	Medication	Dose	Route	Frequency	Supply	GP to continue?
xx/xx/xx	AMOXICILLIN	500 mg	PO	Three times daily	4 days (to complete 7 days)	N
xx/xx/xx	GLICLAZIDE	40 mg	PO	Twice daily	28 days	Y
Notes to patient/GP:						

Common pitfalls

- Unnecessary dual antibiotic therapy prescription in mild CAP.
- Unnecessary IV prescription in moderate severity CAP where oral regimen likely to suffice.
- Failure to consider pleural infection (or other alternative diagnoses) when patients fail to respond to initial adequate therapy.
- Failures in antibiotic stewardship e.g. not narrowing therapy when microbiological diagnosis made, not switching to oral antibiotics at appropriate opportunity.
- Use of NIV in patients profoundly hypoxic with respiratory acidosis – it will not help.
- Remember to arrange follow up to ensure radiological resolution of pneumonia, and ensure no underlying pathology, e.g. neoplasm (mandatory in smokers and patients aged >40).

🔑 Key learning points

- Core aspects of management of CAP involves oxygen, adequate hydration/ resuscitation and antibiotics.
- Severity assessment is key in determining prognosis and antibiotic strategy.
- Mild (CURB-65 0/1) and moderate (CURB-65 2) CAP can usually be managed with oral antibiotics, with monotherapy in mild CAP.
- Severe CAP will need broader-spectrum antibiotic cover and IV therapy.
- Remember the principles of antibiotic stewardship in ongoing management on the wards.

FURTHER READING

BTS Pneumonia guidelines published in 2009 are still valid, with recent NICE guidance published in 2014 (CG191) concentrating more on the core factors of assessment and initial management. The BTS has also produced a summary of where the 2009 BTS guideline remains valid, and where overlaps exist. Available at: www.brit-thoracic.org.uk/guidelines-and-quality-standards/community-acquired-pneumonia-in-adults-guideline/annotated-bts-guideline-for-the-management-of-cap-in-adults-2015/ (accessed Dec. 2015).

- BTS guidelines (Lim *et al.*, 2009).
- NICE. *Pneumonia in Adults: Diagnosis and Management*, CG191, 2014. Available at: www.nice.org.uk/guidance/cg191 (accessed Dec. 2015).

Prescribing in other respiratory infections

Prescribing in bronchiectasis

Exacerbations of bronchiectasis are characterised by increased sputum purulence, increased sputum volume, increased dyspnoea and (when measured in clinic) a decline in lung function, along with systemic features of infection (fever, raised inflammatory markers), although these latter features are often less prominent. CXR may not show much in the way of dramatic new changes as infection is usually limited to the airways (may be prominent bronchial wall thickening, but often a subtle sign) rather than the alveoli and lung parenchyma to cause consolidation.

Management depends on the degree of symptoms. Mild exacerbations can often be managed in the community with oral antibiotics but if this fails or there is significant symptoms burden or systemic

upset at presentation, admission for IV antibiotics may be necessary. In prescribing antibiotics the following principles should be followed:

- Always send sputum for culture to inform management.
- Initial empirical therapy should be based on either last sputum culture result or ,if not available, what has been effective previously.
- Antibiotic use should be guided by antibiotic sensitivity.
- Low doses of antibiotics are not effective.
- Antibiotic courses need to be 14 days long as standard, in contrast to other respiratory infections (e.g. infectious exacerbation of COPD/ pneumonia) where shorter courses will be adequate.
- IV therapy should usually cover the possibility of *Pseudomonas aerginosa* infection.

Organisms responsible for exacerbations of bronchiectasis are commonly *Staphylococcus aureus*, *Haemophilus influenzae*, *Moraxella catarhalis* and *Pseudomonas aerginosa*. Pseudomonas tends to colonise the airways and cause exacerbations in more severe disease, and *S. aureus* earlier in the timecourse of the disease. Some strains of *H. influenzae* can produce β-lactamase and so negate the efficacy of amoxicillin – be guided by sputum culture and sensitivity.

Initial antibiotic regimes should cover these organisms and the following are suggested. As above, consideration must be given to culture and sensitivity results. Sometimes, however (especially in relation to pseudomonas), the *in vitro* sensitivity may not reflect *in vivo* sensitivity and if clinical improvement has occurred with the instituted regimen it is not unreasonable to continue.

✓ DRUGS checklist for bronchiectasis – mild/ moderate exacerbations where oral therapy appropriate

	Amoxicillin/ ampicillin	Co-amoxiclav	Ciprofloxacin	Doxycycline
Dose	500 mg	625 mg	500–750 mg	200 mg stat then 100 mg
Route	PO	PO	PO	PO
Units	mg	mg	mg	mg
Given	TDS	TDS	BD	OD
Special situations	Should cover: *H. influenzae* *S. pneumoniae* *M. catarrhalis*. 1 g TDS sometimes used if failure to improve with lower doses.	Should cover: *H. influenzae* *M. catarrhalis* *S. aureus*.	Use lower dose in milder exacerbations only. Should cover *Pseudomonas* and coliforms (more unusual), although risk of resistance with recurrent use.	Should cover *H. influenzae* *S. pneumoniae* *M. catarrhalis*

✓ DRUGS checklist for bronchiectasis – moderate/ severe exacerbations/ failure of oral therapy where IV therapy required

	Ceftazidime	Tazocin	Meropenem
Dose	2 g	4.5 g	2 g
Route	IV	IV	IV
Units	g	g	G
Given	TDS	TDS	TDS
Special situations	Give 1 g TDS if eGFR <50 mL/min, or if age >80 years.	BD dosing if eGFR <20 mL/min	Dose also reduced in renal impairment as follows: eGFR 26–50 dose 2 g BD eGFR 10–25 dose 1 g BD eGFR < 10 dose 1 g OD

Some units will combine the above IV therapy with gentamicin (5–7 mg/kg once daily) but there are no RCTs confirming benefit of this combination in non-CF (cystic fibrosis) bronchiectasis and given the potential ototoxicity, especially in the elderly, it is increasingly common practice to not use gentamicin in this group of patients.

Other drugs used in bronchiectasis

In addition to antibiotics, adjuncts to physiotherapy to aid sputum expectoration are often employed. The decision to use these is usually made on an individual basis dependent on how much difficulty the patient is having in managing their secretions, and often on the advice of physiotherapists. Nebulised normal saline (0.9%) has been shown to improve sputum yield, viscosity and sputum expectoration in addition to an active cycle of breathing physiotherapy techniques, but it is not as effectively as hypertonic (7%) saline (Kellet *et al.*, 2005), although this was in relatively stable, outpatient management of bronchiectasis. There are no trials of the use of hypertonic saline in the context of exacerbations. Recombinant DNase, while effective in CF has not been shown to be of benefit in non-CF bronchiectasis (Wills *et al.*, 1996). Carbocysteine (750 mg TDS) may also improve sputum viscosity and is often used, but again there are no clinical trials showing benefit. There is evidence that long-term (at least 3 months) macrolide therapy (azithromycin 500 mg three times weekly or 250 mg daily, or erythromycin 250 mg BD) reduces the risk of exacerbations in patients with bronchiectasis (Haworth *et al.*, 2014).

Prescribing in tuberculosis

The overwhelming majority of patients treated for tuberculosis (TB) are commenced on treatment in the outpatient setting. If a patient is commenced on antituberculous therapy as an inpatient, or is admitted for another reason while taking TB treatment, the main thing that causes confusion, and potentially drug errors,

is the terminology of combination agents used. It is uncommon for patients to be prescribed drugs as individual components, unless on some directly observed therapy (DOT) regimes. Standard treatment consists of four drugs for 2 months (rifampicin, isoniazid, pyrazinamide and ethambutol) and then two drugs (rifampicin and isoniazid) for a further 4 months.

In the initial phase RIFATER is usually used – this contains rifampicin, isoniazid and pyrazinamide. In the continuation phase RIFINAH is usually used. This contains both rifampicin and isoniazid. Clearly, if patients are mistakenly given the wrong product at the wrong phase of their treatment they are either at risk of under treatment and inherent risks of developing drug resistance, or over treatment and risk of side effects.

Other key points in prescribing in TB are:

- Dose of TB medications (both number and strength of RIFATER/ RIFINAH and ethambutol) is dependent on weight and individual patient prescriptions must be checked in the BNF (BMA/RPS, 2015).
- Rifampicin will cause discolouration of urine (pinky orangey colour) and patients must be warned about this.
- Baseline LFT and U&E need to be checked but if normal these do not need to be monitored during treatment.
- Patients must be warned about side effects of drugs, especially hepatotoxicity, and should be told to contact their doctor for urgent LFT checking if they develop itching, jaundice or abdominal discomfort.
- Pyridoxine (vitamin B_6) 10 mg once daily should be prescribed alongside isoniazid to reduce the risk of developing peripheral neuropathy.
- Ethambutol does carry a risk of optic neuritis but this is rare in patients only taking the standard regimen. Patients needing prolonged treatment (e.g. drug resistance/ non-tuberculous mycobacterium treatment) need monitoring of visual acuity.

Now visit **www.wileyessential.com/pharmacology** to test yourself on this chapter.

References

Austrian R, Gold J (1964). Pneumococcal bacteraemia with especial reference to bacteraemia pneumococcal pneumonia. *Ann Intern Med* 60: 759–76.

Barbera JA, Reyes A, Roca J *et al.* (1992). Effect of intravenously administered aminophylline on ventilation/perfusion inequality during recovery from exacerbations of chronic obstructive pulmonary disease. *Am Rev Respir Dis* 145: 1328–33.

Birtles RJ, Harrison TG, Samuel D *et al.* (1990). Evaluation of urinary antigen ELISA for diagnosing Legionella pneumophila serogroup 1 infection. *J Clin Pathol* 43: 685–90.

British Medical Association and Royal Pharmaceutical Society of Great Britain (BMA/RPS) (2015). *British National Formulary 69*, 69th edn. BMJ group and Pharmaceutical Press, London. Available at: www.bnf.org (accessed Dec. 2015).

British Thoracic Society Scottish Intercollegiate Guidelines Network (BTS SIGN) (2014). British guideline on the management of asthma. *Thorax* 69 (Suppl. 1): i1–i192.

Cole JM, Sheehan AH, Jordan JK (2012). Concomitant use of ipratropium and tiotropium in chronic obstructive pulmonary disease. *Ann Pharmacother* 46: 1717–21.

Duffy N, Walker P, Diamantea F *et al.* (2005). Intravenous aminophylline in patients admitted to hospital with non-acidotic exacerbations of chronic obstructive pulmonary disease: a prospective randomised controlled trial. *Thorax* 60: 713–7.

Davies L, Angus RM, Calverley PM (1999). Oral corticosteroids in patients admitted to hospital with exacerbations of chronic obstructive pulmonary disease: a prospective randomised controlled trial. *Lancet* 354: 456–60.

Edwards L, Shirtcliffe P, Wadsworth K *et al.* (2013). Use of nebulised magnesium sulphate as an adjuvant in the treatment of acute exacerbations of COPD in adults: A randomised double-blind placebo-controlled trial. *Thorax* 68: 338–43.

Etminan M, Jafari S, Carleton B *et al.* (2012). Beta-blocker use and COPD mortality: a systematic review and meta-analysis *BMC Pulmonary Medicine* 12: 48.

Goodacre S, Cohen J, Bradburn M *et al.* (2013). Intravenous or nebulised magnesium sulphate versus standard therapy for severe acute asthma (3Mg trial): a double-blind, randomised controlled trial. *Lancet Respir Med* 1: 293–300.

Hardinge M, Annandale J, Bourne S *et al.* (2015). British Thoracic Society guidelines for home oxygen use in adults. *Thorax* 70(Suppl. 1): 1–43.

Haworth CS, Bilton D, Elborn JS (2014). Long-term macrolide maintenance therapy in non-CF bronchiectasis: evidence and questions. *Respir Med* 108: 1397–408.

Kellett F, Redfern J, Niven RM (2005). Evaluation of nebulised hypertonic saline (7%) as an adjunct to physiotherapy in patients with stable bronchiectasis. *Respir Med* 99: 27–31.

Kew KM, Kirtchuk L, Michell CI (2014). Intravenous magnesium sulfate for treating adults with acute asthma in the emergency department. *Cochrane Database Syst Rev* (5): CD010909.

Leuppi JD, Schuetz P, Bingisser R *et al.* (2013). Short-term vs. conventional glucocorticoid therapy in acute exacerbations of chronic obstructive pulmonary disease: the REDUCE randomized clinical trial. *JAMA* 309: 2223–31.

Lightowler JV, Wedzicha JA, Elliott MW *et al.* (2003). Non-invasive positive pressure ventilation to treat respiratory failure resulting from exacerbations of chronic obstructive pulmonary disease: Cochrane systematic review and meta-analysis. *BMJ* 326: 185–7.

Lim WS, Baudouin SV, George RC *et al.* (2009). BTS guidelines for the management of community acquired pneumonia in adults: update 2009. *Thorax* 64 (Suppl. 3): iii1–55.

Lim WS, van der Eerden MM, Laing R *et al.* (2003). Defining community acquired pneumonia severity on presentation to hospital: an international derivation and validation study. *Thorax* 58: 377–82.

McCrory DC, Brown CD (2002). Anti-cholinergic bronchodilators versus beta 2 sympathomimetic agents for acute exacerbations of chronic obstructive pulmonary disease. *Cochrane Database Syst Rev* (4): CD003900.

McFadden ER Jr. (1986). Critical appraisal of the therapy of asthma–an idea whose time has come. *Am Rev Respir Dis* 133: 723–4.

Monso E, Ruiz J, Rosell A *et al.* (1995). Bacterial infection in chronic obstructive pulmonary disease. A study of stable and exacerbated outpatients using the protected specimen brush. *Am J Respir Crit Care Med* 152: 1316–20.

Nair P, Milan SJ, Rowe BH (2012). Addition of intravenous aminophylline to inhaled beta(2)-agonists in adults with acute asthma. *Cochrane Database Syst Rev* (12): CD002742.

Niewoehner DE, Erbland ML, Deupree RH *et al.* (1999). Effect of systemic glucocorticoids on exacerbations of chronic obstructive pulmonary disease. Department of Veterans Affairs Cooperative Study Group. *N Engl J Med* 340: 1941–7.

O'Driscoll BR, Howard LS, Davison AG, British Thoracic Society (2008). BTS guideline for emergency oxygen use in adult patients. *Thorax* 63 (Suppl. 6): vi1–68.

Parameswaran K, Belda J, Rowe BH (2000). Addition of intravenous aminophylline to beta2-agonists in adults with acute asthma. *Cochrane Database Syst Rev* (4): CD002742.

Rodrigo G, Rodrigo C, Burschtin O (1999). A meta-analysis of the effects of ipratropium bromide in adults with acute asthma. *Am J Med* 107: 363–70.

Rowe BH, Bretzlaff JA, Bourdon C *et al.* (2000). Magnesium sulfate for treating exacerbations of acute asthma in the emergency department. *Cochrane Database Syst Rev* (2): CD001490.

Rowe BH, Spooner C, Ducharme FM *et al.* (2001a). Early emergency department treatment of acute asthma with systemic corticosteroids. *Cochrane Database Syst Rev* (1): CD002178.

Rowe BH, Spooner CH, Ducharme FM *et al.* (2001b). Corticosteroids for preventing relapse following acute exacerbations of asthma. *Cochrane Database Syst Rev* (1): CD000195.

Shivanthan MC, Rajapakse S (2014). Magnesium for acute exacerbation of chronic obstructive pulmonary disease: A systematic review of randomised trials. *Ann Thoracic Med* 9: 77–80.

Short PM, Lipworth SIW, Elder DHJ *et al.* (2011). Effect of β blockers in treatment of chronic obstructive pulmonary disease: a retrospective cohort study. *BMJ* 342: d2549.

Smith MD, Derrington P, Evans R *et al.* (2003). Rapid diagnosis of bacteremic pneumococcal infections in adults by using the Binax NOW Streptococcus pneumoniae urinary antigen test: a prospective, controlled clinical evaluation. *J Clin Microbiol* 41: 2810–3.

Soler N, Torres A, Ewig S *et al.* (1998). Bronchial microbial patterns in severe exacerbations of chronic obstructive pulmonary disease (COPD) requiring mechanical ventilation. *Am J Respir Crit Care Med* 157: 1498–505.

Stockley RA, O'Brien C, Pye A *et al.* (2000). Relationship of sputum color to nature and outpatient management of acute exacerbations of COPD. *Chest* 117: 1638–45.

Stoodley RG, Aaron SD, Dales RE (1999). The role of ipratropium bromide in the emergency management of acute asthma exacerbation: a metaanalysis of randomized clinical trials. *Ann Emerg Med* 34: 8–18.

Tomar RP, Vasudevan R (2012). Metabolic acidosis due to inhaled salbutamol toxicity: A hazardous side effect complicating management of suspected cases of acute severe asthma. *Med J Armed Forces India* 68: 242–4.

Wills PJ, Wodehouse T, Corkery K *et al.* (1996). Short-term recombinant human DNase in bronchiectasis. Effect on clinical state and in vitro sputum transportability. *Am J Respir Crit Care Med* 154: 413–7.

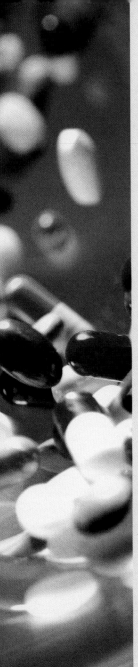

CHAPTER 5
Gastroenterology
Georgia Woodfield

Key topics:

Learning objectives

By the end of this chapter you should…

■ …be able to write a prescription for patients with acute presentations of gastrointestinal problems, taking into account relevant contraindications, cautions and side effects.

■ …be able to talk about the mechanisms of action of the key drugs used to treat these conditions.

■ …be able to describe the pharmacological strategies employed in the long-term management of inflammatory bowel disease and hepatitis.

■ …be aware of some of the key trials that underpin the management of these conditions.

Essential Practical Prescribing, First Edition. Georgia Woodfield, Benedict Lyle Phillips, Victoria Taylor, Amy Hawkins and Andrew Stanton. © 2016 by John Wiley & Sons, Ltd. Published 2016 by John Wiley & Sons, Ltd.

Upper gastrointestinal haemorrhage

> ## Mr WIlliam Bower
> ## Age: 60
> ## Hospital number: 123456

🔍 Case study

Presenting complaint: *A 60-year-old man presents to A&E with epigastric pain and profuse coffee-ground vomiting.*

Background: *He lives alone, recently retired lawyer. He is an ex-smoker (20 pack years) and drinks 35 units of alcohol per week.*

PMH: *Hypertension, gastro-oesophageal reflux, neck pain*

PHARMACY STAMP	AGE 60	FORENAME, SURNAME William Bower
	D.O.B. xx/xx/xxxx	ADDRESS Redfern Drive
		NHS NUMBER

AMLODIPINE 5 mg oral once daily.

RANITIDINE 150 mg oral twice daily.

IBUPROFEN 400 mg oral three times daily as required.

| SIGNATURE OF PRESCRIBER | DATE |

SP21000

Allergies: *Codeine (causes nausea)*

FH: *Father had an MI age 50*

Examination:
Pulse 110, BP 90/62, Sats 97% on air, RR 25, BM 5

CVS: *Capillary refill time 3 seconds, pulse feels regular, JVP not seen, no oedema, HS I + II + 0*

RS: *Equal expansion with air entry to both bases and no added sounds*

Abdo: *Soft, tender epigastrium, no masses palpated, bowel sounds present, no ascites, no jaundice*

Neuro: *Moving all 4 limbs, alert, mobile*

PR exam: *Melaena*

ECG: *Sinus tachycardia*

Bloods: *Hb 100, Plt 150, WCC 8.9, Na 136, K 4,3, Urea 9.0, Creat 100, INR 1.1
ALT 55, ALkP 110, alb 38, amylase 70*

Diagnosis

Acute upper GI bleed. In light of his history of gastroesophageal reflux disease (GORD) and the fact he is on an non-steroid anti-inflammatory drug (NSAID) and has epigastric pain, the most likely diagnosis is bleeding peptic ulcer. Other causes could be gastritis, oesophagitis or malignancy. However, he also has a history of high alcohol with a raised alanine transaminase (ALT) and low platelets, both of which support the possibility of liver disease. Therefore chronic liver disease with a variceal bleed should be in the differential diagnosis, and the examination must incorporate looking for signs of chronic liver disease.

Acute GI bleed is a medical emergency where the initial focus is to stabilise the patient to enable urgent upper GI endoscopy.

This patient has adverse signs because he is hypotensive and tachycardic, with a low Hb. He has a Blatchford Score of 10. Some centres may use the Rockall Score instead, but full scoring can only be done postendoscopy, hence the Blatchford Score is largely considered to be

(Continued)

Case study (Continued)

more appropriate in acutely presenting inpatients (Stanley *et al.*, 2009).

Glasgow–Blatchford Score

- Hb men (g/L): Hb <130 +1, Hb <120 +3, Hb <100 +6;
- Hb women (g/L): Hb <120 +1, Hb <100 +6
- Urea (mmol/L) urea>6.5 +2, urea >8 +3, urea>10 +4, urea >25 +6
- Systolic BP (mmHg): SBP <110 +1, SBP <100 +2, SBP <90 +3
- Heart rate >100 beats/min +1
- Melaena +1
- Syncope +2
- Hepatic disease +2
- Heart failure +2

This is a screening tool to assess the likelihood that a patient will need an intervention (blood transfusion or endoscopic therapy).

Those with a score of 0 are low risk and could be discharged with treatment in an outpatient setting. Scores of >6 were associated with 50% risk of needing an intervention (Blatchford *et al.*, 2000).

NICE guidelines recommend that endoscopy be offered to unstable patients with severe acute upper gastrointestinal bleeding immediately after resuscitation (NICE, 2012a).

Initial measures

This patient should be managed with the standard ABCD approach for haemorrhagic shock, usually in the resuscitation bay of the emergency department, or in a high-dependency environment.

Most importantly, he needs urgent wide-bore IV access with blood sent for cross match of 3–6 units of packed red cells (depending on hospital policy). The NSAID must be stopped and fluid resuscitation initiated with IV crystalloids. He should be placed on a cardiac monitor with 15-minute observations. Arrangements should be made for urgent endoscopy as per hospital protocol.

 Guidelines

- The National Institute of Clinical Excellence (NICE) has complete guidelines on the managements of acute upper GI bleeding: *Acute Upper Gastrointestinal Bleeding in over 16s: Management*, CG141, 2012. Available at: www.nice.org.uk/guidance/cg141 (accessed Dec. 2015).
- The British Society of Gastroenterology has guidelines on variceal haemorrhage: Jalan R, Hayes P (2000). *UK Guidelines on the Management of Variceal Haemorrhage in Cirrhotic Patients*. British Society of Gastroenterology. Available at: www.bsg.org.uk/images/stories/docs/clinical/guidelines/liver/vari_hae.pdf (accessed May 2015).

Prescribing for acute upper GI bleed

All causes of upper GI bleed need resuscitation, as shown in the charts.

FLUID CHART

Date	Fluid	Dose	Route	Time to be given	Signature	Print name
xx/xx/xx	SODIUM CHLORIDE 0.9%	500 ml	IV	STAT	A. Doctor	A. Doctor

AS REQUIRED MEDICATION

DRUG OXYGEN				Date	
				Time	
Dose Aim sats 94–98%	Route INH	Max freq		Start date xx/xx/xx	Dose
					Route
Signature/Bleep A. Doctor		Max dose in 24 hrs	Review		Given
Additional instructions					Check

If they are on warfarin or have deranged clotting due to liver disease, this needs to be reversed with prothrombin complex concentrate. This is available from the haematology lab.

Those with major bleeding may require both blood and fresh frozen plasma infusions.

Local guidelines may vary on when to transfuse in GI bleed, as over-transfusion can worsen GI bleeds by increasing the blood pressure too quickly. Most Trusts permit anaemia of 75 g/L before transfusion for this reason, instead of the 'standard' 80 g/L cut off.

Those without major haemorrhage but who have either a fibrinogen level of less than 1 g/L, or a prothrombin time (International Normalised Ratio) or activated partial thromboplastin time greater than 1.5 times normal should also be given fresh frozen plasma.

For variceal bleeds, medications should be given as shown in the drug chart.

ONCE ONLY PRESCRIPTIONS					Prescriber	
Date	Time to be given	DRUG	Dose	Route	Signature	Bleep
xx/xx/xx	08.00	TERLIPRESSIN	2 mg	IV	A. Doctor	
xx/xx/xx	08.00	CIPROFLOXACIN*	400 mg	IV	A. Doctor	

*Choice of antibiotic may vary according to local hospital policy. Tazocin is a common alternative

For UGI bleeds acid-suppression drugs (proton pump inhibitors [PPIs] or H$_2$ receptor antagonists) are often given before endoscopy for patients with suspected non-variceal upper GI bleeding. NICE guidelines recommend that these should be offered only where there are stigmata of recent haemorrhage shown at endoscopy, where evidence supports the use of IV PPI. However, in reality, there may be uncertainty about cause of bleeding and/or a delay in endoscopy, hence it is often given straightaway.

Terlipressin: rationale and evidence

Terlipressin is recommended for treatment of patients with suspected variceal bleeding at presentation. Treatment should be given for 72 hours (maximum 5 days) or until definitive haemostasis has been achieved endoscopically or otherwise (NICE, 2012a). Terlipressin is an analogue of vasopressin, used as a vasoactive drug in the management of hepatorenal syndrome, oesophageal varices and in hypotension as a result of septic shock where norepinephrine has been ineffective. It works by reducing portal blood flow, portal systemic collateral blood flow and variceal pressure (Jalan and Hayes, 2000). This decreases bleeding from the site of variceal rupture. However, it does have significant systemic side effects. These include an increase in peripheral resistance, a reduction in cardiac output with a reduction in heart rate and coronary blood flow. For these reasons it is not used in patients with ischaemic heart disease unless it is an emergency.

Evidence

Terlipressin for acute variceal haemorrhage
A number of randomised trials have shown that terlipressin reduces failure to control variceal bleeding when compared with no active treatment. However, mortality was unaffected in these (Jalan and Hayes, 2000).

Terlipressin has been shown to reduce mortality rate when compared to placebo, with a 34% relative risk reduction in mortality rate (Ioannou et al., 2003a, 2003b).

DRUGS checklist for TERLIPRESSIN

Dose	2 mg initial dose
Route	IV
Units	mg
Given	Every 4 hours until bleeding controlled
	Dose can be reduced to 1 mg after initial dose if side effects develop or if patient is <50 kg
	Normal duration of treatment is for 72 hours (or until haemostasis is achieved)
Special situations	Can cause hypertension and hypotension, which may already be present in a patient with haemorrhagic shock. This limits its use.
	Caution in patients with heart disease (due to it decreasing cardiac output).
	Can cause prolonged QT interval.

Terlipressin: essential pharmacology

Terlipressin is a prodrug that is cleaved *in vivo* into vasopressin by endo- and exopeptidases in the liver and kidneys. This process occurs over 4–6 hours, hence the need for repeated injections of terlipressin for oesophageal bleeds. Vasopressin (and terlipressin) stimulate vascular V_{1a} and V_{1b} receptors and V_2 receptors in the renal tubules, causing vasoconstriction, increased left ventricular afterload and decreased splanchnic blood flow. The vasopressin receptor V_{1a} is responsible for initiating vasoconstriction, liver gluconeogenesis, platelet aggregation and release of factor VIII. The vasopressin receptor V_{1b} is responsible for mediating corticotrophin release from the pituitary gland. The V_2 vasopressin receptor controls free water resorption in the renal medulla. The overall result is of vasoconstriction and increased free water resorption, however, because terlipressin has a relative specificity for the splanchnic circulation, it causes vasoconstriction in these vessels. This results in a reduction in portal pressure, hence a reduction in the amount of bleeding from a varix (Kam *et al.*, 2004).

Problems with terlipressin arise when patients are haemodynamically unstable, which is often the case in variceal bleed. It can cause both hypertension and hypotension, which may already be present in a patient with haemorrhagic shock, which can limit its use. For this reason, the initial 2 mg dose is given but may have to be reduced to 1mg subsequently if the patient does not tolerate it. Because of vasoconstriction and increase in afterload, patients with pre-existing heart disease may experience a reduction in cardiac output. This makes it potentially a dangerous drug in these circumstances, and a senior should be consulted.

Ciprofloxacin: rationale and evidence

Ciprofloxacin is a broad-spectrum fluoroquinolone antibiotic particularly effective for infections caused by Gram-negative bacteria. These include *Escherichia coli*, *Haemophilus influenzae*, *Klebsiella pneumoniae*, *Legionella pneumophila*, *Moraxella catarrhalis*, *Proteus mirabilis* and *Pseudomonas aeruginosa*. It is therefore often used for urinary tract infections, sexually transmitted diseases (gonorrhoea and chancroid), skin and bone infections, gastrointestinal infections, intra-abdominal infections (combined with an antianaerobic agent), some lower respiratory tract infections (particularly in pseudomonal infections), febrile neutropenia (combined with a Gram-positive bacterial agent) and malignant external otitis. It also is effective for some Gram-positive bacterial infections. It has good tissue penetration (Davis *et al.*, 1996).

All patients with suspected or confirmed variceal bleeding should be offered prophylactic antibiotic therapy at presentation. This is because bacterial infections occur within 48 hours in about 20% of patients who have upper gastrointestinal bleeding in the presence of liver cirrhosis (Jalan and Hayes, 2000).

Evidence

Antibiotics for the prevention of bacterial infections in cirrhotic patients with gastrointestinal bleeding

A meta-analysis published in *Hepatology* (Bernard *et al.*, 1999) showed that short-term antibiotic prophylaxis significantly increases the mean percentage of patients free of infection and significantly increases short-term survival rate in cirrhotic patients with gastrointestinal bleeding.

The choice of the antibiotic varies according to the hospital, and you should follow the policy of the unit where the patient is being treated. However, most of the present studies have used fluoroquinolones, and therefore ciprofloxacin has the greatest evidence base (Jalan and Hayes, 2000).

DRUGS checklist for CIPROFLOXACIN

Dose	500 mg
Route	PO
Units	mg

Given	Twice daily
Special situations	Can be given IV at a dose of 400 mg. However, as it is the GI tract that is the target in this instance and additionally it is very irritant to veins, the oral route is preferential.

Ciprofloxacin: essential pharmacology

Ciprofloxacin works by inhibiting the enzymes DNA gyrase (a type II topoisomerase) and topoisomerase IV enzymes. These are necessary for separation of bacterial DNA in cell division, hence ciprofloxacin inhibits this process (Drlica *et al.*, 1997).

Ciprofloxacin inhibits the drug-metabolising enzyme cytochrome P450. This is important if patients are on warfarin or any other drugs using this pathway as drug concentrations may be affected.

Side effects include GI disturbance, abnormal liver function tests and rash. However, ciprofloxacin-specific effects include an increased risk of tendinitis and tendon rupture, where there is a 1.9-fold increase in risk (van der Linden, 2002). This is particularly of concern in patients on steroids or immunosuppressants for organ transplants. Patients with myasthenia gravis may have exacerbation of their muscle weakness.

Proton pump inhibitors: rationale and evidence

PPIs such as omeprazole, lansoprazole and pantoprazole are very common medications used for decreasing stomach acid secretion, thereby slowing the progression of peptic ulcer disease. PPIs have been shown to be very effective for healing of peptic ulcers and give good results in reflux oesophagitis. PPIs are combined with antibiotics for eradication of *Helicobacter pylori* in peptic ulcer disease.

PPIs are also used in gastrointestinal bleeding. This is because gastric acid prevents cessation of bleeding from a peptic ulcer by inhibition of clot formation, promotion of clot lysis and by ongoing tissue damage (Kolkman and Meuwissen,

1996). Also, haemostasis is unlikely to occur at a pH of less than 5.4 (Green *et al.*, 1978). For this reason PPIs and H_2 receptor antagonists are given to inhibit gastric acid secretion and therefore increase pH.

Acute upper GI bleed patients are very commonly prescribed IV PPIs in an attempt to acutely decrease bleeding from a potential peptic ulcer. However, this practice is not evidence based and in fact both NICE and SIGN guidelines (see Guidelines) advise against giving IV PPIs prior to endoscopy. They should, however, be prescribed in non-variceal gastrointestinal bleeds where stigmata of recent haemorrhage is shown at endoscopy. They are therefore a postendoscopy therapy. This recommendation against IV PPIs before endoscopy may be due to the small amount of evidence that PPI treatment initiated prior to endoscopy reduces the proportion of patients with stigmata of recent haemorrhage at the index endoscopy. PPIs have no role in the management of variceal haemorrhage.

Evidence

PPI treatment in upper GI bleeding
A review of multiple systematic reviews showed that there was no evidence that PPI treatment reduces mortality following upper GI bleeding, whether treatment is initiated prior to endoscopy or after endoscopic confirmation that the bleed originates from a peptic ulcer (PU).

However, in the situation of an endoscopically confirmed PU, PPI therapy has been shown to reduce re-bleeding rates. This is the case whether the PPI is administered orally or intravenously and whether or not endoscopic haemostatic treatment is first administered (Leontiadis *et al.*, 2007).

PPI versus H_2 receptor antagonists for prevention of re-bleeding
A meta-analysis of RCTs reported superiority of PPI therapy over H_2RA therapy in preventing ulcer re-bleeding (Gisbert *et al.*, 2001).

✓ **DRUGS checklist for OMEPRAZOLE**

Dose	20–40 mg
Route	PO, can be given IV (if active bleeding ulcer seen at oesophagogastroduodenoscopy)
Units	mg
Given	OD
Special situations	Generally given at the higher dose in this situation of confirmed peptic ulcer on endoscopy. In situations of severe recurrent ulceration, e.g. Zollinger–Ellison syndrome, the dose can be up to 120 mg per day (divided doses).

✓ **DRUGS checklist for LANSOPRAZOLE**

Dose	15–30 mg
Route	PO
Units	mg
Given	OD
Special situations	Generally given at the higher dose in this situation of confirmed peptic ulcer on endoscopy. May be used instead of omeprazole where there are intolerances or known drug interactions, e.g. omeprazole and clopidogrel (should be switched to lansoprazole if on clopidogrel).

✓ **DRUGS checklist for PANTOPRAZOLE**

Dose	80 mg stat then 8 mg/h for 72 hours
Route	IV then IV infusion
Units	mg
Given	Stat then as an infusion over (up to) 72 hours
Special situations	This is given after acute GI bleed where the patient is still obtunded or shocked, and therefore would not tolerate oral medication. Can also be given orally as a tablet 40–80 mg.

Proton pump inhibitors: essential pharmacology

Proton pump inhibitors irreversibly bind to the hydrogen/ potassium adenosine triphosphatase (H^+/ K^+ ATPase) enzyme system of the gastric parietal cells. This is the gastric proton pump responsible for secreting H^+ ions into the gastric lumen (Zajac et al., 2013). This is the last stage of gastric acid production. The PPIs are prodrugs, and in order to become active require an acidic environment. When in contact with gastric acid, the compound is protonated and converted to the active sulphenamide or sulphenic acid that binds to the gastric proton pump and blocks gastric acid secretion (Shin and Sachs, 2008). All PPIs except tenatoprazole have short half-lives (about 1 hour) but, because of irreversible binding, acid secretion can be affected for up to 72 hours.

Omeprazole, lansoprazole, rabeprazole and pantoprazole show equivalent efficacy in acid suppression studies, as well as for healing of reflux esophagitis and duodenal ulcers. However, esomeprazole and tenatoprazole have stronger acid suppression, with a longer period of intragastric pH greater than 4.

Other medications used in upper GI haemorrhage

After the initial resuscitation, most upper GI haemorrhages will require an endoscopy to definitively treat the bleed by banding the varix or injecting/ clipping/ heat-treating the bleeding peptic ulcer. After GI bleed there are, however, a number of pharmacological considerations. Ongoing PPI therapy for prevention of rebleeding has already been discussed.

Propranolol

Beta blocker therapy is given to all patients who have had a variceal bleed as secondary prophylaxis, once haemodynamic stability has been achieved and the patient has improved. It is also given as primary prophylaxis to those who have had varices seen on an endoscopy, but who have never bled from them (Jalan and Hayes, 2000). The aim of therapy is to reduce the hepatic venous pressure gradient to less than 12 mmHg. This is because, in most cases, portal pressure reflects intravariceal pressure and a hepatic venous pressure gradient greater than 12 mmHg is necessary for the development of, and bleeding from, oesophageal varices (Lebrec et al., 1980).

Propranolol has been shown to reduce the portal pressure gradient, reduce azygos blood flow and reduce variceal pressure. It achieves this by causing splanchnic vasoconstriction and reducing cardiac output (Jalan and Hayes, 2000).

Evidence

Propranolol as primary prevention of variceal bleeds
A meta-analysis showed that the risk of rebleeding was significantly lower with propranolol use in patients who had had a variceal bleed. Mortality was also reduced, but with only borderline significance detected (Hayes et al., 1990).

DRUGS checklist for PROPRANOLOL for variceal bleed

Dose	40 mg
Route	PO
Units	mg

Given	BD
	Increase to 80 mg BD if blood pressure will allow
Special situations	Long-acting propranolol at either 80 or 160 mg OD can be used to improve compliance.

Where propranolol can't be used due to contraindications or intolerance, variceal band ligation is the treatment of choice. Where neither can be used, carvedilol can be used an alternative to propranolol. Isosorbide mononitrate is another choice (20 mg twice daily), but there is limited evidence for its use.

Guidelines

The British Society of Gastroenterology has guidelines on variceal haemorrhage. Available at: www.bsg.org.uk/images/stories/docs/clinical/guidelines/liver/vari_hae.pdf (accessed Dec. 2015).

Lactulose

In patients with liver cirrhosis, upper GI bleeds are a well-known trigger for decompensation of chronic liver disease. This can manifest with jaundice, ascites and encephalopathy.

See Section Acute Hepatitis for the treatment of alcohol encephalopathy.

Alcohol withdrawal medications

Patients with high alcohol intake are at risk of withdrawal. Please see Chapter 2 for details about treatment of alcohol withdrawal.

Further aspects of upper GI bleed

Another consideration in a very unstable patient who continues to bleed from a variceal haemorrhage is a Sengstaken Blakemore tube. This is an oesophageal device with a gastric and oesophageal balloon, which can be inflated in order to apply direct pressure to a bleeding varix. It is a specialist piece of equipment and should be inserted by a senior. It can cause oesophageal perforation if used incorrectly. This intervention is rarely employed as evidence supports terlipressin as being just as efficacious.

Endoscopy is the mainstay of diagnosis and treatment in upper GI bleeds of any cause. It should be offered to unstable patients with severe acute upper GI bleeding immediately after resuscitation, or within 24 hours of admission to all other patients with upper GI bleeding. Endoscopic treatments for bleeding peptic ulcers include adrenaline injection, thermal probe treatment, thrombin injection and clipping. Oesophageal varices are banded and gastric varices can be treated with endoscopic injection of *N*-butyl-2-cyanoacrylate (sclerotherapy).

Where bleeding cannot be controlled endoscopically, surgical input may rarely be required (e.g. oversewing ulcers, partial gastrectomy).

For patients with varices (gastric or oesophageal) that cannot be controlled by band ligation, transjugular intrahepatic portosystemic shunts (TIPSs) can be offered to decrease variceal pressure and decrease bleeding.

Case outcome and discharge

Mr Bower had an endoscopy, which revealed a bleeding gastric ulcer as well as gastritis. The ulcer was treated with adrenaline injection and clipping. He was advised to stop ibuprofen treatment and to avoid all other NSAIDs. He was commenced on 40 mg omeprazole to aid ulcer healing and for treatment of gastritis, and advised to stop drinking alcohol. Ranitidine was stopped because, although effective for many people, he has had a bleed whilst taking this, hence a PPI is a better alternative. He was informed of the fact that his liver function was deranged and platelets were low, revealing heavy alcohol consumption with evidence of organ damage as a result. This is reversible at this stage with alcohol cessation. He was therefore referred to the alcohol liaison nurse as a source of information and support post-discharge from hospital. The GP was informed of

this, as a liver ultrasound scan may be required in the future if liver function tests (LFTs) do not improve with cessation of alcohol.

Because gastric ulcers have malignant potential, Mr Bower was scheduled for a repeat endoscopy in 4–6 weeks, with biopsies intended if the ulcer had not healed. Had Mr Bower been found to have varices, he would have required a repeat endoscopy for rebanding of varices at 2–4 weeks. When the varices had been successfully obliterated, he would then need endoscopic surveillance at 3 months, 6 months and then yearly. He would have been started on propranolol and given a course of ciprofloxacin in this instance, as well as been referred to the alcohol liaison team.

Mr Bower's new prescription is shown. Note ibuprofen has been stopped and ranitidine substituted for omeprazole.

DISCHARGE MEDICATION						
Date	Medication	Dose	Route	Frequency	Supply	GP to continue?
xx/xx/xx	AMLODIPINE	5 mg	PO	Once daily	14 days	Y
xx/xx/xx	OMEPRAZOLE	40 mg	PO	Once daily	14 days	Y

Notes to patient/GP:
Ranitidine changed to omeprazole for treatment of peptic ulcer.

Common pitfalls

- Permissive hypotension and permissive anaemia. Patients who are bleeding out from a peptic ulcer or varix may be difficult to resuscitate to their normal blood pressure. This can be because where a higher blood pressure is reached, this encourages further bleeding. Some centres therefore allow systolic pressure to be >90 mmHg rather than >100 mmHg, and allow Hb to be 75 g/L rather than 80 g/L before transfusion is commenced. This very much depends on the stability of the patient, their other co-morbidities, the time until endoscopy and the trust's policy.

- Patients with liver cirrhosis often have chronically low blood pressure. If possible, it is useful to look back through old notes to get an idea of a patient's usual parameters. Clinical acumen must also be used to detect whether the patient has signs of shock aside from low blood pressure, as this will guide as to the chronicity of the BP readings.

- Remember to calculate the Blatchford or Rockall score in patients who have had a GI bleed, and then had endoscopy, as it is useful for predicting risk of adverse events and mortality.

SUMMARY

Acute upper gastrointestinal bleeding is a common medical emergency that has a 10% hospital mortality rate (NICE, 2012a). Despite changes in management, mortality has not significantly improved over the past 50 years.

Endoscopy is the primary diagnostic and therapeutic investigation in patients with acute upper GI bleeding. However, this does not reveal a cause in approximately 20% of patients presenting with apparent acute GI bleed. The most common causes are peptic ulcer and oesophagogastric varices.

Bleeding from the upper gastrointestinal tract (GIT) is about four times as common as bleeding from the lower GIT.

🔑 Key learning points

Acute GI bleed
- The primary focus is resuscitation in order to stabilise the patient for endoscopy.
- This may require fluid, blood and fresh frozen plasma.
- Urgent endoscopy is required for all unstable bleeding patients, after resuscitation.

Bleeding peptic ulcers
- IV PPIs are not recommended by NICE prior to endoscopy, but you will see these being given in many hospitals anyway.
- Once peptic ulcer disease is confirmed on endoscopy, give regular PPI to aid ulcer healing.
- Consider other causes such as NSAIDs, alcohol and steroid use.

Bleeding varices
- Reverse coagulopathy with vitamin K and prothrombin complex concentrate if clotting is deranged.
- Give IV terlipressin.
- Start antibiotics early.
- Propranolol for prevention of rebleeding once patient is stable.

FURTHER READING

- The British Society of Gastroenterology has very useful website with guidelines, information, learning resources and teaching days. Available at: www.bsg.org.uk (accessed Dec. 2015).
- The British Liver Trust has information for patients and doctors. Available at: www.britishlivertrust.org.uk (accessed Dec. 2015).
- American Gastroenterology Association. Available at: www.gastro.org (accessed Dec. 2015).
- American Liver Foundation. Available at: www.liverfoundation.org (accessed Dec. 2015).

Acute inflammatory bowel disease

> **Miss Priya Patel**
>
> **Age: 20**
>
> **Hospital number: 123456**

Case study

Presenting complaint: *A 20-year old woman presents to A&E with 48 hours of bloody diarrhoea 8 times per day and abdominal cramps. She has had no recent travel and no recent antibiotics.*

Background: *Miss Patel is at university, usually independent and active, she is a non-smoker*

PMH: *Ulcerative pancolitis, one flare in the past, no surgery*

Allergies: *None*

FH: *Mother had a malignant colon polyp removed age 40*

Examination:
Pulse 110, BP 100/62, Sats 97% on air, RR 25, BM 5, temp. 37°C

CVS: *Capillary refill time 1 second, pulse feels regular, JVP not seen, no oedema, HS I + II + 0*

RS: *Equal expansion with air entry to both bases and no added sounds*

Abdo: *Soft, generally tender epigastrium particularly left iliac fossa, no masses palpated, bowel sounds present, no peritonism*

Neuro: *Moving all 4 limbs, alert, mobile*
No iritis
No rashes

ECG: *Sinus tachycardia*

Bloods: *Hb 120, Plt 400, WCC 12.9, Na 138, K 4.3, Urea 6.0, Creat 100, INR 1.1, ALT 35, AlkP 90, alb 38, amylase 70*

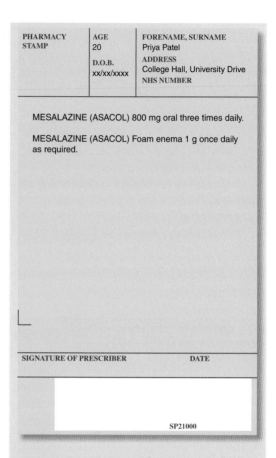

| PHARMACY STAMP | AGE 20 | FORENAME, SURNAME Priya Patel |
| | D.O.B. xx/xx/xxxx | ADDRESS College Hall, University Drive NHS NUMBER |

MESALAZINE (ASACOL) 800 mg oral three times daily.

MESALAZINE (ASACOL) Foam enema 1 g once daily as required.

SIGNATURE OF PRESCRIBER   DATE

SP21000

Diagnosis

Acute severe flare of ulcerative colitis.

Other causes of acute bloody diarrhoea include infective diarrhoea (including *Clostridium difficile* infection), ischaemic bowel and drug-induced colitis. A thorough history needs to be taken regarding recent travel, recent antibiotics (within 8 weeks) or new medications and any contacts with diarrhoeal illness (see Section Acute Infective Diarrhoea). Stool needs to be sent for culture regardless, as *C. difficile* infection has a higher prevalence in patients with inflammatory bowel disease (IBD) through unknown mechanisms and is associated with increased mortality (Mowat *et al.*, 2011). Other differential diagnoses include colonic Crohn's disease. If this patient did not have a previous confirmed diagnosis of ulcerative colitis, this might be difficult to differentiate. A thorough examination is needed looking for signs of Crohn's disease – fistulae, iritis, erythema nodosum and oral involvement. Cytomegalovirus (CMV) colitis should be considered in severe or refractory colitis, as reactivation can occur in patients with IBD on immunosuppression (Mowat *et al.*, 2011).

An acute severe flare of IBD is a medical and potentially surgical emergency, as toxic megacolon (colonic diameter >5.5 cm, or caecum >9 cm) and perforation can occur from severe inflammation of the colon. The natural history of untreated severe ulcerative colitis carries a mortality of 24%. This was reduced to 7% with the introduction of intravenous corticosteroids and subsequently to <1% with timely and expert surgical input (Truelove and Witts, 1955; Rice-Oxley and Truelove, 1950).

Likelihood of requirement for surgery increases if stool frequency is more than six per day, pyrexia or tachycardia are present, an abdominal X-ray shows colonic dilatation, of if there is anaemia or high erythrocyte sedimentation rate (ESR) (>45 mm/h). Having low albumin indicates poor nutritional state and probably less reserve, therefore is a predictor of poorer prognosis.

Severity of colitis can be quickly and easily assessed using the Truelove and Witts severity Index (Table 5.1). Immediate admission to hospital is warranted for all patients fulfilling criteria for severe colitis.

Initial measures

This patient fulfils the criteria for severe colitis and should first be managed with the standard ABCD approach for an unwell patient. Priorities for her need to be getting IV access and sending a full set of bloods, including ESR, clotting and group and save, and getting an abdominal X-ray. If she has toxic megacolon or perforation this is a surgical emergency. Regardless of this, prompt referral to both gastroenterology and surgical teams is required. This is to allow early discussions to take place, as if the stool frequency is ≥6 per 24 hours or 3–6 per 24 hours but with a C-reactive protein (CRP) >45 on day 3 of IV hydrocortisone, this predicts an 85% likelihood of requiring a colectomy during the admission (Travis *et al.*, 1996). Early surgical and stoma care nurse involvement allows early initiation of discussions regarding surgery and the potential need for a stoma. This gives the patient time to come to a decision should their medical management fail, and prevents delays in decision making later in the admission.

All anticholinergics, antidiarrhoeal agents and opioid drugs should be stopped as these can increase risk of colonic dilatation as they are constipating agents.

Table 5.1 Truelove and Witts Colitis Severity Index.

	Mild	Moderate	Severe
Bowel frequency per day	<4	4-6	>6 stools per day
Blood in stools	Small	moderate	Visible frank blood
Pyrexia >37.8°C	No	No	Yes
Heart rate >90 bpm	No	No	Yes
Anaemia <10 g/100 mL	No	No	Yes
ESR	<30	<30	>30

Source: Truelove SC, Witts LJ (1955). Cortisone in ulcerative colitis: final report on a therapeutic trial. *Br Med J* ii:1041.

ⓘ Guidelines

- NICE has complete guidelines on the managements of ulcerative colitis. *Ulcerative Colitis: Management*, CG166, 2013. Available at: www.nice.org.uk/guidance/cg166 (accessed Dec. 2015).
- The British Society of Gastroenterology has guidelines on IBD (acute and chronic management considerations). Available at: www.bsg.org.uk/images/stories/docs/clinical/guidelines/ibd/ibd_2011.pdf (accessed Dec. 2015).

Prescribing for acute severe colitis in IBD

Management of acute severe colitis is the same for ulcerative colitis and Crohn's colitis. Subsequent management may differ according to gastroenterologist opinion. The mainstay of initial treatment is steroids, which are completely effective in around 40% (Jakobovits and Travis, 2005).

ONCE ONLY PRESCRIPTIONS					Prescriber	
Date	Time to be given	DRUG	Dose	Route	Signature	Bleep
xx/xx/xx	08.00	HYDROCORTISONE	100 mg	IV	A. Doctor	
xx/xx/xx	08.00	PARACETAMOL	1 g	IV/PO	A. Doctor	
xx/xx/xx	08.00	ENOXAPARIN	40 mg	S/C	A. Doctor	

FLUID CHART						
Date	Fluid	Dose	Route	Time to be given	Signature	Print name
xx/xx/xx	SODIUM CHLORIDE 0.9%	500 ml	IV	Over 4 hours	A. Doctor	A. Doctor

If the patient is due to have an imminent colectomy (in <24 hours), discuss with surgeons before giving prophylactic enoxaparin (or any thromboprophylaxis agent) due to possible increased bleeding risk. However, in the vast majority of cases prophylactic low molecular weight heparin (LMWH) is needed, as surgery may not be done straightaway and they are at high risk of deep vein thrombosis and pulmonary embolus (PE).

Patients with Hb <8 g/L as a result of significant bloody diarrhoea may require blood transfusion.

Hydrocortisone: rationale and evidence

Corticosteroids are potent anti-inflammatory agents. They ideally have no role in maintenance therapy for either ulcerative colitis or Crohn's disease, but are important for moderate to severe relapses of these conditions, aiming to induce remission.

They act by suppressing inflammation, which is the key component of these conditions. Corticosteroids used for IBD include oral prednisolone, prednisone, budesonide or intravenous hydrocortisone and methylprednisolone. For acute severe exacerbations, IV therapy is used for maximum systemic absorption. This route, however, means a higher chance of steroid side effects, and is therefore for short-term use only.

> **[TOP TIP]** The anti-inflammatory dose equivalence of steroids (mineralocorticoid effects differ):
>
> prednisolone 5 mg = betamethasone 0.75 mg
> methylprednisolone 4 mg
> hydrocotisone 20 mg

Evidence

Corticosteroids for mild/moderate active ulcerative colitis

Oral prednisolone (starting at 40 mg daily) induced remission in 77% of 118 patients with mild-to-moderate disease within 2 weeks, compared to 48% treated with 8 g/day sulfasalazine. A combination of oral and rectal steroids is better than either alone.

Adverse events are significantly more frequent at a dose of 60 mg/day compared to 40 mg/day, without added benefit, so 40 mg appears optimal for outpatient management of acute ulcerative colitis.

Too rapid reduction in the dose of steroids can be associated with early relapse and doses of prednisolone <15 mg day are ineffective for active disease (Truelove et al., 1962; Baron et al., 1962; Lennard-Jones et al., 1960).

Corticosteroids for mild/moderate active Crohn's disease

The European Cooperative Crohn's Disease Study on 105 patients achieved 83% remission on prednisone 1 mg/kg/day compared to 38% on placebo (number needed to treat 1/42) over 18 weeks.

The high placebo response rate should be noted, because disease activity in Crohn's disease (and ulcerative colitis) fluctuates spontaneously (Malchow et al., 1984).

✓ DRUGS checklist for HYDROCORTISONE

Dose	100 mg
Route	IV
Units	mg
Given	QDS
Special situations	Higher doses of steroids offer no greater benefit, but lower doses are less effective (Mowat *et al.*, 2011). Intravenous steroids are generally given for up to 5 days. There is no benefit beyond 7–10 days (Turner *et al.*, 2007).

Adverse effects of steroids

There are numerous side effects of steroids. They cause thin skin, redistribution of fat (buffalo hump and moon face) as well as retention of fluid leading to oedema. They also cause sleep and mood disturbance (very common side effect). Hormonal effects lead to acne and steroid-induced diabetes. Steroids also cause dyspepsia and can exacerbate stomach ulcers. They are given to suppress inflammation, where the mechanism is immunosuppression. Patients are therefore more prone to infections. This is relevant for acute colitis patients who may undergo a colectomy during their admission, as they have increased risk of postoperative infection.

Long-term use has additional effects, including increased risk of posterior subcapsular cataracts, osteoporosis, osteonecrosis of the femoral head and myopathy.

Patients must be aware that they cannot withdraw steroid treatment suddenly, particularly if on high doses. Steroid withdrawal can be severe, in the form of an addisonian crisis, or can cause a corticosteroid withdrawal syndrome of myalgia, malaise and arthralgia.

Hydrocortisone: essential pharmacology

Hydrocortisone is a synthetic glucocorticosteroid hormone, which binds to glucocorticoid receptors present in most cells. Steroids have many functions but are used therapeutically because of their role in immune system feedback in up-regulating the expression of anti-inflammatory proteins and down-regulating the expression of proinflammatory proteins. This occurs via inhibition of several inflammatory pathways: suppression of interleukin transcription, suppression of arachidonic acid metabolism and stimulation of apoptosis of lymphocytes within the lamina propria of the gut. Glucocorticoids repress the expression of proinflammatory proteins by preventing the translocation of transcription factors from the cytoplasm of a cell into the nucleus. Proinflammatory proteins include interleukins IL-1B, IL-4, IL-5 and IL-8, chemokines, cytokines, GM-CSF and tumour necrosis factor-α (TNFα) genes (Newton, 2000).

Other medications used in IBD

For an acute severe flare of colitis, prophylactic LMWH should be given in the vast majority of cases. Other medications that should be considered in the short term are ciclosporin or infliximab as rescue therapy, if steroids are not working.

Enoxaparin

Crohn's disease and ulcerative colitis flares create a proinflammatory and prothrombogenic state in patients, regardless of age, mobility and otherwise low thrombus risk. LMWH subcutaneous injection is therefore essential to reduce the risk of thromboembolism. This is easily forgotten but is very important. Both NICE and the BSG recommend this, and it has been shown to decrease thromboembolism risk in IBD (Irving *et al.*, 2005). Enoxaparin is widely used, but dalteparin or tinzaparin are used in some Trusts.

If the patient is going for imminent colectomy, be guided by surgical advice before giving enoxaparin. This is because enoxaparin will increase bleeding risk. However, because surgery itself is a thromboembolism risk (postoperatively), the decision may depend on timing of surgery and other risk factors.

✓ **DRUGS checklist for ENOXAPARIN**

Dose	40 mg
Route	SC
Units	mg
Given	OD
Special situations	Dose needs reduction in renal failure to 20 mg OD, or where CrCl is very low, 50 units BD heparin SC may be substituted.

See Section Venous Thrombosis Prophylaxis in Chapter 7.

Ciclosporin

IV ciclosporin A can be given on specialist gastroenterology advice as an alternative to IV corticosteroids where steroids are contraindicated, or where patients cannot tolerate them or decline them. IV ciclosporin may also be considered as an additional therapy (rescue therapy) where patients have little or no improvement within 72 hours of IV steroid therapy, or whose symptoms are worsening during this time. These patients remain on intravenous steroids alongside rescue therapy. Patients fulfilling these criteria need also to be considered for surgery (NICE, 2013a). Ciclosporin would normally be given at 2 mg/kg/day.

Following induction of remission, oral ciclosporin is often continued for up to 3–6 months (Mowat *et al.*, 2011), during which time a maintenance drug such as azathioprine may need to be initiated with the intention of stopping the ciclosporin.

Contraindications to ciclosporin include Mg^{2+} <0.5 mmol/L or cholesterol <3.0 mmol/L, so these must be checked first and measurements repeated within 48 hours of commencing therapy. Ciclosporin is nephrotoxic, limiting treatment in patients with pre-existing renal disease (Naesens *et al.*, 2009). Creatinine must be closely monitored throughout treatment, as ciclosporin toxicity can occur with hyperkalaemia and acute renal failure. It is also neurotoxic and can cause paraesthesia, confusion and convulsions. It is classed as an International Agency for Research on Cancer

(IARC) Group 1 carcinogen due to the fact that it increases the risk of squamous cell carcinoma, particularly of the skin.

Infliximab

Infliximab can be used for acute exacerbations of ulcerative colitis where there is no improvement by day 3 or there is subsequent deterioration, where conventional therapy has failed or is unsuitable. This means it may be used instead of ciclosporin (NICE, 2015). Alternatives to infliximab include adalimumab and golimumab (also monoclonal antibody therapies), which are also approved by NICE.

Giving infliximab is a senior decision, where funding has to be applied for, and in this situation NICE recommends an induction course of three doses of infliximab only. This is generally 5 mg/kg at 0, 2 and 6 weeks, and is intended as a bridge to longer-term immunosuppression such as azathioprine. If there is no response to rescue therapy seen within 4–7 days, colectomy is recommended. Infliximab should not be given with ciclosporin, it is an alternative treatment.

For Crohn's disease, anti-TNF therapy such as infliximab or adalimumab are considered earlier for induction of remission, and a clinician can apply for funding for longer-term use to retain remission.

Contraindications to anti-TNF include demyelinating disease, optic neuritis, malignancy and congestive cardiac failure. Patients must have a full tuberculosis (TB) history and TB risk assessment with a TB Elispot (or equivalent IGRA blood assay) as anti-TNF causes reactivation of latent TB due to immunosuppression. If positive, these patients need a course of TB preventative chemoprophylaxis prior to anti-TNF therapy. Patients must also be checked for evidence of active viral hepatitis.

Further aspects of inflammatory bowel disease management

Endoscopy in the acute phase

In cases where the patient has a history of confirmed inflammatory bowel disease, diagnosis may be more straight forward. However, often an acute severe presentation of colitis may be the first presentation. For this reason flexible sigmoidoscopy and biopsy should be available within 72 h (ideally within 24 h) so that a histological diagnosis can be gained within 5 days. This confirms the diagnosis and excludes CMV (Mowat *et al.*, 2011).

Colonoscopy is contraindicated in acute colitis due to theoretical risk of perforation.

Maintaining remission (NICE, 2013a)

One of the major challenges of IBD is prevention of acute flares and maintenance of remission, ideally without surgery.

A number of different medications are used for ulcerative colitis:

- For patients with proctitis and proctosigmoiditis, topical aminosalicylates (daily or as required) are effective. They can be combined with an oral aminosalicylates for greater symptom control. Oral aminosalicylates taken alone are less effective than combined treatment. Aminosalicylates are 5-aminosalicylic acid (5-ASA) compounds. The usual first-line regimen is oral mesalazine 1.2–2.4 g daily (numerous preparations of mesalazine are available). Topical mesalazine dose is 1 g. Patients on maintenance aminosalicylates should have annual measurement of creatinine, where aminosalicylates should be stopped if renal function deteriorates.
- For patients with more extensive ulcerative colitis, a low maintenance dose of an oral aminosalicylate is usually required.
- Patients with all extents of disease may require oral azathioprine or oral mercaptopurine to maintain remission, in addition to aminosalicylates. These are considered where a patient has two or more inflammatory exacerbations in 12 months that require corticosteroid treatment or where remission is not maintained by aminosalicylates.
- If these are ineffective, methotrexate or anti-TNF therapy is considered.
- In patients who have a single episode of acute severe ulcerative colitis, oral azathioprine or oral mercaptopurine should be considered earlier before oral aminosalicylates are commenced.

These are effective for maintaining establishing and maintaining remission after an acute severe episode.

The maintenance of remission in Crohn's disease is slightly different, particularly as Crohn's disease is more varied in its presentation site, severity and pattern of disease.

- Aminosalicylates can reduce Crohn's disease activity; however, there is less evidence for their efficacy than in ulcerative colitis. It helps some patients but there is no evidence that 5-ASA is superior to placebo for the maintenance of medically induced remission (Akobeng and Gardener, 2005).
- Anti-TNF drugs such as infliximab and adalimumab are considered early for those with severe active disease or those who are steroid dependent as a steroid alternative. They are effective for maintaining remission in Crohn's disease.
- Azathioprine, mercaptopurine and methotrexate are efficacious in inducing remission, but each therapy is limited by time to response, side effects and difficulties surrounding drug withdrawal.

Colonoscopic surveillance

Patients with inflammatory colitis have an increased risk of developing colon cancer. All patients with ulcerative colitis (unless proctitis alone) or Crohn's colitis involving more than one segment of colon should therefore have a colonoscopy 10 years after their symptoms first started and at regular intervals after this.

Patients at low risk of cancer are those with disease confined to the left colon and those with quiescent IBD. Patients with intermediate risk include those with: extensive ulcerative or Crohn's colitis with mild active inflammation, inflammatory polyps or a family history of colorectal cancer in a first-degree relative aged 50 or over.

High-risk patients are those with: extensive ulcerative or Crohn's colitis with moderate or severe active inflammation, primary sclerosing cholangitis (including after liver transplant), a colonic stricture in the past 5 years, a history of any grade of dysplasia in the past 5 years or a family history of colorectal cancer in a first-degree relative aged under 50.

Patients at low risk require a colonoscopy (with chromoscopy) every 5 years, patients with intermediate risk require a colonoscopy every 3 years and those with high risk require yearly colonoscopy.

Case outcome and discharge

Miss Patel received IV hydrocortisone for acute severe colitis, and after 48 hours greatly improved with a stool frequency of three per day and no fever or pain. Flexible sigmoidoscopy and biopsy confirmed non-infective colitis of the sigmoid and descending colon. She had discussions with the surgical team and stoma care nurse, but did not require colectomy on this occasion. Steroids were converted to oral after 72 hours, and the dose weaned from 40 mg oral prednisolone to zero over 8 weeks. As her flare had been severe, she was started on azathioprine as maintenance therapy in addition to the aminosalicylates that she had been taking. She remained in remission for the months after admission. Supplementation with calcium and vitamin D was started to provide bone protection whilst on steroids, and because her levels were found to be on the low side in the community (Homik *et al.*, 2000).

Miss Patel was fortunate in that she reached complete remission after steroids were weaned. However, it is quite common for this not to occur, where around 50% of those who do not enter complete remission with steroids will require colectomy within 1 year (Bojic *et al.*, 2009).

Miss Patel's new prescription is shown. For frequent and prolonged courses of steroids, omeprazole should be given as gastric protection.

Azathioprine for IBD is generally given at a maximum dose of 2–2.5 mg/kg. Miss Patel weighs 65 kg.

DISCHARGE MEDICATION						
Date	Medication	Dose	Route	Frequency	Supply	GP to continue?
xx/xx/xx	PREDNISOLONE	40 mg	PO	Once daily	14 days	Y
xx/xx/xx	ADCAL D3	1 tablet	PO	Once daily	14 days	Y
xx/xx/xx	AZATHIOPRINE	150 mg	PO	Once daily	14 days	Y
xx/xx/xx	MESALAZINE (ASACOL)	800 mg	PO	Three times daily	14 days	Y
xx/xx/xx	MESALAZINE (ASACOL) FOAM ENEMA	1 g	PR	Once daily	14 days	Y

Notes to patient/GP:
Prednisolone wean 5 mg every week, until zero. Mesalazine PR to be taken at times of ulcerative colitis flare, please stop when patient is stable.

Common pitfalls

- NSAIDs are contraindicated in IBD. This is because many studies have found an adverse effect of NSAIDs in precipitating *de novo* IBD or exacerbating pre-existing disease, although the evidence is not always clear (Kefalakes *et al.*, 2009). This is thought to because mucosal damage is mediated by dual inhibition of COX-1 and COX-2. However, selective inhibition with COX-2 inhibitors, or COX-1 inhibition with low-dose aspirin, seems to be safe, particularly where treatment is short term (Takeuchi *et al.*, 2006).
- All anticholinergics, antidiarrhoeal agents and opioid drugs should be stopped in all patients with acute diarrhoea. This is because they are all constipating agents and can increase risk of colonic dilatation.
- Don't forget thromboprophylaxis with LMWH.
- Many patients with IBD (particularly ulcerative colitis) are on 5-ASA preparations to maintain remission. 5-ASA compounds include mesalazine, sulfasalazine, balsalazide and olsalazine. Mesalazine is the most commonly used and is given under lots of different trade names. It is important to get the preparation right as patients are often stable on one type. Mesalazine preparations include Asacol, Salofalk, Ipocol, Mezavant (these all have pH-dependent release) and Pentasa (this is a time-controlled release preparation). Balsalazide and olsalazine release 5-ASA after being split by bacterial enzymes in the large intestine (Mowat *et al.*, 2011).
- It is useful to consider taking the following blood tests in addition to the usual acute bloods, around the time of admission:
  - glucose before steroids are commenced to measure baseline
  - magnesium and cholesterol in case ciclosporin is required
  - thiopurine methyltransferase (TPMT) in case thiopurines such as mercaptopurine or azathioprine are being considered
  - if anti-TNF drugs or azathioprone are being considered, HIV, viral hepatitis and TB need to be tested for before commencement.

An acute severe flare of IBD is a medical and potentially surgical emergency, as toxic megacolon (colonic diameter >5.5 cm or caecum >9 cm) and perforation can occur from severe inflammation of the colon. Ulcerative colitis is the most common type of inflammatory disease of the bowel yet its cause is unknown. It can develop at any age, but peak incidence is between the ages of 15 and 25 years, with a second, smaller peak between 55 and 65 years. Crohn's disease can also affect the colon and cause acute colitis.

Untreated severe ulcerative colitis has a mortality of 24%, but this is reduced to 7% with intravenous corticosteroids and to <1% with timely and expert surgical input (Truelove and Witts, 1955; Rice-Oxley and Truelove, 1950).

Likelihood of requirement for surgery increase if stool frequency is more than eight per day, pyrexia or tachycardia are present, an abdominal X-ray shows colonic dilatation, low albumin, anaemia, high platelets or high CRP (>45 mg/L) are present (Travis *et al.*, 1996).

Admission to hospital is required for all patients fulfilling Truelove and Witts' criteria for severe colitis.

SUMMARY

Key learning points

Acute severe colitis
- The primary focus is resuscitation and exclusion of a surgical emergency such as toxic megacolon/perforation with an erect CXR and AXR.
- Send bloods including CRP, ESR, clotting and group and save.
- Send stool sample for microscopy and culture, as well as for *C. difficile*.
- Severity of colitis should be assessed with the Truelove and Witts' severity index, where any severe criteria require immediate admission.
- Commence IV hydrocortisone.
- Commence low molecular weight heparin for thromboprophylaxis.
- Antibiotics may be given if diagnosis is questioned or infective diarrhoea may be present in addition.
- Early referral to surgeons is required, as colectomy may be recommended if there is no response to IV steroids after 72 hours.
- Expert gastroenterology and surgical advice is required from the beginning of the admission, as induction and maintenance of remission requires specialist decision making and patient consideration.

FURTHER READING

- A very good summary of the management of acute colitis is: Jakobovits SL, Travis SPL (2005). Management of acute severe colitis. *Br Med Bull* 75–76: 131–44.
- The British Society of Gastroenterology has a very useful website with guidelines, information, learning resources and teaching days. Available at: www.bsg.org.uk (accessed Dec. 2015).
- American Gastroenterology Association. Available at: www.gastro.org (accessed Dec. 2015).
- Crohn's and Colitis UK. Available at: www.nacc.org.uk (accessed Dec. 2015).
- Crohn's and Colitis Foundation of America. Available at: www.ccfa.org (accessed Dec. 2015).
- CORE (Digestive Disorders Foundation). Available at: www.corecharity.org.uk (accessed Dec. 2015).
- NHS Choices. Available at: www.nhs.uk (accessed Dec. 2015).
- NHS Evidence. Available at: www.evidence.nhs.uk (accessed Dec. 2015).
- UK Clinical Research Network portfolio (gastrointestinal). Available at: http://public .ukcrn.org.uk (accessed Dec. 2015).

Acute infective diarrhoea

> **Mr Georgios Kosovitsas**
>
> **Age: 38**
>
> **Hospital number: 123456**

🔍 Case study

Presenting complaint: *A 38-year-old man presents to A&E with 48 hours of acute watery diarrhoea 8 times per day and abdominal cramps. He has recently travelled to Morocco. He has had no recent antibiotics and no contact with anyone else unwell.*

Background: *Mr Kosovitsas is a banker, usually independent and active, smokes 15 cigarettes per day*

PMH: *Gastro-oesophageal reflux disease, no known abdominal pathology, appendicitis age 12*

Allergies: *None*

FH: *Nil*

Examination:
Pulse 110, BP 110/62, Sats 97% on air, RR 18, BM 5, temp 38°C

CVS: *Capillary refill time 1 seconds, pulse feels regular, JVP not seen, no oedema, HS I + II + 0*

RS: *Equal expansion with air entry to both bases and no added sounds*

Abdo: *Soft, generally tender, no masses palpated, bowel sounds present, no peritonism*

Neuro: *Moving all 4 limbs, alert, mobile
No rashes*

ECG: *Sinus tachycardia*

Bloods: *Hb 120, Plt 400, WCC 12.9, Na 138, K 4.3, Urea 6.0, Creat 100, INR 1.1 ALT 35, AlkP 90, alb 38, amylase 70*

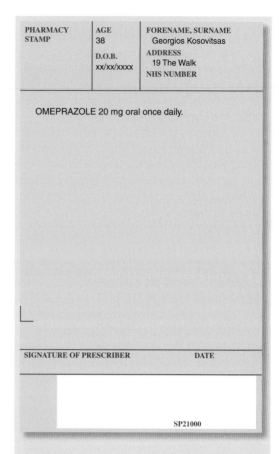

| PHARMACY STAMP | AGE 38 | FORENAME, SURNAME Georgios Kosovitsas |
| | D.O.B. xx/xx/xxxx | ADDRESS 19 The Walk NHS NUMBER |

OMEPRAZOLE 20 mg oral once daily.

SIGNATURE OF PRESCRIBER   DATE

SP21000

Diagnosis

Acute travellers diarrhoea is the most likely cause given the short history, recent travel and fever. This is likely to be a viral, bacterial or protozoal infection from contaminated food or water. Common bacterial infections include *Escherichia coli*, *Salmonella* species, *Shigella* species and *Campylobacter* species (Table 5.2). Common enteroviruses include norovirus and rotavirus. Common protozoal infections include *Cryptosporidium* species, *Giardia lamblia*, *Entamoeba histolytica* and *Cyclospora* species. Forty percent of travellers' diarrhoea cases never have a causative pathogen identified (Peltola and Gorbach, 1997). Serious bacterial infections include *Escherichia coli* 0157 (enterotoxigenic *E. coli*) and *Shigella* (bacterial dysentery), as these can cause profound dehydration and systemic effects such as hae-molytic uraemic syndrome in the case of *E. coli* 0157. However, any cause of diarrhoea can be serious in a vulnerable patient such as the very young or old. If there had been recent antibiotic use or the patient has been in hospital recently, *C. difficile* should be considered. This can be life-threatening in the elderly, immunosup-pressed or those with multiple co-morbidities.

Other differentials for diarrhoea include IBD first presentation, irritable bowel syn-drome and bile salt malabsorption. Infection can also occur in addition to these pathologies.

Travellers' diarrhoea

Classic travellers' diarrhoea is defined as three or more unformed stools within 24 hours, often accompanied by one or more of: fever, nausea, vomiting, cramps, tenesmus or bloody stools (dysentery). Symptoms usually start during or shortly after foreign travel (Al Abri *et al.*, 2005). The illness is often mild and self-limit-ing, usually lasting 3–5 days; however, illness severity varies depending on the individual and causative pathogen.

Clostridium difficile infection

Clostridium difficile is a Gram-positive obligate anaerobe that can form spores. These spores can survive outside the body on clothes and

surfaces, and facilitate spread and antibiotic resistance. *C. difficile* is the most important cause of hospital-acquired diarrhoea. It col-onises where the natural bacterial flora of the bowel has been cleared by recent antibiotic therapy, in patients who are vulnerable with other infections or where patients are immu-nocompromised, for example from recent chemotherapy. It produces exotoxins A and B. Particular antibiotics that lead to increased risk of *C. difficile* infection include clindamy-cin, amoxicillin and cephalosporins. Other risk factors include extremes of age (over 80% of *C. difficile* infections occur in those over 65 years), recent GI surgery, prolonged hospital stays and malignancy.

Treatment for *C. difficile* differs according to classification of mild/moderate or severe. However, there is no widespread consensus definition for severe infection. The Society for Healthcare Epidemiology of America (SHEA) and the Infectious Diseases Society of America (IDSA) guidelines, as recommended by the Centres for Disease Control and Prevention (CDC), classify 'severe' as a white cell count of 15 000 cells/mL or higher, or a serum cre-atinine level greater than or equal to 1.5 times the premorbid level (see Guidelines). These criteria are based on expert opinion and are therefore not prospectively validated severity scores.

Public Health England (Wilcox, 2013) recommends using the following markers of severity: WCC $>15 \times 10^9$/L, acutely rising blood creatinine (e.g. >50% increase above baseline), temperature >38.5°C, evidence of severe colitis (abdominal signs, radiology) (see Guidelines).

Other definitions for severe *C. difficile* infection have included stool count, albumin and advancing age (Zar *et al.*, 2007; Louie *et al.*, 2006; Pépin *et al.*, 2004; Loo *et al.*, 2005).

Please refer to individual Trust guidelines for the specific hospital policy on this, as it will guide treatment decisions.

Please also see Chapter 11 regarding *C. dif-ficile* infection and treatment.

Table 5.2 Incubation periods for common infections.

	Incubation period
Campylobacter	Up to 10 days
Cryptosporidium	1–12 days
E. coli 0157	1–14 days
Giardia	7–10 days
Salmonella	6–72 hour
Shigellosis (bacterial dysentery)	1–7 days

Source: Public Health England. Available at: www.hpa.org.uk.

(*Continued*)

Case study (Continued)

Initial measures

This patient should be assessed with the standard ABCD approach for an unwell patient, with a thorough history taken. He is young with no serious co-morbidities, and if he is haemodynamically stable with no biochemical signs of dehydration, he may be able to go home to be managed as an outpatient. Priorities for him need to be sending a full set of bloods including CRP and sending a stool sample for microscopy and culture. As he is febrile and tachycardic in an ED setting, IV fluids for correction of dehydration could be given whilst he is waiting for results.

If he had any signs of peritonism, an abdominal X-ray should be ordered and admission arranged.

If the presentation was different, for example if he were elderly, had had recent antibiotics or a recent hospital stay, or was admitted from another healthcare institution, *C. difficile* should be considered. All inciting antibiotics should be stopped.

! Guidelines

- The Health Protection Agency has published a report on *Foreign Travel-Associated Illness: a Focus on Travellers' Diarrhoea*, 2010. This focuses on likely infection aetiologies for different areas, and public health considerations. Available at: http://webarchive .nationalarchives.gov.uk/20140714084352/ http://www.hpa.org.uk/webc/HPAwebFile/ HPAweb_C/1287146380314 (accessed Dec. 2015).
- The Health Protection Agency has published a report *Clostridium Difficile Infection: Guidance on Management and Treatment*, 2013. Available at: www.gov.uk/government/uploads/ system/uploads/attachment_data/file/321891/ Clostridium_difficile_management_and_ treatment.pdf (accessed Dec. 2015).
- The CDC has published: *Clinical Practice Guidelines for Clostridium Difficile Infection in Adults*, 2010. Available at: www.cdc.gov/ HAI/pdfs/cdiff/Cohen-IDSA-SHEA-CDI-guidelines-2010.pdf (accessed Dec. 2015).

- The American College of Gastroenterology has published: *Guidelines for Diagnosis, Treatment, and Prevention of Clostridium difficile Infections*, 2013. Available at: http://gi.org/guideline/diagnosis-and-management-of-c-difficile-associated-diarrhea-and-colitis/ (accessed Dec. 2015).

Prescribing for acute infective diarrhoea

Management of acute diarrhoea differs according to whether it is considered to be travellers diarrhoea/ gastroenteritis, or whether it is thought to be *C. difficile* infection. *C. difficile* infection would be very unlikely in this patient.

Travellers diarrhoea/gastroenteritis with unknown causative pathogen

REGULAR PRESCRIPTIONS

				Circle/enter times below ↓	↘ Enter dates below			
					Day 1	Day 2	Day 3	Day 4
DRUG CIPROFLOXACIN				06				
				(08)				
Dose 500 mg	Route PO	Freq BD for 1 week	Start date xx/xx/xx	12				
Signature A. Doctor		Bleep	Review	16				
Additional instructions				18				
				(22)				
DRUG METRONIDAZOLE				06				
				(08)				
Dose 400 mg	Route PO	Freq TDS for 1 week	Start date xx/xx/xx	12				
Signature A. Doctor		Bleep	Review	(14)				
Additional instructions				18				
				(22)				
DRUG PARACETAMOL				(06)				
				08				
Dose 1 g	Route IV/PO	Freq QDS	Start date xx/xx/xx	(12)				
Signature A. Doctor		Bleep	Review	16				
Additional instructions				(18)				
				(24)				

FLUID CHART

Date	Fluid	Dose	Route	Time to be given	Signature	Print name
xx/xx/xx	SODIUM CHLORIDE 0.9%	500 ml	IV	Over 2 hours	A. Doctor	A. Doctor

If the patient is to be discharged, oral rehydration salts can be recommended instead of IV fluids. These are easily bought over the counter and consist of a salt and sugar powder that is diluted and ingested. Antinausea drugs may also be required for gastroenteritis with a vomiting component.

Suspected C. difficile infection

- Mild–moderate infection: metronidazole should usually be give for 10–14 days.

REGULAR PRESCRIPTIONS

				Circle/enter times below ↓	↘ Enter dates below			
					Day 1	Day 2	Day 3	Day 4
DRUG METRONIDAZOLE				06				
				⑧				
Dose 400 mg	Route PO	Freq TDS	Start date xx/xx/xx	12				
Signature A. Doctor		Bleep	Review	⑭				
Additional instructions				18				
				㉒				
DRUG PARACETAMOL				⑥				
				08				
Dose 1 g	Route IV/PO	Freq QDS	Start date xx/xx/xx	⑫				
Signature A. Doctor		Bleep	Review	16				
Additional instructions				⑱				
				㉔				

FLUID CHART

Date	Fluid	Dose	Route	Time to be given	Signature	Print name
xx/xx/xx	SODIUM CHLORIDE 0.9%	500 ml	IV	Over 2 hours	A. Doctor	A. Doctor

- Severe infection: vancomycin should usually be given for 10–14 days.

FLUID CHART

Date	Fluid	Dose	Route	Time to be given	Signature	Print name
xx/xx/xx	SODIUM CHLORIDE 0.9%	500 ml	IV	Over 4 hours	A. Doctor	A. Doctor

REGULAR PRESCRIPTIONS

				Circle/enter times below ↓	↘ Enter dates below			
					Day 1	Day 2	Day 3	Day 4
DRUG VANCOMYCIN				⑥				
				08				
Dose 125 mg	Route PO	Freq QDS	Start date xx/xx/xx	⑫				
Signature A. Doctor		Bleep	Review	16				
Additional instructions				⑱				
				㉔				
DRUG PARACETAMOL				⑥				
				08				
Dose 1 g	Route IV/PO	Freq QDS	Start date xx/xx/xx	⑫				
Signature A. Doctor		Bleep	Review	16				
Additional instructions				⑱				
				㉔				

FLUID CHART

Date	Fluid	Dose	Route	Time to be given	Signature	Print name
xx/xx/xx	SODIUM CHLORIDE 0.9%	500 ml	IV	Over 2 hours	A. Doctor	A. Doctor

- Severe infection with complications such as hypotension, shock, ileus, toxic megacolon.

REGULAR PRESCRIPTIONS

				Circle/enter times below ↓	↘ Enter dates below			
					Day 1	Day 2	Day 3	Day 4
DRUG METRONIDAZOLE				06				
				⑧				
Dose 500 mg	Route IV	Freq TDS	Start date xx/xx/xx	12				
Signature A. Doctor		Bleep	Review	⑭				
Additional instructions				18				
				㉒				
DRUG VANCOMYCIN				⑥				
				08				
Dose 500 mg	Route PO/NG	Freq QDS	Start date xx/xx/xx	⑫				
Signature A. Doctor		Bleep	Review	16				
Additional instructions				⑱				
				㉔				
DRUG PARACETAMOL				⑥				
				08				
Dose 1 g	Route IV/PO	Freq QDS	Start date xx/xx/xx	⑫				
Signature A. Doctor		Bleep	Review	16				
Additional instructions				⑱				
				㉔				

FLUID CHART

Date	Fluid	Dose	Route	Time to be given	Signature	Print name
xx/xx/xx	SODIUM CHLORIDE 0.9%	500 ml	IV	Over 2 hours	A. Doctor	A. Doctor

These treatment guidelines vary between trusts, particularly as definitions for mild, moderate and severe infection differ.

Metronidazole: rationale and evidence

Metronidazole is a nitroimidazole antibiotic drug with high activity against anaerobic bacteria and protozoa. It is therefore used for trichomonal vaginitis, bacterial vaginosis, *Entamoeba histolytica* and *Giardia lamblia* infections as well as *C. difficile* infections. It is also used in surgical and gynaecological sepsis because of its activity against colonic anaerobes such as *Bacteroides fragilis*.

For infective diarrhoea including *C. difficile* infections, oral metronidazole is preferable; however, IV treatment is also effective.

🔍 Evidence

Metronidazole for mild C. difficile
Metronidazole has been shown to be as effective as oral vancomycin in mild to moderate *C. difficile* (Zar et al., 2007; Louie et al., 2007; Bouza et al., 2008).

✓ DRUGS checklist for METRONIDAZOLE

Dose	400 mg
Route	PO
Units	mg
Given	TDS
Special situations	Can be given IV (500 mg TDS) if oral is not tolerated. Causes nausea and taste disturbances. Has a disulfiram-like reaction with alcohol. Metronidazole is an enzyme inhibitor and may therefore interact with other medications, notably warfarin. Dose reduction in severe hepatic impairment: give 400 mg (PO) or 500 mg (IV) **once daily**.

Metronidazole: essential pharmacology

Metronidazole works by inhibition of nucleic acid synthesis by disrupting the DNA of microbial cells. It is bactericidal, amoebicidal and trichomoncidal. Metronidazole is only effective once it is partially reduced by low-redox-potential electron transfer proteins (e.g. nitroreductases such as ferredoxin). The reduction product is cytotoxic with antimicrobial effects. Reduction of metronidazole only occurs in anaerobic cells; this is why it has relatively little effect upon aerobic bacteria.

Metronidazole distributes widely in body tissues; it crosses the blood–brain barrier, crosses the placenta and appears in the saliva and breast milk of lactating mothers at plasma concentration. It also reaches therapeutic concentrations in the bile and the cerebrospinal fluid. It is considered one of the main essential antibiotics by the World Health Organisation.

Metronidazole is metabolised by hepatic oxidation and caution is advised in patients with severe hepatic insufficiency. No dose reduction is needed in patients with renal impairment.

Ciprofloxacin: rationale and evidence

Ciprofloxacin is a broad-spectrum fluoroquinolone antibiotic, particularly effective for infections caused by Gram-negative bacteria, including *Salmonella, Shigella, Campylobacter, Neisseria* and *Pseudomonas*. It is therefore often used for urinary tract infections, sexually transmitted diseases (gonorrhoea and chancroid), skin and bone infections, gastrointestinal infections, intra-abdominal infections (combined with an antianaerobic agent), some lower respiratory tract infections (particularly in pseudomonal infections), febrile neutropenia (combined with Gram-positive bacterial agent) and malignant external otitis. It also is effective for some Gram-positive bacterial infections, such as those caused by *Streptococcus pneumoniae* and *Enterococcus faecalis*. It has good tissue penetration (Davis *et al.*, 1996).

✓ DRUGS checklist for CIPROFLOXACIN

Dose	500 mg
Route	PO
Units	mg
Given	Twice daily, continued for 10–14 days
Special situations	Can be given IV at a dose of 400 mg. However, as it is the GI tract that is the target in this instance, and additionally it is very irritant to veins, the oral route is preferential.

Ciprofloxacin: essential pharmacology

Please see ciprofloxacin in Section Upper Gastrointestinal Haemorrhage.

Vancomycin: rationale and evidence

Vancomycin is an aminoglycoside antibiotic with bactericidal activity against aerobic and anaerobic Gram-positive bacteria, including multiresistant staphylococci. It is therefore used IV for Gram-positive infections such as endocarditis and methicillin-resistant *Staphylococcus aureus* (MRSA) infections. It is also effective for *C. difficile* diarrhoea when used orally. This is an ineffective route for other types of infection as there is little systemic absorption of vancomycin from the gut.

For patients with severe *C. difficile* infection, oral vancomycin is used instead of metronidazole due to the relatively high failure rates of metronidazole seen in recent reports. Vancomycin also gives a faster clinical response compared to metronidazole (Wilcox and Howe, 1995; Musher *et al.*, 2005; Lahue and Davidson, 2007; Zar *et al.*, 2007).

🔍 Evidence

Vancomycin for severe *Clostridium difficile* infection

Two double-blind randomised studies reported that vancomycin is superior to metronidazole in severe cases of *C. difficile* infection (Louie *et al.*, 2007; Bouza *et al.*, 2008). A pooled analysis of these two phase 3 studies has shown that metronidazole was overall inferior to vancomycin (Johnson *et al.*, 2012).

✓ DRUGS checklist for VANCOMYCIN

Dose	125 mg
Route	PO/NG
Units	mg
Given	QDS
Special situations	Dose can be increased to 500 mg QDS in patients who are worsening or have signs of severe colitis.
	Intracolonic vancomycin (500 mg in 100–500 mL saline 4–12 hourly) can be given as a retention enema. This involves administering the drug via a Foley catheter per rectum with the 30 mL balloon inflated and catheter clamped. After 60 minutes the balloon is deflated and catheter removed (Apisarnthanarak *et al.*, 2002).
	The make-up of this prescription is an IV powder for reconstitution; however, it is licensed to give this compound orally for *C. difficile* treatment.

Vancomycin: essential pharmacology

Vancomycin acts by inhibiting cell wall synthesis in Gram-positive bacteria. It does this by forming hydrogen bonds with peptides in the cell wall, preventing synthesis of *N*-acetylmuramic acid (NAM) and *N*-acetylglucosamine (NAG). These are long polymers that are essential for formation of the backbone structure of the bacterial cell wall. Without these proteins the cell wall structure is compromised.

Gram-negative bacteria have a different cell wall synthesis mechanism, hence vancomycin is not active against most of these (one exception being some non-gonococcal species of *Neisseria*).

Cautions with vancomycin

Vancomycin has a narrow therapeutic window, where different plasma concentrations are sought depending on severity of infection. Vancomycin trough levels should be taken before the third dose, and then subsequently depending on levels and individual hospital policy. Even at therapeutic levels, vancomycin is a well known nephrotoxin. Patients with pre-existing reduced creatinine clearance will accumulate vancomycin more quickly and exacerbate their renal failure. This is why levels are so important, as much harm can be done with vancomycin.

Aminoglycosides are also ototoxic, where the risk is likely to increase if plasma levels are high. Tinnitus and reduced hearing warrant immediate cessation of vancomycin.

When given by fast IV, vancomycin has a high incidence of 'red man syndrome'. This consists of pain, thrombophlebitis, flushing and red rash around 10 minutes after completion of the infusion. This is an allergic reaction due to non-specific mast cell degranulation and is not IgE-mediated. Occasionally, anaphylaxis can occur.

For this reason vancomycin must be given by slow IV infusion over at least 60 minutes (maximum rate of 10 mg/min for doses >500 mg). This reduces the incidence of problems, but in sensitive individuals antihistamines can be given as treatment and prevention or red man syndrome.

Other medications used in infective diarrhoea

There are a number of other medications considered in patients with diarrhoea, particularly in *C. difficile*. This is because about 20% of patients treated initially with either metronidazole or vancomycin for *C. difficile* will have a recurrence, so there is much focus on prevention of a repeat episode (Teasley *et al.*, 1983; Bartlett, 1985; Wenisch *et al.*, 1996).

Probiotics

The rationale behind giving probiotics is that they will help to replenish more quickly the natural commensal bacterial flora of the gut, thus preventing colonisation of *C. difficile* and harmful pathogens. There is, however, no convincing evidence that this is effective in treating or preventing *C. difficile* infection.

One randomised, double-blind, placebo-controlled trial showed a beneficial effect of using yoghurt as prophylaxis in patients receiving antibiotics (Hickson *et al.*, 2007). However, the study had major methodological flaws threatening the validity and generalisability of the study (Wilcox and Sandoe, 2007). A systematic review and meta-analysis found that more research is needed to determine which probiotics are most efficacious, for which patients and in relation to which antibiotics (Hempel *et al.*, 2012).

Fidaxomicin

Fidaxomicin is a macrocyclic antibacterial that exerts its activity in the gastrointestinal tract, as it is very poorly absorbed into the systemic circulation. It has a narrow spectrum of antibacterial activity, mainly directed against *C. difficile,* with some moderate activity against other Gram-positive species.

Oral fidaxomicin was approved for the treatment of *C. difficile* infection in Europe in 2012 (Johnson and Wilcox, 2012; Wilcox, 2012).

It should be considered for patients with *C. difficile* infection who have had recurrent infection or are considered at high risk for recurrence, as it is superior for prevention of recurrent infection (see Evidence). Those at risk of recurrence include elderly patients with multiple co-morbidities who are receiving concomitant antibiotics (Hu *et al.*, 2009; Wilcox, 2012).

It should also be considered for severe infection where symptoms are not improving on initial treatment, depending on local policy and expertise.

Evidence

Fidaxomicin for *Clostridium difficile* infection
Evidence from two double-blind, randomised controlled trials indicated that fidaxomicin is non-inferior to vancomycin in curing patients with mild to severe *C. difficile* infection. Its side-effect profile appears similar to that of oral vancomycin and it may have advantages in reducing the rate of recurrence. The cost is considerably higher than vancomycin (Louie *et al.*, 2011; Cornely *et al.*, 2012).

A 2011 systematic review concluded that no antimicrobial agent is clearly superior for the initial cure of *C. difficile* infection, but that recurrence is less frequent with fidaxomicin than with vancomycin (Drekonja *et al.*, 2011).

✓ DRUGS checklist for FIDAXOMICIN

Dose	200 mg
Route	PO
Units	mg
Given	Twice daily
Special situations	Give for 10–14 days.

Guidelines

NICE. *Clostridium difficile Infection: Fidaxomicin*, ESNM1, 2012. Available at: www.nice.org.uk/Advice/ESNM1 (accessed Dec. 2015).

Further aspects of acute infective diarrhoea management

Faecal transplant for C. difficile infection

Faecal transplant has been trialled as a method of restoring natural gut bacterial flora to patients with *C. difficile* infection, to help treat infection and prevent recurrence. A systematic review concluded that faecal transplant by infusion of fresh faeces in normal saline via enema was highly effective at achieving resolution of recurrent *C. difficile* infection (92% resolved), with few adverse effects (Gough *et al.*, 2011).

A randomised study of faecal transplantation for recurrent *C. difficile* infection showed significantly less chance of recurrence compared to vancomycin with or without bowel lavage (van Nood *et al.*, 2013).

This is generally used as a last resort due to practical difficulty, aesthetic concerns, patient reluctance and lack of a cost-effectiveness evaluation. Costs are due to complexity of the procedure (donor testing, consenting, sample processing and endoscopy).

Prevention of spread

Patients with any diarrhoeal or vomiting illness need to be advised to stay off work, school or nursery until they have been free from any symptoms for at least 48 hours. Patients or anyone in contact with someone with diarrhoea and vomiting must not prepare food or visit healthcare establishments during this time.

Those with diarrhoeal symptoms who are inpatients must be isolated in side rooms or designated bays, with standard infection control precautions taken (glove, aprons, handwashing).

Meticulous hand and equipment hygiene is required, as *C. difficile* spores can survive on surfaces and are not killed by alcohol gel.

Other drugs implicated in C. difficile infection

See HPA guidance (Wilcox, 2013).

There is increasing evidence that acid-suppressing medications may be a risk factor for *C. difficile* infection, including H_2 receptor antagonists and in particular PPIs (Dial *et al.*, 2005, 2006; Howell *et al.*, 2010; Janarthanan *et al.*, 2012).

This association is not proven, as it may have been confounded by other *C. difficile* infection risk factors (Cohen *et al.*, 2010). However, these findings warrant review of PPI therapy to ensure that it is still required, particularly in those with or at high risk of *C. difficile* infection.

Case outcome and discharge

Mr Kosovitsas was discharged with oral antibiotics and oral rehydration salts and made a full recovery within 3 days. Stool culture came back as a *Salmonella* (non-typhoid) species. Treated travellers diarrhoea is unlikely to recur, unless reinfection occurs.

If Mr Kosovitsas had had *C. difficile* infection, he would have been at higher risk of recurrence, as recurrent *C. difficile* infection occurs in around 15–30% of patients treated with metronidazole or vancomycin (Teasley *et al.*, 1983; Bartlett, 1985; Wenisch *et al.*, 1996). Some of these recurrences are reinfections (20–50%), and some are relapses due to the same strain (where relapses tend to occur in the first 2 weeks after treatment cessation)(Wilcox *et al.*, 1998). After a first recurrence, the risk of another infection increases to 45–60% (McFarland *et al.*, 1999).

Even though Mr Kosovitsas did not have *C. difficile* infection, his prescription for omeprazole was reviewed and decided that he should stop taking this due to resolution of GORD symptoms.

There is no evidence that metronidazole or vancomycin are effective in preventing *C. difficile* infection, and in fact this therapy may actually increase risk.

Mr Kosovitsas's new prescription is shown. Note omeprazole has been stopped.

DISCHARGE MEDICATION						
Date	Medication	Dose	Route	Frequency	Supply	GP to continue?
xx/xx/xx	CIPROFLOXACIN	500 mg	PO	Twice daily	1 week	N
xx/xx/xx	METRONIDAZOLE	400 mg	PO	Three times daily	1 week	N

Notes to patient/GP:
Omeprazole stopped as no longer required.

Common pitfalls

- Metronidazole causes severe nausea and vomiting (disulfiram reaction) with alcohol; patients need to be aware of this.

- Vancomycin given orally is actually a preparation for injection (powder for reconstitution) which is given by mouth. This can be confusing if nursing staff are not familiar with *C. difficile* treatment.
- *C. difficile* testing consists of antigen and toxin testing. Those with antigen positivity need treatment; however, if *C. difficile* toxin is positive but antigen is negative and the patient is well, they do **not** require treatment.

- *C. difficile* spores are not killed by alcohol gel, hence hand washing with soap is vital to prevent spread.
- Constipating agents such as loperamide and opiates are generally avoided in *C. difficile* due to theoretical increased risk of colonic dilation and toxic megacolon. However, there is not convincing evidence that these therapies cause harm (Wilcox and Howe, 1995).

SUMMARY

Acute travellers diarrhoea commonly presents with a short history of diarrhoea and/or vomiting, recent travel and fever. It is generally due to a viral, bacterial or protozoal infection from contaminated food or water. Estimates as to the causative pathogen can be made according to the area of travel. Although it is usually self-limiting, any cause of diarrhoea can be serious in a vulnerable patient such as the very young or old.

If there had been recent antibiotic use, a recent hospital/residential home stay, previous *C. difficile* infection or general frailty in a vulnerable patient then *C. difficile* should be considered. This can be life-threatening in the elderly, immunosuppressed or those with multiple co-morbidities.

Other differentials for diarrhoea include IBD first presentation, irritable bowel syndrome and bile salt malabsorption. Infection can also occur in addition to these pathologies.

Key diagnostic aids include the taking of careful history including a travel, sexual and contact history, taking stool cultures, monitoring of symptoms and disease progression, blood tests for infection and inflammatory markers and flexible sigmoidoscopy.

🔑 Key learning points

Acute travellers' diarrhoea

- This is usually self-limiting. If the patient is dehydrated or frail and needs admission, then IV fluids with monitoring of renal function and CRP is required.
- Give oral ciprofloxacin and metronidazole for 7-10 days.
- Send stool for culture, as *E .coli* 0157 and typhoid can be more serious, as well as to rule out *Clostridium difficile*.

Suspected *Clostridium difficile* diarrhoea

- If this is suspected due to recent antibiotic use, prolonged hospital stay, previous infection or general frailty in a vulnerable patient then this needs treatment.
- Send stool sample for culture, as well as for *C. difficile*.
- Mild *C. difficile* symptoms can be treated with oral metronidazole.
- Severe symptoms should be treated with oral vancomycin.
- If it is recurrent or severe infection, fidaxomycin may be considered according to local gastroenterology team opinion.
- As in all forms of colitis, flexible sigmoidoscopy may be recommended by the gastroenterology team. In the case of *C. difficile* infection this would show pseudomembranous colitis.
- Surgical input may be required if signs of colonic dilatation or toxic megacolon develop.
- All patients with infective diarrhoea must be isolated away from other patients, with meticulous hand hygiene and infection control measures in place.

Acute hepatitis

Mr Gerald de Souza

Age: 42

Hospital number: 123456

🔍 Case study

Presenting complaint: *A 42-year-old man presents to A&E with a week's history of nausea and anorexia, he has now noticed jaundiced sclera and skin. His friend says he is more drowsy than usual*

Background: *Mr de Souza is from Portugal and is unemployed at present living in a hostel for the homeless. He is usually independent and active, he smokes 15 cigarettes per day and denies illicit drug use but admits 'heavy' alcohol consumption with a recent intake of more than usual over the past week (1 bottle of vodka per day)*

PMH: *Gastro-oesophageal reflux disease, nil else diagnosed. Liver function tests done at the GP 6 months ago showed an ALT in the normal range.*

Allergies: *None*

FH: *Unknown*

Examination:
Pulse 110, BP 95/62, Sats 97% on air, RR 18, BM 5, temp 36°C

CVS: *Capillary refill time 1 second, pulse feels regular, JVP not seen, no oedema, HS I + II + 0*

RS: *Equal expansion with air entry to both bases and no added sounds*

Abdo: *Soft, tender RUQ, no guarding, no masses palpated, bowel sounds present*

Neuro: *Moving all 4 limbs, drowsy but easily rousable with GCS 15. Mobile*
No rashes. No focal neurology.
Sweating with some signs of alcohol withdrawal

ECG: *Sinus tachycardia*

Bloods: *Hb 120, Plt 300, WCC 10.9, Na 138, K 4,3, Urea 6.0, Creat 100, PT 18 seconds, Bili 40, ALT 300, AST 465, AlkP 90, alb 25, amylase 70*
Paracetamol blood level 0
USS liver: no gallstones seen, common bile duct non-dilated, heterogeneous inflammation of liver with evidence of cirrhosis, no ascites, no masses

PHARMACY STAMP	AGE 42	FORENAME, SURNAME Gerald de Souza
	D.O.B. xx/xx/xxxx	ADDRESS Hillside House, Castle Street NHS NUMBER

OMEPRAZOLE 20 mg oral once daily.

SIGNATURE OF PRESCRIBER   DATE

SP21000

(Continued)

Case study (*Continued*)

Diagnosis

Acute alcoholic hepatitis. This specific aetiology of the hepatitis diagnosis is most likely given the relatively short history of illness in the context of recent very high alcohol consumption. The patient has acutely raised transaminases (AST>ALT is a common feature of alcoholic hepatitis) with no signs of common bile duct obstruction on ultrasound scan. Worryingly, however, he also signs of synthetic dysfunction of the liver (low albumin and prolonged PT) raising concern about underlying cirrhosis and development of liver failure. He is drowsy, suggesting early/ grade 1 encephalopathy but alternative causes of this must be considered. Specifically subdural haemorrhage (enquire about history of falls), sepsis and deranged electrolytes must be considered.

Other less likely possibilities include acute viral hepatitis, drug-related hepatitis (always consider paracetamol), autoimmune hepatitis, ischaemic hepatitis (unlikely if no pain) and malignancy.

Initial assessment must therefore include a thorough history including sexual and drug history, family history, recent medications and over the counter medications as well as mental health state.

Alcoholic liver disease is a large burden on healthcare resources; alcohol related disorders may account for as much as 9.2% of all disability-adjusted life years according to the World Health Organization's Global Information System on Alcohol and Health (WHO, 2013).

Hepatic Encephalopathy Score (West Haven criteria)

- Grade 1 – General lack of awareness; euphoria or anxiety; shortened attention span; impaired performance of addition or subtraction
- Grade 2 – Lethargy or apathy; minimal disorientation for time or place; subtle personality change; inappropriate behaviour
- Grade 3 – Somnolence to semistupor, but responsive to verbal stimuli; confusion; gross disorientation
- Grade 4 – Coma (unresponsive to verbal or noxious stimuli)

(Cash *et al.*, 2010; Ferenci *et al.*, 2002).

Initial measures

This patient should be assessed with the standard ABCD approach for an unwell patient, with a thorough history taken. Priorities are IV access with a full set of 'liver screen' bloods (including viral hepatitis screen , paracetamol levels, autoimmune screen, ferritin and caeruloplasmin). CT head would exclude an intracranial haemorrhage as a cause for his drowsiness.

⊘ Guidelines

- The American College of Gastroenterology has guidelines on alcoholic liver disease management (O'Shea *et al.*, 2010).
- European Association for the Study of the Liver has guidelines on alcoholic liver disease: *EASL Clinical Practical Guidelines: Management of Alcoholic Liver Disease* (EASL, 2012). Available at: www.easl.eu/research/our-contributions/clinical-practice-guidelines/detail/management-of-alcoholic-liver-disease/report/1 (accessed Dec. 2015).

Prescribing for acute hepatitis

Management of hepatitis is supportive in all cases, with more specific medications depending on the aetiology of hepatitis. In this case the patient probably has alcoholic hepatitis with encephalopathy and alcohol withdrawal.

REGULAR PRESCRIPTIONS

DRUG LACTULOSE				Circle/enter times below ↓	Day 1	Day 2	Day 3	Day 4
				06				
				⑧				
Dose 2 ml	Route PO	Freq BD	Start date xx/xx/xx	12				
Signature A. Doctor		Bleep	Review	16				
Additional instructions				⑳				
				22				

DRUG VITAMIN K					06				
				⑧				
Dose 10 mg	Route IV	Freq OD	Start date xx/xx/xx	12				
Signature A. Doctor		Bleep	Review	16				
Additional instructions Give for 3 days				18				
				22				

DRUG PABRINEX					06				
				⑧				
Dose 2 pairs	Route IV	Freq BD	Start date xx/xx/xx	12				
Signature A. Doctor		Bleep	Review	16				
Additional instructions Give for 3 days				⑱				
				22				

DRUG CHLORDIAZEPOXIDE					⑥				
				08				
Dose 4 mg	Route PO	Freq QDS	Start date xx/xx/xx	⑫				
Signature A. Doctor		Bleep	Review	16				
Additional instructions Wean dose daily				⑱				
				㉒				

✓ **DRUGS checklist for LACTULOSE for hepatic encephalopathy**

Dose	10–30 mL
Route	PO
Units	mg
Given	BD
Special situations	Titrate up to keep bowels moving twice daily.

Lactulose: essential pharmacology

Lactose is metabolised in the colon by bacteria in the stool. This results in lactic and acetic acid production, which acidifies the stool, encouraging absorption of ammonia into the colon. The ammonia is then excreted, lowering the amount absorbed into the blood stream.

Vitamin K: rationale and evidence

Vitamin K is a group of fat-soluble vitamins of similar structure. They are all 2-methyl-1,4-naphthoquinone (3-) derivatives. They are required in the body as a crucial element in the functioning of the coagulation cascade. As vitamin K is lipid soluble it is stored in fat tissue with other lipid-soluble vitamins A, D and E.

The importance of vitamin K in clotting is shown by the large effect that warfarin (a vitamin K antagonist) has on the ability of a patient to form clots. Warfarin blocks recycling of vitamin K and creates a deficiency of the active vitamin. This causes powerful inhibition of the coagulation cascade and has been used therapeutically for many years (see Chapter 16).

In liver disease there is prolongation of the INR due to hepatic synthetic dysfunction. The pathogenesis is not vitamin K deficiency. Therefore giving vitamin K may have zero effect on the INR. However, some articles describe a vitamin K deficiency state in cirrhosis due to mechanisms including bile salt deficiency, bile salt secretory failure and the use of broad-spectrum antibiotics (Amarapurkar and Amarapurkar, 2011). It also becomes much easier to interpret an increasing INR if vitamin K is

Lactulose: rationale and evidence

Lactulose is a disaccharide and osmotic laxative. It is used for hepatic encephalopathy because it reduces plasma ammonia concentrations, which are likely to be a key component in causing encephalopathy in patients with liver cirrhosis. The effectiveness of lactulose in encephalopathy is controversial (Als-Nielsen *et al.*, 2004; Shawcross and Jalan, 2004).

🔍 **Evidence**

Lactulose for hepatic encephalopathy
A Cochrane review concluded that there was insufficient evidence to determine whether lactulose and lactitol are of benefit for hepatic encephalopathy. It remains first-line treatment despite this (Cash *et al.*, 2010). For acute liver failure, it is also unclear whether lactulose is beneficial (Als-Nielsen *et al.*, 2004).

replaced. This is important because if vitamin K has been replaced, any further deterioration in INR can be attributed to worsening liver disease. This is especially important in, for example, paracetamol overdose when consideration for referral to transplant is made on the basis of liver failure development, one indicator of which is increasing INR.

Additionally, alcoholic patients may often also have poor diets low in green vegetables, hence a degree of their coagulopathy may be due to vitamin K deficiency resulting from malnutrition.

Evidence

Vitamin K for coagulopathy in liver disease
Vitamin K therapy does not cause significant improvements in the majority of coagulation parameters and hence does not seem to be routinely indicated in patients with liver disease (Saja *et al.*, 2013).

✓ DRUGS checklist for VITAMIN K

Dose	10 mg
Route	IV
Units	mg
Given	Usually given for 3 consecutive days to ensure adequate replacement (Amarapurkar and Amarapurkar, 2011)
Special situations	None

Vitamin K: essential pharmacology

Vitamin K modifies proteins required for blood coagulation by allowing them to bind calcium ions. This is via carboxylation of glutamate residues in proteins to form gamma-carboxyglutamate (Gla) residues. Gla residues are usually involved in binding calcium, and are essential for the biological activity of all known Gla proteins (Furie *et al.*, 1999). Gla proteins are essential for blood coagulation for the synthesis of prothrombin (factor II), factors VII,

IX and X and proteins C, S and Z (Mann, 1999). Clotting factors II, VII, IX and X are therefore the 'vitamin K-dependent clotting factors'. Gla proteins also have a role in bone metabolism.

Other medications used for acute hepatitis: alcoholic hepatitis

Alcohol abstinence

This is the cornerstone of treatment for all alcohol-related illness.

Steroids or pentoxifylline

In this case of likely alcoholic hepatitis, Maddrey's Discriminant Function can be used to predict prognosis (short-term mortality in particular) and for determining suitability for steroid treatment. This is a specialist gastroenterology decision.

At the time of writing the STOPAH trial (STeroids of Pentoxifylline for Alcoholic Hepatitis) results have been published. This is a multicentre randomised controlled trial in the UK (Thursz *et al.*, 2015) comparing steroids, pentoxifylline and placebo in terms of mortality in alcoholic hepatitis. Steroids were previously recommended for consideration in severe alcoholic hepatitis where Maddrey's score was greater than or equal to 32. The trial showed that prednisolone had a benefit on mortality at 28 days (however, this did not reach statistical significance) but there was no benefit at 90 days or 1 year. Pentoxifylline (a TNFα antagonist) was shown to have no benefit.

Maddrey's score for alcoholic hepatitis

The modified Maddrey's Discriminant Function can be calculated with the following formula (Maddrey *et al.*, 1978; Haber *et al.*, 2003):

$$(4.6 \times (PT \text{ test} - \text{control})) + \text{serum bilirubin in mg/dL}$$

To calculate Maddrey's discriminant function using SI units – micromol/L (i.e. not US) divide bilirubin value by 17.

Prospective studies have shown that, it is useful in predicting short-term prognosis especially mortality within 30 days (Sheth *et al.*, 2002).

Patients with a score of 32 are at the highest risk of dying, with a 1-month mortality as high as 30–50 % (Mathurin *et al.*, 1996).

Guidelines

The American College of Gastroenterology guidelines (Jan 2010) define severe alcoholic hepatitis as a modified Discriminant Function (mDF) ≥ 32 and/or hepatic encephalopathy.

This guideline recommends a 4-week course of prednisolone (40 mg/day for 28 days, usually followed by a 2-week taper) in these severe alcoholic hepatitis patients.

It also recommends that pentoxifylline therapy (400 mg orally three times daily for 4 weeks) be considered, especially if there are contraindications to steroid therapy (O'Shea *et al.*, 2010; Whitfield *et al.*, 2009).

These results have been largely superseded by the STOPAH trail (Thursz, 2015) which found no significant survival benefit for either of these treatments.

Evidence

Corticosteroids for severe alcoholic hepatitis
A large meta-analysis showed a significant increase in short-term survival among the steroid-treated patients with Maddrey's score greater or equal to 32 compared with the control patients (84.6% vs. 65% survival) (Rambaldi *et al.*, 2008).

Pentoxifylline for severe alcoholic hepatitis
A double-blinded randomised controlled trial in 2000 showed that pentoxifylline improves short-term survival, where the the benefit appeared to be related to decreased risk of hepatorenal syndrome.

A subsequent Cochrane review of five trials concluded that there is not enough evidence to confirm the effect of pentoxifylline on patients with alcoholic hepatitis (Akriviadis *et al.*, 2000; Whitfield *et al.*, 2009).

These results have been largely superseded by the STOPAH trail (Thursz *et al.*, 2015) which found no significant survival benefit for either of these treatments.

Other TNFα antagonist therapies for alcoholic hepatitis

Infliximab and etanercept have been trialled in a number of studies (Spahr *et al.*, 2002; Naveau *et al.*, 2004; Mookerjee *et al.*, 2004; Boetticher *et al.*, 2008). These have found no benefit on mortality and in some cases adverse outcomes. These are therefore not recommended for use for alcoholic hepatitis, and further studies are being done.

Alcohol withdrawal medications

Patients with alcoholic hepatitis are likely to have had a recent heavy alcohol consumption history and are high risk for alcohol withdrawal. All patients drinking over the recommended alcohol allowance should be prescribed Pabrinex (an IV form of vitamin B_1 or thiamine) in order to help prevent Wernicke's encephalopathy and progression to Korsakoff's dementia. They should also be prescribed chlordiazepoxide, a benzodiazepine, to help with alcohol withdrawal symptoms and prevent withdrawal seizures.

Please see Chapter 1 for details about both these prescriptions.

Nutrition as a treatment for alcoholic liver disease patients

Significant protein malnutrition is common in alcoholics (Mezey, 1991) and severity of malnutrition has been shown to correlate with disease severity and outcomes (Mendenhall *et al.*, 1984). In one study, the mortality rate was 3.3% in patients achieving a positive nitrogen balance compared to 58% mortality in those who weren't (Calvey *et al.*, 1985). Many patients also have significant vitamin deficiencies.

Dietician review with oral or parenteral supplements is therefore recommended for patients with alcoholic hepatitis at risk of undernutrition, with recommendation of high calorie and high protein diets (Plauth *et al.*, 2006).

Liver transplantation

In deteriorating patients not responding to therapy, transplant may be their final option. This is huge decision and involves complete patient understanding and cooperation as well as commitment to alcohol abstinence.

🔍 Evidence

Liver transplant for acute alcoholic hepatitis
A prospective multicentre study showed that early transplantation improves the probability of 6-month survival among patients with severe alcoholic hepatitis in whom medical therapy failed.

The report challenges the previous rule that alcoholics must be abstinent for 6 months pretransplant and argues that because the risk of early death is very high, it is necessary consider all available treatment options including transplantation in targeted patients (Lucey *et al.*, 2009; Mathurin *et al.*, 2011).

Overall, liver transplants for acute alcoholic hepatitis are uncommon: 71% of transplants are done for cirrhosis, 11% hepatocellular carcinoma, 10% for acute liver failure, 6% for metabolic disease. Outcome is worse when patients have acute liver failure, as they are likely to have coexisting multiorgan failure: survival is 65% at 1 year versus 80–90% 1-year survival post-transplant.

Contraindications to transplant include sepsis, extrahepatic malignancy, active alcohol use and marked cardiological or respiratory dysfunction.

Other medications used for acute hepatitis: hepatitis B

The treatment of acute hepatitis B is a specialist area where decisions would be made by a hepatologist. Acute infection can cause malaise, jaundice, itching and in around 1% of cases, acute liver failure (Shiffman, 2010). The majority of individuals resolve the acute infection and develop life-long immunity, and some may not know that they were ever infected. For this reason, acute hepatitis B is often not treated. However, if there is liver failure, an antiviral may be commenced (Shiffman, 2010).

For patients with chronic hepatitis B (HbsAg positive), decision to treat is based on level of detectable viral DNA in the bloodstream, as well as presence or absence of cirrhosis, age and ALT level.

Antiviral treatment is generally offered to adults above the age of 30 years who have a persistently elevated HBV DNA (greater than 2000 IU/mL) and persistently abnormal ALT (above 30 IU/mL in males and above to 19 IU/mL in females). This is generally the case on two consecutive tests conducted 3 months apart. Patients who are under 30 years of age and have the above criteria are considered for treatment if they also have necroinflammation/ fibrosis on a liver biopsy, or an elastography score greater than 6 kPa.

Any patient should be considered for treatment if their HBV DNA is greater than 20 000 IU/mL and ALT is abnormal, regardless of age or extent of disease on biopsy/elastography. Any patient should also be considered for treatment if they have evidence of cirrhosis with a detectable viral load.

Medication options are (NICE, 2013b):

- **Peginterferon alfa-2a.** This is for people with compensated liver disease (either HBeAg-positive or HBeAg-negative) and should not be given to those with decompensated disease. Peginterferon alfa-2a should not be given in pregnancy unless the potential benefit outweighs risk.
- **Entecavir.** This is for people with either HBeAg-positive or HBeAg-negative chronic hepatitis B infection. It is used first line instead of peginterferon in those with decompensated liver disease.
- **Tenofovir.** This is for people with either HBeAg-positive or HBeAg-negative chronic hepatitis B infection. It is used second line instead of peginterferon in those with decompensated liver disease, where the patient has a history of lamivudine resistance. The dose must be adjusted in renal failure.

ⓘ Guidelines

- NICE guidelines (2013): *Hepatitis B (Chronic): Diagnosis and Management*, CG165, 2013. Available at: www.nice.org.uk/ guidance/CG165 (accessed Dec. 2015).

This has partially updated previous treatment-specific guidelines:

- NICE. *Adefovir Dipivoxil and Peginterferon alfa-2a for the Treatment of Chronic Hepatitis*

B, TA96, 2006. Available at: www.nice.org
.uk/guidance/ta96 (accessed Dec. 2015).
- NICE. *Entecavir for the Treatment of
  Chronic Hepatitis B*, TA153, 2008.
  Available at: www.nice.org.uk/guidance/
  ta153 (accessed Dec. 2015).
- NICE. *Tenofovir Disoproxil for the Treatment
  of Hepatitis B*, TA173, 2009. Available at:
  www.nice.org.uk/guidance/ta173 (accessed
  Dec. 2015).

Other medications used for acute hepatitis: hepatitis C

The treatment of acute hepatitis C is a specialist area where decisions would be made by a hepatologist. In the majority of patients, the acute phase of the infection has no symptoms and they may be unaware that they have it. It is therefore rarely treated in the acute phase. Symptoms occur in only 15% of patients (Maheshwari *et al.*, 2008), and these may comprise of a non-specific illness of malaise, lethargy and decreased appetite. Jaundice and acute hepatitis are rare (Bailey, 2010). Around 80% of individuals exposed to the virus will develop a chronic infection defined as where the virus persists in the blood 6 months postinfection (Nelson *et al.*, 2011).

For patients with chronic hepatitis C patients treatment is based on the presence of viral DNA in the bloodstream and evidence of liver damage on biopsy (with or without abnormal LFTs). Those with mild disease may be monitored for a period without treatment, whereas those with moderate or severe treatment should be treated early. Treatment decisions will also change as newer antivirals become available and affordable. Duration of treatment is based on the genotype of the virus, the viral load at the start of treatment and the response to treatment (as shown by change in viral load).

The mainstay of treatment for chronic hepatitis C up until 2011 was combination therapy with peginterferon alpha and ribavirin (NICE, 2010). In 2011, telaprevir and boceprevir were licensed for use in addition to the above regimen for genotype 1 disease (either one drug or the other in addition) (NICE, 2012b, 2012c).

New hepatitis C direct-acting antivirals sofosbuvir, simeprevir and daclatasvir were approved by the EU in 2014 and NICE, as well as combination therapies containing ledipasvir, paritaprevir, ombitasvir and dasabuvir in 2015 (EASL, 2015). These have all shown efficacy in reaching sustained virological resistance.

The choice of agent, when to treat and who to treat are specialist decisions by a hepatologist.

ⓘ Guidelines

Updated guidelines on management of hepatitis C
- The European Association of the Study of the Liver has guidelines on the management of hepatitis C: *EASL Clinical Practice Guidelines*, 2015. Available at: www.easl.eu/research/our-contributions/clinical-practice-guidelines/detail/recommendations-on-treatment-of-hepatitis-c-2015/report/2 (accessed Dec 2015).
- NICE. *Sofosbuvir for Treating Chronic Hepatitis C*, TA330, 2015. Available at: www.nice.org.uk/guidance/TA330 (accessed December 2015).
- NICE. *Simeprevir in Combination with Peginterferon alfa and Ribavirin for Treating Genotypes 1 and 4 Chronic Hepatitis C*, TA331, 2015. Available at: www.nice.org.uk/guidance/ta331 (accessed December 2015).
- NICE. *Daclatasvir for Treating Chronic Hepatitis C*, TA364, 2015. Available at: www.nice.org.uk/guidance/TA364 (accessed December 2015).
- NICE. *Ledipasvir-Sofosbuvir for Treating Chronic Hepatitis C*, TA363, 2015. Available at: www.nice.org.uk/guidance/TA363 (accessed December 2015).
- NICE. *Ombitasvir–Paritaprevir–Ritonavir with or without Dasabuvir for Treating Chronic Hepatitis C,* TA365, 2015. Available at: www.nice.org.uk/guidance/TA365 (accessed December 2015).

Any combination of hepatitis C drugs is limited by side-effects, particularly of interferon. In addition, all regimens involves adherence and close monitoring. This limited some patient's suitability for treatment (Booth *et al.*, 2001).

The risk of developing cirrhosis as a result of chronic hepatitis C ranges from 5% to 25% over 25 to 30 years (Seeff, 2002; Liang *et al.*, 2000). Development of cirrhosis increases the risk of hepatocellular carcinoma.

Further aspects of acute hepatitis management

This chapter has discussed the treatment options for acute alcoholic hepatitis and viral hepatitis B and C. There are numerous other causes of hepatitis such as autoimmune hepatitis and drug-induced hepatitis, which have not been discussed.

Further aspects of management to consider in alcoholic hepatitis include:

- Discussion and explanation to the patient regarding the reality of the very poor prognosis of alcoholic hepatitis and need for alcohol cessation.
- This difficult subject should be approached via a dedicated alcohol care team that should be present in some form in every hospital.
- This includes an alcohol liaison nurse with links to mental health teams and community services, with follow up after discharge from hospital.
- Other complications of alcohol related liver disease need to be managed, e.g. ascites, GI bleed risk.

Further aspects of management to consider in viral hepatitis include:

- Counselling about implications of the disease, including safe sex and IV drug use discussions, with appropriate support put in place.
- Counselling about the treatment regimens, which may be difficult due to length of time and side-effect profile, with the possibility of ineffectiveness in terms of clearing the virus.

Case outcome and discharge

Mr de Souza was treated with lactulose for hepatic encephalopathy, vitamin K for deranged coagulation and alcohol withdrawal medications. His liver screen came back negative for viral hepatitis and HIV, with no evidence of autoimmune hepatitis. He was seen by the gastroenterology team, but did not qualify as severe alcoholic hepatitis as

his Maddrey's score was 25. He was therefore not given steroids or pentoxifylline. He was managed supportively, with the main focus of his care being prevention of future admissions by discussions surrounding alcohol cessation and healthy lifestyle. He was referred to the alcohol liaison nurse who arranged follow up in the community, with a contact number for any questions or difficulties that may arise. Over the next 3 days Mr de Souza improved clinically and liver function started to improve slightly. He was put in touch with social services considering his difficult housing situation, and they arranged a hostel for him to stay in until more permanent accommodation could be arranged. On discharge, his thiamine was changed from IV Pabrinex to oral thiamine, and lactulose was titrated down as he was passing three stools per day.

Mr de Souza's new prescription is shown. Note omeprazole has been stopped.

DISCHARGE MEDICATION						
Date	Medication	Dose	Route	Frequency	Supply	GP to continue?
xx/xx/xx	THIAMINE	100 mg	PO	Three times daily	14 days	Y
xx/xx/xx	LACTULOSE	10 mL	PO	Once daily	14 days	Y
xx/xx/xx	VITAMIN B CO-STRONG	1 tablet	PO	Once daily	14 days	Y

Notes to patient/GP:
Omeprazole stopped as no longer required.

Common pitfalls

- Do not immediately attribute drowsiness to hepatic encephalopathy without considering other causes such as sepsis, cerebral haemorrhage and postictal state.
- Don't forget Pabrinex (thiamine), as if encephalopathy progresses to Korsakoff's syndrome, this becomes irreversible. This is relevant for a heavy alcohol consumer presenting with any pathology.
- Acute liver failure is a life-threatening emergency and generally requires intensive care input due to the multiorgan failure that ensues.
- Encephalopathy itself increases risk of aspiration and threatened airways, in which case intensive care input is required.

Acute hepatitis is a broad diagnosis where further management depends on the aetiology. Given the short history of symptoms, AST/ALT rise and jaundice with high alcohol consumption, alcoholic hepatitis is the most likely diagnosis in this case.

Other possibilities include acute viral hepatitis, drug induced hepatitis and autoimmune hepatitis.

Initial assessment must therefore include a thorough history, including sexual and drug history, family history, recent medications and over the counter medications as well as mental health state.

Alcoholic liver disease is a large burden on healthcare resources: alcohol-related disorders may account for as much as 9.2% of all disability-adjusted life years according to the World Health Organisation's Global Information System on Alcohol and Health (WHO, 2013).

SUMMARY

🔑 Key learning points

Alcoholic hepatitis
- Treatment is mainly supportive, with alcohol cessation being the cornerstone.
- Lactulose is given for hepatic encephalopathy, aiming for three stools per day.
- Vitamin K is given to at least partly correct coagulopathy.
- Pabrinex IV then oral thiamine are given to prevent Korsakoff's dementia.
- Where Maddrey's score is greater or equal to 32, disease specific therapies may be considered (steroids or pentoxifylline), although evidence is weak.
- Alcohol liaison nurses and community support is important for maintaining health, alcohol cessation and prevention of future admissions.

Hepatitis B
- Acute hepatitis B is often not treated, as the majority of people clear the virus spontaneously.
- Of those who become chronically infected, decision for antiviral treatment is based on age, ALT level, viral load and evidence of liver damage.
- Treatment options include peginterferon alfa-2a, entecavir and tenofovir.
- This is always under specialist hepatology guidance.
- Counselling needs to include information on prevention of transmission.

Hepatitis C
- Acute hepatitis C may not be detected, as many people are asymptomatic of initial infection.
- Treatment decisions for chronic hepatitis C are based on detection of viral DNA and evidence of liver damage, not necessarily ALT level.
- Duration of treatment is based on the genotype of the virus, the viral load at the start of treatment and the response to treatment.
- The specific antiviral used would be decided by a hepatologist.
- Counselling needs to include information on prevention of transmission.
- All forms of hepatitis have the possible option of liver transplant as a final attempt at curative treatment. However, the criteria are strict and not all patients will benefit therefore this is a careful specialist decision based on each individual's specific circumstances.

FURTHER READING

- Haber PS, Warner R, Seth D *et al.* (2003). Pathogenesis and management of alcoholic hepatitis. *J Gastroenterol Hepatol* 18: 1332–44.
- American Gastroenterology Association. Available at: www.gastro.org (accessed Dec. 2015).
- European Association for the Study of the Liver. Available at: www.easl.eu/(accessed Dec. 2015).
- NHS Choices. Available at: www.nhs.uk (accessed Dec. 2015).
- NHS Evidence. Available at: www.evidence.nhs.uk (accessed Dec. 2015).

Constipation

Mrs Sarah Batty

Age: 68

Hospital number: 123456

Case study

Presenting complaint: *A 68-year-old woman presents to the GP with difficulty passing stool for 2 years. It is now worsening and causing her to have generalised abdominal pain.*

Background: *She lives with her husband and is his carer. She is independent and mobile*

PMH: *2 caesarean sections, longstanding neck pain due to osteoarthritis*

Allergies: *none*

FH: *Father had an MI age 50*

Examination:
Pulse 80, BP 136/82, Sats 97% on air, RR 12, BM 5.4

CVS: *Capillary refill time <2 seconds, pulse feels regular, JVP not seen, no oedema, HS I + II + 0*

RS: *Equal expansion with air entry to both bases and no added sounds*

Abdo: *Soft, mildly tender abdomen with fullness around the sigmoid, bowel sounds present PR reveals impacted hard stool, no blood*

Neuro: *Moving all 4 limbs, alert, mobile*

ECG: *Sinus rhythm*

Bloods: *Hb 130, Plt 350, WCC 8.9, Na 136, K 4.3, Urea 6.0, Creat 100, INR 1.1 ALT 35, AlkP 110, alb 42, amylase 70*

PHARMACY STAMP	AGE 68	FORENAME, SURNAME Sarah Batty
	D.O.B. xx/xx/xxxx	ADDRESS Flat 4, 21 Farley Road
		NHS NUMBER

PARACETAMOL 1g oral four times daily as required.

IBUPROFEN 400 mg oral three times daily as required.

CODEINE PHOSPHATE 30–60 mg oral three times daily as required.

SIGNATURE OF PRESCRIBER	DATE

SP21000

CXR: No free air under diaphragm, clear chest

AXR: Faecally loaded colon

Diagnosis

Chronic constipation. This is extremely common, particularly in patients on constipating medications such as codeine or any opioid. It is also more common in sedentary patients, or in those who have poor diets low in fibre or little water. Constipation is more common in older patients, partly due to the increased incidence of diverticular disease.

Initial measures

It is important to rule out worrying causes for constipation such as small or large bowel obstruction, or a colonic mass such as colorectal cancer. The history is therefore very important, and if suspected, further investigations should be organised such as an abdominal and erect-chest X-ray, CT abdomen, CT pneumocolon, or a colonoscopy, depending on suspicion. Blood tests can also be done for medical causes of constipation and abdominal pain such as hypercalcaemia or hypothyroidism.

The first advice for anyone with constipation is to remove the cause, in this case codeine is likely to be exacerbating things. Dietary advice is also key. Fibre together with fluids may be enough in itself to solve the problem. The recommended amount of dietary fibre is 20–35 g/day. Dietician referral may be required.

Laxatives can then be trialled, the choice of which depends on patient preference, previous experience and severity of the problem. Different classes of laxatives can be used in combination, as well as suppositories and enemas if required.

Prescribing for constipation

REGULAR PRESCRIPTIONS					Circle/enter times below ↓	Enter dates below			
						Day 1	Day 2	Day 3	Day 4
DRUG ISPAGULA HUSK (FYBOGEL®)					06				
					(08)				
Dose 1 sachet	Route PO	Freq OD	Start date xx/xx/xx		12				
Signature A. Doctor		Bleep	Review		16				
					18				
Additional instructions					22				
DRUG LACTULOSE					06				
					(08)				
Dose 10 ml	Route PO	Freq BD	Start date xx/xx/xx		12				
Signature A. Doctor		Bleep	Review		16				
					(20)				
Additional instructions					22				
DRUG SENNA					06				
					08				
Dose 1 tablet	Route PO	Freq ON	Start date xx/xx/xx		12				
Signature A. Doctor		Bleep	Review		16				
					18				
Additional instructions					(22)				

The choice of laxative depends on patient preference, previous experience and severity of the problem. Different classes of laxatives can be used in combination, as well as suppositories and enemas if required.

Bulk-forming laxatives: rationale and evidence

Bulk-forming laxatives include ispaghula husk (Fybogel or Ispagel), psyllium seed, methylcellulose and wheat dextrin (Benefiber). They have few side effects and are safe in pregnancy. They can be used in patients with stomas, as well as those with diverticular disease or IBD (BMA/RPS, 2015).

🔍 Evidence

Fibre and water for constipation
There is a dose response between fibre intake, water intake and faecal output (Voderholzer *et al.*, 1997; Anti *et al.*, 1998).

🔍 Evidence

Bulk-forming laxatives
There is much anecdotal evidence that these are effective laxatives. A systematic review found that psyllium increases stool frequency (Bharucha *et al.*, 2013).

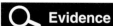

DRUGS checklist for ISPAGHULA HUSK (Fybogel®)

Dose	1–2 sachets, containing 3.5 g of ispaghula husk granules
Route	PO
Units	Sachets
Given	Up to four sachets per day
Special situations	Can cause flatulence and abdominal distension. Laxatives should not be given in cases of bowel obstruction.

Bulk-forming laxatives: essential pharmacology

The aforementioned bulk-forming laxatives are natural or synthetic polysaccharides, which work by absorbing water and thereby increasing faecal mass. This stimulates peristalsis. They increase frequency of stool passage and soften the stool, making it easier to pass.

Stimulant laxatives: rationale and evidence

Stimulant laxatives include senna, bisocodyl, docusate sodium, glycerine suppositories and sodium picosulphate.

Evidence

Stimulant laxatives in constipation
A randomised trial of sodium picosulphate used over 4 weeks in 45 patients demonstrated improved bowel function versus placebo (Mueller-Lissner et al., 2010).

DRUGS checklist for SENNA

Dose	1–2 tablets
Route	PO
Units	Tablets
Given	Best taken at night but can be twice daily
Special situations	Takes 8–12 hours to work, hence night-time regimen is best.

Stimulant laxatives: essential pharmacology

Stimulant laxatives work by causing increased intestinal motility. They do this by altering electrolyte transport in the intestinal mucosa, as well as increasing intestinal motor activity. For this reason they can cause abdominal cramps and must be avoided in intestinal obstruction. Glycerine suppositories work because glycerol is a mild irritant to the rectal mucosa. Sodium picosulpate is a strong stimulant used to evacuate bowels prior to radiological or endoscopic procedures.

Stimulant laxatives can cause hypokalaemia, protein losing enteropathy and sodium overload if taken chronically, so should be used with caution.

Osmotic laxatives: rationale and evidence

Osmotic laxatives include polyethylene glycol (also called macrogols) and semisynthetic disaccharides such as lactulose. Phosphate enemas are also in this category. Phosphate enemas are useful for severe constipation where a rapid effect is needed. This includes cleansing the distal bowel for a flexible sigmoidoscopy procedure.

Evidence

Polyethylene glycol and lactulose for constipation
Systematic reviews have found that polyethylene glycol and lactulose are effective in improving stool consistency and frequency (Bharucha et al., 2013).

✓ DRUGS checklist for LACTULOSE

Dose	10–30 mL
Route	PO
Units	mL
Given	Up to TDS
Special situations	Takes 24–48 hours to exert its effect.

✓ DRUGS checklist for POLYETHYLENE GLYCOL (Movicol ®)

Dose	1–3 sachets
Route	PO
Units	Sachets
Given	Up to TDS
Special situations	Movicol comes in lemon or chocolate flavour.
	1 sachet is dissolved in half a glass of water (approximately 125 mL).
	8 sachets can be given in 1 day for faecal impaction, this should be for short-term use only at this high dosage.

Osmotic laxatives: essential pharmacology

Osmotic laxatives increase the amount of water in the large bowel. This is done by drawing water from the body or by retaining the water that they were ingested with. This then liquefies and softens the stool, allowing easier passage. Lactose in particular is metabolised in the colon by bacteria in the stool. This results in lactic and acetic acid production, which acidifies the stool, encouraging absorption of ammonia into the colon. The ammonia is then excreted, lowering the amount absorbed into the blood stream. For this reason, lactulose is also used to reduce hepatic encephalopathy.

Other medications used in constipation

Normal bowel function is dependent on a healthy and balanced diet. This advice should be delivered to patients. Food diaries may be used to highlight unhealthy behaviours. Referral to nutritionist is of great benefit in the education of patients.

For difficult-to-control constipation, acute relief or where a patient cannot tolerate oral laxatives, suppositories and enemas can be used. Glycerine suppositories are glycerol-filled capsules, which are inserted at night. Throughout the night the softening effect takes place aiming for a stool in the morning.

Phosphate enemas are a rectal flush of sodium dihydrogen phosphate dehydrate or sodium acid phosphate, which provides quick relief from impacted stool. These are very effective and can be used prior to flexible sigmoidoscopy for bowel preparation.

Faecal softeners are another class of laxative, which are used less often in modern hospitals. Arachis (peanut oil) can lubricate faecal passage, particularly when given as an enema. Liquid paraffin is a traditional lubricant but has fallen out of favour.

Severe and long-term constipation can be treated, in rare cases, with surgery. Colectomy with end ileostomy is the final treatment in cases of severe long-term constipation, when all medical treatment options have been exhausted (Wofford and Verne, 2000).

Further aspects of constipation management

Bowel preparation prior to colonoscopy or CT pneumocolon is a common prescription as a junior doctor, as frail or elderly patients may be admitted for these procedures specifically for monitored bowel preparation. Common agents used for bowel preparation are Moviprep, Citramag or picosulphate. They are also given before colonic surgery.

These are prescribed in a regimen that varies at different trusts. Also, for colonic surgery it very much depends on the surgeon as to whether bowel preparation is wanted or not.

Caution must be taken with those with renal failure, as dehydration and electrolyte disturbance may be more pronounced in these patients. Hypovolaemia can be corrected with IV fluids concurrently.

a patient has significant co-morbidities such as renal or heart failure. These patients may have the senna omitted, or may have moviprep (a polyethylene glycol solution) instead of Citramag.

Categories of bowel prep agent include:
- Macrogols: Moviprep and Klean Prep
- Magnesium citrate preparations: Citramag
- Sodium picosulpahte: Citrafleet.

Case outcome and discharge

Mrs Batty stopped taking codeine for neck pain and increased her water and fibre intake. This improved her bowel habit but she still required lactulose and Fybogel around twice per week. She may well have diverticular disease given her age and how common it is, so it is important to aim for regular soft stools in order to prevent diverticulitis (infection in the diverticulae).

Mrs Batty's new prescription is shown. Note codeine has been stopped.

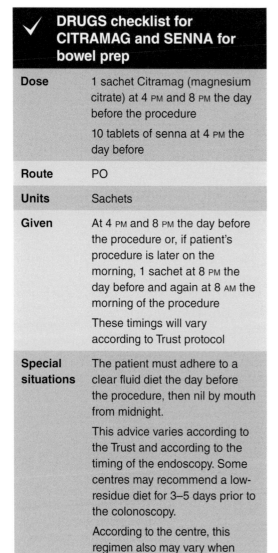

DRUGS checklist for CITRAMAG and SENNA for bowel prep

Dose	1 sachet Citramag (magnesium citrate) at 4 PM and 8 PM the day before the procedure 10 tablets of senna at 4 PM the day before
Route	PO
Units	Sachets
Given	At 4 PM and 8 PM the day before the procedure or, if patient's procedure is later on the morning, 1 sachet at 8 PM the day before and again at 8 AM the morning of the procedure These timings will vary according to Trust protocol
Special situations	The patient must adhere to a clear fluid diet the day before the procedure, then nil by mouth from midnight. This advice varies according to the Trust and according to the timing of the endoscopy. Some centres may recommend a low-residue diet for 3–5 days prior to the colonoscopy. According to the centre, this regimen also may vary when

DISCHARGE MEDICATION

Date	Medication	Dose	Route	Frequency	Supply	GP to continue?
xx/xx/xx	PARACETAMOL	1 g	PO	Four times a day, as required	14 days	Y
xx/xx/xx	IBUPROFEN	400 mg	PO	Three times a day, as required	14 days	Y
xx/xx/xx	MOVICOL	1 sachet	PO	Once daily	14 days	Y
xx/xx/xx	SENNA	1 tablet	PO	Once per night	14 days	Y

Notes to patient/GP:
Codeine stopped as contributing to constipation.

Common pitfalls

- Laxative overuse can result in diarrhoea, but more importantly electrolyte disturbances due to GI losses. The most common is hypokalaemia. Doses should therefore be tailored to an individual's specific requirements.
- Laxatives, like many other drugs, can be abused. Watch out for laxative overuse in people with eating disorders.

Laxatives are a common prescription for any junior doctor, both in hospital and in the community. Laxatives with different mechanisms of action can be combined, but there is little benefit to be gained from using two of the same class.

SUMMARY

🔑 Key learning points

The best management for a patient with constipation is lifestyle and dietary advice. If this is ineffective, laxatives can be prescribed.

Classes of laxatives
- Bulk forming: methylcellulose, ispaghula husk
- Stimulants: senna, bisacodyl, sodium picosulfate
- Osmotic agents: lactulose, Movicol (polyethylene glycol) glycerine suppository, magnesium sulfate and magnesium citrate
- Stool softeners: sodium docusate.

Now visit **www.wileyessential.com/pharmacology** to test yourself on this chapter.

References

Akobeng AK, Gardener E (2005). Oral 5-aminosalicylic acid for maintenance of medically induced remission in Crohn's disease. *Cochrane Database Syst Rev* (1): CD003715.

Akriviadis E, Botla R, Briggs W *et al.* (2000). Pentoxifylline improves short-term survival in severe acute alcoholic hepatitis. *Gastroenterology* 199: 1637–48.

Al-Abri S, Beeching NJ, Nye FJ (2005). Travellers' diarrhoea. *Lancet Infect Dis* 5: 349–60.

Als-Nielsen B, Gluud LL, Gluud C (2004). Nonabsorbable disaccharides for hepatic encephalopathy. *Cochrane Database Syst Rev* (2): CD003044.

Amarapurkar P, Amarapurkar D (2011). Management of coagulopathy in patients with decompensated liver cirrhosis. *Int J Hepatol* 2011: 695470.

Anti M, Pignataro G, Armuzzi A *et al.* (1998). Water supplementation enhances the effect of high-fiber diet on stool frequency and laxative consumption in adult patients with functional constipation. *Hepatogastroenterology* 45: 727.

Apisarnthanarak A, Razavi B, Mundy LM (2002). Adjunctive intracolonic vancomycin for severe Clostridium difficile colitis: case series and review of the literature. *Clin Infect Dis* 35: 690–6.

Bailey C (2010). Hepatic failure: an evidence-based approach in the emergency department. *Emerg Med Pract* 12 (4).

Baron JH, Connell AM, Kanaghinis TG *et al.* (1962). Out-patient treatment of ulcerative colitis. Comparison between three doses of oral prednisone. *Br Med J* 2: 441.

Bartlett JG (1985). Treatment of Clostridium difficile colitis. *Gastroenterology* 89: 1192–5.

Bernard B, Grangé J-D, Nguyen Khac E, *et al.* (1999). Antibiotic prophylaxis for the prevention of bacterial infections in cirrhotic patients with gastrointestinal bleeding: A meta-analysis. *Hepatology* 29: 655–61.

Bharucha A, Pemberton J, Locke G (2013). 3rd American Gastroenterological Association technical review on constipation. *Gastroenterology* 144: 218.

Blatchford O, Murray W, Blatchford M (2000). A risk score to predict need for treatment for upper gastrointestinal haemorrhage. *Lancet* 356: 1318–21.

Boetticher NC, Peine CJ, Kwo P *et al.* (2008). A randomized, double-blinded, placebo-controlled multicenter trial of etanercept in the treatment of alcoholic hepatitis. *Gastroenterology* 135: 1953–60.

Bojic D, Radojicic Z, Nedeljkovic-Protic M *et al.* (2009). Long-term outcome after admission for acute severe ulcerative colitis in Oxford: the 1992–1993 cohort. *Inflamm Bowel Dis* 15: 823–8.

Booth J, O'Grady J, Neuberger J (2001). Clinical guidelines on the management of hepatitis C. *Gut* 49 (Suppl.): 1–21.

Bouza E, Dryden M, Mohammed R *et al.* (2008). Results of a phase III trial comparing tolevamer, vancomycin and metronidazole in patients with Clostridium difficile-associated diarrhoea. 18th European Congress of Clinical Microbiology and Infectious Diseases. *Clin Microbiol Infect* 14 (Suppl. s7).

British Medical Association and Royal Pharmaceutical Society of Great Britain (BMA/RPS) (2015). *British National Formulary 69*, 69th edn. BMJ group and Pharmaceutical Press, London.

Calvey H, Davis M, Williams R (1985). Controlled trial of nutritional supplementation, with and without branched chain amino acid enrichment, in treatment of acute alcoholic hepatitis. *J Hepatol* 1: 141–51.

Cash WJ, McConville P, McDermott E *et al.* (2010). Current concepts in the assessment and treatment of hepatic encephalopathy. *Q J Med* 103: 9–16.

Cohen SH, Gerding DN, Johnson S *et al.* (2010). Society for Healthcare Epidemiology of America; Infectious Diseases Society of America. Clinical practice guidelines for Clostridium difficile infection in adults: 2010 update by the society for healthcare epidemiology of America (SHEA) and the Infectious Diseases Society of America (IDSA). *Infect Control Hosp Epidemiol* 31: 431–55.

Cornely OA, Crook DW, Esposito R *et al.* OPT-80-004 Clinical Study Group (2012). Fidaxomicin versus vancomycin for infection with Clostridium difficile in Europe, Canada, and the USA: a double-blind, non-inferiority, randomised controlled trial. *Lancet Infect Dis* 12: 281–9.

Davis RI, Markham A, Balfour JA (1996). Ciprofloxacin. An updated review of its pharmacology, therapeutic efficacy and tolerability. *Drugs* 51: 1019–74.

Dial S, Delaney JA, Barkun AN *et al.* (2005). Use of gastric acid-suppressive agents and the risk of community-acquired Clostridium difficile associated disease. *JAMA* 294: 2989–95.

Dial S, Delaney JA, Schneider V *et al.* (2006). Proton pump inhibitor use and risk of community-acquired Clostridium difficile-associated disease defined by prescription for oral vancomycin therapy. *Can Med Associ J* 175: 745–8.

Drekonja DM, Butler M, MacDonald R *et al.* (2011). Comparative effectiveness of Clostridium difficile treatments: a systematic review. *Ann Intern Med* 155: 839–47.

Drlica K, Zhao X (1997). DNA gyrase, topoisomerase IV, and the 4-quinolones. *Microbiol Mol Biol Rev* 61: 377–92.

European Association for the Study of the Liver (2012). EASL clinical practical guidelines: management of alcoholic liver disease. *J Hepatol* 57: 399–420.

European Association for the Study of the Liver (2015). EASL clinical practical guidelines: recommendations on treatment of hepatitis C. *J Hepatol* 63: 199–236.

Ferenci P, Lockwood A, Mullen K *et al.* (2002). Hepatic encephalopathy-definition, nomenclature, diagnosis, and quantification: final report of the working party at the 11th World Congresses of Gastroenterology, Vienna, 1998. *Hepatology* 35: 716–21.

Furie B, Bouchard BA, Furie BC (1999). Vitamin K-dependent biosynthesis of gamma-carboxyglutamic acid. *Blood* 93: 1798–808.

Gisbert JP, Gonzalez L, Calvet X *et al.* (2001). Proton pump inhibitors versus H2-antagonists: a meta-analysis of their efficacy in treating bleeding peptic ulcer. *Aliment Pharmacol* 15: 917–26.

Gough E, Shaikh H, Manges AR (2011). Systematic review of intestinal microbiota transplantation (fecal bacteriotherapy) for recurrent Clostridium difficile infection. *Clin Infect Dis* 53: 994–1002.

Green FJ, Kaplan MM, Curtis LE *et al.* (1978). Effects of acid and pepsin on blood coagulation and platelet aggregation. A possible contributor to prolonged gastro duodenal mucosal haemorrhage. *Gastroenterology* 74: 38–43.

Haber PS, Warner R, Seth D *et al.* (2003). Pathogenesis and management of alcoholic hepatitis. *J Gastroenterol Hepatol* 18: 1332–44.

Hayes PC, Davis JM, Lewis JA *et al.* (1990). Metaanalysis of the value of propranolol in the prevention of variceal haemorrhage. *Lancet* 336: 153–6.

Hempel S, Newberry SJ, Maher AR *et al.* (2012). Probiotics for the prevention and treatment of antibiotic-associated diarrhea: a systematic review and meta-analysis. *JAMA* 307: 1959–69.

Hickson M, D'Souza AL, Muthu N *et al.* (2007). Use of probiotic Lactobacillus preparation to prevent diarrhoea associated with antibiotics: randomised double blind placebo controlled trial. *BMJ* 335: 80.

Homik J, Suarez-Almazor ME, Shea B *et al.* (2000). Calcium and vitamin D for corticosteroid-induced osteoporosis. *Cochrane Database Syst Rev* (2): CD000952.

Howell MD, Novack V, Grgurich P *et al.* (2010). Iatrogenic gastric acid suppression and the risk of nosocomial Clostridium difficile infection. *Arch Intern Med* 170: 784–90.

Hu MY, Katchar K, Kyne L *et al.* (2009). Prospective derivation and validation of a clinical prediction rule for recurrent Clostridium difficile infection. *Gastroenterology* 136: 1206–14.

Ioannou GN, Doust J, Rockey DC (2003a). Systematic review: Terlipressin in acute oesophageal variceal haemorrhage. *Aliment Pharmacol Ther* 17: 53–64.

Ioannou G, Doust J, Rockey DC (2003b). Terlipressin for acute esophageal variceal hemorrhage. *Cochrane Database Syst Rev* (1) CD002147.

Irving PM, Pasi KJ, Rampton DS (2005). Thrombosis and inflammatory bowel disease. *Clin Gastroenterol Hepatol* 3: 617–28.

Jakobovits S, Travis SP (2005). Management of acute severe colitis. *Br Med Bull* 75–76: 131–44.

Jalan R, Hayes P (2000). UK Guidelines on the Management of Variceal Haemorrhage in Cirrhotic Patients. British Society of Gastroenterology. Available at: http://www.bsg.org.uk/pdf_word_docs/vari_hae.pdf (accessed Dec 2015).

Janarthanan S, Ditah I, Adler DG *et al.* (2012). Clostridium difficile-associated diarrhea and proton pump inhibitor therapy: a meta-analysis. *Am J Gastroenterol* 107: 1001–10.

Johnson AP, Wilcox MH (2012). Fidaxomicin: a new option for the treatment of Clostridium difficile infection. *J Antimicrob Chemother* 67: 2788–92.

Johnson S, Gerding D, Davidson D *et al.* (2012). Efficacy and safety of oral vancomycin versus oral metronidazole for treatment of Clostridium difficile associated diarrhea (CDAD): pooled results from two randomized clinical trials. ID Week 2012, Infectious Diseases Society of America. San Diego, USA; abstract 818.

Kam P, Williams S, Yoong F (2004). Vasopressin and terlipressin: pharmacology and its clinical relevance. *Anaesthesia* 59: 993–1001.

Kefalakes H, Stylianides TJ, Amanakis G *et al.* (2009). Exacerbation of inflammatory bowel diseases associated with the use of nonsteroidal anti-inflammatory drugs:myth or reality? *Eur J Clin Pharmacol* 65: 963–70.

Kolkman JJ, Meuwissen SGM (1996). A review on treatment of bleeding peptic ulcer: a collaborative task of gastroenterologist and surgeon. *Scand J Gastroenterol* 31: 16–25.

Lahue BJ, Davidson DM (2007). Metronidazole and vancomycin outcomes for Clostridium difficile-associated diarrhoea in a US hospital database. *European Conference on Clinical Microbiology and Infectious Diseases*, Munich.

Lebrec D, De Fleury P, Rue VB *et al.* (1980). Portal hypertension, size of esophageal varices, and risk of gastrointestinal bleeding in alcoholic cirrhosis. *Gastroenterology* 79: 1139–44.

Lennard-Jones JE, Longmore AJ, Newell AC *et al.* (1960). An assessment of prednisone, salazopyrin, and topical hydrocortisone hemisuccinate used as out-patient treatment for ulcerative colitis. *Gut* 1: 217–22.

Leontiadis GI, Sreedharan A, Dorward S *et al.* (2007). Systematic reviews of the clinical effectiveness and cost-effectiveness of proton pump inhibitors in acute upper gastrointestinal bleeding. *Health Technology Assessment* 11: iii–iv, 1–164.

Liang TJ, Rehermann B, Seeff LB *et al.* (2000). Pathogenesis, natural history, treatment, and prevention of hepatitis C. *Ann Intern Med* 132: 296–305.

Loo VG, Poirier L, Miller MA *et al.* (2005). A predominantly clonal multi- institutional outbreak of Clostridium difficile-associated diarrhea with high morbidity and mortality. *N Engl J Med* 353: 2442–9.

Louie T, Gerson M, Grimard D *et al.* (2007). Results of a phase III trial comparing tolevamer, vancomycin and metronidazole in patients with Clostridium difficile associated diarrhea. *47th Interscience Conference on Antimicrobial Agents and Chemotherapy*, Chicago.

Louie TJ, Miller MA, Mullane KM *et al.* OPT-80-003 Clinical Study Group (2011). Fidaxomicin versus vancomycin for Clostridium difficile infection. *N Engl J Med* 364: 422–31.

Louie TJ, Peppe J, Watt CK *et al.* (2006). Tolevamer, a novel non antibiotic polymer, compared with vancomycin in the treatment of mild to moderately severe Clostridium difficile-associated diarrhea. *Clin Infect Dis* 43: 411–20.

Lucey MR, Mathurin P, Morgan TR (2009). Alcoholic hepatitis. *N Engl J Med* 360: 2758–69.

Maddrey WC, Boitnott JK, Bedine MS *et al.* (1978). Corticosteroid therapy of alcoholic hepatitis. *Gastroenterology* 75: 193–9.

Maheshwari A, Ray S, Thuluvath PJ (2008). Acute hepatitis C. *Lancet* 372: 321–32.

Malchow H, Ewe K, Brandes JW *et al.* (1984). European Cooperative Crohn's Disease Study (ECCDS): results of drug treatment. *Gastroenterology* 86: 249–66.

Mann KG (1999). Biochemistry and physiology of blood coagulation. *Thromb Haemost* 82: 165–74.

Mathurin P, Duchatelle V, Ramond MJ *et al.* (1996). Survival and prognostic factors in patients with severe alcoholic hepatitis treated with prednisolone. *Gastroenterology* 110: 1847–53.

Mathurin P, Moreno C, Samuel D *et al.* (2011). Early liver transplantation for severe alcoholic hepatitis. *N Engl J Med* 365: 1790–800.

McFarland LV, Surawicz CM, Rubin M *et al.* (1999). Recurrent Clostridium difficile disease: epidemiology and clinical characteristics. *Infect Control Hosp Epidemiol* 20: 43–50.

Mendenhall CL, Anderson S, Weesner RE *et al.* (1984). Protein-calorie malnutrition associated with alcoholic hepatitis. Veterans Administration Cooperative Study Group on Alcoholic Hepatitis. *Am J Med* 76: 211–22.

Mezey E (1991). Interaction between alcohol and nutrition in the pathogenesis of alcoholic liver disease. *Semin Liver Dis* 11: 340–8.

Mookerjee RP, Tilg H, Williams R *et al.* (2004). Infliximab and alcoholic hepatitis *Hepatology* 40: 499–500.

Mowat C, Cole A, Windsor A *et al* On behalf of the IBD Section of the British Society of Gastroenterology (2011). Guidelines for the management of inflammatory bowel disease in adults. *Gut* 60: 571–607.

Mueller-Lissner S, Kamm M, Wald A *et al.* (2010). Multicenter, 4-week, double-blind, randomized, placebo-controlled trial of sodium picosulfate in patients with chronic constipation. *Am J Gastroenterol* 105: 897.

Musher DM, Aslam S, Logan N *et al.* (2005). Relatively poor outcome after treatment of Clostridium difficile colitis with metronidazole. *Clin Infect Dis* 40: 1586–90.

Naesens M, Kuypers DR, Sarwal M (2009). Calcineurin inhibitor nephrotoxicity. *Clin J Am Soc Nephrol* 4: 481–509.

National Institute of Health and Care Excellence (NICE) (2010). *Peginterferon alfa and Ribavirin for the Treatment of Chronic Hepatitis C*, TA200. Available at: www.nice.org.uk/Guidance/ TA200 (accessed Dec. 2015).

National Institute of Health and Care Excellence (NICE) (2012a). *Acute Upper Gastrointestinal Bleeding in over 16s: Management*, CG141.

Available at: www.nice.org.uk/guidance/cg141 (accessed Dec. 2015).

National Institute of Health and Care Excellence (NICE) (2012b). *Bocepravir for the Treatment of Genotype 1 Chronic Hepatitis C*, TA253. Available at: www.nice.org.uk/guidance/TA253 (accessed Dec. 2015).

National Institute of Health and Care Excellence (NICE) (2012c). *Telapravir for the Treatment of Genotype 1 Chronic Hepatitis C*, TA252. Available at: www.nice.org.uk/guidance/TA252 (accessed Dec. 2015).

National Institute of Health and Care Excellence (NICE) (2013a). *Ulcerative Colitis: Management*, CG166. Available at: www.nice.org.uk/guidance/cg166 (accessed Dec. 2015).

National Institute of Health and Care Excellence (NICE) (2013b). Hepatitis B (chronic): diagnosis and management, CG165. Available at: www.nice.org.uk/Guidance/CG165 (accessed Dec. 2015).

National Institute of Health and Care Excellence (NICE) (2015). *Infliximab, Adalimumab and Golimumab for Treating Moderately to Severely Active Ulcerative Colitis after the Failure of Conventional Therapy*, TA329. Available at: www.nice.org.uk/guidance/ta329 (accessed Dec. 2015).

Naveau S, Chollet-Martin S, Dharancy S *et al.* (2004). A double-blind randomized controlled trial of infliximab associated with prednisolone in acute alcoholic hepatitis. *Hepatology* 39: 1390–7.

Nelson PK, Mathers BM, Cowie B *et al.* (2011). Global epidemiology of hepatitis B and hepatitis C in people who inject drugs: results of systematic reviews. *Lancet* 378: 571–83.

Newton R (2000). Molecular mechanisms of glucocorticoid action: what is important? *Thorax* 55: 603–13.

O'Shea R, Dasarathy S, McCullough A (2010). Alcoholic liver disease: ACG practice guidelines. *Am J Gastroenterol* 105: 14–32.

Peltola H, Gorbach SL (1997). Travelers' diarrhea – epidemiology and clinical aspects. In: DuPontHL, SteffenR (eds). *Textbook of Travel Medicine and Health*. BC Decker, Hamilton.

Pépin J, Valiquette L, Alary ME *et al.* (2004). Clostridium difficile-associated diarrhea in a region of Quebec from 1991 to 2003: a changing pattern of disease severity. *Can Med Assoc J* 171: 466–72.

Plauth M, Cabre E, Riggio O *et al.* (2006). ESPEN guidelines on enteral nutrition: liver disease. *Clin Nutr* 25: 285–94.

Rambaldi A, Saconato HH, Christensen E *et al.* (2008). Systematic review: glucocorticosteroids for alcoholic hepatitis – a Cochrane Hepatobiliary Group systematic review with meta-analyses and trial sequential analyses of randomized clinical trials. *Aliment Pharmacol Ther* 27: 1167–78.

Rice-Oxley JM, Truelove SC (1950). Ulcerative colitis: course and prognosis. *Lancet* 255: 663–6.

Saja MF, Abdo AA, Sanai FM *et al.* (2013). The coagulopathy of liver disease: does vitamin K help? *Blood Coagul Fibrinolysis* 24: 10–7.

Seeff LB (2002). Natural history of chronic hepatitis C. *Hepatology* (Suppl.): S35–S46.

Shawcross DL, Jalan R (2004). Treatment of hepatic encephalopathy: it's not lactulose. *BMJ* 329: 112.

Sheth M, Riggs M, Patel T (2002). Utility of the Mayo End-Stage Liver Disease (MELD) score in assessing prognosis of patients with alcoholic hepatitis. *BMC Gastroenterology* 2: 2.

Shiffman ML (2010). Management of acute hepatitis B. *Clin Liver Dis* 14: 75–91.

Shin JM, Sachs G (2008). Pharmacology of proton pump inhibitors. *Curr Gastroenterol Reports* 10: 528–34.

Spahr L, Rubbia-Brandt L, Frossard JL *et al.* (2002). Combination of steroids with infliximab or placebo in severe alcoholic hepatitis: a randomized controlled pilot study. *J Hepatol* 37: 448–55.

Stanley AJ, Ashley D, Dalton HR *et al.* (2009). Outpatient management of patients with low-risk upper-gastrointestinal haemorrhage: multicentre validation and prospective evaluation. *Lancet* 373: 42–7.

Takeuchi K, Smale S, Premchand P *et al.* (2006). Prevalence and mechanism of nonsteroidal anti-inflammatory drug-induced clinical relapse in patients with inflammatory bowel disease. *Clin Gastroenterol Hepatol* 4: 196–202.

Teasley DG, Gerding DN, Olson MM *et al.* (1983). Prospective randomised trial of metronidazole versus vancomycin for Clostridium difficile-associated diarrhoea and colitis. *Lancet* 2: 1043–6.

Thursz M, Richardson P, Allison M (2015). Prednisolone or pentoxifylline for alcoholic hepatitis. *N Engl J Med* 372: 1619–28.

Travis SPL, Farrant JM, Ricketts C *et al.* (1996). Predicting outcome in severe ulcerative colitis. *Gut* 38: 905.

Truelove SC, Watkinson G, Draper G (1962). Comparison of corticosteroid and sulphasalazine therapy in ulcerative colitis. *Br Med J* 2: 1708–11.

Truelove SC, Witts LJ (1955). Cortisone in ulcerative colitis: final report on a therapeutic trial. *Br Med J* 2: 1041–8.

Turner D, Walsh CM, Steinhart AH *et al.* (2007). Response to corticosteroids in severe ulcerative colitis: a systematic review of the literature and a meta-regression. *Clin Gastroenterol Hepatol* 5: 103–10.

van der Linden PD, Sturkenboom MC, Herings RM *et al.* (2002). Fluoroquinolones and risk of Achilles tendon disorders: case-control study. *BMJ* 324: 1306–7.

van Nood E, Vrieze A, Nieuwdorp M *et al.* (2013). Duodenal infusion of donor feces for recurrent Clostridium difficile. *N Engl J Med* 368: 407–15.

Voderholzer W, Schatke W, Muhldorfer B *et al.* (1997). Clinical response to dietary fiber treatment of chronic constipation. *Am J Gastroenterol* 92: 95.

Wenisch C, Parschalk B, Hasenhundl M *et al.* (1996). Comparison of vancomycin, teicoplanin, metronidazole, and fusidic acid for the treatment of Clostridium difficile associated diarrhea. *Clin Infect Dis* 22: 813–18.

Whitfield, K, Rambaldi A, Wetterslev J *et al.* (2009). Pentoxifylline for alcoholic hepatitis. *Cochrane Database Syst Rev* (4): CD007339.

Wilcox MH (2012). Progress with a difficult infection. *Lancet Infect Dis* 12: 256–7.

Wilcox M for Public Health England (2013). Available at: www.gov.uk/government/uploads/system/uploads/attachment_data/file/321891/Clostridium_difficile_management_and_treatment.pdf (accessed Dec 2015).

Wilcox MH, Fawley WN, Settle CD *et al.* (1998). Recurrence of symptoms in Clostridium difficile infection – relapse or reinfection? *J Hosp Infect* 38: 93–100.

Wilcox MH, Howe R (1995). Diarrhoea caused by Clostridium difficile: response time for treatment with metronidazole and vancomycin. *J Antimicrob Chemother* 36: 673–9.

Wilcox MH, Sandoe JA (2007). Probiotics and diarrhea: data are not widely applicable. *BMJ* 335: 171.

Wofford SA, Verne GN (2000). Approach to patients with refractory constipation. *Curr Gastroenterol Rep* 2: 389.

World Health Organisation (WHO). *Global Information System on Alcohol and Health* (GISAH), 2013. Available at: www.who.int/gho/alcohol/en/ (accessed Aug. 2014).

Zajac P, Holbrook A, Super ME *et al.* (2013). An overview: Current clinical guidelines for the evaluation, diagnosis, treatment, and management of dyspepsia. *Osteopathic Family Physician* 5: 79–85.

Zar FA, Bakkanagari SR, Moorthi KM *et al.* (2007). A comparison of vancomycin and metronidazole for the treatment of Clostridium difficile-associated diarrhea, stratified by disease severity. *Clin Infect Dis* 45: 302–7.

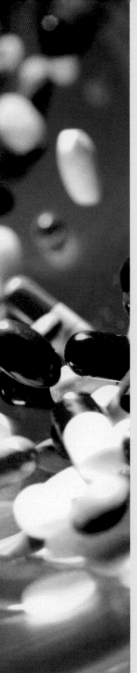

CHAPTER 6
Neurology
Victoria Taylor

Key topics:

Learning objectives

By the end of this chapter you should…

- …be able to write a prescription for patients with acute ischaemic stroke, acute seizures or bacterial meningitis, taking into account relevant contraindications, cautions and side effects.

- …be able to talk about the mechanisms of action of the key drugs used to treat these conditions.

- …be able to describe the pharmacological strategies employed in the long-term management of stroke, epilepsy and Parkinson's disease.

- …be aware of some of the key trials that underpin the management of these conditions.

Essential Practical Prescribing, First Edition. Georgia Woodfield, Benedict Lyle Phillips, Victoria Taylor, Amy Hawkins and Andrew Stanton. © 2016 by John Wiley & Sons, Ltd. Published 2016 by John Wiley & Sons, Ltd.

Stroke

Mr Robert Morrison
Age: 72
Hospital number: 123456

 Case study

Presenting complaint: *A 72-year-old man presents to A&E having woken up with right arm and leg weakness and muddled speech.*

Background: *He lives with his wife in a house and mobilises with a stick. He is an ex-smoker (20 pack years) and drinks 5–6 units of alcohol per week*

PMH: *Hypertension, myocardial infarction (7 years ago), osteoarthritis, right knee-replacement (3 years ago)*

Allergies: *Oxytetracycline (causes a rash)*

Examination:
HR 80, BP 146/76, Sats 97% on air, RR 16, BM 5.2
CVS: Capillary refill time <2 seconds, pulse feels regular, JVP not seen, no pitting oedema, HS I + II + 0
RS: Equal expansion with air entry to both bases and no added sounds

Abdo: *Soft, non-tender, no masses palpated, bowel sounds present*

Neuro:
Higher function and speech: An expressive dysphasia is found with preserved ability to follow instructions
Cranial nerves: A swallow test leads to coughing
Limbs: MRC grade 2 weakness in right arm and MRC grade 3 weakness in right leg with an extensor plantar response on the right

ECG: *Normal sinus rhythm*

Bloods: *Hb 13.6, Plt 324, WCC 8.9, Na 136, K 4.3, Urea 6.5, Creat 136, INR 1.1*

CT brain: *No evidence of acute bleeding.*

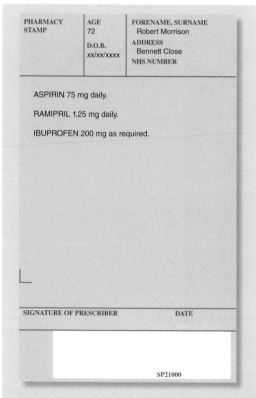

| PHARMACY STAMP | AGE 72 | FORENAME, SURNAME Robert Morrison |
| | D.O.B. xx/xx/xxxx | ADDRESS Bennett Close NHS NUMBER |

ASPIRIN 75 mg daily.

RAMIPRIL 1.25 mg daily.

IBUPROFEN 200 mg as required.

SIGNATURE OF PRESCRIBER   DATE

SP21000

Diagnosis

Left-hemisphere stroke (partial anterior circulation infarct).

The patient has developed sudden-onset neurological symptoms restricted to a particular vascular territory, that is the left MCA territory. He does not have evidence of intracranial bleeding or any of the 'stroke mimics' such as a space-occupying lesion (e.g. tumour), hypoglycaemia or a history of epilepsy or migraine. He has known risk factors for stroke including ischaemic heart disease, hypertension and being an ex-smoker.

Initial measures

Patients presenting with a suspected stroke must be urgently assessed on arrival in the Emergency Department regarding their suitability for thrombolysis. This patient also needs to be made 'nil by mouth' (NBM) until he can undergo a formal assessment of his swallow. Hydration should be maintained with intravenous fluids until an enteral feeding tube (e.g. a nasogastric tube) can be sited. This should happen within 24 hours (NICE, 2008).

Thrombolysis

The management of ischaemic stroke depends on the time of onset of symptoms and the degree of disability caused. Where it is *known* that symptoms started within the last 4.5 hours, where the degree of disability is neither too severe nor too mild (according to the National Institutes of Health Stroke Scale [NIHSS] scale) and where there are no other contraindications, intravenous thrombolysis may be used. Alteplase, a recombinant tPA (tissue plasminogen activator), is the main agent used for thrombolysis. This decision needs to be made by a senior clinician (usually a stroke physician) as the risks of thrombolysis, such as intracerebral haemorrhage, are not insignificant (NICE, 2008; SIGN, 2008).

In this case, the patient awoke with the symptoms. The time of onset of his symptoms is therefore *not known*. Where thrombolysis is not appropriate, aspirin is the main pharmacological intervention. Much of the management of stroke is non-pharmacological and current evidence shows that patients do better if they are transferred directly to a specialist stroke unit (Stroke Unit Trialists' Collaboration, 1997).

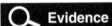 **Evidence**

Thrombolytic therapy
In 1995, the National Institute of Neurological Disorders and Stroke (NINDS) group showed that r-tPA improved functional outcomes after stroke if given within 3 hours of acute stroke (NINDS and rtPA Study Group, 1995). Hacke *et al.* (2008) subsequently showed that this could be extended to 4.5 hours. However, a pooled analysis of trials (Hacke *et al.*, 2004) has shown that outcomes are better the earlier r-tPA is administered. A recent meta-analysis did not show any effect of age on outcome within 4.5 hours (Emberson *et al.*, 2014).

 Guidelines

Having taken into account recent trial outcomes, NICE updated its guidance in 2012 to extend the period in which alteplase treatment can be given from up to 3 hours postsymptom onset to 4.5 hours.

Prescribing for strokes not amenable to thrombolysis

Prescribing

ONCE ONLY PRESCRIPTIONS						
Date	Time to be given	DRUG	Dose	Route	Prescriber	
					Signature	Bleep
xx/xx/xx	xx:xx	ASPIRIN	300 mg	PR	A. Doctor	

Aspirin 300 mg as a stat dose is given as soon as an intracerebral haemorrhage has been excluded (using brain imaging) where thrombolysis is not an option. This can be given per rectum or via an enteral feeding tube for patients with an unsafe swallow (up to half of patients who suffer a stroke have dysphagia) (Singh and Hamdy, 2006).

Aspirin: rationale and evidence

Aspirin 300 mg should be given for 14 days following the stroke. For patients intolerant of aspirin clopidogrel 75 mg daily should be used instead (NICE, 2008). If the patient is at high risk of gastrointestinal bleeding, a proton pump inhibitor (e.g. omeprazole) should be given as well.

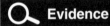 **Evidence**

Aspirin in acute stroke
A Cochrane review (Sandercock *et al.*, 2008) supports the use of aspirin in acute stroke. The review looked at over 43 000 patients in 12 randomised trials. Although other antiplatelet agents were used in some trials, 94% of the data came from two large trials using aspirin, 160–300 mg, within 48 hours of an acute stroke. The data showed that aspirin decreases the risk of death or dependency after stroke (maximum follow-up: 6 months) with a number needed to treat in order to benefit one person (NNTB) of 79. There was a small increase in the risk of intracranial haemorrhage, which was felt to be outweighed by the benefits of aspirin treatment.

✓	**DRUGS checklist for ASPIRIN**
Dose	300 mg in acute stroke
	75 mg in primary/secondary prevention of thromboembolic disease
Route	PO or PR; can also be given via nasogastric tube
Units	milligrams (mg)
Given	Once daily
Special situations	May predispose to GI bleeding. Can cause a hypersensitivity reaction with bronchospasm, rhinorrhoea, urticaria and angioedema.

Aspirin: essential pharmacology

How does it work?

Aspirin has two main clinical effects: at low doses it inhibits platelet aggregation and at higher doses it has anti-inflammatory properties (it has been classed as a non-steroidal anti-inflammatory drug [NSAID]) (Vane and Botting, 1998). In current clinical practice, it is used mainly as an antiplatelet agent in the prevention and treatment of arterial thromboses, for example MI and stroke. Aspirin works by irreversibly inhibiting the cyclo-oxygenase (COX) enzyme, which is present in nearly all tissues. This leads to decreased production of inflammatory mediators called 'prostanoids'. Its antiplatelet effect can be explained by its actions on a particular prostanoid called thromboxane A_2 (TXA_2). This is usually synthesised in platelets in response to endothelial damage and promotes platelet aggregation. This in turn initiates haemostasis, clot formation and endothelial repair (but also thrombosis). By irreversibly inhibiting COX in platelets, aspirin reduces TXA_2 levels and therefore reduces platelet aggregation. Interestingly, although low-dose aspirin has a short half-life (minutes to hours), it only needs to be given once a day. This is because platelets lack nuclei and therefore cannot synthesise new proteins, including COX (Pantano, 1994). Therefore the antiplatelet effect of aspirin persists until more platelets are produced (the lifespan of a platelet is 8–10 days).

Unwanted effects

The side effects of aspirin are also related to its ability to deplete prostanoids. Certain prostanoids, namely prostacyclin and prostaglandin E2, inhibit gastric acid production and promote gastric mucus production, both of which protect the mucosa from erosions and ulcers (Miller, 2006). Therefore the depletion of these prostanoids, caused by the inhibition of COX by aspirin, leads to an increased risk of gastric erosions and ulcers. Because of aspirin's antiplatelet activity, the risk of bleeding from these ulcers and erosions is also increased.

Aspirin hypersensitivity is caused by an imbalance between prostanoids and leukotrienes. These are both inflammatory mediators produced from the same precursor, arachidonic acid. When aspirin inhibits COX, more arachidonic acid is available for conversion into leukotrienes by the enzyme lipoxygenase (LOX). The imbalance between the prostanoids and the leukotrienes leads to leukotriene-mediated inflammation in the airways and upper respiratory tract (Szczeklik *et al.*, 2004). In some people, this leads to symptoms of rhinitis, angioedema, bronchospasm and urticaria, especially if they already have asthma. This also explains why leukotriene *antagonists* such as 'montelukast' are used to treat asthma (see Chapter 4).

Other drugs used in stroke

Acute stroke

Oxygen: Similar to acute myocardial infarction, oxygen therapy is only indicated in acute stroke if the patient is hypoxic (i.e. if the oxygen saturations are outside the target range of 94–98%) (NICE, 2008; SIGN, 2008).

Antihypertensives: Hypertension is not usually treated in acute ischaemic stroke unless there is evidence of a hypertensive emergency such as encephalopathy. This is because of the risk of cerebral hypoperfusion. Under normal circumstances a phenomenon known as 'cerebral autoregulation' protects the brain from hypoperfusion when the systemic blood pressure is lowered. However, after a stroke, this may not work as well (Sprigg and Bath, 2005), putting patients at risk of further ischaemic brain injury if their systemic blood pressure is lowered. There is no clear evidence as to whether patients should continue previously prescribed antihypertensive agents.

Statins: Although it is recommended that all patients who have had an ischaemic stroke should be given a statin (see Evidence), this treatment should not be initiated until 48 hours after the onset of the stroke. However, if the patient is already on a statin, this should be continued (NICE, 2008; SIGN, 2008).

Thromboprophylaxis: Although intuitively, inpatients with a stroke would seem to be at increased risk of venous thromboembolism, anticoagulants are *not* usually recommended in this group, in the acute phase at least (SIGN, 2008). This is because of concerns that these medications may provoke haemorrhage into the infarcted brain tissue. Therefore close attention should be paid to providing adequate hydration and nutrition alongside intensive physiotherapy and early mobilisation. Mechanical prophylaxis in the form of intermittent pneumatic compression devices or similar is often used; this needs to be started within the first 48 hours.

Secondary prevention

Antiplatelets: Clopidogrel is usually recommended for secondary prevention after ischaemic stroke, once patients have received 14 days of aspirin 300 mg. The combination of dipyridamole and aspirin was previously more popular but dipyridamole is often not tolerated due to its propensity to cause headaches (see Evidence).

Antihypertensives: Antihypertensives should be considered in all patients who have suffered an ischaemic stoke. One trial in particular showed a reduction in stroke recurrence in patients given perindopril and indapamide. It is likely, however, that this is a 'class effect'; that is, the outcome would be similar if any ACE-I or any thiazide diuretic were

used. There is also some data that calcium channel antagonists (such as amlodipine) and diuretics have an advantage because they also address blood pressure fluctuations (see Evidence).

Cholesterol-lowering drugs: A statin should be prescribed after an ischaemia stroke regardless of the cholesterol level. Atorvastatin 80 mg was shown in one trial to reduce stroke recurrence (see Evidence) but again, it is likely that this is a class effect and that other statins would have similar benefits. A starting dose of atorvastatin 20 mg or simvastatin 40 mg is commonly used, unless using simvastatin in combination with amlodipine, in which case a reduced dose of simvastatin 20 mg should be used, according to recent MHRA advice (MHRA, 2014).

🔍 Evidence

Antiplatelet agents

The ESPRIT trial (Halkes *et al.*, 2006) showed that using aspirin *and* dipyridamole is more effective than aspirin alone in the secondary prevention of stroke. However, a significant number of patients stopped therapy due to side effects (mainly headaches). A further trial called PRoFESS (Sacco *et al.*, 2008) showed clopidogrel monotherapy to have equal efficacy to the combination of aspirin and dypiridamole in preventing further strokes. There seems to be no benefit of using clopidogrel and aspirin together (Diener *et al.*, 2004).

Antihypertensive agents

In 2001, it was shown that the combination of perindopril and indapamide reduced stroke risk (PROGRESS Collaborative Group, 2001). Rashid *et al.* (2003) later performed a systematic review of RCTs which confirmed that lowering blood pressure is effective in preventing vascular events (including stroke) following a stroke. Webb *et al.* (2014) showed that calcium channel antagonists and diuretics reduced blood pressure variability and maximum systolic blood pressure after stroke or TIA.

(Continued)

Evidence (Continued)

Cholesterol-lowering agents

The SPARCL trial (Amarenco *et al.*, 2006) showed that atorvastatin, 80 mg daily, reduced the incidence of fatal or non-fatal stroke with a NNTB of 45 over 5 years, irrespective of baseline cholesterol. However, there was a slight increased risk of intracranial haemorrhage with a NNTH of 107.

Other considerations

Diabetes: A fasting blood glucose level or Hb_{A1C} should be checked to ensure that the patient is not diabetic.

ECG/ prolonged ambulatory ECG recording: If atrial fibrillation (AF) is diagnosed, it should be treated as for AF in any other situation (see Chapter 3 Cardiology) with the caveat that warfarin, if indicated, should not be commenced until 14 days has elapsed to avoid the risk of haemorrhage into the infarcted brain tissue (NICE, 2008).

Stroke in young patients: This is less likely in young patients is less likely to be caused by atherosclerosis or AF and so further investigations should be performed to look for an underlying cause such as a thrombotic tendency, patent foramen ovale or a vasculitic process.

Case outcome and discharge

Mr Morrison had a CT scan, which confirmed an area of infarction in the left cerebral hemisphere (internal capsule). Because the precise timing of onset of symptoms could not be determined he did not meet the criteria for thrombolysis. He was moved to the acute stroke unit. Over the next 3 weeks, his expressive dysphasia and weakness improved. He underwent physiotherapy as well as speech and language therapy and, after 3 weeks of rehabilitation, was able to walk with a stick and communicate as normal. He had a 72-hour ECG recording, which did not show evidence of AF although a fasting glucose was raised and his fasting lipids were also above the desired range. He was started on a statin, as well as metformin, after receiving advice from the diabetes specialist nurse. His blood pressure control was optimised by increasing his ramipril dose. He was discharged with the medications listed.

DISCHARGE MEDICATION						
Date	Medication	Dose	Route	Frequency	Supply	GP to continue?
xx/xx/xx	ATORVASTATIN	80 mg	PO	Once daily at night	14 days	Y
xx/xx/xx	METFORMIN	500 mg	PO	Twice daily with meals	14 days	Y
xx/xx/xx	RAMIPRIL	2.5 mg	PO	Once daily	14 days	Y
xx/xx/xx	CLOPIDOGREL	75 mg	PO	Once daily	14 days	Y

Notes to patient/GP: Atorvastatin started for secondary prevention of stroke. Metformin started for new diagnosis of diabetes mellitus. Ramipril dose increased to improve blood pressure control. Aspirin stopped and clopidogrel started for secondary prevention of stroke.

Common pitfalls

- An inability to swallow doesn't preclude acute treatment with aspirin, as this medication can also be given per rectum (PR).
- Prophylactic low molecular weight heparin (LMWH) is not recommended in patients with an acute stroke due to the risk of haemorrhagic transformation.

SUMMARY

There are a number of pharmacological interventions that can improve the outcome and prognosis in stroke. As with all medical interventions there are risks as well as benefits and the decision to administer a potentially harmful treatment should be supported by good evidence where possible. It is important to recognise that pharmacological intervention represents only one facet of treatment and this is certainly the case in stroke. Many of the improved outcomes in stroke care over recent years have resulted from good nursing care in a specialised stroke unit with access to intensive treatment from allied professionals such as physiotherapists, nutritionists and speech and language therapists.

Key learning points

Acute stroke
- Oxygen is recommended only if the patient is hypoxic.
- Consider thrombolysis if the time of onset of symptoms is clear and was within the last 4.5 hours. The decision to thrombolyse should be made by a senior physician.
- For ischaemic stroke, give aspirin 300 mg for 14 days.

Secondary prevention
- Consider: antiplatelet agents, antihypertensive medications, cholesterol-lowering drugs, as well as considering the treatment of contributory conditions such as diabetes, hypercholesterolaemia and atrial fibrillation.

FURTHER READING

- SIGN and NICE guidelines give excellent guidance about the treatment of stroke and are regularly updated.
- A comprehensive review of recent stroke trials is: Rothwell PM, Algra A, Amarenco P (2011). Medical treatment in acute and long-term secondary prevention after transient ischaemic attack and ischaemic stroke. *Lancet* 377: 1681–92.
- A good review of secondary prevention measures after stroke is: Schulz UG (2013). Drug treatments in the secondary prevention of ischaemic stroke. *Maturitas* 76: 267–71.

Bacterial meningitis

Mrs Hayley Jones
Age: 38
Hospital number: 123456

Case study

Presenting complaint: Mrs Jones is brought in by ambulance having been found at home, collapsed. Her husband comes in with her and says she had complained of a headache and a stiff neck earlier that day and has vomited once but that she was previously fit and well. He does not think she has taken any illicit substances or been exposed to any toxins. He is not aware of any recent head injuries and they have not been abroad in the last 6 months. She had been well over the weekend but stayed at home today feeling unwell. The rest of the family is well.

PMH: Nil

DH: Microgynon 30 (combined oral contraceptive pill)

Allergies: None known

SH: Mrs Jones lives with her husband and 10-year-old daughter and works as a primary school teacher.

Weight: 57 kg

O/E:
Looks unwell; lying in bed quite still with her eyes closed; seems unaware of her surroundings.
GCS: 10 (E: 3, V: 2, M: 5)
Febrile 39.2°C
Airway: Patent
Breathing: RR 16; Sats 98% OA
Air entry to both lung bases, no added sounds
Circulation: HR: 118; BP: 105/65
CRT 3 seconds; HS I+II+O
Disability: Blood sugar 4.0
Neurology: The pupils are equal and reactive to light. Although she is not compliant with a full

(Continued)

🔍 Case study (Continued)

neurological examination, she has a positive Kernig's sign; her plantar responses are downgoing
Exposure: No meningococcal rash seen. NB. Leg pain and cold hands and feet can precede the rash in meningococcal meningitis.

Bedside tests: urine dip negative, CXR clear lung fields
ABG on air: pH 7.35, Pao_2 11, Pco_2 4.5, BE −1.8, HCO_3 22.8, lactate 5.

PHARMACY STAMP	AGE 38	FORENAME, SURNAME
	38	Hayley Jones
	D.O.B. xx/xx/xxxx	ADDRESS 79 Airedale Road
		NHS NUMBER

MICROGYNON 30; take as directed.

SIGNATURE OF PRESCRIBER   DATE

SP21000

Diagnosis

Possible bacterial meningitis but, with a low GCS, a viral meningoencephalitis cannot be excluded. The differential diagnosis also includes viral meningitis, although patients are not typically as unwell with this.

Initial measures

The priority here is to gain venous access, take blood samples including blood cultures and then administer empirical antibiotics/antiviral medications as soon as possible. She also needs a lumbar puncture as soon as possible, assuming a CT head does not suggest raised intracranial pressure (this is impossible to exclude clinically given the decreased GCS) but this should not delay antibiotic administration. As this patient has evidence of systemic sepsis (HR >100, temp >38, raised lactate), other measures are also required as detailed in Chapter 11, Section Sepsis and Antibiotics.

A CT scan is normal and lumbar puncture is performed, which shows a cloudy CSF.

Prescribing for suspected bacterial meningitis

FLUID CHART

Date	Fluid	Dose	Route	Rate/ duration	Signature	Print name
xx/xx/xx	SODIUM CHLORIDE 0.9%	500 ml	IV	STAT	A. Doctor	A. Doctor

REGULAR PRESCRIPTIONS

	Circle/enter times below	Day 1	Day 2	Day 3	Day 4
DRUG CEFTRIAXONE	06				
	(08)				
Dose 2 g / Route IV / Freq BD / Start date xx/xx/xx	12				
Signature A. Doctor / Bleep / Review	16				
Additional instructions	(20)				
	22				
DRUG DEXAMETHASONE	(06)				
	08				
Dose 8 mg / Route IV / Freq QDS / Start date xx/xx/xx	(12)				
Signature A. Doctor / Bleep / Review	16				
Additional instructions 0.15 mg/kg	(18)				
	(24)				
DRUG ACICLOVIR	06				
	(08)				
Dose 570 mg / Route IV / Freq TDS / Start date xx/xx/xx	12				
Signature A. Doctor / Bleep / Review	(14)				
Additional instructions 10 mg/kg	18				
	(22)				

The mainstay of treatment for bacterial meningitis comprises antibiotics and supportive measures such as fluid therapy. Some guidelines recommend using dexamethasone 0.15 mg/kg every 6 hours for the first 2–4 days (Tunkel *et al.*, 2004). Antibiotics should be administered promptly. Even with treatment, bacterial meningitis has a mortality rate of 13–27% (Fitch and van de Beek, 2007). Cover has also been provided in case of a viral meningo-encephalitis with aciclovir, at a dose of 10 mg/kg every 8 hours.

The commonest organisms implicated in bacterial meningitis in all age groups are *Streptococcus pneumonia* ('pneumococcal' meningitis), *Neisseria meningitides* ('meningococcal' meningitis) and *Haemophilus influenza* (Durand *et al.*, 1993) (although with the vaccination programme, *Haemophilus* has almost disappeared). A typical regimen for suspected meningitis, which would cover these organisms, would be ceftriaxone 2 g BD. However, antibiotic regimens vary from area to area according to local bacterial prevalences and sensitivities and you should consult your local antibiotics guidelines. For example, in the USA and parts of Europe, vancomycin is added to the regimen in recognition of the growing incidence of multidrug-resistant *Streptococcus pneumonia* (Fitch and van de Beek, 2007). The antibiotics you use will also depend on the likely organism, which varies with the age of the patient and the presence of other risk factors such as recent travel or immunosuppression. In patients over the age of 50 years, pregnant women and children under 1 month old, antibiotics should cover *Listeria monocytogenes* and you should add ampicillin to your regimen (Tunkel *et al.*, 2004). In immunosuppressed patients, you need to consider unusual organisms such as *Cryptococcus*, *Toxoplasma* or *Mycobacterium tuberculosis*. If you are unsure or if there are atypical features, your local microbiologist will be able to provide further advice.

Ceftriaxone: rationale and evidence

The third-generation cephalosporins are generally used as first-line empirical treatment in cases of suspected acute bacterial meningitis in an inpatient setting, although you are, as always, referred to your local guidelines. Common choices include ceftriaxone or cefotaxime. There is a rationale rather than any reliable evidence (see Evidence Newer Versus older Antibiotic Regimens in Bacterial Meningitis)

for using these newer broad-spectrum antibiotics. However, probably more important than the choice of antibiotic is the speed with which it is administered (see Evidence Do Not Delay Treatment) and if the patient has evidence of sepsis, as in this case, you should aim to start antibiotic therapy within an hour of diagnosis.

🔍 Evidence

Newer versus older antibiotic regimens in bacterial meningitis

A systematic review from the Cochrane database (Prasad *et al.*, 2007) looked at whether newer third-generation cephalosporins show any advantage over older penicillin/ampicillin/chloramphenicol-based regimens for acute bacterial meningitis. No difference in rates of death or long-term disability was found. However, most of the studies reviewed were more than 20 years old and therefore may not reflect emerging resistance patterns. A current trial would be difficult to justify given the life-threatening nature of this condition.

✓ DRUGS checklist for CEFTRIAXONE in bacterial meningitis

Dose	2 g
Route	Slow IV injection or IM (Do not give more than 1 g at any one IM site)
Units	Milligrams (mg)
Given	Twice daily (BD)
Special situations	Ceftriaxone should **not** be mixed with, or given in the same line as, calcium-containing solutions (e.g. Hartmann's solution).
	A proportion of patients who are allergic to penicillin may also be allergic to cephalosporins.
	For side effects, see Chapter 11 Microbiology.

🔍 Evidence

Do not delay treatment

A retrospective cohort study of 123 adults with proven bacterial meningitis showed an 8.4 times greater risk of mortality where the 'door-to-antibiotic' time was >6 hours (Proulx *et al.*, 2005). A subsequent prospective observational study of 156 adult patients admitted to ICU with pneumococcal meningitis showed a delay in administration of antibiotics of >3 hours from hospital admission to be the strongest predictor of 3 month mortality (Auburtin *et al.*, 2006).

Although these studies do not represent the highest grade of evidence, similar results are reflected elsewhere in the literature and the principle of early antibiotics treatment in sepsis is also endorsed by the Surviving Sepsis guidelines (Dellinger *et al.*, 2013).

Ceftriaxone: essential pharmacology

As discussed in Chapter 11, the cephalosporins are broad-spectrum beta-lactam antibiotics. The key features that make ceftriaxone suitable in this situation include its ability to cross the blood–brain barrier (especially in the presence of meningeal inflammation) and its activity against the organisms which typically cause the condition, even in the presence of bacterial beta-lactamases. Only 4–17% of the plasma concentration of ceftriaxone is attained in the CNS and therefore higher doses than those used for other conditions are required to achieve sufficient concentrations in the CNS.

For further details of cephalosporin pharmacology, please refer to Chapter 11, Section Cephalosporins.

Dexamethasone: rationale and evidence

Potential long-term complications in survivors of bacterial meningitis include hearing loss and other neurological deficits. It may seem counter-intuitive to administer an immunosuppressive agent in the context of an acute infection but as is often the case in infectious diseases, a proportion of the damage caused by the infection is due to the body's immune response and the associated inflammation and corticosteroids have been suggested as a way of limiting this inflammatory damage. In animal models, dexamethasone has been shown to attenuate some of the changes in the CNS associated with meningitis, including brain oedema, raised intracranial pressure, raised CSF lactate (Tauber *et al.*, 1985) and there is also some evidence of clinical benefit in humans (see Evidence). It is highlighted that this treatment must be given alongside antibiotic therapy.

✓ DRUGS checklist for DEXAMETHASONE in bacterial meningitis

Dose	0.15 mg/ kg
Route	IV
Units	milligrams (mg)
Given	Four times per day (QDS) for 4 days
	The first dose should be given with or prior to the first dose of antibiotics
Special situations	Steroid side effects are discussed elsewhere (Chapter 12), although the short-term use of corticosteroids is associated with very few adverse outcomes.
	The efficacy of coumarins such as warfarin may be enhanced.
	The efficacy of the contraceptive pill may also be affected.
	Some experts recommend stopping treatment if an organism other than *Streptococcus pneumonia* is cultured.

🔍 Evidence

Corticosteroids in bacterial meningitis
A systematic review (Brouwer et al., 2013)
including 25 RCTs and a total of 4121
participants (adults and children) suggests
that corticosteroids given in bacterial
meningitis significantly reduce mortality for
cases of pneumococcal meningitis but there
was no significant reduction in mortality found
for cases caused by N. meningitides,
H. influenza or other organisms. It also showed
a significant decrease in hearing loss,
which only held true for cases caused by
H. influenza. The only significant adverse effect
of corticosteroid treatment was found to be an
increased incidence of recurrent fever.

Dexamethasone: essential pharmacology

Dexamethasone is a glucocorticoid, with potent anti-inflammatory effects. Dexamethasone is approximately seven times as potent as prednisolone and 30 times as potent as hydrocortisone. It is lipophilic and diffuses through cell membranes. As discussed in the section on hydrocortisone (see Chapter 2, Section Anaphylaxis), glucocorticoids acts on the intracellular glucocorticoid receptor to modulate gene transcription, although other, less well-defined, shorter-term effects are also produced via interaction with cell-surface receptors. Downstream effects of glucocorticoid therapy include inhibition of prostaglandin production via several mechanisms, including suppressing transcription of cyclo-oxygenase 2 (COX-2) and inducing transcription of annexin-1 and MAPK phosphatase 1. The glucocorticoid-receptor complex also blocks the transcriptional activity of another transcription factor (NF-κB) which would otherwise promote transcription of cytokines, chemokines, cell adhesion molecules and complement factors, all of which are involved in the inflammatory or immune response (Rhen and Cidlowski, 2005).

Whilst dexamethasone has potent actions following interactions with *glucocorticoid* receptors, it only has very minor effects on *mineralocorticoid* receptors and causes only minimal sodium retention. It is therefore especially useful where water retention would be deleterious, for example in cases where there is potential cerebral oedema (Rang et al., 2003). Excretion is mainly renal but the effects of glucocorticoids persist beyond the duration of their presence in the body, due to their effects on gene transcription (Datapharm, 2015).

Further aspects of meningitis management

Escalation

Patients with bacterial meningitis often need care in a high dependency or intensive care (ICU) setting. Where there is evidence of severe sepsis, neurological sequelae or the patient's conscious level is impaired, early discussion with the ICU team is recommended.

Notification

Bacterial meningitis is a notifiable disease and your local health protection officer should be informed (in the USA, the equivalent organisation is the Centres for Disease Control and Prevention or CDC). Prophylaxis is usually provided to close contacts of the primary case, that is people who live with them and anyone exposed to respiratory droplets/ secretions. Options for prophylaxis usually include ciprofloxacin, rifampicin or IM ceftriaxone but your health protection officer will advise. See the Public Health England (PHE) website for further details.

A note on viral meningitis

Meningitis can also be caused by a variety of other pathogens (viruses, fungi and parasites) as well as a number of non-infectious causes such as cancer, sarcoidosis and drugs. Viral meningitis is fairly common, usually caused by an enterovirus and is generally self-limiting. It is worthwhile noting that aciclovir is of *no benefit* in viral meningitis and is only indicated in cases of suspected viral encephalitis or meningoencephalitis, where herpes simplex virus or varicella zoster virus might be implicated (Chadwick, 2005). In this case the patient had a reduced GCS and so aciclovir was provided in case of viral meningoencephalitis.

Case outcome and discharge

Mrs Jones was transferred to ICU and intubated. Five days later, she started to recover. Her blood cultures grew *Streptococcus pneumoniae*, which was sensitive to ceftriaxone. After discussion with the local microbiology team, it was decided to continue antibiotics for 14 days. She was left without any significant neurological deficits. Her family was given prophylaxis although it was not deemed necessary for prophylaxis to be given out at the school where she worked.

Mrs Jones did not require any medications on discharge.

Common pitfalls

■ Don't delay antibiotics. Antibiotics must be administered as early as possible. Whilst it is ideal to obtain CSF samples prior to antibiotics, this vital treatment should not be delayed. If performing a lumbar puncture is going to incur a significant delay, for example where a CT scan is required, antibiotics should be given prior to the CT and lumbar puncture.

■ Don't forget to take blood cultures. There is no excuse for not taking blood cultures immediately and it is often the blood cultures which yield the offending organism, 53% of the time in one study (Proulx *et al.*, 2005).

SUMMARY

Bacterial meningitis is a serious and life-threatening infection. It should be suspected and treated where there is evidence of meningism in conjunction with fever or other signs of sepsis. Antibiotics are the mainstay of treatment and there is some evidence to support the use of dexamethasone too.

🔑 Key learning points

Meningitis management
- Do not delay antibiotic treatment in cases of suspected meningitis but remember to take blood cultures and ideally CSF samples first.
- Consider the addition of dexamethasone when giving the first dose or prior to the first dose of antibiotics.
- Try to obtain information that might help determine which organism is involved.
- Discuss the case early on with the microbiology and ICU teams.
- Meningitis is a notifiable disease.

FURTHER READING

■ A good article outlining the diagnosis and treatment of bacterial meningitis is: Fitch MT, van de Beek, D (2007). Emergency diagnosis and treatment of adult meningitis. *Lancet Infect Dis* 7: 191–200.

■ NICE produces guidelines for the management of meningitis in children: NICE. *Meningitis (Bacterial) and Menigococcal Septicaemia in Under 16s: Recognition, Diagnosis and Management*, CG102, 2010. Available at: www.nice.org.uk/guidance/cg102 (accessed Dec. 2015).

Seizures and epilepsy

> ## Ms Penny Haversham
> ## Age: 23 years
> ## Hospital number: 123456

🔍 Case study

PC : A 23-year-old woman is brought in to A&E by ambulance. She is having a generalised seizure. It started approximately 15 minutes ago. Prior to the seizure she had been watching TV with her boyfriend. She is afebrile and has not been unwell recently.

PMH: Epilepsy

Allergies: None

Examination:
HR 100 reg, RR 20, BP 160/70, Sats 95% on air, afebrile, BM 6.5, warm peripheries, capillary refill time 2 seconds
Ongoing seizure activity: alternating contraction and relaxation of all 4 limbs with eyes rolled back. Further examination is difficult but there is air entry at both bases. There are no obvious injuries externally. She is unresponsive to voice or pain. Her trousers are wet with urine.

Estimated weight: 60 kg

Diagnosis

This patient is having a seizure and is heading towards status epilepticus. Status epilepticus is formally defined as epileptic activity continuing for more than 30 minutes, either as ongoing seizure activity or intermittent seizure activity without regaining consciousness in between. That said, it is clearly not appropriate to wait for 30 minutes before treating an ongoing seizure, especially as it is recognised that the longer a seizure continues for, the poorer the outcome. Treatment should be initiated in generalised tonic–clonic activity lasting more than 5 minutes (Kelso and Cock, 2005).

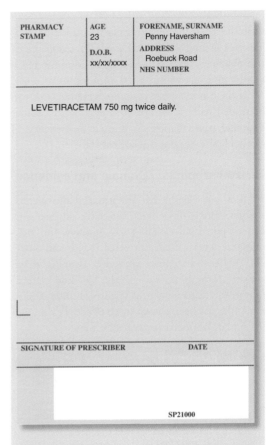

| PHARMACY STAMP | AGE 23 | FORENAME, SURNAME Penny Haversham |
| | D.O.B. xx/xx/xxxx | ADDRESS Roebuck Road NHS NUMBER |

LEVETIRACETAM 750 mg twice daily.

| SIGNATURE OF PRESCRIBER | DATE |

SP21000

Initial measures

It is recommended that treatment be initiated in seizures that do not terminate after 5 minutes (NICE, 2012; SIGN, 2005). ABC measures are a priority. The airway should be secured with an oropharyngeal ('Guedel') or nasopharyngeal airway and high-flow-oxygen given. In practice, a nasopharyngeal airway is generally used as there is often trismus of the master muscle and the jaw is clenched shut. The pulse, BP and respiratory function should be assessed. It is important to secure IV access, check glucose levels and get senior help.

Prescribing for acute seizures

ONCE ONLY PRESCRIPTIONS					Prescriber	
Date	Time to be given	DRUG	Dose	Route	Signature	Bleep
xx/xx/xx	xx:xx	OXYGEN	15 L/min	Reservoir mask	A. Doctor	
xx/xx/xx	xx:xx	LORAZEPAM	4 mg	IV	A. Doctor	

In the hospital setting, where IV access has been established, IV lorazepam 4 mg is considered first-line treatment (NICE, 2012; SIGN, 2005; Cock and Shapira, 2002). This can be re-administered if there is no effect within 5–10 minutes.

If there is evidence of hypoglycaemia, this can be treated with 50 mL of 50% dextrose. Consider thiamine (see Chapter 5) if there is evidence of alcohol abuse or poor nutritional state.

Benzodiazepines: rationale and evidence

Seizures are caused by abnormal neuronal discharges. This over-activity can have adverse outcomes, potentially leading to cognitive and neurological deficits if left untreated (Kelso and Cock, 2005). Benzodiazepines work by damping down activity in the brain and are the first-line medication in the management of seizures. Lorazepam, in particular has been shown to be effective, although IM midazolam is also equally effective.

🔍 Evidence

A Cochrane review (Prasad *et al.*, 2005) showed that lorazepam was more effective than diazepam or phenytoin in the immediate treatment of status epilepticus. A study (Silbergleit *et al.*, 2012), showed non-inferiority of IM midazolam as compared to IV lorazepam.

✓ DRUGS checklist for LORAZEPAM

Dose	4 mg (or 0.1 mg/kg) in acute seizures
Route	IV
Units	mg
Given	As required
Special situations	Lorazepam is kept in the fridge. There is a risk of respiratory depression if mixed with other CNS depressants. Lorazepam does *not* have an active metabolite and so has a shorter duration of action than diazepam.

Alternatives to lorazepam

IV diazepam (10 mg) would be a second-line choice. If it is not possible to get IV access, IM midazolam (10 mg) or buccal midazolam (5–10 mg) can be used. Rectal diazepam (10–20 mg) is also available for use in the community.

Benzodiazepines: essential pharmacology

How do they work?

Seizures are caused by excessive excitatory activity in the central nervous system. The benzodiazepines work by binding at an allosteric site and enhancing the effects of the major inhibitory neurotransmitter: GABA, at the $GABA_A$ receptor (Rudolph *et al.*, 2001). This results in a general 'dampening-down' of brain activity.

Unwanted effects

Other effects (these may be helpful or unwanted) include sedation, decreased anxiety, anterograde amnesia and impaired coordination. The benzodiazepines have also been noted to cause paradoxical reactions including agitation and aggression (Datapharm, 2015).

Tolerance: Benzodiazepines exhibit the phenomenon of tolerance which means that larger and larger doses are required to produce the same clinical effect.

Dependence: Benzodiazepines exhibit 'dependence', which means that the patient experiences symptoms of withdrawal when the drug is stopped abruptly.

Flumazenil: There is a specific antidote to benzodiazepines called 'flumazenil', but this is only licensed for very specific indications as it carries a risk of convulsions, especially if the patient has also taken tricyclic antidepressants (TCAs).

Prescribing for prolonged seizures

What if the seizure continues despite two doses of benzodiazepines?

FLUID CHART						
Date	Infusion fluid/ Volume	Additive/ Dose	Rate/ Duration	Time to be given	Signature	Print name
xx/xx/xx	SODIUM CHLORIDE 0.9%, 250 ml	PHENYTOIN 1200 mg	30 minutes	xx:xx	A. Doctor	A. Doctor

If there is no improvement after two doses of a benzodiazepine, the anaesthetics and ICU teams need to be made aware of the situation. In terms of medications, the next line of treatment is a phenytoin (or phenobarbital) infusion. The loading dose for a patient not already taking phenytoin is 20 mg/kg, which in this patient would be 1200 mg (20 mg × 60 kg).

Phenytoin: rationale and evidence

Phenytoin selectively inhibits very active neurons and is therefore used to treat status epilepticus. It is a second-line agent, as it has been found to be less effective than the benzodiazepines (see Evidence) and has a number of side effects. It remains, however, a useful drug in resistant seizures and is also non-sedating. You may also come across fosphenytoin, a phenytoin precursor, which has some advantages over phenytoin but is much more expensive.

✓	DRUGS checklist for PHENYTOIN
Dose	Loading dose: 15–20 mg/kg Maintenance: 100 mg TDS (or 300 mg OD)
Route	IV (maintenance doses can be given PO)
Units	milligrams (mg)
Given	Diluted in 0.9% saline (concentration not more than 10 mg/mL) and given at a rate not exceeding 50 mg/min
Special situations	Phenytoin must be given via a large-bore cannula in the antecubital fossa or above. The patient should be on a cardiac monitor as it can cause hypotension and arrhythmias. Phenytoin is administered by weight and so the dose is specific to the individual patient. Phenytoin is an enzyme inducer and may interact with other medications.

Phenytoin: essential pharmacology

How does it work?

Phenytoin is thought to work by inhibiting voltage-dependent sodium channels. It selectively inhibits very active neurons without too much of an effect on normally functioning neurons (Kwan *et al.*, 2001). It has unpredictable pharmacokinetics and a narrow therapeutic window (40–80 micromole/L or 10–20 mg/L). Above 80 micromole/L manifestations of toxicity include ataxia, horizontal nystagmus and slurred speech (Datapharm, 2015).

Phenytoin should be administered via a wide-bore cannula in a large vein (antecubital fossa or proximal). This is because of its high pH, which can lead to cellulitis if it extravasates (Datapharm, 2015). It should not be administered in the same intravenous line as other medications. A cardiac monitor is required as phenytoin can cause cardiac arrhythmias and hypotension, especially if given quickly. It should not be used in patients with second or third-degree heart block. Long-term side effects of phenytoin include gum hypertrophy, hirsutism, rashes and hepatitis (Datapharm, 2015). Phenytoin is not generally recommended in pregnancy as it can cause fetal malformations (so-called 'hydantoin syndrome') but this risk must be weighed up against the risk to the fetus from a seizure, which may lead to significant hypoxia. This is especially true in status epilepticus, where senior advice should be sought.

Phenytoin is an enzyme inducer, increasing the activity of liver enzymes and speeding up the metabolism of other medications (Lynch and Price, 2007). This is of little relevance in the acute situation but should be taken into account when it is used in the long-term management of epilepsy (see Section Pharmacological Management of Epilepsy).

Further aspects of seizure management

Other issues

It is important to look for the underlying cause for the seizure.

- If this is a first seizure, the differential diagnosis includes hypoglycaemia, electrolyte disturbances, alcohol withdrawal, infection, toxic substances, underlying structural brain lesions and autoimmune causes.

- If the patient has known epilepsy, the above differentials are still valid but it may be that the patient has not taken their usual antiepileptic drug (AED), or has started a new medication which has interacted with their AEDs resulting in subtherapeutic levels (see Section Pharmacological Management of Epilepsy). It is possible to check AED levels for some medications, although these results take a while to come back. In practical terms, it is important to ensure that a person with epilepsy receives their usual AEDs and to check for interactions.

Refractory seizures

If the above treatment doesn't abate the seizure, further management usually involves general anaesthesia, EEG monitoring and specialist care in an intensive care setting.

Case outcome and discharge

Ms Haversham's seizure was controlled with two doses of lorazepam. She admitted to stopping her epilepsy medications as she had wanted to conceive and was worried about the effects antiepileptic medications might have on a potential baby. She was counselled by the epilepsy nurse specialist as to the risks of omitting antiepileptic medications and managing epilepsy in pregnancy. She agreed to continue with her medications and to come back to neurology clinic for further discussion about pregnancy planning and epilepsy.

DISCHARGE MEDICATION						
Date	Medication	Dose	Route	Frequency	Supply	GP to continue?
xx/xx/xx	LEVETIRACETAM	750 mg	PO	Twice daily	14 days	Y

Notes to patient/GP:
No changes to regular medications.

Pharmacological management of epilepsy

Antiepileptic drugs

The long-term management of epilepsy is complex. Epilepsy should always be treated by a specialist but it is important to have some understanding of the potential side effects and interactions of AEDs.

The AED used depends on the type of seizure. Current NICE (2012) recommendations are given in Table 6.1.

It is also important to be aware that AEDs are not uncommonly referred to by their trade names rather than their generic names, as different preparations may vary in their bioavailability or pharmacokinetics. A few examples are:

Emeside is ethosuximide
Epanutin is phenytoin
Epilim and Epival are sodium valproate
Keppra is levetiracetam
Tegretol is carbamazepine

Unwanted effects

AEDs are a particularly troublesome group of drugs in terms of side effects, although newer drugs with

Table 6.1 Antiepileptic drug recommendations (NICE, 2012).			
	Generalised tonic–clonic epilepsy	**Focal seizures**	**Absence epilepsy**
First line	Sodium valproate *For women of childbearing age:* Levetiracetam Lamotrigine	Carbamazepine Lamotrigine	Ethosuxamide Sodium valproate
Second line	Lamotrigine Carbamazepine Oxcarbazepine	Levetiracetam Oxcarbazepine Sodium valproate	Lamotrigine

Table 6.2 Side effects of common antiepileptic drugs (Datapharm, 2015).

Sodium valproate	Nausea, diarrhoea, liver injury, tremor, nystagmus, confusion, hyponatraemia, anaemia, thrombocytopenia, alopecia, weight gain
Carbamazepine	Nausea and vomiting, ataxia, dizziness, fatigue, headache, dry mouth, rash, raised γ-glutamyl transferase, leukopenia
Lamotrigine	Headache, rash, tremor, irritability, insomnia, nausea, diarrhoea, arthralgia, rash

fewer or less debilitating side effects are being developed. Because of these side effects, a single agent is used wherever possible. Some of the side effects of common AEDs are listed in Table 6.2.

Drug monitoring: Routine blood monitoring of AED levels is not recommended unless there is a particular concern such as suspected toxicity, the need for dose adjustment or an episode of status epilepticus. Not all AEDs have a defined therapeutic window. AED levels are mainly used with phenytoin, carbamazepine and phenobarbitone.

⊘ Guidelines

NICE produces regularly updated clinical guidance about the management of epilepsy. NICE CG137 offers particularly useful advice about AEDs in pregnancy (NICE, 2012):

- Many AEDs carry a risk of malformations or neurodevelopmental impairment in the unborn child: women of child-bearing age should be warned of this.
- Sodium valproate and combinations of AEDs carry the highest risk.
- Seizures during pregnancy also potentially carry a risk to the fetus as well as the mother.

- When used in pregnancy, AEDs should be given at the lowest effective dose and should be given as monotherapy wherever possible.
- Folic acid 5 mg daily should be offered to women planning a pregnancy. It should ideally be started 3 months prior to conception and should be continued during pregnancy.

Common pitfalls

Drug interactions: enzyme inducers and inhibitors

A particular problem with AEDs is their propensity to interact with other medications. A number of the AEDs are either enzyme inducers or enzyme inhibitors (Lynch and Price, 2007). The enzymes referred to here are the cytochrome P450 enzymes (the 'P' is for pink as these enzymes combine with carbon monoxide to form a compound with peak absorption at 450 nm). They participate in phase I metabolism (i.e. the initial handling of a drug in the liver once it has been absorbed in the gut) to form an active or inactive metabolite; an essential step towards drug elimination. Induction of these enzymes leads to increased drug metabolism and inhibition leads to decreased drug metabolism.

A number of the AEDs are enzyme inducers, namely phenytoin, carbamazepine and phenobarbital. They up-regulate an important CYP450 enzyme isoform called CYP3A4 (amongst others) which is usually responsible for the metabolism of commonly used drugs such as simvastatin, amlodipine, oestradiol-containing contraceptives and ciclosporin (an immunosuppressant used after organ transplant). These drugs can potentially have a diminished clinical effect when taken alongside phenytoin, carbamazepine or phenobarbitone as they are metabolised and eliminated more quickly (Lynch and Price, 2007). Enzyme *inhibitors* probably cause more interactions in practice and are discussed in Chapter 11.

Clinical correlate: AEDs and contraception

Of particular note, is the potential interaction between AEDs and the oral contraceptive pill (OCP). Enzyme inducers will speed up the metabolism of the OCP thereby lessening its contraceptive efficacy. The current guidance is to use a pill with a minimum of 50 micrograms of oestrogen daily and provide advice about alternative methods of contraception (NICE, 2012). It is important to look out for these and similar interactions.

[TOP TIP] Always ask about herbal remedies! Similar to phenytoin, a popular herbal remedy called St John's Wort (used for depression) seems to act as an enzyme inducer and can reduce the efficacy of the oral contraceptive pill (Hall *et al.*, 2003) as well as other prescribed medications, including medications for HIV and immunosuppressant medications used after organ transplantation, with important clinical consequences (Schwarz *et al.*, 2003; Mannel, 2004).

SUMMARY

Status epilepticus is a medical emergency and every doctor should be aware of the initial steps in its management. An ABC approach is warranted, as is early senior input. Although junior doctors would not be expected to initiate long-term treatment for epilepsy, an awareness of the treatments available, along with their side effects and interactions is important, as all junior doctors will encounter these medications at some point in their career.

🔑 Key learning points

Pharmacological management of status epilepticus
- Oxygen and IV lorazepam
  - → Repeat IV lorazepam
  - → Phenytoin infusion
  - → ITU/anaesthetics input.

Epilepsy medications (AEDs)
- Epilepsy should be managed by a specialist.
- Different AEDs are used according to the specific type of epilepsy.
- AEDs have a number of important side effects and many are teratogenic.
- Many AEDs are enzyme inducers and may alter the effectiveness of medications taken concurrently, notably the oral contraceptive pill.

FURTHER READING

- There is a good review of status epilepticus which can be found in the journal *Practical Neurology*: Kelso ARC, Cock HR (2005). Status epilepticus. *Pract Neurol* 5: 322–33.
- SIGN and NICE guidelines about epilepsy are available and are regularly updated according to the latest evidence.
- For further information about drug side effects, see the British National Formulary (British Medical Association and Royal Pharmaceutical Society of Great Britain (BMA/RPS) (2015). *British National Formulary 69*, 69th edn. BMJ group and Pharmaceutical Press, London) or Datapharm eMC. Available at: www.medicines. org.uk (accessed Dec. 2015).

Parkinson's disease

> **Mr Harry Carter**
>
> **Age: 73 years**
>
> **Hospital number: 123456**

🔍 Case study

A 73-year-old man is transferred to your ward from the emergency department. He was admitted yesterday with pneumonia. Today, he remains unwell with difficulty communicating and seems to move very little. He is receiving antibiotics and fluids via an intravenous drip. His wife tells you he has been deteriorating at home for a few days, with fevers, vomiting, cough and confusion and has been unable to take any of his usual medications. She has brought along his medication list to show you.

PMH: *Parkinson's disease, hypertension, benign prostatic hypertrophy, MI (3 years ago)*

DH: *See FP10*

His wife also brings a piece of paper with the times he usually takes his Sinemet: 6 AM, 11 AM, 4 PM and 9 PM

Allergies: *None*

Salient examination findings:
Sats 95% on air, RR 23, T 37.7°C
Coarse crepitations heard at the left lung base
Bedside swallow test – coughing
Weight: 65 kg

Investigations:
CXR: opacification with air-bronchograms at the left base
WCC 15.6, CRP 103

Diagnosis
Community acquired pneumonia, leading to inability to take medications, deterioration in

| PHARMACY STAMP | AGE 73 | FORENAME, SURNAME Harry Carter |
| | **D.O.B.** xx/xx/xxxx | **ADDRESS** 29 Yewtree Close **NHS NUMBER** |

SINEMET 187.5 mg four times daily.

RAMIPRIL 1.25 mg once daily.

ASPIRIN 75 mg once daily.

TAMSULOSIN 400 micrograms once daily.

SIGNATURE OF PRESCRIBER   DATE

SP21000

underlying Parkinson's disease (PD) and aspiration risk.

Initial management
Consider the following:
- Which medications here is it most important that Mr Carter receives?
- What are the options for giving these medications if a patient can't swallow?
- What medication(s) are safe to use if there is ongoing nausea?

Prescribing in Parkinson's disease

AS REQUIRED MEDICATION					
DRUG METOCLOPRAMIDE				Date	
				Time	
Dose 10 mg	Route PO/IM/IV	Max freq TDS	Start date xx/xx/xx	Dose	
				Route	
Signature/Bleep A. Doctor		Max dose in 24 hrs 30 mg	Review	Given	
Additional instructions				Check	

REGULAR PRESCRIPTIONS

		Circle/enter times below ↓	↴ Enter dates below			
			Day 1	Day 2	Day 3	Day 4
DRUG SINEMET		06				
Dose 187.5 mg / Route PO / Freq QDS / Start date xx/xx/xx		08	4			
		12				
Signature A. Doctor / Bleep / Review		16				
Details on chart		18				
		22				
DRUG RAMIPRIL		06				
Dose 1.25 mg / Route PO / Freq OD / Start date xx/xx/xx		08	4			
		12				
Signature A. Doctor / Bleep / Review		16				
Details on chart		18				
		22				
DRUG ASPIRIN		06				
Dose 75 mg / Route PO / Freq OD / Start date xx/xx/xx		08	4			
		12				
Signature A. Doctor / Bleep / Review		16				
Details on chart		18				
		22				
DRUG TAMSULOSIN		06				
Dose 400 micrograms / Route PO / Freq OD / Start date xx/xx/xx		08	4			
		12				
Signature A. Doctor / Bleep / Review		16				
Details on chart		18				
		22				

On many drug charts, nurses will use a code to explain why a medication was omitted, e.g. 1 = patient refused, 2 = patient unavailable, 3 = doctor request, 4 = patient nil by mouth, etc.

What is wrong with his drug chart?

1. Mr Carter's PD medications have been omitted by nursing staff as he is 'nil by mouth'. It is unlikely he will come to any harm from temporary omission of his ACE-I/ beta-blocker or aspirin as his blood pressure is probably lower than usual due to the presence of infection but the consequences of omitting PD medications can be serious.

2. The timings of the PD medications do not correlate to when the patient receives them at home, which may worsen his PD control even if he does receive his medications.

3. The antiemetics prescribed may further worsen his PD.

Medications used in Parkinson's disease

The treatment of PD is usually managed by experts: geriatricians, neurologists or GPs with a specialist interest. However, a good understanding of the various medications used is essential to any general physician as (1) PD is a common condition and (2) the consequences of omitting or misprescribing can be catastrophic for the patient. Furthermore, studies have shown that patients with PD are hospitalised 1.5 times more frequently than patients without PD (Gerlach et al., 2011) and in one retrospective single-centre audit, 74% of patients with PD who were admitted to hospital had their PD medications stopped, omitted or inappropriately prescribed (Magdalinou et al., 2007).

PD is a neurodegenerative disorder that results in the core signs of: bradykinesia, tremor, rigidity and postural instability (Gelb et al., 1999). There is no cure for the disease and no medication that can prevent further degeneration but medications can control the symptoms in the following ways:

- Replace dopamine (levodopa, dopamine agonists)
- Prevent dopamine breakdown (MAO B inhibitors: selegiline, rasagiline)
- Stimulate dopamine release (amantadine).

Another treatment you may hear about is deep brain stimulation (DBS), where electrodes are implanted in the thalamus, subthalamic nucleus or globus pallidus. This is currently only available in specialist centres.

The primary pathological deficit is degeneration of dopaminergic neurons in the substantia nigra of the basal ganglia, part of the 'extrapyramidal' system responsible for refining the movements initiated within the 'pyramidal' system. Therefore it seems logical that the most widely used treatments act to replace the dopamine.

Levodopa (L-DOPA): rational and evidence

Levodopa is the precursor of dopamine and has been used clinically in Parkinson's disease since the 1960s (Barbeau, 1969). It works by increasing dopamine levels in the CNS to alleviate symptoms. As discussed below, levodopa requires conversion to dopamine by the enzyme dopa-decarboxylase to exert its effects. Because dopamine has both peripheral as well as central actions, levodopa is combined with a *peripherally acting* dopa-decarboxylase *inhibitor*

(DDC-I) to prevent the levodopa being converted to dopamine outside the CNS and causing peripheral side effects.

Treatment is usually started at the point when the symptoms start to interfere with the patient's life. Either levodopa or a dopamine agonist are usually used as first-line treatment, although in younger patients a dopamine agonist is sometimes preferred as initial treatment to delay the development of motor side effects that come with prolonged use of levodopa. However, these medications come with their own set of side effects (see Evidence) and the vast majority of patients with PD will need to start taking levodopa at some point along the disease course. Low doses are used initially and are titrated upwards to achieve symptom control (NICE, 2006).

✓ DRUGS checklist for LEVODOPA (L-DOPA)

Dose	50–800 mg daily in divided doses
Route	PO; can also be given via nasogastric tube
	NB. Duodopa, a newer gel formulation of levodopa/ carbidopa can be given via an intestinal pump.
Units	milligrams (mg)
Given	Usually 2–4 times daily
Special situations	Side effects include: nausea, headache, hypotension, hallucinations, dyskinesias. The therapeutic effects may 'wear-off' in between doses leading to fluctuation in symptoms. Furthermore, the response to levodopa lessens with time, necessitating increasing doses to achieve symptom control.

As levodopa/dopa-decarboxylase inhibitors come as combination tablets, they can be prescribed by their *trade names* rather than their *generic names* (Table 6.3). Doses for co-careldopa and/or co-beneldopa are generally as in Table 6.4.

NB. Modified-release (MR) or controlled-release (CR) preparations also exist; equivalent doses

🔍 Evidence

Levodopa/ DDC-I versus placebo

The ELLDOPA trial (Fahn *et al.*, 2004), although aiming to look at the question of whether levodopa affects the progression of PD, represents the only RCT which proves the efficacy of levodopa/DDC-I versus placebo in PD. Early trials in the 1960s and 70s which used levodopa alone are not representative of the way levodopa is currently used, that is in combination with a DDC-I.

In the ELLDOPA trial, a total of 361 patients with early PD (diagnosed within the previous 2 years) were randomised to receive either placebo or one of three dosing regimens of levodopa/ carbidopa over a period of 40 weeks. Their symptoms were assessed using the standardised UPDRS scale of PD symptoms, with a group of these patients also undergoing neuroimaging (SPECT). Results showed that levodopa significantly reduced the symptoms of PD in a dose-dependent fashion as compared to placebo. The side effects of dyskinesia, hypertonia, infection, headache and nausea were also found to be dose dependent.

Table 6.3 Levodopa preparations.

Name	Contains
Co-careldopa (Sinemet)	Levodopa + carbidopa
Co-beneldopa (Madopar)	Levodopa + benserazide
Stalevo	Levodopa + carbidopa + entacapone[a]

[a]Entacapone is a COMT-inhibitor (See Section Other drugs used in Parkinson's Disease) which helps prolong the duration of action of levodopa.

Table 6.4 Doses for co-careldopa and/or co-beneldopa.

Strength of tablet (mg)	Levodopa dose (mg)	DDC-I dose (mg)
62.5	50	12.5
110	100	10
125	100	25
187.5	150	37.5
250	200	50
275	250	25

DDC-I, dopa-decarboxylase inhibitor.

for these medications are lower than for immediate-release preparations.

Finally, levodopa can also be administered via an intestinal pump as Duodopa, for patients who have severe difficulties with motor fluctuations.

Enhancing the actions of levodopa

You may come across levodopa being used in combination with other medications, namely COMT-inhibitors (e.g. entacapone, tolcapone) and MAOB-inhibitors (e.g. selegiline, rasagiline), both of which inhibit enzymes that breakdown dopamine, enhancing the effects of levodopa.

Levodopa: essential pharmacology

Dopamine is a naturally occurring compound found in the body. It has actions both in the central and peripheral nervous systems. In the central nervous system, dopamine plays a role in several pathways, including in motor control pathways (as seen in Parkinson's disease), as well as motivations and reward pathways amongst others (Rang *et al.*, 2003). It is one of several neurotransmitters which are synthesised from the amino acid L-tyrosine. Levodopa is the precursor of dopamine and is converted to dopamine by the enzyme dopa-decarboxylase within dopaminergic neurons, as well as elsewhere in the body. The reason that levodopa rather than dopamine is administered is that dopamine cannot cross the blood–brain barrier whilst levodopa can (Pardridge, 2003). The levodopa is usually given with a peripherally acting dopa-decarboxylase inhibitor, which prevents the levodopa being converted to dopamine before it crosses the blood–brain barrier. The advantages of this are twofold: (1) this decreases the dose of levodopa required to achieve the desired effects in the CNS and (2) it reduces the peripheral side effects. These agents include:

- **carbidopa** (a component of co-careldopa)
- **benserazide** (a component of co-beneldopa).

Dopamine agonists: rationale and evidence

An alternative or additional group of agents used in Parkinson's disease are the dopamine agonists. Their main advantage is that they tend to cause fewer motor complications. This means they have often been used as first-line agents in younger patients, in order to delay the onset of levodopa-associated complications. However, they are less effective than levodopa, usually requiring the addition of levodopa at some point in the disease course.

There are two main groups of dopamine agonists (listed in Table 6.5). The non-ergoline-derived

Table 6.5 Main groups of dopamine agonists.

Dopamine agonists	Specific features
Non-ergoline derivatives	
Ropinirole	Tablets
Pramipexole	Tablets
Rotigotine	Transdermal patch
Apomorphine	Given subcutaneously, usually via a pump. Highly potent, but also emetogenic
Ergoline derivatives	
Bromocriptine	Tablets; the ergot-derived dopamine agonists can cause vasospasm and rarely, fibrotic reactions (cardiac valve fibrosis, peritoneal fibrosis etc.)
Pergolide	
Lisuride	

dopamine agonists are preferred as the ergoline-derived dopamine agonists require regular monitoring and can, rarely, cause serious fibrotic reactions (NICE, 2006).

The dopamine agonists have a number of side effects that you should be aware of including confusion and hallucinations, making them less suitable in the elderly population. They can also cause impulse control disorders, which patients should be made aware of (see Box).

Medicine and Law

In 2008, $8.2 million was awarded to a patient who claimed to have developed a gambling addiction whilst taking Mirapex (pramipexole), gambling away $260 000. It was claimed that the drug companies were aware of this side effect but had failed to issue warnings to patients. This was the first of a number of cases to go to trial in re. Mirapex Product Liability Litigation, case number 07-md-01839, in the US District Court for the District of Minnesota.

Evidence

Levodopa versus dopamine agonists
The CALM-PD trial (Parkinson Study Group, 2000) was a double blind RCT of 301 patients comparing pramipexole with levodopa for the initial treatment of PD symptoms. The study showed that whilst the dopamine agonist group suffered significantly fewer motor complications, the levodopa group had significantly more improvement in their symptoms.

Dopamine agonists: essential pharmacology

Dopamine agonists work by acting directly at the dopamine receptor and unlike levodopa, do not require metabolism to reach their active form. They also tend to be longer acting, which perhaps contributes to the lower frequency of motor complications seen with this group.

Other aspects of Parkinson's disease

Non-pharmacological management

As with any chronic disease, pharmacological therapy is only one aspect of management. Management involves patient education and input from members of the multidisciplinary team, which may include specialist nurses, speech and language therapists, physiotherapists and occupational therapists. In advanced disease, it may become appropriate to involve the palliative care team (NICE, 2006).

Treating Parkinson's disease in patients who are nil by mouth

The most frequently used option for giving PD medications in patients who are nil by mouth is to give therapy enterally but via a nasogastric tube. An alternative is to give therapy parenterally via a transdermal patch, but this involves using different drugs to the patient's usual medication.

Nasogastric tube: Most medications for Parkinson's disease can be crushed and delivered by nasogastric tube. Your local pharmacist will be able to advise further or you can visit www.medicines.org.uk for details of each drug.

Transdermal preparations: Rotigotine is a dopamine agonist that is delivered transdermally. The patch is changed every 24 hours and comes in a range of strengths. Advice should be sought from the local Parkinson's specialist nurse or Parkinson's consultant if you are changing someone's PD medications but Table 6.6 gives a rough guide to approximately equivalent doses.

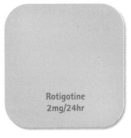

Rotigotine
2mg/24hr

Table 6.6 Levodopa and rotigotine equivalent doses.

Levodopa total daily dose	Rotigotine dose
100 mg	2 mg/24 hours
150 mg	4 mg/24 hours
300 mg	8 mg/24 hours

The maximum dose of rotigotine is 16 mg/24 hours. Calculated using algorithm as per Brennan and Genever, 2010.

Detailed algorithms are available to calculate a rotigotine dose for patients using modified release preparations, dopamine agonists, combinations of levodopa and dopamine agonists and COMT-inhibitors, which are especially useful for patients with PD who are undergoing surgery (Brennan and Genever, 2010). **It is advised that you consult a PD specialist and/ or a pharmacist before attempting to switch to rotigotine.** Guidance is also available on the Parkinson's UK website.

Be aware: According to www.medicines.org.uk, rotigotine patches contain aluminium and should be removed during MRI or planned cardioversion to avoid skin burns.

Other drugs used in Parkinson's disease

Treatments for Parkinson's disease

Mono-amine oxidase B (MAO B) inhibitors: selegiline, rasagiline. MAO B metabolises dopamine and therefore MAO B inhibitors prolong the actions of dopamine by preventing this. They can be used as initial monotherapy although are more often combined with other treatments. As monotherapy they are only effective for mild symptoms.

Catechol-O-methyl-transferase (COMT) inhibitors: entacapone, tolcapone. COMT is another enzyme that breaks down dopamine. COMT inhibitors are used as an adjunct to enhance the effects of levodopa (see Section Levodopa (L-dopa): Rational and Evidence).

Amantadine: Amantidine's mechanism of action is unclear. It can be helpful in lessening the dyskinesias associated with PD treatment.

Anticholinergics: Trihexyphenidyl. Anticholinergic medications (to be specific: muscarinic antagonists) reduce the relative cholinergic excess which results from depletion of dopamine and can help reduce symptoms of tremor and rigidity; they may also help with sialorrhoea (excessive saliva production). However, the side effects of anticholinergic medications are well documented (constipation, dry mouth, urinary retention, nausea and vomiting, dizziness, confusion, angle-closure glaucoma (rarely)) and should be used with caution in the elderly.

Treatment for complications of PD

REM-sleep behaviour disorder (RBD): You may come across patients who are taking **clonazepam** or **melatonin** for RBD.

Orthostatic hypotension: Patients may need to increase their salt intake or take **fludrocortisone** or **midodrine** for symptomatic orthostatic hypotension.

Depression: Patients with Parkinson's disease may also be taking **antidepressant medications**. Beware the interaction between MAO inhibitors and certain antidepressants.

Constipation: Patients with PD are prone to constipation and may be taking **laxatives**. Even if not, hospitalisation and the associated decrease in mobility may well precipitate constipation in this group. This should be treated promptly.

Case outcome and discharge

The PD specialist nurse reviewed Mr Carter and recommended giving his medications via an naso-gastric tube. This was inserted and an explanation given to the nurses on the ward as to why it was important that he receive his PD medications at specific times. His antiemetic was also changed to domperidone. Once he started to receive his Sinemet again he felt much better. His cough improved, which helped him to expectorate sputum from his chest. The sputum was cultured and grew a streptococcus, sensitive to amoxicillin and so his antibiotics were rationalised. He was discharged home to complete his course of antibiotics and follow up was booked for 6 weeks time with a repeat chest X-ray to ensure that the pneumonia had cleared completely and that there were no underlying pulmonary abnormalities.

DISCHARGE MEDICATION						
Date	Medication	Dose	Route	Frequency	Supply	GP to continue?
xx/xx/xx	AMOXICILLIN	500 mg	PO	Three times daily	To complete a 7 day course, i.e. until xx/xx/xx	N
xx/xx/xx	SINEMET	187.5 mg	PO	Four times daily (06.00, 11.00, 16.00, 21.00)	14 days	Y
xx/xx/xx	ASPIRIN	75 mg	PO	Once daily	14 days	Y
xx/xx/xx	RAMIPRIL	1.25 mg	PO	Once daily	14 days	Y
xx/xx/xx	TAMSULOSIN	400 micrograms	PO	Once daily	14 days	Y

Notes to patient/GP:
No changes to regular medications.

Common pitfalls

Drugs to avoid in Parkinson's disease

Any drug that depletes or opposes the actions of dopamine is likely to cause deterioration in symptoms or in extreme circumstances can cause neuroleptic malignant syndrome. These include:

- Metoclopramide
- Prochlorperazine
- Haloperidol
- Levomepromazine.

If antiemetics are required, domperidone is the agent of choice as, although it is a dopamine antagonist, it acts *peripherally* to oppose the action of dopamine; it does not readily cross the blood–brain barrier. Cyclizine and ondansetron may also be used safely.

Parkinson's disease and surgery

Careful planning is required for patients with PD who need to undergo a surgical procedure. The PD nurse specialist or consultant should be involved and patients should be placed first on the operating list. Problems include: missed medication doses and problems with enteral absorption postoperatively. If doses of PD medications are likely to be missed, alternative preparations may need to be used, such as transdermal patches (Brennan and Genever, 2010).

Neuroleptic malignant-like syndrome

Be aware: Suddenly stopping dopaminergic medication can cause a form of neuroleptic malignant syndrome, a 'dopamine withdrawal syndrome', which manifests as hyperpyrexia, rigidity and confusion (Keyser and Rodnitzky, 1991; Serrano-Dueñas, 2003).

Serotonin syndrome

Be aware: Depression is a common complication of PD. However, combination of MAO inhibitors with certain antidepressants can precipitate serotonin syndrome. Serotonin syndrome comprises the triad of autonomic hyperactivity (e.g. tachycardia, hyperpyrexia), neuromuscular abnormalities (e.g. tremor, hyperreflexia) and changes in mental status (e.g. agitation, anxiety) (Boyer and Shannon, 2005).

A note on drug-induced parkinsonism

There are a number of drugs that can cause parkinsonism:

- Antipsychotics
- Antiemetics
- Calcium antagonists
- Sodium valproate
- Methyldopa.

Symptoms should resolve once the medication is stopped but this often takes several months and the patients should be followed up as a small proportion will later develop idiopathic PD (in these cases it is thought that the episode of parkinsonism represents a transient unmasking of subclinical PD) (Taylor and Counsell, 2006).

SUMMARY

Parkinson's disease is a chronic, degenerative condition whose symptoms are controlled with an often complicated regimen of medications. It is of paramount importance that patients with PD who are in hospital for any reason receive their medications and that they receive them at the time when normally take them at home and that if changes are required, a specialist in PD is consulted.

🔑 Key learning points

Prescribing in Parkinson's disease
- Treatment is initiated by a specialist.
- It is of the utmost importance that patients receive their medications at their usual times when they come into hospital.
- Do not abruptly withdraw Parkinson's disease medications.
- A nasogastric tube should be considered early on in patients made 'nil by mouth'.
- Advice should be sought from the PD specialist nurse or a specialist physician as well as from your ward pharmacist when considering a change in PD medications.
- There are a number of (in particular antiemetic) medications that are contraindicated in patients with Parkinson's disease.

FURTHER READING

- A good summary of the diagnosis and management of Parkinson's disease can be found in the *New England Journal of Medicine*:
  - Nutt JG, Wooten FW (2005). Diagnosis and initial management of Parkinson's disease. *N Engl J Med* 353: 1021–7.
- A good leaflet about the emergency management of PD is available from Parkinson's UK (www. parkinsons.org.uk), which includes a detailed algorithm for converting various preparations to transdermal patches: www.parkinsons.org.uk/sites/default/files/publications/download/english/pk0135_emergencymanagement.pdf

---

Now visit **www.wileyessential.com/pharmacology**
to test yourself on this chapter.

References

Amarenco P, Bogousslavsky J, Callahan A *et al.* (2006). High-dose atorvastatin after stroke or transient ischemic attack. Stroke Prevention by Aggressive Reduction in Cholesterol Levels (SPARCL). *N Engl J Med* 355: 549–59.

Auburtin M, Wolff M, Charpentier J *et al.* (2006). Detrimental role of delayed antibiotic administration and penicillin-nonsusceptible strains in adult intensive care unit patients with pneumococcal meningitis: The PNEUMOREA prospective multicenter study. *Crit Care Med* 34: 2758–65.

Barbeau A (1969). L-dopa therapy in Parkinson's disease: a critical review of nine years' experience. *Canad Med Ass J* 101: 59–68.

Boyer EW, Shannon M (2005). The serotonin syndrome. *N Engl J Med* 352: 1112.

Brennan KA, Genever RW (2010). Managing Parkinson's disease during surgery. *BMJ* 341: 990–3.

Brouwer MC, McIntyre P, Prasad K et al. (2013). Corticosteroids for acute bacterial meningitis. *Cochrane Database Syst Rev* (6): CD004405.

Chadwick DR (2005). Viral meningitis. *Br Med Bull* 75–76: 1–14.

Cock HR, Schapira AH (2002). A comparison of lorazepam and diazepam as initial therapy in convulsive status epilepticus. *Q J Med* 95: 225–31.

Datapharm (2015). *Electronic Medicines Compendium (eMC) Summaries of Product Characteristics (SPC)*. Available at: www.medicines.org.uk (accessed Dec. 2015).

Dellinger RP, Levy MM, Rhodes A et al. (2013). Surviving sepsis campaign: international guidelines for management of severe sepsis and septic shock: 2012. *Crit Care Med* 41: 580–637.

Diener HC, Bogousslavsky J, Brass LM et al.; MATCH Investigators (2004). Aspirin and clopidogrel compared with clopidogrel alone after recent ischaemic stroke or transient ischaemic attack in high-risk patients (MATCH): randomised, double-blind, placebo-controlled trial. *Lancet* 364: 331–7.

Durand ML, Calderwood SB, Weber DJ et al. (1993). Acute bacterial meningitis in adults – a review of 493 episodes. *N Engl J Med* 328: 21–8.

Emberson J, Lees KR, Lyden P et al. for the Stroke Thrombolysis Trialists' Collaborative Group (2014). Effect of treatment delay, age, and stroke severity on the effects of intravenous thrombolysis with alteplase for acute ischaemic stroke: a meta-analysis of individual patient data from randomised trials. *Lancet* 384: 1929–35.

Fahn S, Oakes D, Shoulson I et al.: Parkinson's Study Group (2004). Levodopa and the progression of Parkinson's disease (ELLDOPA trial). *N Engl J Med* 351: 2498–508.

Fitch MT, van de Beek D (2007). Emergency diagnosis and treatment of adult meningitis *Lancet Infect Dis* 7: 191–200.

Gelb DJ, Oliver G, Gilman S (1999). Diagnostic criteria for Parkinson's disease. *Arch Neurol* 56: 33–9.

Gerlach OHH, Winogrodzka A, Weber WEJ (2011). Clinical problems in the hospitalised Parkinson's disease patient: systematic review. *Mov Disorder* 26: 197–208.

Hacke W, Donnan G, Fieschi C et al., ATLANTIS Trials Investigators, ECASS Trials Investigators, NINDS rt-PA Study Group Investigators (2004). Association of outcome with early stroke treatment: pooled analysis of ATLANTIS, ECASS, and NINDS rt-PA stroke trials. *Lancet* 363: 768–74.

Hacke W, Kaste M, Bluhmki E et al.; ECASS Investigators (2008). Thrombolysis with alteplase 3 to 4.5 hours after acute ischemic stroke. *N Engl J Med* 359: 1317–29.

Halkes PH, van Gijn J, Kappelle LJ et al. ESPRIT Study Group (2006). Aspirin plus dipyridamole versus aspirin alone after cerebral ischaemia of arterial origin (ESPRIT): randomised controlled trial. *Lancet* 367: 1665–67.

Hall SD, Wang Z, Huang SM et al. (2003). The interaction between St John's wort and an oral contraceptive. *Clin Pharmacol Ther* 74: 525–35.

Kelso ARC, Cock HR (2005). Status epilepticus. *Pract Neurol* 5: 322–33.

Keyser DL, Rodnitzky RL (1991). Neuroleptic malignant syndrome in Parkinson's disease after withdrawal or alteration of dopaminergic therapy. *Arch Intern Med* 151: 794–6.

Kwan P, Sills GJ, Brodie MJ (2001). The mechanisms of action of commonly used antiepileptic drugs. *Pharmacol Ther* 90: 21–34.

Lynch T, Price A (2007). The effect of cytochrome P450 metabolism on drug response, interactions, and adverse effects. *Am Fam Physician* 76: 391–6.

Magdalinou KN, Martin A, Kessel B (2007). Prescribing medications in Parkinson's disease (PD) patients during acute admissions to a District General Hospital. *Parkinsonism Relat Disord* 13: 539–40.

Mannel M (2004). Drug interactions with St John's wort : mechanisms and clinical implications. *Drug Saf* 27: 773–97.

Medicines and Healthcare Products Regulatory Agency (MHRA) (2014). *Drugs safety update: Statins benefits and risks*. Available at: www.gov.uk/drug-safety-update/statins-benefits-and-risks (accessed April 2015).

Miller SB (2006). Prostaglandins in health and disease: an overview. *Semin Arthritis Rheum* 36: 37–49.

National Institute for Health and Care Excellence (NICE) (2006). *Parkinson's Disease: Diagnosis and Management in Primary and Secondary care*, CG35. Available at: www.nice.org.uk/guidance/cg35 (accessed Sept. 2014). *CG35 is currently referred to as 'Parkinson's disease in the over-20s: diagnosis and management'*.

National Institute for Health and Care Excellence (NICE) (2008). *Stroke: National Clinical Guideline for Diagnosis and Initial Management of Acute Stroke and Transient Ischaemic Attack (TIA)*, CG68. Available at: www.nice.org.uk/guidance/cg68 (accessed Feb. 2014). *CG35 is currently referred to as 'Parkinson's disease in the over-20s: diagnosis and management'*.

National Institute for Health and Care Excellence (NICE) (2012). *The Epilepsies: the Diagnosis and Management of the Epilepsies in Adults and Children in Primary and Secondary Care*, CG137. Available at: www.nice.org.uk/guidance/cg137 (accessed Jan. 2014).

National Institute of Neurological Disorders and Stroke rt-PA Stroke Study Group (NINDS and rtPA Study Group) (1995). Tissue plasminogen activator for acute ischemic stroke. *N Engl J Med* 333: 1581–8.

Pantano C (1994). Aspirin as an antiplatelet. *N Engl J Med* 330: 1287–94.

Pardridge WM (2003). Blood-brain barrier drug targeting: the future of brain drug development *Mol Interv* 3: 290–105.

Parkinson Study Group (2000). Pramipexole vs levodopa as initial treatment for Parkinson Disease. *JAMA* 284: 1931.

Prasad K, Al-Roomi K, Krishnan PR *et al.* (2005) Anticonvulsant therapy for status epilepticus. *Cochrane Database Syst Rev* (9): CD003723.

Prasad K, Kumar A, Singhal T *et al.* (2007). Third generation cephalosporins versus conventional antibiotics for treating acute bacterial meningitis. *Cochrane Database Syst Rev* (4): CD001832.

PROGRESS Collaborative Group (2001). Randomised trial of a perindopril-based blood-presure lowering regimen among 6105 individuals with previous stroke or transient ischaemic attack. *Lancet* 358: 1033–41.

Proulx N, Fre'chette D, Toye B *et al.* (2005). Delays in the administration of antibiotics are associated with mortality from adult acute bacterial meningitis. *Q J Med* 98: 291–8.

Rashid P, Leonardi-Bee J, Bath P (2003). Blood pressure reduction and secondary prevention of stroke and other vascular events: a systematic review. *Stroke* 34: 2741–8.

Rang HP, Dale MM, Ritter JM *et al.* (2003): *Pharmacology*, 5th edn. Churchill Livingstone.

Rhen T, Cidlowski JA (2005). Antiinflammatory action of glucocorticoids – new mechanisms for old drugs. *N Engl J Med* 353: 1711–23.

Rudolph U, Crestani F, Möhler H (2001). $GABA_A$ receptor subtypes: dissecting their pharmacological functions. *Trend Pharmacol Sci* 22: 188–94.

Sacco RL, Diener HC, Yusuf S *et al.*: the PRoFESS Study Group (2008). Aspirin and extended-release dipyridamole versus clopidogrel for recurrent stroke. *N Engl J Med* 359: 1238–51.

Sandercock PA, Counsell C, Gubitz GJ *et al.* (2008). Antiplatelet therapy for acute ischaemic stroke. *Cochrane Database Syst Rev* (3): CD000029.

Schwarz UI, Büschel B, Kirch W (2003). Unwanted pregnancy on self-medication with St John's wort despite hormonal contraception. *Br J Clin Pharmacol* 55: 112–3.

Scottish Intercollegiate Guideline Network (SIGN) (2005). *Diagnosis and Management of Epilepsy in Adults*, SIGN 70. Available at: www.sign.ac.uk/guidelines/ (accessed April 2013).

Scottish Intercollegiate Guideline Network (SIGN) (2008). *Management of Patients with Stroke or TIA: Assessment, Investigation, Immediate Management and Secondary Prevention*, SIGN 108. Available at: www.sign.ac.uk/guidelines/ (accessed April 2013).

Serrano-Dueñas M (2003). Neuroleptic malignant syndrome-like, or–dopaminergic malignant syndrome–due to levodopa therapy withdrawal.

Clinical features in 11 patients. *Parkinsonism Relat Disord* 9: 175–8.

Silbergleit R, Durkalski V, Lowenstein D *et al.*; NETT Investigators (2012). Intramuscular versus intravenous therapy for prehospital status epilepticus. *N Engl J Med* 366: 591–60.

Singh S, Hamdy S (2006). Dysphagia in stroke patients. *Postgrad Med J* 82: 383–91.

Sprigg N, Bath PMW (2005). Management of blood pressure in acute stroke. *Pract Neurol* 5: 218–23.

Stroke Unit Trialists' Collaboration (1997). Collaborative systematic review of the randomised trials of organised in-patient (stroke unit) care after stroke. *BMJ* 314: 1151–9.

Szczeklik A, Sanak M, Nizankowska–Mogilnicka E *et al.* (2004). Aspirin intolerance and the cyclooxygenase–leukotriene pathways. *Current Op Pulm Med* 10: 51–6.

Tauber MG, Khayam-Bashi H, Sande MA (1985). Effects of ampicillin and corticosteroids on brain water content, cerebrospinal fluid pressure, and cerebrospinal fluid lactate levels in experimental pneumococcal meningitis. *J Infect Dis* 151: 528–34.

Taylor KSM, Counsell C (2006). Is it Parkinson's disease, and if not, what is it? *Pract Neurol* 6: 154–65.

Tunkel AR, Hartman BJ, Kaplan SL *et al.* (2004). Practice guidelines for the management of bacterial meningitis. *Clin Infect Dis* 39: 1267–84.

Vane JR, Botting RM (1998). Mechanism of action of non-steroidal anti-inflammatory drugs. *Am J Med* 104: 2S–8S.

Webb AJ, Wilson M, Lovett N *et al.* (2014). Response of day-to-day home blood pressure variability by antihypertensive drug class after transient ischemic attack or nondisabling stroke. *Stroke* 45: 2967–73.

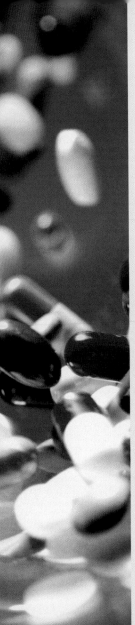

CHAPTER 7
Surgery
Benedict Lyle Phillips

Key topics:

Learning objectives

By the end of this chapter you should…

- …be able to write a safe IV fluid prescription for patients in both maintenance and resuscitation situations.
- …be able to prescribe blood products safely and identify complications.
- …be able to safely prescribe antiemetics in the treatment of nausea and vomiting.
- …be able to safely prescribe analgesia in postoperative patients.
- …be able to assess patient risk factors for venous thromboembolism and begin prophylactic treatment if appropriate.
- …be able to safely prescribe laxatives.

Essential Practical Prescribing, First Edition. Georgia Woodfield, Benedict Lyle Phillips, Victoria Taylor, Amy Hawkins and Andrew Stanton. © 2016 by John Wiley & Sons, Ltd. Published 2016 by John Wiley & Sons, Ltd.

Fluid management

> ## Miss Yemi Oluwajobi
> ## Age: 28
> ## Hospital number: 123456

🔍 Case study

Presenting complaint: *A fit and well 28-year-old lady attends the emergency department unit with a painful discharging pilonidal abscess.*

Background: *This patient noticed a lump in the natal cleft that has increased in size and become painful. Her general practitioner has referred the patient to the general surgical department for consideration for an incision and drainage under general anaesthetic. She weighs 65 kg.*

PHARMACY STAMP	AGE 30	FORENAME, SURNAME
		Yemi Oluwajobi
	D.O.B. 2/10/1984	ADDRESS Riverside Place
		NHS NUMBER

MICROGYNON 30 orally, once daily as directed.

SIGNATURE OF PRESCRIBER	DATE

SP21000

PMH: *She is well and has no co-morbidities. She will be 'nil-by-mouth' for the next few hours as she waits to have her operation on the emergency list.*

Allergies: *None*

FH: *Nil relevant*

Examination, observations and tests: *Pulse 80, BP 120/80, Sats 100% on room air, RR 14, BM 5.9*

BMI: *24*

CVS: *Capillary refill time <2 second, pulse regular, HS I + II + 0*

RS: *Equal expansion with air entry to both bases and no added sounds*

Regular medications: *See FP10*

Diagnosis

Pilonidal abscess requiring incision and drainage operation under general anaesthetic. The patient is euvolaemic (see Box Terminology). The patient will be placed nil-by-mouth for several hours whilst she waits for the procedure. She will therefore require intravenous maintenance fluids.

Prescribing maintenance fluids

Many patients in hospital need intravenous (IV) fluid in order to maintain or correct hydration and electrolyte concentration. The challenges of safe prescribing are:

- Choosing the correct fluid, as each has different ingredients
- Deciding on the rate of infusion
- Recognising complications of IV fluid.

Broadly speaking, IV fluid management can be divided into:

- **Maintenance:** a patient who has normal hydration and electrolyte levels, but will not be able to take or absorb fluid orally for a period of time. For example, before general anaesthetic patients need an empty stomach to avoid aspiration of gastric contents. The doctor must therefore maintain their hydration and electrolytes during this period.

■ **Resuscitation:** a patient is deficient in fluid and has signs of volume depletion, or has deranged electrolytes. Fluid is therefore needed to correct this. Once corrected, the patient can either drink orally or have ongoing maintenance fluid as above.

A typical maintenance fluid chart prescription is shown. Remember that IV fluids come in set sizes of bags. These are typically 1000 mL and 500 mL bags. So the prescription should state the size of the fluid bag (1000 mL in this case). This means that the IV fluid would last for a maximum of approximately 12 hours in this case, if required.

FLUID CHART							
Date	Infusion fluid			Drug to be added		Signature	Print name
	Name and strength	Volume	Rate	Approved name	Dose		
01/12/ 2014	DEXTROSE 4%/ SALINE 0.18%	500 ml	81 ml per hour	None	None	A. Doctor	A. Doctor

Maintenance fluids: rationale and evidence

Water is a major component of cells in the body. Adequate hydration is therefore required to maintain normal cellular activity. Maintenance fluid is required in patients who are not expected to eat or drink normally for a prolonged period. Maintenance fluid is given intravenously to preserve water and electrolyte balance (Sterns, 2014).

In this case, Yemi Oluwajobi is euvolaemic, and therefore does not need resuscitation fluid. She is not allowed to eat or drink prior to having a general anaesthetic. Intravenous fluids will prevent her from getting dehydrated during this period of abstinence from food and drink. The patient's fluid requirements will be based on her weight of 65 kg.

According to NICE Guidelines on IV fluid therapy in adults (NICE, 2013), water requirements in adults is 25–30 mL/kg/day.

She therefore needs (30×65 kg)

= 1950 mL of fluid per day (24-hour period)

Rate of infusion (per hour) = 1950 mL / 24

= 81 mL per hour as an initial prescription

However, following this initial prescription, the rate of infusion can be increase or decreased based on a fluid balance assessment of the patient.

Remember that IV fluid prescription should be based on patients' ideal body weight. Patients rarely need more than 3000 mL of fluid per day. Patients who have a body mass index (BMI) of greater than 40 kg/m^2 should be discussed with an expert (such as an anaesthetist or intensive care doctor) before prescribing fluids.

Consider providing less fluid in patients at risk of fluid overload (20–25 mL/kg/day). Patients who are at risk of fluid overload:

■ are older or frail people
■ have renal or cardiac failure.

Fluid balance assessment should be based on:

■ Patient history: Thirst may indicate that the patient is in need of water (though thirst may also be a symptom of conditions such as diabetes mellitus, diabetes insipidus and hypercalcaemia)
    Fluid balance assessment:
    ● Mucosal surfaces: dry surfaces such as the tongue indicates fluid depletion
    ● Skin turgor: loss of skin elasticity indicates fluid depletion
    ● Jugular venous pressure (JVP): absent or low JVP indicates fluid depletion. High JVP may indicate fluid overload, but is a pathological finding in other conditions as well
    ● Auscultation of lung fields: pulmonary oedema or pleural effusions may indicate fluid overload
    ● Pitting oedema: may indicate fluid overload
■ Bedside measures:
    ● Heart rate: raised in fluid depletion
    ● Blood pressure: low in fluid depletion
    ● Fluid balance charts: negative daily balance indicates that the patient fluid requirements are not being met.

The NICE guidelines on IV fluid prescription in adults recommend that IV fluid prescriptions are assessed at least every 24 hours. Maintenance IV fluid should be given during daylight hours and, if possible, suspended at night. This allows patients to have undisturbed sleep.

✓	**DRUGS checklist for CRYSTALLOIDS**
	Crystalloids: 0.9% saline, 5% dextrose, dextrose 4%/saline 0.18%, Hartmann's solution
Dose	1950 mL (based on patient weight of 65 kg)
Route	IV
Units	mL
Given	Over 24 hours
Special sitituations	Used as maintenance fluid. Some crystalloids are used as resuscitation fluid (see Evidence Choice of IV Fluid in Resuscitation). NICE guidelines suggest that dextrose 4%/saline 0.18% would be the most appropriate maintenance fluid.

Maintenance fluids: essential pharmacology

The action of intravenous fluids is dependent on the fluid content. Whilst the main ingredient of fluid is water, added ingredients alter the way in which the fluid distributes itself. Therefore it is of fundamental importance to choose the correct fluid for a given situation (Rose and Post, 2001).

Intravenous fluids can be broadly categorised into crystalloids and colloids.

Crystalloids

Crystalloids are fluids that are water-soluble electrolytes in water.

0.9% Saline (or 0.9% sodium chloride): This is water containing sodium chloride (NaCl) and contains 150 mmol/L of sodium (Na). It is therefore also known as 'saline'. The normal level of sodium in the blood is 135–145 mmol/L and so 0.9% saline is approximately isotonic (the same osmolar concentration as blood). 0.9% saline can be used as a maintenance or as a resuscitation fluid.

Avoid its use when patients are hypernatraemic (have high sodium in the blood). It must not be used as maintenance fluid in isolation as it will provide over and above the maintenance requirement for sodium and chloride (1 mmol/kg/day) and risk hyperchloraemic metabolic acidosis (see Section Hyperchloraemic Acidosis). Most regimens will alternate the use of 0.9% saline with 5% dextrose.

5% Dextrose: This is water containing glucose (50 mg/mL). The small amount of glucose in the water is quickly metabolised by the liver, but is important in providing enough glucose to avoid patients developing starvation ketosis if nil-by-mouth for significant periods (50–100 g/day required). It is used only as a maintenance fluid, and not in resuscitation. 5% dextrose is also isotonic.

Dextrose/saline solution: This is a mixture of both dextrose and sodium chloride. Although dextrose/saline solutions may come in different concentrations, a commonly used formula is sodium chloride 0.18% in dextrose 4% (containing 31 mmol/L of sodium, and 40 g/L of dextrose). Potassium 20–40 mmol is often added to dextrose/saline (maintenance electrolytes are discussed in Section Maintenance Electrolytes). This particular solution has been incorporated into the NICE guidelines (NICE, 2013) on IV fluid therapy in adults in hospital. It is used exclusively as a maintenance fluid (not as a resuscitation fluid). The NICE guidelines recommend prescribing sodium chloride 0.18% in dextrose 4% with 27 mmol/L of potassium on the first day of maintenance fluid, after which the patient's fluid and electrolyte needs should be reassessed. Begin with 25–30 mL/kg/day. Prescribing more than 2.5 litres per day of dextrose/saline increases the risk of hyponatraemia. All of the fluids discussed in this chapter relate to IV fluid therapy in adults only. However, it should be mentioned that dextrose 4%/saline 0.18% is specifically contraindicated in children (aged 16 years or less) as it causes acute hyponatraemic encephalopathy (National Patient Safety Agency, 2007).

Hartmann's solution: This is water with sodium (131 mmol/L), potassium (5 mmol/L), calcium (2 mmol/L) and lactate (29 mmol/L). It is isotonic and can be used as a maintenance or as a resuscitation fluid. Avoid its use when a patient is hyperkalaemic (high potassium) because potassium is one of its components. Likewise lactate can worsen a lactic acidosis if used.

Colloids

Colloids are never used as maintenance fluids, but will be discussed here to provide a comparison with crystalloids. Colloids are fluids that contain insoluble large molecules in water. Theoretically, colloids preserve osmotic pressure within the intravascular space. This is because the molecules are large, and diffuse out of blood vessels very slowly. Water is therefore forced to travel into the blood vessels instead.

Gelofusin: This is saline containing gelatin, a large insoluble molecule. As gelatin is a large molecule, it diffuses across membranes very slowly and remains within the intravascular space for 4 hours. It is therefore intended to be used as a resuscitation fluid. However, the use of Gelofusin is dwindling due to strong evidence against its benefits. Evidence indicates that patient outcomes are not significantly different compared to using 0.9% saline. There is further evidence that the use of colloids in critically ill patients may increase mortality (Perel and Roberts, 2013). The authors do not recommend using colloids such as Gelofusin.

Human albumin solution 4% (HAS): This is human albumin solution in water. It is most commonly used for IV fluid replacement in patients with portal hypertension during paracentesis. For every 2 litres of ascites removed, 1 unit (approximately 100 mL) of human albumin solution 4% is given IV. This is to avoid dangerous fluid shifts that may occur when removing ascites from the peritoneal cavity. According the NICE guidelines (NICE, 2013) on IV fluid therapy in adults in hospital, HAS 4–5% may be used as a resuscitation fluid for patients with severe sepsis.

However, this should be discussed with an intensive care consultant first.

Terminology

Fluid status – this is the state of a person's hydration. Fluid status can be assessed clinically, by history, examination and by bedside tests.

Euvolaemia – this describes a state of normal fluid status. If a euvolaemic patient needed IV fluids (e.g. during a period where they are fasting) they would be given maintenance fluid only.

Hypervolaemia – this describes a state of excessive circulating fluid in the body.

Hypovolaemia – this describes a state of reduced circulating fluid in the body.

Nil-by-mouth – is an instruction given to patients indicating that they should not eat or drink (taking nothing orally). This is commonly abbreviated to NBM. A typical reason for a patient being NBM is prior to surgery, where there is a risk of aspirating gastric contents during a general anaesthetic. Patients who are NBM for long periods are given maintenance IV fluid.

Case outcome and discharge

Yemi Oluwajobi received maintenance fluids during the preoperative period of 8 hours. She was able to eat and drink soon after her operation, and had an uneventful recovery. She was discharged later that evening with as-required analgesia only.

DISCHARGE MEDICATION						
Date	Medication	Dose	Route	Frequency	Supply	GP to continue?
xx/xx/xx	PARACETAMOL	1 g	PO	Four times daily (maximum 4 g in 24 hours)	7 days	N
xx/xx/xx	CODEINE PHOSPHATE	30-60 mg	PO	Four times daily	7 days	N
xx/xx/xx	MICROGYNON 30	1 tablet	PO	Once daily	14 days	Y
Notes to patient/GP:						

Common pitfalls

Fluid overload

- The most common pitfall in prescribing IV fluids is fluid overload and failure to prescribe the appropriate volume according to weight. Excessive IV fluid administration can cause fluid overload in any patient. Therefore appropriate and accurate fluid replacement is important. Fluid charts are important in giving clinicians an idea of fluid in and out when prescribing maintenance fluid, and observations are important when prescribing resuscitation fluid. Reassessing your patient's fluid status regularly will help to avoid fluid overload.
- Every patient is different, and IV fluids should be modified according to how patients respond to it.

- There are specific groups of patients who are at higher risk of fluid overload:
  - Cardiac failure
  - Renal failure
  - Liver failure
  - Low protein states
  - Elderly patients.
- These conditions are associated with inappropriate distribution of fluid. Excessive IV fluid can precipitate fluid distribution into the third space.
- The third space is a conceptual space where there is normally insignificant amounts of fluid. Sequestered fluid moves into the third space due to heart-pump failure (cardiac failure) and loss of oncotic pressure within vessels (proteinuria in renal failure, hypoalbuminaemia in liver failure and low protein states).
- Elderly patients are an important demographic to consider as they may have a combination of the conditions that precipitate fluid overload.

SUMMARY

- Humans require hydration and electrolytes for normal cellular and metabolic function. In some instances it is necessary to supplement fluid and electrolytes. IV fluid prescribing can be categorised into two situations: maintenance and resuscitation.
- In maintenance IV fluid, 25–30 mL/kg/day of water is required. Maintenance IV fluid should be initiated according to this 'empirical' formula. However, ongoing IV fluid should be tailored and titrated according to the patient's response and observations. It is therefore important to keep an accurate measure of fluid balance.
- There are various IV fluids to choose from. These can be categorised according to their contents as crystalloids and colloids.

FURTHER READING

- Recommendations from the NICE guidelines *Intravenous Fluid Therapy in over 16s in Hospital* (NICE, 2013).

🔑 Key learning points

Maintenance fluids
- Consider whether the clinical situation requires maintenance or resuscitation fluids.
- If a patient is unable to maintain hydration orally, consider maintenance IV fluid.

(Continued)

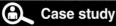 **Key learning points (Continued)**

- If patients need IV fluids for routine maintenance alone, restrict the initial prescription to:
  - 25–30 mL/kg/day of water **and**
  - approximately 1 mmol/kg/day of potassium, sodium and chloride **and**
  - approximately 50–100 g/day of glucose to limit starvation ketosis.
- Assess patients' fluid balance based on history, examination and bedside measures. Titrate the IV fluid prescription based on estimated patient needs.
- IV fluid prescriptions should be assessed at least every 24 hours.
- Crystalloids are the gold standard maintenance fluid of choice – sodium chloride, dextrose 4%/saline 0.18%, Hartmann's solution and dextrose 5%.
- Evidence indicates that colloids may increase mortality in critically unwell patients.

Maintenance electrolytes

Mr Gordon Smith

Age: 48

Hospital number: 123456

Case study

Presenting complaint: A 48-year-old man is recovering from an operation to remove a suspected malignant tumour in his caecum.

Background: He is day 1 postoperative and is only allowed to sip 30 mL of fluid per hour orally. As he recovers, the doctors will allow him to drink and eat more, but for now, his bowels need to be rested. He weighs 80 kg.

PMH: Osteoarthritis

Allergies: None

FH: Nil relevant

Examination, observations and tests:
Pulse 80, BP 120/80, Sats 100% on room air, RR 16, BM 7.0

CVS: Capillary refill time <2 second, pulse regular, HS I + II + 0 . JVP: 3 cm (normally 2–4 cm). Moist mucosal surfaces. Normal skin turgor

RS: Equal expansion with air entry to both bases and no added sounds

Regular medications: None

Postoperative blood tests:
Sodium (Na^+) = 140 mmol/L (Normally 135–145 mmol/L)
Potassium (K^+) = 4.5 mmol/L (Normally 3.5–5.0 mmol/L)

Diagnosis
The patient is day 1 postoperative from an operation. Fluid balance examination indicates that he is currently euvolaemic. He also has normal sodium and potassium. The patient has had an operation on his bowels and will have reduced oral intake in the postoperative period. He will therefore require maintenance fluids and electrolytes.

Prescribing maintenance electrolytes

The two most important electrolytes in the blood are sodium and potassium. There are other electrolytes that are important in certain situations, such as magnesium and calcium. Electrolytes such as sodium are present in certain fluids (such as 0.9% saline and Hartmann's solution). It cannot be added separately to other fluids. Potassium is also present in certain fluids (such as Hartmann's solution and blood). It can be added as a separate ingredient to 0.9% saline, 5% dextrose and saline/dextrose. It is not added separately to any other fluid.

An example of an initial IV fluid prescription for adult patient in the first 24 (based on a patient weight of 80 kg) is shown.

FLUID CHART

Date	Infusion fluid			Drug to be added		Signature	Print name
	Name and strength	Volume	Rate	Approved name	Dose		
01/12/ 2015	DEXTROSE 4%/ SALINE 0.18%	1000 ml bag	100 ml per hour	POTASSIUM CHLORIDE	40 mmol	A. Doctor	A. Doctor
01/12/ 2015	DEXTROSE 4%/ SALINE 0.18%	1000 ml bag	100 ml per hour	POTASSIUM CHLORIDE	40 mmol	A. Doctor	A. Doctor
01/12/ 2015	DEXTROSE 4%/ SALINE 0.18%	1000 ml bag	100 ml per hour	None		A. Doctor	A. Doctor

Prescribing maintenance electrolytes: rationale and evidence

Sodium

For a healthy adult, the NICE guidelines on IV fluid therapy in adults (NICE, 2013) recommend 1 mmol/kg/day of sodium (Na^+). A patient weighing 80 kg would therefore require 80 mmol of sodium per day. This need is satisfied by a 500 mL bag of 0.9% saline (because there is 150 mmol of sodium in 1000 mL of 0.9% saline). For this reason, the remaining water requirement should be gained by using 5% dextrose, which contains no sodium. Repeated prescription of 0.9% saline would result in hypernatraemia (high sodium) if continued for several days. Furthermore, chloride (Cl^-) in the 0.9% saline can result in a metabolic acidosis if given in excess.

Dextrose 4%/ saline 0.18% provides 31 mmol of sodium per litre. Using this solution avoids the risk of hypernatraemia that would occur if 0.9% saline was repeatedly without 5% dextrose. The NICE guidelines (NICE, 2013) support its use on the first day of maintenance fluid.

Potassium

For a healthy adult, the NICE guidelines (NICE, 2013) recommend 1 mmol/kg/day of potassium (K^+). Most IV fluids do not contain potassium or contain only a small amount (Hartmann's solution only contains 5 mmol in 1000 mL). Potassium can be added to 0.9% saline, 5% dextrose or dextrose/saline in the form of potassium chloride (KCl).

Potassium must not be infused at a rate of greater than 10 mmol/hour. The rapid rise in serum potassium of greater than this would result in myocardial instability. This means that a 1000 mL bag of 0.9% saline, dextrose/saline, or 5% dextrose, containing 40 mmol of potassium chlorine (KCl), cannot be infused faster than over 4 hours. If a faster rate of infusion is required, then the crystalloid must not have potassium added.

A complication of potassium replacement is hyperkalaemia. Hyperkalaemia is defined as a serum potassium of >5.5 mmol/L (Chapagain and Ashman, 2012), and is a life-threatening emergency due to cardiac conduction abnormalities. The faster the potassium infusion, the more cardiotoxic it may be (Paice *et al.*, 1983). Therefore, potassium should not be administered faster than 10 mmol/hour outside the intensive care or cardiology units whilst on a cardiac monitor.

In the case described here, 40 mmol of potassium chloride could be added to two out of three bags of fluid to provide a total daily potassium of 80 mmol.

Fluid and electrolyte losses

In normal adults, fluid and electrolytes are lost in multiple ways:

- Urine
- Faeces
- Vomiting
- Surgical drains
- Insensible losses.

Insensible losses describe the loss of water from the skin, such as sweating, and respiratory tract. This is normally 500 mL per day. This means that if our patient has had a total of 2400 mL of fluid **in** (via IV and oral fluid) and there has been 2400 mL **out**, then the patient's fluid balance would be zero. However, given normal insensible losses that cannot be recorded, the patient would in fact be negative 500 mL.

Fluid and electrolyte losses are increased in certain situations:

- Increased urine output – for example diuretic medication or diabetes insipidus
- Increased output from the gastrointestinal tract – for example, vomiting, diarrhoea, ileus or enteric fistulae. A single episode of vomiting results in fluid loss of approximately 200 mL.
- Increased insensible losses – for example fever (typically 700–1000 mL), increased sweating or use of non-humidified oxygen, especially those who are intubated and on a ventilator
- Third-space losses – this describes an interstitial space in the body where fluid does not normally

accumulate in large volumes. Examples of third spaces include the peritoneal or pleural cavity.

Nursing and medical staff should measure, as accurately as possible, the fluid **in** (IV, oral, NG feeding) and the fluid **out** (urine, surgical drains). It is not practical to measure fluid loss from faeces and vomitus unfortunately.

At the end of each day, net fluid balance should be calculated. For a patient to have neutral fluid status, the fluid balance should be positive, of at lease +500 mL, to account for insensible loss.

Prescribing maintenance electrolytes: essential pharmacology

Sodium and potassium are essential electrolytes that are needed for normal cellular function.

Sodium is primarily an extracellular anion. Sodium concentration is maintained by Na/K ATPase pumps on the surface of cells. Sodium balance is essential to maintain the correct osmolality of cells. Sodium is gained through the diet.

Potassium is primarily an intracellular anion. Tissues that are most sensitive to abnormal potassium concentrations are cardiac and skeletal muscles. Potassium concentration within cells is also maintained by Na/K ATPase pumps. Like sodium, potassium is normally gained in the diet.

IV supplementation of both sodium and potassium is required in patients who are unable to obtain their normal potassium requirements from their diet, or in critical illness.

Sodium and potassium loss from the body can occur through various means. However, there are certain bodily fluids that contain high concentrations of electrolytes. These fluids must be identified, and supplementation anticipated:

- Sodium-rich fluid
  - Urine
  - Sweat
- Potassium-rich fluid
  - Urine
  - Vomit
  - Diarrhoea
  - Ileostomy (type of stoma).

Electrolyte maintenance should begin with normal daily requirements and be titrated by the patient's daily serum electrolytes.

Case outcome and discharge

Gordon Smith (80 kg) has both fluid and electrolyte requirements, which should be maintained. Fluid losses should be identified and accounted for. Fluid constituents are explained above, but a calculation is required in order to correctly replace electrolytes according to the patients known requirements and the amount they are drinking.

Maintenance fluid calculation

Water requirements in adults: 25–30 mL/kg/day

His daily requirement is therefore
$(30 \text{ mL} \times 80 \text{ kg}) = 2400 \text{ mL/day}$

If he is drinking small amounts then the IV requirement should be decreased to incorporate this so as not to overload him. Gordon is drinking around 250 mL per day at present.

Additionally, if there are extra losses (vomiting, fever) then extra fluid should be added to this calculation. Gordon has vomited twice (2×200 mL); this also makes him more likely to require potassium supplementation.

Total fluid prescription = 2400 mL – 250 mL
+ 400 mL = 2550 mL per day

Maintenance electrolytes:

Sodium and potassium requirements in adults: 1 mmol/kg/day

His daily requirement is therefore (1 mmol × 80 kg) = 80 mmol of sodium and 80 mmol of potassium

Gordon started to tolerate oral fluids after 24 hours, and was allowed to eat and drink. Fluids were therefore discontinued and he was discharged after 4 days.

Common pitfalls

Hyperchloraemic acidosis

Patients who receive excess 0.9% sodium chloride are at risk of developing hyperchloraemic acidosis. In maintenance fluid replacement, chloride can be limited by giving patients fluids that are low in chloride such as dextrose 4%/saline 0.18%, Hartmann's solution or dextrose 5%.

- The two most important electrolytes in the blood are sodium and potassium. There are other electrolytes that are important in certain situations such as magnesium and calcium.
- For a healthy adult, daily requirements of sodium (Na^+) are 1 mmol/kg/day. Potassium administration should not exceed 10 mmol per hour, to avoid dangerous cardiac arrhythmias.
- Dextrose 4%/ saline 0.18% is the initial maintenance fluid of choice according to the NICE guidelines on IV fluid therapy in adults. It is contraindicated in children.
- To keep up with fluid and electrolyte losses, take into account fluids that contain large amounts of sodium and potassium.

SUMMARY

FURTHER READING

- Read the recommendations from the NICE guidelines *Intravenous Fluid Therapy in over 16s in Hospital* (NICE, 2013).

🔑 Key learning points

Maintenance electrolytes
- Sodium and potassium are the two main electrolytes discussed in this chapter.
- Patients have fluid and electrolyte requirements that must be pre-empted. Replacement of these electrolytes is essential in maintaining homeostasis.
- If patients need IV fluids for routine maintenance alone, restrict the initial prescription to:
  - 25–30 ml/kg/day of water **and**
  - approximately 1 mmol/kg/day of potassium, sodium and chloride **and**
  - approximately 50–100 g/day of glucose to limit starvation ketosis.
- Do not infuse IV potassium faster than 10 mmol/hour as this destabilises the myocardium and can cause cardiac arrhythmias.
- Maintenance IV fluid and electrolytes prescriptions should be assessed at least every 24 hours.

Resuscitation fluids

Ms Camille Rossini
Age: 34
Hospital number: 123456

🔍 Case study

Presenting complaint: *34-year-old lady who has come to the emergency department with severe abdominal pain.*

Background: *4-day history of right upper quadrant pain with fever. She is known to have gall stones and is awaiting laparoscopic cholecystectomy for biliary colic. She is 50 kg in weight*

PMH: *Gall stones*
Observations in triage: BP 79/50, HR 120, Temperature 38.0°C (pyrexial), S_aO_2 99% room air, RR 26. She remains conscious but confused.

ECG: *sinus tachycardia.*

Examination
CVS: Pale and sweaty, capillary refill time 2 seconds, HR regular, HS I+II+0
RS: Chest clear, equal air entry,

Abdomen: *Tender RUQ, positive Murphy's sign, no masses and no peritonism.*

Bloods: *Hb 13.0, Plt 324,* **WCC 16.0, CRP 150,** *amylase 50, Na 136, K 4.0, Urea 8.0, Creat 120, INR 1.1, Bili 20, LFTs normal*

Diagnosis

Biliary sepsis due to cholecystitis (infection of the gall bladder, commonly associated with gall stones) Septic shock requiring urgent resuscitation IV fluid.

Initial measures

Shock is acute circulatory failure leading to inadequate organ perfusion. The degree can be assessed clinically and gives clinicians an idea of how much fluid loss has occurred (Table 7.1). Remember that there are five forms of shock: septic, haemorrhagic, anaphylactic, cardiogenic and neurogenic. Cardiogenic shock should not be treated with IV fluids.

The initial step in the management of septic shock can be summarised as 'the sepsis six', which are a set of fundamental interventions in the treatment of sepsis (see Box The Sepsis Six Steps), but note that IV fluid challenges are a key part.

Table 7.1 Classes of shock and estimated fluid loss.

	Class 1	Class 2	Class 3	Class 4
Approx % fluid volume loss	<15%	15–30%	30–40%	>40%
Heart rate	<100	Tachycardia	Tachycardia	Tachycardia
Systolic BP	Normal	Normal	Reduced	Reduced
Diastolic BP	Normal	Increased	Increased	Increased
Respiration rate	Normal	Increased	Increased	Increased
Urine output	Normal (>0.5 mL/kg/h)	Reduced (<0.5 mL/kg/h)	Oligoanuric	Oligoanuric
Mental status	Anxious	Anxious	Confused	Impaired consciousness

The sepsis six steps

The surviving sepsis campaign has highlighted six key intervention in patients with sepsis (Dellinger *et al.*, 2008)
1. Administration of high-flow oxygen
2. Take blood cultures
3. Give broad-spectrum antibiotics
4. Give intravenous fluid challenges
5. Measure serum lactate and haemoglobin
6. Measure accurate hourly urine output

Prescribing resuscitation fluids

Resuscitation fluids are the mainstay of treatment in hypovolaemia

✓ **DRUGS checklist for 0.9% SODIUM CHLORIDE**

Dose	500 mL
Route	IV
Units	mL
Given	STAT The actual speed depends on the size of the cannula. Speed can be increased by using a pressure device to squeeze the bag (this can also be done manually in an emergency). IV fluid boluses should ideally be given in less than 15 minutes

Special situations	In an emergency situation there is less concern about co-morbidities such as heart failure/old age which may predispose to fluid overload and pulmonary oedema with large fluid volumes. This is because the life-threatening problem of hypotension has to addressed first.

An example of a fluid chart with resuscitation fluid for the first 15 minutes of the patient's stay is shown.

FLUID CHART					
Date	Infusion fluid			Signature	Print name
	Name and strength	Volume	Rate		
01/12/2014	SALINE 0.9%	500 ml	STAT	A. Doctor	A. Doctor

The situation needs to be re-evaluated rapidly, as she may well need further IV crystalloid boluses if her blood pressure has not normalised. In the absence of an improvement after repeated IV crystalloid boluses, the intensive care specialists need to assess the patient for inotropic support for septic shock.

Resuscitation fluids: rationale and evidence

The NICE guidelines on IV fluid therapy in adults (NICE, 2013) recommend that 500 mL of crystalloid should be given as an initial fluid bolus (over less than 15 minutes).

The fluid of choice should be any crystalloid, with a sodium concentration of 130–154 mmol/L. This means than any of the following may be used as a resuscitation fluid:

- 0.9% Sodium chloride
- Hartmann's solution

Colloids such as Gelofusin should no longer be used as they are associated with increased mortality in critically unwell patients (Perel and Roberts, 2013).

Resuscitation fluids: essential pharmacology

To safely prescribe IV fluid in resuscitation, one must understand **fluid distribution** in the body.

Water is the main solvent in the body, therefore fluid and water are used interchangeably when talking about fluid distribution.

The body **normally** has two main spaces where there is fluid:

1. Intracellular fluid (ICF) – this fluid accounts for two-thirds of the total body water, and is within cells.
2. Extracellular (ECF) – this accounts for the remaining third of the total body water, and can be divided into two:
   (a) Intravascular (blood plasma) within blood vessels
   (b) Extravascular (interstitial space) between cells.

There is a third space where fluid can accumulate in large amounts inappropriately. The third-space losses will be discussed later, but includes pathological accumulation of fluid in the pleural space (pleural effusions) and in the peritoneal cavity (ascites).

An average 70-kg man has 42 L of water within his body. Two-thirds of this water is intracellular (28 L), and the remaining one-third is extracellular (14 L). This extracellular fluid includes the water that contributes to blood within circulation (intravascular fluid; approximately 3 L) and water between cells (interstitial fluid; approximately 11 L) (Figure 7.1).

Water is the main ingredient of blood plasma and acts as a solvent to its other constituents, including proteins. Blood circulates within the intravascular space and IV fluid is given directly into this space. However, IV fluid entering via the intravascular space will redistribute throughout the other spaces, depending on the type of fluid. The distribution of fluid is dependent on the oncotic pressure exerted by large proteins such as albumin, and the permeability of blood vessels.

The aim of IV fluid resuscitation is to expand the volume of fluid in the intravascular space, where it can contribute to blood pressure and help to perfuse vital organs. If **5% dextrose** is administered IV, this distributes evenly throughout the fluid compartments (one-third will remain within the extracellular space, and two-thirds will go into the intracellular space). This means that if 1000 mL of 5% dextrose is administered, only 333 mL will

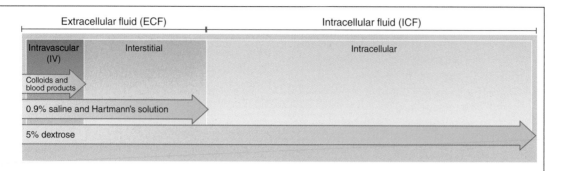

Figure 7.1 The distribution of fluid in the body, with one-third being extracellular and two-thirds being intracellular. The extracellular space includes the intravascular space, where IV fluid enters directly, and the interstitial space.

remain within the intravascular space. It is for this reason that 5% dextrose is not an effective resuscitation fluid. Likewise dextrose/saline will redistribute across the ECF and ICF. Dextrose/saline is therefore not used as a resuscitation fluid either.

The fluids **0.9% saline** and **Hartmann's solution** are more physiological and have an osmolality that is similar to extracellular fluid. This means that these fluids only distribute throughout the ECF, and contribute more to intravascular fluid expansion. The more sodium in a solution, the better it will stay within the ECF.

Colloids are a group of IV fluid that have recently fallen out of favour due to evidence indicating that they are associated with increased mortality in critically unwell patients (Perel and Roberts, 2013). They will be discussed because junior doctors may still encounter centres that use them. However, their use is not recommended by this book. Colloids have been engineered to only remain in the intravascular space in order to be maximally effective in fluid resuscitation. They contain large particles, which cannot easily distribute. Therefore if 1000 mL of colloid is given IV, all of this will remain in the intravascular space in the short term. Figure 7.1 shows the fluid compartments and how the IV fluids discussed distribute. Unfortunately, over a number of hours, the large particles in colloids break down, and cause the fluid to distribute more evenly. Theoretically, colloids should be more effective in resuscitation than crystalloids. However, this has not been reflected in randomised control trials comparing the two (see Evidence).

Evidence

Choice of IV fluid in resuscitation

In 2013, the Cochrane Library performed a meta-analysis of 74 trials comparing crystalloid and colloid fluids in critically unwell patients requiring fluid resuscitation. The authors state that 'there is no evidence from randomised controlled trials that resuscitation with colloids reduces the risk of death, compared to resuscitation with crystalloids, in patients with trauma, burns or following surgery'. Crystalloids are therefore recommended, over colloids, in fluid resuscitation (Perel and Roberts, 2013).

IV fluid resuscitation should be focused on replacing estimated fluid loss. The percentage of total fluid volume loss can be estimated according to basic bedside observations: heart rate, blood pressure, respiratory rate, urine output and mental status. The degree of shock, with its estimated fluid loss, can therefore be categorised according to severity (Table 7.1).

In haemorrhagic shock, the fluid loss is primarily whole blood. It is therefore advised to replace like with like. Up to 2 litres of non-blood fluid can be given but following this, packed red cell transfusion should be arranged. However, patients exhibiting haemorrhagic shock in class 3 and 4 should receive blood preferentially over other non-blood fluids. Transfusion of blood products will be discussed in the Section Blood Products.

Case outcome and discharge

Camille Rossini's presenting observations indicate that she is tachycardic, hypotensive and confused. She is therefore in septic shock, class 3. She was therefore treated according to the 'Sepsis Six', with high-flow oxygen and broad-spectrum antibiotics. Blood cultures, serum lactate and haemoglobin were checked. She also received IV fluid challenges (in boluses) of 500 mL boluses of crystalloid (Hartmann's solution was given in her case).

Camille Rossini responded after the initial 500 mL bolus of Hartmann's solution. Therefore two further boluses were given, without signs of fluid overload.

Once her heart rate and blood pressure stabilised, the patient received maintenance IV fluids. The patient was discharged 3 days later on oral antibiotics. She will attend the day surgery department in 6 weeks time for an elective laparoscopic cholecystectomy to remove her gall bladder.

Common pitfalls

■ **Fluid overload:** Fluid overload is a common pitfall in the prescription of maintenance fluid (see Section Fluid Management). However, it may also occur in the resuscitation situation, where IV fluid administration may be faster and in greater volumes. Reassessing your patient's fluid status regularly will help to avoid fluid overload. Every patient is different, and IV fluids should be modified according to how patients respond to it. Patients with multiple co-morbidities, such as heart failure, it may be advisable to gain central venous pressure monitoring in order to guide fluid administration.

■ **Failure to respond to IV fluids:** Failure to respond successfully to IV fluid may indicate that the patient has a degree of heart failure. Patients who do not respond haemodynamically, or who develop signs of fluid overload (whilst remaining intravascularly depleted) may require positive inotropes. These are given primarily in the intensive care unit; referral to an intensivist is therefore advised. Invasive monitoring, such as central venous pressure, may also guide fluid replacement.

SUMMARY

- There are five forms of shock: septic, haemorrhagic, anaphylactic, cardiogenic and neurogenic. IV fluid is the mainstay of treatment in haemorrhagic and septic shock. The degree of shock can be estimated clinically, and should provide the prescriber with a good idea of fluid loss.
- We recommend that resuscitation fluid should be limited to 0.9% sodium chloride and Hartmann's solution. The use of colloids are not associated with improved survival but are considerably more expensive than crystalloids (Perel and Roberts, 2013).
- Initial IV fluid boluses of 500 mL crystalloid should be given, as fluid challenge (over less than 15 minutes).
- Failure to respond to IV fluids may indicate that inotropic medications are needed, and referral to intensive care is advised.

FURTHER READING

■ NICE guidelines on intravenous fluid therapy in adults in hospital: *Intravenous Fluid Therapy in Over 16s in Hospital*, CG174, 2013. Available at: www.nice.org.uk/guidance/cg174 (accessed Jan. 2015).

Blood products

> **Benjamin Francoise**
>
> **Age: 30**
>
> **Hospital number: 123456**

🔍 Case study

Presenting complaint: A 30-year-old man is brought in to the accident and emergency department by ambulance crew following a road traffic accident.

Background: This usually fit and well gentleman was struck by a vehicle whilst cycling his bicycle. Primary trauma survey performed by the ambulance crew has identified bilateral fractured femurs. He is currently in bilateral Thomas splints.

PMH: Nil relevant

Allergies: None

FH: Nil relevant
The trauma team completed the primary survey examination according to Advanced Trauma Life Support guidelines following the ABCDE structure as follows:

Airway: patent, 15 L/min oxygen via non-rebreathe mask

Breathing: Saturations 100%. Equal air entry. RR 28/min

Circulation: heart rate 150 bpm, blood pressure 90/60, capillary refill 5 seconds, heart sounds I+II+0

IV access is gained in both upper limbs. Bloods are taken for XM 6 units of red cells, FBC, U&Es

Disability: GCS = E4 M6 V5 = 15/15, capillary glucose = 5.8

Exposure: Temperature 35.6. Bilateral open femur fractures in Thomas splints
Pelvis and abdominal examination unremarkable

Diagnosis
Haemorrhagic shock secondary to bilateral femur fractures.

Initial measures
As described above, the initial management of trauma patients follows the Advanced Trauma Life Support (ATLS) guidelines, in an ABCDE structure. The purpose of the primary survey is to identify life-threatening injuries. Whilst haemorrhage is a component of Circulation, it is important to identify and treat injuries pertaining to Airway and Breathing first, as they may kill the patient more quickly. However, it is accepted that a clear point of bleeding should have immediate direct compression to control the haemorrhage.

Heart rate, blood pressure, respiratory rate, mental status and urine output enable the trauma team to estimate the degree of blood loss according to the class of shock (Table 7.1).

Once blood tests have been taken, IV saline should be started as the initial resuscitation fluid. In class 3–4, the resuscitation fluid of choice is packed red cells, which can be urgently arranged whilst IV saline keeps the IV access patent.

Prescribing blood products

The most important message to convey in the safe prescription of blood products is to give the **correct blood** to the **correct patient**:

1. Patient's details are checked prior to taking a cross-matching blood test.
2. Blood bottles should never be prelabelled.
3. Patient's identity is rechecked and cross-examined with the blood product that is to be given.

An example of a prescription for 1 unit of packed red cells is shown.

BLOOD PRESCRIPTION CHART							
Date	Infusion fluid			Drug to be added		Prescriber's signature	Print name
	Name and strength	Volume	Rate	Approved name	Dose		
1st Dec 2014	PACKED RED CELLS	1 unit	3 hours	None added	–	A. Doctor	A. Doctor

The components of blood that can be transfused include:

- Packed red cells
- Platelets
- Fresh frozen plasma (FFP) and cryoprecipitate.

Blood products: rationale and evidence

Packed red cells are red blood cells in a nutrient and anticoagulation solution (containing saline, adenine, glucose and mannitol), and come in transfusion bags of approximately 300 mL. Each 300-mL bag is prescribed as 1 unit. A transfusion of packed red cells is commonly known as a blood transfusion; a transfusion of whole blood is no longer used. Blood transfusions must be ABO and RhD compatible with the recipient in order to avoid an immune-mediated haemolytic crisis. Therefore confirming that the correct blood product is for the correct patient is of paramount importance.

For blood to be prescribed safely, the correct patient details must be checked and observations undertaken before and during the transfusion, in order to detect a transfusion-related reaction. Red cells cannot be out of the fridge for more than 4 hours. It is therefore advised to prescribe red cells over a maximum of 3.5 hours (to account for transport time). Packed red cells can be transfused as quickly as is necessary. Red cells are usually prescribed on a separate blood transfusion prescription chart. One unit of packed red cells should cause an incremental increase in haemoglobin of approximately 10 g/L. For example, transfusing 1 unit of packed red cells to a patient with a haemoglobin of 70 g/L should result in a post-transfusion haemoglobin of around 80 g/L.

Certain blood products, like packed red cells, should be avoid in patients who have a religious belief against blood products, such as 'Jehovah's Witnesses'. These patients must have signed documentation detailing which 'major' and 'minor' fractions of blood they will consider in the event of blood loss. Doctors have been successfully sued for saving adult patients' lives with blood products in this setting.

Blood can contain cytomegalovirus, which can be dangerous for patients who are immunosuppressed – these patients should received specially irradiated blood.

Terminology

Group and save: This is a blood test that requests the transfusion laboratory to identify the patient's ABO group, and save serum so that if blood was required, this could be issued within 15 minutes. It allows anticipation of blood loss without actually issuing units of blood unless it was needed.

Cross match: This is a blood test that requests the transfusion laboratory to identify the patient's ABO group and issue blood immediately. You must specify how many units of red cells you require.

✓ DRUGS checklist for PACKED RED CELLS

Dose	1 unit
Route	IV
Units	units
Given	Infusion of no more than 4 hours
Special situations	Patient identity must be confirmed – always correct product to correct patient. Must be ABO/Rh compatible. Monitor for transfusion reactions.

Platelets are prescribed therapeutically (active bleeding) or prophylactically (to prevent spontaneous bleeding) in patients with thrombocytopenia (low platelets). In the presence of thrombocytopenia of less than 50×10^9/L, platelets should only be transfused if there is active bleeding or if imminent urgent surgery is required. Platelets are prescribed in 'pools'. A single pool of platelets should be infused over 30 minutes. A single pool contains 7×10^{10} platelets (Slichter, 2007) and should increase the platelet count by 30×10^9 within 10 minutes. Platelets do express ABO antigens and should therefore only be prescribed between compatible blood groups.

✓	**DRUGS checklist for PLATELETS**
Dose	1 pool
Route	IV
Units	pools
Given	Infusion over 30 minutes
Special situations	Must be prescribed with permission from a haematologist. Must be ABO/Rh compatible. Monitor for transfusion reactions.

Fresh frozen plasma (FFP) is the liquid constituent of blood, which is collected by centrifugation and is then frozen. It contains clotting factors and is therefore used in coagulopathies:

- Reversal of warfarin
- Replacement of isolated clotting factors II, V, VII, IX, X and XI
- Massive transfusion of packed red cells, to prevent disseminated intravascular coagulation (DIC)
- Treatment of thrombotic thrombocytopenic purpura.

FFP is prescribed in units that contain 200–250 mL of yellow fluid. A single unit of FFP should be infused over 90 minutes (Silvergleid, 2015).

✓	**DRUGS checklist for FRESH FROZEN PLASMA**
Dose	1 unit
Route	IV
Units	units
Given	Infusion over 90 minutes
Special situations	Must be prescribed with permission from a haematologist.

Cryoprecipitate is the liquid that forms when FFP thaws at 4°C into a more concentrated solution of 10–20 mL. Its key ingredients are fibrinogen and factor XIII. It is a highly specialised blood product which should only be prescribed by a haematologist.

Packed red cells: essential pharmacology

Of all the blood products available, red blood cells are the most commonly prescribed. However, in order to safely prescribe red blood cells, one must understand the concept of ABO compatibility.

ABO compatibility

The majority of mortality from blood transfusion is due to avoidable errors in ABO-compatibility (Stainsby *et al.*, 2005). ABO are antigens that are present on red blood cells. Patients are one of four ABO blood groups (Table 7.2).

In addition to the ABO blood group system, there are additional antigens on red cells, which fall into the Rhesus blood group system. In the context of blood transfusion, the most important Rhesus antigen is D, which can either be D-positive or D-negative. If a patient who is Rhesus D-negative is exposed to as little as 0.5 mL of Rhesus D-positive blood, there is a significant counterattack of anti-D antibody production (Kumpel, 2002). Rhesus D is highly immunogenic in healthy patients.

There are other blood group systems that take into account clinically relevant antigens. These include:

- Lewis, P1 and I blood groups
- MNSS blood groups

Table 7.2 ABO blood groups.

Blood group	Antigen on RBC	Antibody in serum	Clinical status
A	A	Anti-B	Can only receive A or O blood Can only donate to A or AB patients
B	B	Anti-A	Can only receive B or O blood Can only donate to B and AB patients
AB	A and B	None	Universal recipient Can only donate to AB patients
O	None	Anti-A and Anti-B	Can only receive O blood Universal donor

- Kell blood groups
- Duffy blood groups
- Kidd blood groups
- Others.

The blood transfusion department in the hospital can provide three forms of packed red cells:

1. Fully cross-matched blood: this is matched to ABO, Rhesus and other clinically relevant blood groups. The risk of a transfusion-related reaction is therefore very low. However, fully cross-matched blood is individually tailored to each patient and can take more than 45 minutes for the transfusion department to provide.

2. Group-specific blood: this is ABO and Rhesus matched blood. The other blood group systems are not included. There is therefore a small risk of a transfusion-related reaction. However, it takes approximately 30 minutes for the transfusion department to provide group-specific blood.

3. O-negative blood: containing red cells with no surface antigens. It can therefore be given to any patient. O-negative blood is a finite resource and is only used in life-threatening haemorrhage.

The choice of packed red cells therefore depends on the estimated time and urgency that the blood product is required.

Patients who have previously provided blood for Group and Save have the advantage of receiving fully cross-matched blood within 15 minutes, provided that they have not had a recent sensitising event, such as a recent blood transfusion.

Case outcome and discharge

Benjamin Francoise had a primary and secondary trauma survey according to ATLS guidelines. IV access was gained and 0.9% saline was started until blood products became available. Six units of packed red cells. Both legs were put in Thomas splints for femoral fractures, and surgery was not required. He was kept in hospital for 4 days whilst he recovered from his injuries and then was discharged with an ongoing physiotherapy regime and simple analgesia.

Common pitfalls

Transfusion-related reactions

Transfusion-related reactions are a complication of giving products that are immunogenic (Roback *et al.*, 2011). The reaction should be categorised according to the signs and symptoms of the patient.

- Category 1 (mild) – localised itchy rash, fever. Slow blood transfusion and give paracetamol and antihistamine.
- Category 2 (moderate) – fever, rigors, tachycardia and tachypnoea. Stop blood transfusion, start IV 0.9% sodium chlorine and treat as per anaphylaxis. Send blood back to lab.
- Category 3 (severe) – fever, rigors, tachycardia, hypotension and tachypnoea, unexplained bleeding. Stop blood transfusion. Treat as per anaphylaxis. Start antibiotics if bacteraemia is suspected. Send blood back to lab.

Fluid overload

Fluid overload may occur in blood transfusion in the same way that it can occur with other IV fluids. The slowest a unit can be given is over 4 hours (logistically over 3.5 hours to account for the time it takes for the blood to be taken from the fridge). IV furosemide can be given between units of packed red cells (20 mg IV in diuretic naïve patients, and 40 mg IV in patients who are already taking a diuretic regularly). However, it is not appropriate to administer furosemide with blood products in patients who are hypovolaemic.

Hyperkalaemia

Packed red cells contain potassium and can cause hyperkalaemia (Simon and Bove, 1971). Treat patients as per hyperkalaemia (see Chapter 10, Section Hyperkalaemia).

Massive transfusion

Massive transfusion is defined as severe haemorrhage requiring the transfusion of 10 units of packed red cells in 24 hours. This posses specific complications, including derangement of coagulation and hyperkalaemia (Collins, 1974).

SUMMARY

- Blood products include packed red cells, platelets, fresh frozen plasma and cryoprecipitate. In order to safely prescribe blood products, one must understand the concept of ABO and rhesus compatibility. The correct blood should be given to the correct patient in order to avoid life-threatening transfusion-related reactions.
- Packed red cells should be prescribed in units, and should be prescribed over a maximum of 4 hours (logistically this is 3.5 hours to account for time between fridge and patient).

☞ Key learning points

Blood products
- Packed red cells are prescribed as units, containing 300 ml of fluid.
- One unit of packed red cells should result in an incremental increase in haemoglobin of 10g/L, if there is no ongoing bleeding.
- Blood products should be ABO and Rh compatible to avoid transfusion-related reactions.
- Platelets are prescribed as 'pools' and should be prescribed as an infusion over 30 minutes.
- Platelets should only be prescribed if there is thrombocytopenia of $>50 \times 10^9$/L in the presence of active bleeding or prior to surgery, and only once agreed with a haematologist.
- FFP contains clotting factors and is commonly used to reverse warfarin and other coagulopathies.
- As with other IV fluids, there is a risk of fluid overload.

FURTHER READING

■ Pandey S, Vyas GN (2012). Adverse effects of plasma transfusion. *Transfusion* **52** (Suppl. 1), 65S–79S.

Nausea and vomiting

> **Mr Claude Mamet**
>
> **Age: 50**
>
> **Hospital number: 123456**

 Case study

Presenting complaint: A 50-year-old gentleman comes to the general surgical clinic with nausea and vomiting.

Background: He underwent a right hemicolectomy for colon cancer disease 9 months ago. Today he is nauseated and has vomited numerous times over 2 days. On further questioning he last passed stool 3 days ago and denies passing flatus subsequently.

PMH: Adenocarcimona of the ascending colon treated by open right hemicolectomy. Previous appendicectomy.

Allergies: None

FH: Nil relevant

Examination, observations and tests:
Pulse 110, BP 120/80, Sats 98% on room air, RR 14, BM 7.0

BMI: 24

CVS: Capillary refill time 3 seconds, pulse regular, HS I + II + 0

RS: Equal expansion with air entry to both bases and no added sounds

Abdo: Distended abdomen which is tense and drum-like. Tympanic to percussion. No shifting dullness. Scars: Midline laparotomy scar, Lanz incision scar Digital examination of the rectum reveals no masses and is empty.

ECG: Sinus tachycardia, WCC: 18, Na 136, K 3.3, Urea 9.0, Creat 100, INR 1.0

Regular medications: Nil regular

Abdominal XR: Dilated loops of small bowel, measuring 4 cm in diameter (normally <3), in a laddered pattern

Chest XR: There is no evidence of pneumoperitoneum (free extraluminal pair in the peritoneum, such as under the diaphragm)

Diagnosis
Probably small bowel obstruction. Given his history of intra-abdominal surgery, this may be caused by adhesions.

Initial measures
The initial measures in small bowel obstruction are traditionally summarised by 'drip and suck'. This means nasograstric tube suction in order to decompress the stomach and bowel (suck) and to place the patient nil-by-mouth with IV fluid replacement (drip). However, symptoms of nausea and vomiting must also be treated, and this will be the focus of the chapter.

Prescribing for nausea and vomiting

Nausea and vomiting (emesis) are common symptoms, which can be treated with antiemetics. The most common settings for using antiemetics in hospital are (Scorza *et al.*, 2007):

- Secondary to a disease process
- Side effect of other medications
- Postoperative nausea and vomiting (PONV)
- Palliative care
- Pregnancy (hyperemesis gravidarum).

Antiemetics can cause dangerous side effects and complications if used in the wrong setting. The correct selection of an antiemetic medication will relieve symptoms more effectively, avoid side effects and gain other bonus effects.

ONCE ONLY PRESCRIPTIONS					Prescriber	
Date	Time to be given	DRUG	Dose	Route	Signature	Bleep
15/1/15	13:00	CYCLIZINE	50 mg	IV	A. Doctor	

Antiemetics: rationale and evidence

In the surgical department postoperative nausea and vomiting (PONV) is a common symptom following emergency and elective surgery. Adequate control of nausea and vomiting is a necessary criterion for discharge from the theatre recovery room (Metz and Hebbard, 2007).

The rational of adequate PONV control extends to beyond the immediate postoperative period. There is strong evidence that patient satisfaction is significantly reduced in the presence of PONV, and can be a cause of unplanned admission into hospital following day surgery (Scorza *et al.*, 2007).

Patient factors associated with higher rates of PONV include:

- Female gender
- Non-smoker status
- Younger age
- History of motion sickness or previous PONV.

Evidence

Reducing the risk of postoperative nausea and vomiting

The IMPACT (International Multicentre Protocol to Assess the single and Combined benefits of antiemetic medication in a controlled clinical Trial) trial is, to date, the largest study of postoperative nausea and vomiting (PONV) prophylactics. Patients who were considered high risk of PONV were enrolled. High risk constituted ≥2 risk factors: female, non-smoker, previous PONV, motion sickness and anticipated need for postoperative opioids; 4123 patients were randomised to one of 64 combinations of six interventions to reduce PONV:

- 4 mg of ondansetron or no ondansetron
- 4 mg of dexamethasone or no dexamethasone
- 1.25 mg of droperidol or no droperidol
- propofol or a volatile anesthetic
- nitrogen or nitrous oxide
- remifentanil or fentanyl.

The study showed that ondansetron, dexamethasone and droperidol are equally effective at reducing PONV by 26%. Because antiemetic interventions are similarly effective and act independently, the safest or least expensive should be used first. The use of propofol and nitrogen reduced the risk of PONV by 19% and 12%, respectively. The study also suggests that patients with a low risk of PONV should not receive prophylactic antiemetics as this is not cost effective. Patients at moderate risk will benefit from a single antiemetic, whilst high-risk patients will benefit from multiple agents (Apfel *et al.*, 2004).

Antiemetics: essential pharmacology

There are five commonly used classes of drugs that antagonise neurotransmitter receptors which are known to cause nausea and vomiting (Egerton-Warburton *et al.*, 2014).

1. **Antihistamines**
   Examples: cyclizine and promethazine
   Actions: antimuscarinic effect
   Indications: opioid analgesia, hyperemesis gravida
   Contraindications: avoid in acute coronary syndromes due to increased risk of arrhythmia. Use with caution in prostatic hypertrophy, urinary retention, angle-closure glaucoma, and pyloroduodenal obstruction due to its antimuscarinic effects.
   Side effects: sedating

2. **Dopamine antagonists** (also known as phenothiazines)
   Examples: prochlorperazine, and chlorpromazine.
   Actions: blocks the neuroendocrine signal dopamine
   Indications: cancer-related nausea and vomiting, including chemotherapy and radiotherapy, nausea and vomiting associated with opioids and anaesthetic agents
   Contraindications: Parkinson's disease, coma and CNS depression, phaeochromocytoma. Caution in the elderly, epilepsy as it reduces the seizure threshold, myasthenia gravis

3. **Prokinetics**
   Example: metoclopramide
   Actions: similar dopamine-blocking effect as the dopamine antagonists
   Indications: gastroduodenal, hepatic and biliary disease. Its prokinetic effect on bowel peristalsis means that it is useful in ileus and pseudo-obstruction

Contraindications: prokinetic effect on the bowel means that it is contraindicated in bowel obstruction

Side effects: dystonic reactions – oculogyric crisis

4. **5HT$_3$-receptor antagonists**

Example: ondansetron

Actions: similar dopamine-blocking effect as the dopamine antagonists

Indications: gastroduodenal, hepatic and biliary disease. Its prokinetic effect on bowel peristalsis means that it is useful in ileus and pseudo-obstruction

Contraindications: prokinetic effect on the bowel means that it is contraindicated in bowel obstruction. Caution should be used when administering ondansetron to patients at rick of cardiac arrhythmias – it causes a dose-dependent prolongation of the QT interval (MHRA, 2012).

5. **Corticosteroid**

Example: dexamethasone is the main corticosteroid used in emesis

Actions: similar dopamine-blocking effect as the dopamine antagonists

Indications: gastroduodenal, hepatic and biliary disease. Its prokinetic effect on bowel peristalsis means that it is useful in ileus and pseudo-obstruction

Contraindications: prokinetic effect on the bowel means that it is contraindicated in bowel obstruction

Side effects: gastroduodenal ulcer and bleeding.

Special situations	Prokinetic effect on bowel
	Therefore contraindicated in bowel obstruction, perforation or bowel surgery within 4 days.
	Extrapyramidal effects, so cannot use in parkinsonism.

✓ DRUGS checklist for CYCLIZINE	
Dose	50 mg
Route	Oral – patient is vomiting
	IV – does the patient have IV access?
	IM – painful route
Units	mg
Given	Given as a bolus
	Maximum TDS (8 hourly)
Special situations	Antimuscarinic – therefore worsens urinary retention.
	Avoided in acute coronary syndrome (arrhythmic).

✓ DRUGS checklist for METOCLOPRAMIDE	
Dose	5–10 mg
Route	Oral – patient is vomiting
	IV – does the patient have IV access?
	IM – painful route
Units	mg
Given	If IV, give over 2 minutes
	Maximum TDS

✓ DRUGS checklist for ONDANSETRON	
Dose	4–8 mg
Route	Oral – patient is vomiting
	IV – does the patient have IV access?
	IM – painful route
Units	mg
Given	Maximum TDS (8 hourly)
Special situations	Prokinetic effect on the bowel means that it is contraindicated in bowel obstruction.

	Antihistamines	Dopamine antagonists	Prokinetics	5HT₃-receptor antagonists	Corticosteroids
Antihistamines		Can be combined but causes increased sedation, and hypoglycemia	Safe combination	Safe combination	Safe combination
Dopamine antagonists	Can be combined but causes increased sedation, and hypoglycemia		Increased extra-pyramidal effects	Safe combination	Safe combination
Prokinetics	Safe combination	Increased extra-pyramidal effects		Safe combination	Safe combination
5HT₃-receptor antagonists	Safe combination	Safe combination	Safe combination		Safe combination
Corticosteroids	Safe combination	Safe combination	Safe combination	Safe combination	

Figure 7.2 Effective and safe combinations of antiemetic classes.

Combining antiemetics

Certain classes of antiemetics can be used together to treat nausea and vomiting if a single agent is not effective alone. However, antiemetics from the same class (for example, cyclizine and promethazine) are not used together, and certain classes of antiemetic cannot be combined with others (Hasler and Chey, 2003). See Figure 7.2 for effective and safe combinations of antiemetic classes.

Case outcome and discharge

Mr Claude Mamet, who was admitted with small bowel obstruction secondary to intra-abdominal adhesions, was treated with antiemetics for nausea and vomiting. Given that the surgical pathology was a mechanical bowel obstruction, prokinetic antiemetics were avoided, as these can increase the risk of bowel perforation. Instead, the patient was treated with one antiemetic:

■ Cyclizine 50 mg QDS intravenous.

The small bowel obstruction was treated with 'suck and drip', in the form of an NG tube and intravenous fluid. He was treated conservatively for 24 hours during which his symptoms ameliorated. He passed flatus, followed by stool. He was discharged once he tolerated an oral diet after 3 days as an inpatient.

Common pitfalls

The most common pitfall in the prescription of antiemetic medication is failure to identify relative and absolute contraindications. Each class of antiemetic has actions that have the potential to cause harm (see Section Antiemetics: Essential Pharmacology). Knowledge of these pathways will prevent morbidity.

Another common pitfall is interaction between antiemetic classes. Two main interactions exist:

1. Dopamine antagonists and antihistamines: this causes sedation as well as hypoglycaemia.
2. Dopamine antagonists and prokinetics: this causes increased risk of extrapyramidal side effects, such as dystonias and oculogyric crises.

There are five main classes of antiemetics, some of which can be used in combination. However, important drug interactions exist when combining dopamine antagonists with prokinetics, or antihistamines. Adequate control of nausea and vomiting improves patient satisfaction and reduces the risk of patients requiring admission following day surgery.

SUMMARY

🔑 Key learning points

Antiemetics
- Nausea and vomiting is common, especially in the postoperative period.
- There are five commonly used classes of drugs which antagonise neurotransmitter receptors that are known to cause nausea and vomiting.
- Drug interactions exist between dopamine antagonists and prokinetics, and dopamine antagonists and antihistamines.

FURTHER READING

- Antiemetics in the context of PONV have been discussed in this chapter. However, further reading is recommended on the use of antiemetics in chemotherapy-induced nausea and vomiting: Hesketh PJ (2008). Chemotherapy-induced nausea and vomiting. *N Engl J Med* **358**: 2482.

Postoperative pain

Mr Rodrick Phelps

Age: 67

Hospital number: 123456

🔍 Case study

Presenting complaint: *A 67-year-old man attends the urology department for an elective prostatectomy.*

Background: *This patient is a retired diplomat who has had biopsy-proven prostate cancer. He has elected for a radical robotic-assisted prostatectomy. As the junior doctor, you will carry out a preoperative* clerking, *examination and tests. You will write a drug chart with his regular medications, as well as his postoperative pain medications.*

PMH: *Gout*

Allergies: *Cyclizine (causes confusion)*

FH: *Nil relevant*

Preoperative examination, observations and tests:
Pulse 90, BP 120/80, Sats 99% on air, RR 14, BM 5.9

CVS: *Capillary refill time 3 seconds, pulse regular, HS I + II + 0*

RS: *Equal expansion with air entry to both bases and no added sounds*

(Continued)

(🔍) Case study (*Continued*)

Abdo: Soft and non-tender

ECG: Sinus rhythm

Bloods: Hb 1, Plt 150, WCC 8.9, Na 136, K 4.3, Urea 9.0, Creat 100, INR 1.1, ALT 55, ALkP 110, alb 38, amylase 70

Regular medications: See form

PHARMACY STAMP	AGE 67	FORENAME, SURNAME
		Roderick Phelps
	D.O.B. 16/03/1947	ADDRESS Acacia Avenue
		NHS NUMBER

ALLOPURINOL 100 mg once daily.

SIGNATURE OF PRESCRIBER	DATE

SP21000

Diagnosis

Elective radical prostatectomy through robotic-assisted ports. Significant postoperative pain should be anticipated. He will require postoperative analgesia.

Initial measures

Pre-emptive analgesia should be been administered by the anaesthetist and/or surgeon.

Pre-emptive analgesia is the administration of analgesia at the induction of anaesthesia by the anaesthetist and/or infiltration of local anaesthetic into the incision during the operation by the surgeon. This reduces the patient's postoperative analgesic requirements.

On return from theatre a postoperative assessment should be carried out, usually by surgical registrar and/or anaesthetist.

The first postoperative assessment should involve looking at the surgeon's postoperative note and instructions, as well as circulatory and respiratory examination. The output of surgical drains should be examined. However, an assessment of the patient's pain is also important.

The magnitude and site of the operation will determine the anticipated postoperative pain, though there is variability between patients.

Abdominal, pelvic surgery and thoracic surgery causes pain that affects muscles of respiration. Patients in pain are at higher risk of developing lower respiratory tract infection due to basal atelectasis and an ineffective cough. Effective pain management allows patients to recruit collapsed alveoli, generate an effective cough to remove secretions, as well as comply with chest physiotherapy.

Prescribing for postoperative pain

The WHO developed the concept of a three-step analgesic ladder in pain management, which was originally developed in the context of palliative care, but is applicable to pain management in general. The first step is to prescribe simple non-opioid analgesia, namely paracetamol and NSAIDs. As pain severity increases, further analgesics are added. The second step is the addition of mild opioids, such as codeine preparations or tramadol. The third step is to add strong opioids, such as morphine preparations.

Step 1 (mild pain): a non-opioid, e.g. paracetamol, NSAIDs

Step 2 (moderate pain): weak opioid, e.g. codeine, tramadol

Step 3: (severe pain): strong opioid, e.g. morphine sulphate, oxycodone.

In postoperative patients, pain will be ongoing, persisting for several days, depending of the magnitude and location of the operation. Analgesia should therefore be prescribed *regularly*, such that there will be no lapse in their effect. 'Breakthrough pain' is a sudden increase in pain over and above the baseline pain expected following an operation. Breakthrough pain is often exacerbated by movement, voiding and passing stool. It is therefore recommended to have PRN analgesia for breakthrough pain, in the form of mild or strong opioids. These are prescribed on the 'when required' section of the drug chart, and the patient is informed that they need to ask for these if they expect or experience breakthrough pain. Nursing staff may also give the prescribed PRN analgesia prior to mobilising the patient.

REGULAR PRESCRIPTIONS

				Circle/enter times below ↓	Enter dates below			
					Day 1	Day 2	Day 3	Day 4
DRUG PARACETAMOL				06				
Dose 1g	Route PO/IV	Freq QDS	Start date 1/1/15	08				
				12				
Signature A. Doctor		Bleep	Review	16				
Additional instructions				18				
				22				

AS REQUIRED MEDICATION

DRUG CODEINE PHOSPHATE				Date	
				Time	
Dose 30–60 mg	Route PO	Timing PRN	Start date 1/1/15	Dose	
				Route	
Signature/Bleep A. Doctor		Max dose in 24 hrs QDS	Review	Given	
Additional instructions				Check	

DRUG ORAMORPH				Date	
				Time	
Dose 5–10 mg	Route PO	Timing PRN up to every 2 hours according to pain	Start date 1/1/15	Dose	
				Route	
Signature/Bleep A. Doctor		Max dose in 24 hrs	Review	Given	
Additional instructions				Check	

Paracetamol: rationale and evidence

Paracetamol is a non-opioid analgesic. It constitutes the first step of the analgesic ladder, along with NSAIDs. However, unlike NSAIDs, paracetamol has very few adverse effects at its therapeutic dose. Paracetamol is therefore commonly used in postoperative pain relief.

DRUGS checklist for PARACETAMOL

Dose	1 g
Route	PO or IV
Units	grams
Given	QDS (maximum daily dose 4 g in adults weighing >50 kg)
Special situations	Some analgesics already contain paracetamol and should not be taken with paracetamol as this would exceed the maximum dosage, e.g. co-codamol (containing paracetamol and codeine phosphate) and co-dydramol (paracetamol and dihydrocodeine).

Paracetamol may be given orally or intravenously. It is therefore possible to prescribe the IV route if the patient has postoperative nausea or vomiting. Furthermore, the IV route offers an advantage over the oral route because of its faster onset of action.

A Cochrane review concluded IV paracetamol reduces opioid consumption (see Evidence). This emphasises the importance of prescribing paracetamol as a background analgesic in combination with opioids. However, the reduction in opioid consumption does not appear to be sufficient to reduce opioid-induced side effects.

Evidence

IV paracetamol reduces opioid consumption postoperatively when combined with opioid analgesia. Patients required 30% less opioids over 4 hours compared to those receiving a placebo. However, this reduction in opioid consumption was not sufficient to reduce opioid-induced side effects (Tzortzopoulou *et al.*, 2011).

Paracetamol and NSAIDs: essential pharmacology

The mechanism of action of paracetamol, also known as acetaminophen, is not fully understood. However, there is evidence supporting paracetamol's action as a cyclooxygenase (COX) inhibitor (Greco et al., 2003). COX enzymes convert arachidonic acid into prostaglandins (Graham et al. 2013), and can be broadly categorised into two main groups: COX-1 and COX-2 (a COX-3 has also been described and is a variant of COX-1) (Lee et al., 2007). COX-1 is involved in the maintenance of the gastric mucosa. Its inhibition is therefore undesirable. COX-2 is involved in the production of prostanoids, which mediate an inflammatory response. NSAIDs like ibuprofen and aspirin are not selective between COX-1 and COX-2 (Patrgnani and Patrono, 2014), which is why unwanted gastric erosions and ulceration are possible adverse effects. Evidence indicates that paracetamol is likely to be act as a selective COX-2 inhibitor. It therefore selectively reduces inflammation, without the unwanted effect of gastric irritation.

Paracetamol also has clinically useful antipyretic actions – it helps to bring down a fever. Leukocytes produce pyrogens, which induce a fever by stimulating the secretion of prostaglandin E which then acts centrally on the anterior hypothalamus to increase body temperature. Paracetamol and NSAIDs therefore inhibit prostaglandin E.

Paracetamol is rapidly absorbed in the GI tract when administered orally. It is then metabolised by the liver. Metabolism of paracetamol in the liver involves three main pathways, namely glucuronidation, sulphation and finally by cytochrome P450, in which a toxic metabolite is produced, called *N*-acetyl-*p*-benzoquinoneimine (NAPQI) (Bessems and Vermeulen, 2001). NAPQI is responsible for the toxic effect of paracetamol. However, at doses used clinically (adult dose 1 g QDS) NAPQI is quickly detoxified. When paracetamol is taken in excess of the usual dose, toxicity does occur, resulting in acute hepatic failure. The antidote for paracetamol toxicity is acetylcysteine, which acts by replenishing hepatic

glutathione, and promoting the metabolism of NAPQI into non-toxic products.

Weak opioids – codeine preparations and tramadol: rationale and evidence

The addition of weak opioids to non-opioid analgesia provides adequate postoperative pain relief in the setting of day surgery (day surgery indicates that the patient is admitted on the day of a minor operation and is expected to be discharged on the same day).

Oral codeine preparations may contain paracetamol, and it is therefore important not to provide the patient with additional paracetamol. Table 7.3 lists common examples of oral codeine preparations that contain paracetamol, though many others exist.

Table 7.3 Examples of oral codeine preparations that contain paracetamol.

Co-codamol 8/500	Each tablet containing 8 mg codeine and 500 mg of paracetamol Adult dose is two tablets given QDS
Co-codamol 30/500	Each tablet containing 30 mg codeine and 500 mg of paracetamol Adult dose is two tablets given QDS
Co-dydramol 10/500	Each tablet containing 10 mg dihydrocodeine and 500 mg of paracetamol Adult dose is two tablets given QDS

✓ DRUGS checklist for CO-CODAMOL (combined codeine and paracetamol preparation)

Dose	2 tablets (30/500 strength)
Route	PO
Units	mg

Given	QDS
Special situations	Constipation may occur with any weak or strong opioid. In the context of surgery, it may be advisable to begin a pre-emptive laxative. Codeine is renally excreted, caution in renal dysfunction.

✓ DRUGS checklist for TRAMADOL

Dose	100 mg
Route	PO
Units	mg
Given	QDS
Special situations	10% of Caucasians have no analgesic benefit from tramadol due to genetic polymorphism of CYP2D6. Tramadol is renally excreted, but is commonly used in patients with renal dysfunction at a reduced dose (such as tramadol 50 mg PO, TDS).

Weak opioids – codeine and tramadol: essential pharmacology

Weak opioids act through similar pathways to strong opioids such as morphine. Weak opioids bind as agonists to μ-opioid receptors in the CNS resulting in analgesia and sedation. Likewise, respiratory depression may occur through the same pathway if used at higher doses. μ-opioid receptors are also present in the mesenteric plexus of the bowel. Weak opioids may cause reduced bowel transit time if used long term. This effect may be desirable or undesirable. For instance, codeine phosphate may be used in patients with chronic non-infective diarrhoea, high output stoma or short gut syndrome to avoid ongoing fluid and electrolyte loss from the GI tract.

Tramadol is metabolised by a member of the cytochrome p450 enzyme called CYP2D6, in the liver (Stamer *et al.*, 2003). Due to genetic polymorphisms, there is no CYP2D6 enzyme activity in 10% of the Caucasian population. This means that 1 in 10 Caucasians will have no significant analgesic effect from tramadol. Indeed, patients with reduced CYP2D6 activity require more breakthrough analgesia during the postoperative period. This should be considered in patients who do not appear to have adequate pain control with tramadol.

Ultimately, opioids (including tramadol) are excreted by the kidneys. Therefore caution should be used in renal impairment – the doses are reduced according the patient's estimated glomerular filtration rate (eGFR). Analgesia in renal impairment is explored in Chapter 10.

Strong opioids – morphine: rationale and evidence

Morphine is the first-line strong opioid of choice in patients without known allergy or significant renal impairment. Morphine is commonly used in cancer treatment and palliative care (see Chapter 9) and in low doses in acute heart failure due to its effect of preload (see Chapter 3).

Morphine comes in many preparations and can be a source of confusion for medical students and junior doctors. Commonly used morphine preparations are:

- **Oramorph** is an oral morphine liquid, which comes in varying strengths. Oramorph should not be prescribed in terms of millilitres (mL), because this depends of the concentration of the preparation. A commonly used concentration is 10 mg/5 mL. A prescription should be made in milligrams (mg) to avoid a dangerous drug error.
- **MST continus** is a long-acting oral preparation that is given every 12 hours (BD).
- **Morphine sulphate** is a preparation that is given intravenously.
- **Hydromorphone** is a morphine derivative that is mainly used in the IV route. Bioavailability of hydromorphone is low orally, but

is still occasionally used. Hydromorphone is particularly useful in patient with end-stage kidney disease (ESKD) because its active metabolite is effectively removed during haemodialysis. It is therefore safe to use in patients undergoing regular haemodialysis, but not in patients with eGFR <30 who have yet to begin haemodialysis.

Other strong opioid preparations are:

- **Oxycodone** is a semisynthetic strong oral opioid. Although it is more expensive than other morphine preparations, it has a more favourable side-effect profile (reduced nausea and vomiting). It is therefore favoured in patients who are intolerant to morphine. It comes in tablet form, as well as IV, IM and S/C. OxyNorm is the immediate release formulation, and OxyContin is the modified release preparation.
- **Fentanyl** is a synthetic opioid used in the IV and S/C routes in the postoperative period. It can be used as a transdermal patch for chronic pain. It is commonly used in patient with eGFR <30 as there is no significant accumulation.

✓	DRUGS checklist for ORAMORPH as an analgesic
Dose	Initial starting dose of immediate release oral morphine in an opioid-naïve patient is 2.5–5 mg
	For anticipatory prescribing at end of life, the starting dose is 2.5 mg SC
Route	Oral
Units	mg (avoid prescribing in mL)
Given	The initial oral dose is usually given 4-hourly, with the PRN dose equal to the 4-hourly dose
	For anticipatory end of life prescribing, the dose is when required, at a maximum of 1 hourly

Special situations	Constipation and nausea are common side effects. Signs of toxicity include increasing drowsiness, vivid dreams and hallucinations, pinpoint pupils and jerking (myoclonus). Dose reduction or other drugs should be used in renal impairment.

Strong opioids – morphine: essential pharmacology

Morphine binds to μ–δ-opioid receptors as an agonist, and thus mimics endogenous endorphins. The analgesic effect of morphine occurs primarily through μ-opioid receptors in the central nervous system resulting in analgesia, sedation and respiratory depression. The development of physical dependence also occurs through this pathway.

μ-opioid receptors are also present on the mesenteric plexus of the GI tract. Morphine acts by inhibiting gastric emptying, causing nausea and vomiting. Reduced peristalsis causes constipation. It is therefore important to provide a pre-emptive antiemetic for nausea and vomiting, and if required, laxatives.

When administered orally, peak plasma concentrations of morphine occur within an hour, with an analgesic effect lasting approximately 4 hours. This is the rationale for 4-hourly dosing.

Modified release oral preparations have a peak concentration within 2–6 hours, with an analgesic effect lasting 12–24 hours. Therefore, when dose requirements are uncertain or unstable, it is more appropriate to use immediate-release formulations. This dose can be switched to a modified-release preparation once analgesia requirements have been established and are at a steady state.

Drugs administered via parenteral routes do not undergo first-pass metabolism. As a result, the relative potency of different formulations vary. Doses must be adjusted accordingly when switching between one dose formulation and another. When converting from oral to subcutaneous morphine, the dose should be divided by 2 (so for example 10 mg oral morphine is equivalent to 5 mg SC morphine).

Patient-controlled analgesia (PCA): rationale and evidence

Patient-controlled analgesia (PCA) is a system that allows a patient to request as-required analgesia at the click of a button. An infusion pump will deliver a bolus of IV analgesia on demand. This allows patients to have greater influence over their pain management. Indeed meta-analyses indicated that patient satisfaction is higher with PCA compared to as-required intramuscular opioids (Ballantyne *et al.*, 1993). This has been attributed to a 'perceived control' over their analgesia, whereas in fact safety mechanisms will not give the patient full control of the delivery of opioid analgesia. To avoid overdose, the system will only provide a bolus within a predetermined time interval, known as the lockout time. Due to meta-analyses supporting the benefits of PCAs they have become a common form of postoperative analgesia, which junior doctors will have to be comfortable with.

A safe PCA prescription must include four main components:

1. Opioid of choice: this may be morphine sulphate, oxycodone or fentanyl.
2. Bolus dose: this is the dose of analgesia that will be delivered if the button is pressed. Common starting doses are:
   (a) morphine 1 mg IV bolus (Owen *et al.*, 1989)
   (b) fentanyl 40 microgram IV bolus (Camu *et al.*, 1998)
3. Lockout time: this is the time between delivery of one bolus and the delivery of another bolus. No bolus will be delivered within the lockout time in order to prevent repeated demands within a short period of time. A common lockout time used for morphine and fentanyl PCA is 5 minutes (Ginsberg *et al.*, 1995). A lockout time of 5 minutes will only allow the patient to receive successful boluses 5 minutes apart.
4. Maximum dosage: this is the maximum dose that the PCA will deliver over a defined period of time, e.g. 1 hour.

On the PCA pump, many models have a 'patient history' button, which will display the number of times the patient has demanded a dose relative to the number of successful deliveries. This allows you to determine whether the analgesic requirements are appropriate for the patient. However, there are other factors for apparent high demands from the patient, such as patient confusion, anxiety or intentional overuse.

Changing any of the four main components to a PCA prescription should be discussed with the anaesthetics or pain team.

PCA prescriptions are often put on a different part of the drug chart. Some hospitals have a sticker that is added to the drug chart given that there are more parameters to define, compared to other prescriptions.

An example of PCA prescription for morphine is shown.

ONCE ONLY PRESCRIPTIONS							Prescriber	
Date	Time to be given	DRUG	IV bolus dose	Route	Lockout time	Maximum dose	Signature	Bleep
xx/xx/xx	xx:xx	MORPHINE SULPHATE PCA	1 mg	IV	5 minutes	10 mg in 1 hour	A. Doctor	

Drug errors relating to the PCA can be classified into two sources: human error (81%) and equipment error (19%)(Schein *et al.*, 2009). Human errors are possible due to the complex process of setting up and programming the PCA. Equipment errors can be caused by infusion pump malfunction from fraying wires or from loss of the integrity of the drug cartridge.

Epidural analgesia: rationale and evidence

Epidural analgesia is initiated before anaesthetic induction by an anaesthetist and should not prescribed by foundation doctors. However, it is useful for junior doctors to be comfortable caring for patients with epidural analgesia postoperatively.

An epidural involves a continuous infusion of local anaesthetic into the epidural space via an epidural catheter. Occasionally, an opioid is also added to the infusion.

A common epidural infusion is 0.1% bupivacaine (long-acting local anaesthetic agent) with 2 mg/mL fentanyl, running at a rate of 16 mL per hour.

Epidural analgesia is used most commonly in abdominal surgery (such as laparotomy) and lower limb surgery.

A common complication of epidural analgesia is mild hypotension.

Case outcome and discharge

Rodrick Phelps underwent an uneventful robotic-assisted prostatectomy. Preoperatively he was prescribed:

- Paracetamol 1 g QDS regularly
- Tramadol 100 mg QDS regularly

He was discharged from theatre recovery with morphine sulphate patient-controlled analgesia (PCA): 1 mg with a 5-minute lockout. The PCA history indicated that patient requests roughly matched successful delivery. Mr Phelps liked to use the PCA prior to mobilising into the chair.

Postoperatively his pain was well controlled, though he had episodes of nausea with no vomiting. Antiemetics were given as required. On the second postoperative day, the PCA was removed. Oramorph 5 mg 4-hourly was started on the as-required section of the drug chart, which he used with decreasing frequency over 24 hours. He was discharged on the third postoperative day.

He was discharged with a prescription as shown.

DISCHARGE MEDICATION

Date	Medication	Dose	Route	Frequency	Supply	GP to continue?
xx/xx/xx	PARACETAMOL	1 g	PO	Four times daily (maximum 4 g in 24 hours)	7 days	N
xx/xx/xx	TRAMADOL	100 mg	PO	Four times daily	7 days	N
xx/xx/xx	LACTULOSE	15 mL	PO	Twice daily	7 days	N

Notes to patient/GP:

Common pitfalls

- Surgical patients with pain that is beyond the level expected for the operation may have a complication of the procedure. Whilst pain must be managed, the surgeon should be informed immediately.
- Remember that some codeine preparations also contain paracetamol.
- Patients who develop lower respiratory tract infection following abdominal, pelvic or thoracic operations may have ineffective pain relief.
- Remember to consider whether a patient has renal impairment when prescribing opioid analgesia. Adjust the choice and dose of analgesia appropriately.

SUMMARY

The magnitude and site of the operation will determine the anticipated postoperative pain, though there is variability between patients. For postoperative pain, the WHO analgesic ladder should be followed, with stepwise analgesic requirements starting with non-opioids, weak opioids and finally strong opioids.

Analgesia should be prescribed on the regular section of the drug chart, with the option of adding as-required analgesia for 'breakthrough pain'. Adequate pain management increases patient satisfaction and reduces the risk of postoperative complications such as lower respiratory tract infections. All weak and strong opioids are renal excreted. Their dose should therefore be determined by the patient's renal function and whether they are on dialysis or not. Patient-controlled analgesia is a common form of postoperative analgesia and requires clear instructions regarding: analgesic used, bolus dose, lockout time and maximum dose. Pain which is out with the expected magnitude indicate a surgical complication. Patients with pain which is difficult to control should be discussed with the pain team.

🔑 **Key learning points**

Postoperative pain
- The magnitude and site of the operation will determine the anticipated postoperative pain, though there is variability between patients.
- The WHO analgesic ladder should be followed, with stepwise analgesic requirements starting with non-opioids, weak opioids and finally strong opioids.
- Analgesia should be prescribed on the regular section of the drug chart, with the option of adding as-required analgesia for 'breakthrough pain'.
- Adequate pain management increase patient satisfaction and reduces the risk of postoperative complications such as lower respiratory tract infections.
- Patient-controlled analgesia is a common form of postoperative analgesia and requires clear instructions regarding: analgesic used, bolus dose, lockout time and maximum dose.
- Pain which is outwith the expected magnitude may indicate a surgical complication.
- Patients with pain that is difficult to control should be discussed with the pain team.

FURTHER READING

- To read more about postoperative pain, see the systematic review carried out by the Cochrane library on analgesia following surgery: Moore RA, Derry S, McQuay HJ *et al.* (2011). Single dose oral analgesics for acute postoperative pain in adults. *Cochrane Database Syst Rev* (9) CD008659.

Venous thromboprophylaxis

Ms Kathryn Greenwood

Age: 44

Hospital number: 123456

🔍 **Case study**

Presenting complaint: *A 44-year-old lady presents to the emergency department with severe epigastric pain.*

Background: *This patient is civil servant who is known to have alcohol dependency. The patient has had multiple episodes of acute pancreatitis in the past and has refused a referral to alcohol liaison services.*

PMH: *Acute pancreatitis secondary to alcohol excess.*

Allergies: *None*

FH: *Nil relevant*

Examination, observations and tests:
Pulse 110, BP 120/80, Sats 96% on 2 L oxygen, RR 14, BM 5.9

BMI: *24*

CVS: *Capillary refill time 3 seconds, pulse regular, HS I + II + 0*

RS: *Equal expansion with air entry to both bases and no added sounds*

Abdo: *Tender epigastrium with no involuntary guarding or peritonism*

ECG: *Sinus tachycardia, WCC 15, Na 136, K 3.3, Urea 9.0, Creat 100, INR 1.1, ALT 80, AlkP 120, GGT 200, alb 32, amylase 1400 USS abdomen: no free fluid. Common bile duct not dilated. Homogenous liver, no lesions. Pancreas obscured by dilated bowel loops*

CT abdomen and pelvis with contrast: acute inflammation of the pancreas with no signs of necrosis or pseudocyst

Regular medications: *Nil regular*

Diagnosis

Patient has acute pancreatitis secondary to alcohol excess. The patient is treated with supportive measures and an alcohol withdrawal regimen.

Initial measures

Virchow described a triad of factors that contribute to thrombosis: stasis, hypercoagulability of blood and endothelial injury.

Whilst in hospital, patients are at risk of thrombosis primarily through venous stasis and hypercoagulability. Immobilisation due to infirmity, pain or subconsciousness results in venous stasis. Inflammation, infection and the physiological stress of surgery puts patients in a hypercoagulable (Kahn *et al.*, 2012). Indeed, venous thromboembolism (VTE) is the second most common complication of inpatient treatment and carries a burden of significant cost to the service (Zhan and Miller, 2003). For these reasons all hospitalised patients are at risk of VTE. Despite this, VTE prophylaxis is under prescribed, leading to preventable morbidity and mortality (Zhan and Miller, 2003).

The initial measure is to carry out a VTE risk assessment for every patient being admitted into hospital, both electively or as an emergency. All hospitals make the VTE risk assessment available to doctors, and many place a visual cue on the drug chart. Patients require VTE assessment on admission and at 48 hours.

The aim of VTE risk assessment is to identify risks for a deep venous thrombosis and/or pulmonary embolus, as well as the risks of bleeding (Shojania *et al.*, 2001). A clinical judgment is made as to whether a patient is at greater risk of VTE than they are of bleeding (Heit *et al.*, 2000), in which case VTE prophylaxis is prescribed.

- Risks of VTE:
  - Age>60
  - Active cancer or receiving cancer treatment
  - Lower limb surgery
  - Dehydration
  - Immobilisation expected >3 days
  - Thrombophilia
  - Obesity
  - Personal history or first-degree family relative with history of DVT/PE
  - Hormone replacement therapy
  - Oral contraceptive pill (if containing oestrogen)
  - Acute surgical admission with inflammatory or intra-abdominal condition
  - Significant medical co-morbidity (cardiorespiratory disease, infection or inflammatory condition)
- Risks of bleeding:
  - Active bleeding
  - Acquired bleeding disorder such as acute liver failure
  - Untreated bleeding disorder
  - Current use of therapeutic-level anticoagulation (such as warfarin with INR >2.0)
  - Thrombocytopenia
  - Spinal or epidural anaesthesia within previous 4 hours or expected within 12 hours
  - Acute stroke (ischaemic or haemorrhagic)
  - Hypertensive crisis (systolic BP >230 mmHg).

Prescribing for venous thromboembolism prophylaxis

There are two main forms of VTE prophylaxis: mechanical and medical.

Mechanical VTE prophylaxis is with the use of thromboembolic deterrent stockings (TEDS), which are graduated compression socks or pneumatic compression stockings which intermittently inflate in order to improve venous return from the lower limbs. Pneumatic compression stockings are primarily used intraoperatively or following lower limb orthopaedic surgery.

TEDS are one of the few medical devices that *are* expected to be prescribed on the drug chart. Although not defined on the prescription, TEDS must be appropriately sized according to the patient's calf diameter. They come in two lengths: knee length and thigh length; the former is most commonly used. There are contraindication to TEDS:

- Peripheral vascular disease: acute or chronic limb ischaemia is exacerbated by TEDS. Indeed, patients with ankle–brachial pulse index (ABPI) of <0.9 should not be given TEDS.
- Recent skin graft or flap: the delicate blood supply to a recent skin graft or flap will be compromised by TEDS.
- Evidence of dermatitis or allergy
- Open wounds.

Medical VTE prophylaxis is the use of heparin preparations for VTE prevention, at a dose that is lower than that needed for full anticoagulation. Therapeutic doses of heparin are based on a patient's weight, whereas prophylactic doses are standardised for all adults. A number of different agents can be used, and this depends on the trust guidelines. A careful assessment must be made prior to prescribing these, as the benefits of preventing potential VTE must outweigh the bleeding risks associated with these agents. VTE prophylactic injections are generally given at 18.00 by convention, as this standardises practice across the hospital and helps prevent it being missed.

REGULAR PRESCRIPTIONS									
				Circle/enter times below ↓	⊠ Enter dates below				
					Day 1	Day 2	Day 3	Day 4	
DRUG TED stockings				06					
				08					
Dose 1 pair	Route TOP on both legs	Freq OD	Start date 1/1/15	12					
Signature A. Doctor		Bleep	Review	16					
Additional instructions				18					
				22					
DRUG TINZAPARIN				06					
				08					
Dose 3500 units	Route SC	Freq OD	Start date 1/1/15	12					
Signature A. Doctor		Bleep	Review	16					
Additional instructions				⑱					
				22					

Graduated compression stockings: rationale and evidence

TEDS work by providing many graduated compression to the venous system of the lower limb. In doing so, they reduce venous stasis, which is one of the three triggers of thrombosis. They are a popular form of VTE prophylaxis as they have few contraindications, few adverse effects and are inexpensive.

✓ DRUGS checklist for TED stockings

Dose	1
Route	Worn medical device
Units	pair
Given	Throughout inpatient stay
Special situations	Contraindicated in peripheral vascular disease (ABPI <0.9), skin graft or flap, allergy, wounds.

🔍 Evidence

Graduated compression stockings are effective in reducing the risk of DVT, especially when combined with another form of VTE prophylaxis (Sachdeva et al., 2010).

Heparin and pentasaccharide preparations for VTE prophylaxis: rationale and evidence

There are three main heparin preparations used in VTE prophylaxis. These are:

1. Low-molecular weight heparin (LMWH) – used for the majority of cases, in patients who have an eGFR of greater than 30. The most commonly used LMWHs are:
   (a) Tinzaparin
   (b) Enoxaparin (trade name Clexane)
   (c) Dalteparin (trade name Fragmin)
   (d) Others LMWH preparations exist but are not commonly used in the UK for VTE prophylaxis.
2. Unfractionated heparin – used mainly in patients with acute or chronic renal dysfunction with an eGFR <30. However, for VTE prophylaxis the preferred route is *subcutaneous bolus*, rather than intravenous.
3. Synthetic pentasaccharide – the most commonly use is fondaparinux. Whilst pentasaccharides are mainly being used in acute coronary syndrome, these may also be used at a lower dose in VTE prophylaxis.

The choice of LMWH preparation is usually made by the hospital or trust. Therefore, before prescribing LMWH always check which preparation is used. Currently, there is little evidence supporting one LMWH preparation over another (Kahn *et al.*, 2013).

Patients who are already being treated with anticoagulants such as heparin, warfarin, dabigatran or rivaroxaban at a *therapeutic* level should not have further medical VTE prophylaxis.

✓ DRUGS checklist for TINZAPARIN (in VTE prophylaxis only)	
Dose	3500 units
Route	Subcutaneous
Units	units
Given	Daily injection, throughout inpatient stay
Special situations	Given once VTE/bleeding risk assessment performed. Should not be used if eGFR <30. If eGFR <30, give unfractionated heparin 5000 units SC BD instead.

✓ DRUGS checklist for ENOXAPARIN (in VTE prophylaxis only)	
Dose	20–40 mg
Route	Subcutaneous
Units	mg
Given	Daily injection, throughout inpatient stay
Special situations	Given once VTE/bleeding risk assessment performed. If eGFR <30, give unfractionated heparin 5000 units SC BD instead. Alternatively reduce dose and monitor factor Xa levels.

✓ DRUGS checklist for DALTEPARIN (in VTE prophylaxis only)	
Dose	5000 units
Route	Subcutaneous
Units	units
Given	Daily injection, throughout inpatient stay
Special situations	Given once VTE/bleeding risk assessment performed. If eGFR <30, give unfractionated heparin 5000 units SC BD instead. Alternatively reduce dose and monitor factor Xa levels.

Common patient safety issues that arise when prescribing medical VTE prophylaxis are:

- Lack of VTE prophylaxis prescribed in a patient who goes on to develop a DVT or PE.
- Incorrect dosage of heparin preparation (such as prescribing LMWH at *therapeutic* dose, rather than *prophylactic* dose).
- Prescribing VTE prophylaxis when it is contraindicated, such as active bleeding.
- Neglecting to stop the heparin preparation once a patient has developed active bleeding.
- Neglecting to change LMWH to unfractionated heparin (subcutaneous) once a patient's eGFR has fallen to less than 30.
- Neglecting a identify heparin-induced thrombocytopenia (HIT), which is an uncommon adverse event of heparin.

Patients admitted into hospital for an acute illness have an eightfold increase in VTE risk (Kahn *et al.*, 2013). There is high-quality evidence in the form of meta-analyses indicating that medical prophylaxis with LMWH, low-dose unfractionated heparin or fondaparinux is associated with a reduction in symptomatic DVT and in fatal pulmonary embolus. VTE risk assessment in all patients, and prescription of mechanical and medical VTE prophylaxis, where not contraindicated, is supported by the NICE guidelines (see Guideline).

Heparin and pentasaccharide preparations for VTE prophylaxis: essential pharmacology

Heparin is an indirect thrombin inhibitor. It binds with antithrombin, and together they inactivate thrombin, clotting factor Xa and to a lesser extent clotting factors XIIa, XIa and IXa (Hirsh *et al.*, 2008). It therefore inhibits the clotting cascade and prevents thrombus formation.

Five percent of patients exposed to heparin develop heparin-induced thrombocytopenia (HIT), which results in a fall in platelet concentration. This complication occurs regardless of the dose or route of administration. It is therefore important to monitor platelet concentration in patients on heparin (Coutre, 2015).

Fondaparinux is a synthetic pentasaccharide, which is used as a heparin-like medication. Like heparin, fondaparinux binds to antithrombin, which results in the inactivation of clotting factor Xa. Fondaparinux is therefore effective as an anticoagulant (Nijkeuter and Huisman, 2004).

Other forms of VTE prophylaxis

In orthopaedic surgery, there are other agents that are commonly used for VTE prophylaxis. Elective hip and knee replacement, and hip fracture, have been identified as high risk for VTE events. This is due to the immobilisation of the lower limb and hypercoagulability of blood postoperatively. Currently, there are two anticoagulants that are in favour following elective orthopaedic surgery:

1. Dabigatran – started 1–4 hours following surgery and may continue to up to 1 month postoperatively whilst in the community. Dabigatran is an oral anticoagulant, which acts as a direct thrombin inhibitor. An initial dose of 110 mg is started within 4 hours of surgery, then increased to 220 mg 12–24 hours later, given once a day. The dose is reduced to 150 mg in patients on amiodarone or verapamil.
2. Rivaroxaban – started 6–10 hours postsurgery. Rivaroxaban is an oral anticoagulant, which acts as a direct factor Xa inhibitor. The dose of rivaroxaban is 10 mg once daily (starting 6–10 hours after surgery). The duration of treatment is dependent on the type of surgery but may continue for between 2 and 5 weeks postsurgery.

Case outcome and discharge

Kathryn Greenwood was diagnosed with acute pancreatitis secondary to alcohol excess. Her risks of VTE and bleeding were assessed on admission and at 48 hours. The VTE risk assessment was documented in the patient's notes.

This patient's VTE risks included acute surgical/inflammatory condition and dehydration. The patient did not have any identified bleeding risks. The patient received TEDS, and tinzaparin 3500 units daily SC injection.

The patient was discharged after 4 days in hospital, with no further VTE prophylaxis. The patient will be followed up in the alcohol clinic and the general surgery clinic.

Common pitfalls

- All patients being admitted into hospital require VTE risk assessment. Day surgery and day procedures are often forgotten about.
- TEDS can do harm in certain patients; be aware of their contraindications.
- Patients with not apparent bleeding risks will be started on medical VTE prophylaxis. However, do not forget to stop anticoagulants in the event of significant bleeding.
- Medical VTE prophylaxis with LMWH, unfractionated heparin and pentasaccharides is at a lower dose (prophylactic dose) relative to therapeutic anticoagulation.

SUMMARY

Venous thromboembolism is a common and preventable cause of morbidity and mortality. All inpatients should be assessed for VTE risk factors. TEDS provide an inexpensive form of VTE prophylaxis with few contraindications. However, TEDS are best used in combination with medical VTE prophylaxis in the form of with LMWH, unfractionated heparin and pentasaccharides, depending on your hospital's preference.

🔑 Key learning points

Venous thromboembolism

- Venous thromboembolism is a common and preventable cause of morbidity and mortality.
- All inpatients should be assessed for VTE risk factors. TEDS provide an inexpensive form of VTE prophylaxis with few contraindications.
- TEDS are best used in combination with medical VTE prophylaxis in the form of with LMWH, unfractionated heparin and pentasaccharides, depending on your hospital's preference.

Constipation

> **Mr Ron Fergusson**
> **Age: 79**
> **Hospital number: 123456**

🔍 Case study

Presenting complaint: *A 79-year-old man presents to the colorectal clinic with constipation. The patient usually passes stool once every 2 days, but has recently been troubled by hard stools.*

Background: *This patient is a retired physician and is otherwise fit and well. His GP has referred him to the colorectal clinic as he has a family history of colorectal cancer*

PMH: *Nil*

Regular medications: *Nil regular*

Allergies: *None*

FH: *Father and brother both had colorectal cancer.*

Examination, observations and tests:
BMI: *24*

CVS: *Capillary refill time 3 seconds, pulse regular, HS I + II + 0 .*

RS: *Equal expansion with air entry to both bases and no added sounds*

Abdo: *Soft and non-tender. No masses or organomegaly*

Per rectal examination: *hard stool in rectum*

Rigid sigmoidoscopy: *No masses, examined to 15 cm*

Colonoscopy is arranged to rule out colorectal cancer: no mucosal lesions found.

Diagnosis
Likely idiopathic constipation.

Initial measures
The initial measure in adults with constipation is to investigate for secondary aetiologies. Common causes of chronic constipation are listed in the Box Common Causes Of Chronic Constipation.

General practitioners will also refer patients to the colorectal clinic with a change in bowel habit (constipation or diarrhoea).

Red flag features for colorectal cancer are:

- Change in bowel habit for more than 6 weeks
- Rectal bleeding if aged >40
- Iron-deficiency anaemia in men or postmenopausal women
- Rectal mass on per rectal examination.

The gold standard investigation is colonoscopy, although CT colonogram is an alternative for patients who are frail or immobile.

The cause of the chronic constipation should be treated if possible. For instance, treatment of hypothyroidism may reverse the chronic constipation. However, laxatives can be used to alleviate constipation.

The term 'absolute constipation' refers to the inability to pass stool or flatus, which occurs in bowel obstruction. This should be treated as a separate entity.

Common causes of chronic constipation.

- Medications
  - Opioids
  - Anticholinergics e.g. antihistamines, antispasmodics, antidepressants, antipsychotics
  - Iron supplements
  - Antacids
  - Calcium channel blockers
- Neurogenic disorders
  - Intestinal pseudo-obstruction
  - Hirschsprung's disease
  - Autonomic neuropathies e.g. diabetes mellitus
  - Multiple sclerosis
  - Parkinson's disease
- Non-neurogenic disorders
  - Pregnancy
  - Myotonic dystrophy
  - Hypokalaemia
  - Hypothyroidism
- Idiopathic constipation
  - Normal colonic transit constipation
  - Slow transit constipation

Prescribing for constipation

The choice of laxative very much depends on cause of constipation and therefore desired mechanism of action, patient preference, what they have already tried and severity of symptoms. Laxatives can be combined to give an initial effect, then decreased as required. Please also see Chapter 5, Section Constipation.

REGULAR PRESCRIPTIONS					Circle/enter times below ↓	↘ Enter dates below			
						Day 1	Day 2	Day 3	Day 4
DRUG MOVICOL					06				
Dose 1 sachet	Route PO	Freq OD	Start date 16/1/15		08				
					✗ 1300				
Signature A. Doctor		Bleep	Review		16				
Additional instructions					18				
					22				
DRUG SENNA					06				
Dose 15 mg	Route PO	Freq ON	Start date 16/1/15		08				
					12				
Signature A. Doctor		Bleep	Review		16				
Additional instructions					⑱				
					22				

Laxatives: rationale and evidence

Broadly speaking, there are four groups of laxatives (Tramonte *et al.*, 1997):

1. Softeners (surfactants): sodium docusate
2. Osmotic agents: lactulose, Movicol (polyethylene glycol) glycerine suppository, magnesium sulfate and magnesium citrate
3. Stimulants : senna, bisacodyl, sodium picosulfate
4. Bulk-forming laxatives: methylcellulose, Ispaghula Husk.

The choice of which laxative to use is based on patient preference, ease of use and cost. There are no adverse interactions between the four groups, with the exception of diarrhoea if over used (Ramkumar and Rao, 2005).

There is little evidence supporting the use of softener laxatives. Whilst they have few side effects, their efficacy is also low. A systematic review indicated that stool softeners are less effective than bulk laxatives (American College of Gastroenterology Chronic Constipation Task Force, 2005).

The efficacy of sodium picosulfate, a stimulant laxative, was investigated in a randomised control trial, compared to placebo (Mueller-Lissner *et al.*, 2010). Fifty-one percent of patients receiving sodium picosulfate reached a mean number of at least three complete spontaneous bowel movements per week. This was significantly more than the placebo ($P <0.0001$). There were also reported improvements in quality of life.

✓ DRUGS checklist for SODIUM DOCUSATE

Dose	200 mg
Route	Oral
Units	mg
Given	BD
Special situations	None

✓ DRUGS checklist for LACTULOSE

Dose	10–20 mL
Route	Oral
Units	mL
Given	BD
Special situations	Lactulose is used as the laxative of choice in those with hepatic encephalopathy as it aids removal of ammonia, which helps with this condition.

✓ DRUGS checklist for SENNA

Dose	2–4 tablets (1 tablet = 7.5 mg)
Route	Oral
Units	Tablets
Given	Usually at night
Special situations	Stimulant laxatives are contraindicated in mechanical bowel obstruction. Stimulating peristalsis in bowel obstruction increases the risk of bowel perforation.

✓ DRUGS checklist for GLYCERINE suppository

Dose	1–2 suppositories
Route	Per rectum (PR)
Units	As individual suppositories
Given	Up to four daily
Special situations	None

Laxatives: essential pharmacology

Softeners (surfactants): These act by decreasing the surface tension of stool, thus allowing water to rehydrate the stool. Softeners are well tolerated and have few side effects.

Osmotic agents: These act by stimulating intestinal water secretion, and increase stool frequency. Excessive use of osmotic laxatives can result in electrolyte or fluid disturbances, especially in patients with renal or cardiac dysfunction. Lactulose is a synthetic disaccharide, which exerts high osmotic pressure within the bowel lumen, thus drawing water into he bowel lumen. Glycerine suppositories exert the osmotic pressure within the rectum where faecal impaction is common. Side effects of osmotic agents include abdominal bloating, nausea and cramping. Caution in renal failure.

Prokinetics: These act by increasing the motor activity of the bowel. Stimulating peristalsis therefore promotes the transit of stool. Stimulant laxatives are contraindicated in mechanical bowel obstruction. Stimulating peristalsis in bowel obstruction increases the risk of bowel perforation. Senna can cause a benign pigmentation of the bowel, called melanosis coli.

Bulk forming laxatives: These are polysaccharides or cellulose derivative, which promote the absorption of water into the stool and thus hydrating and softening the stool. Side effects include increased flatulence and bloating. Trade names include Ispaghula Husk.

Other medications used in constipation

Normal bowel function is dependent on a healthy and balanced diet. This advice should be delivered to patients. Food diaries may be used to highlight unhealthy behaviours. Referral to nutritionist is of great benefit in the education of patients.

Severe and long-term constipation can be treated, in rare cases, with surgery. Colectomy with end ileostomy is the final treatment in cases of severe long-term constipation, when all medical treatment options have been exhausted (Wofford and Verne, 2000).

Further aspects of constipation management

Strong laxatives are needed for bowel preparation prior to some colonic surgery or colonoscopy procedures. For details on how to prescribe bowel preparation see detailed constipation of the gastroenterology chapter.

Case outcome and discharge

Ron Fergusson was seen in the colorectal clinic with constipation. Due to his age, and alteration in bowel habit, he underwent a colonoscopy. This was normal to the point of insertion. He was diagnosed with idiopathic constipation.

Initial advice was given to the patient. This included encouraging oral fluid and fibre intake. Due to patient preference, lactulose was started (15 mL BD oral). This took over 48 hours to improve stool consistency. He was discharged from follow-up.

DISCHARGE MEDICATION						
Date	Medication	Dose	Route	Frequency	Supply	GP to continue?
xx/xx/xx	LACTULOSE	15 mL	PO	Twice daily	7 days	N
Notes to patient/GP:						

Common pitfalls

- Consider medications that cause constipation, and start laxatives prophylactically.
- Consider the easily reversible causes of constipation before starting laxatives.
- Most laxative take up to 48 hours to work, so be patient.
- Altered bowel habit should be investigated in older patients, as colorectal cancer is a cause.

SUMMARY

- Constipation is a common complain for patients in and out of the hospital. It is important to differentiate between constipation and other causes of difficulty in passing stool.
- An array of laxatives exist; however, there is only weak evidence supporting a hierarchy of their use. Current use of laxatives is dependent on physician and patient preference. Caution should be used in patients with acute and chronic renal failure, as fluid loss from the stool can exacerbate renal dysfunction. It is important to understand that laxatives can take up to 48 hours to work.

🔑 Key learning points

Laxatives
- There are four types of laxative: softeners, prokinetics, bulk forming and osmotic laxatives.
- The choice of oral laxative is based on patient and physician preference.

FURTHER READING

- Please see Chapter 5, Section Constipation in this text.
- Tramonte SM, Brand MB, Mulrow CD *et al.* (1997). The treatment of chronic constipation in adults. A systematic review. J Gen Intern 12: 15.

Now visit **www.wileyessential.com/pharmacology** to test yourself on this chapter.

References

American College of Gastroenterology Chronic Constipation Task Force (2005). An evidence-based approach to the management of chronic constipation in North America. *Am J Gastroenterol* 100: S1.

Apfel CC, Korttila K, Abdalla M *et al.* (2004). A factorial trial of six interventions for the prevention of postoperative nausea and vomiting. *N Engl J Med* 350: 2441.

Ballantyne JC, Carr DB, Chalmers TC *et al.* (1993). Postoperative patient-controlled analgesia: meta-analyses of initial randomized control trials. *J Clin Anesth* 5: 182–9.

Bessems JG, Vermeulen NP (2001). Paracetamol (acetaminophen)-induced toxicity: molecular and biochemical mechanisms, analogues and protective approaches. *Crit Rev Toxicol* 31: 55.

Camu F, Van Aken H, Bovill JG (1998). Postoperative analgesic effects of three demand-dose sizes of fentanyl administered by patient-controlled analgesia. *Anesth Analg* 87: 890–5.

Chapagain A, Ashman N (2012). Hyperkalaemia in the age of aldosterone antagonism. *QJM* 105: 1049–57.

Collins JA (1974). Problems associated with the massive transfusion of stored blood. *Surgery* 75: 274.

Coutre S (2015). Management of heparin-induced thrombocytopenia. In: LeungLL (ed). *UpToDate*, Wolters Kluwer: Waltham, MA.

Dellinger RP, Levy MM, Carlet JM *et al.* (2008). Surviving Sepsis Campaign: international guidelines for management of severe sepsis and septic shock. *Crit Care Med* 36: 296–327.

Egerton-Warburton D, Meek R, Mee MJ *et al.* (2014). antiemetic use for nausea and vomiting in adult emergency department patients: randomized controlled trial comparing ondansetron, metoclopramide, and placebo. *Ann Emerg Med* 64: 526–32.

Ginsberg B, Gil KM, Muir M *et al.* (1995). The influence of lockout intervals and drug selection on patient-controlled analgesia following gynecological surgery. *Pain* 62: 95–100.

Graham GG, Davies MJ, Day RO *et al.* (2013). The modern pharmacology of paracetamol: therapeutic actions, mechanism of action, metabolism, toxicity and recent pharmacological findings. *Inflammopharmacology* 21: 201–32.

Greco A, Ajmone-Cat MA, Nicolini A *et al.* (2003). Paracetamol effectively reduces prostaglandin E2 synthesis in brain macrophages by inhibiting enzymatic activity of cyclooxygenase but not phospholipase and prostaglandin E synthase. *J Neurosci* 71: 844–52.

Hasler WL, Chey WD (2003). Nausea and vomiting. *Gastroenterology* 125: 1860–7.

Heit JA, Silverstein MD, Mohr DN *et al.* (2000). Risk factors for deep vein thrombosis and pulmonary embolism: a population-based case-control study. *Arch Intern Med* 160: 809–15.

Hesketh PJ (2008). Chemotherapy-induced nausea and vomiting. *N Engl J Med* 358: 2482–94.

Hirsh J, Bauer KA, Donati MB *et al.* (2008). Parenteral anticoagulants: American College of Chest Physicians Evidence-Based Clinical Practice Guidelines, 8th edn. *Chest* 133: 141S.

Kahn SR, Lim W, Dunn AS *et al.*; American College of Chest Physicians (2012). Prevention of VTE in nonsurgical patients: antithrombotic therapy and prevention of thrombosis, 9th edn: American College of Chest Physicians Evidence-Based Clinical Practice Guidelines. *Chest* 141 (2 Suppl.): e195S–226S

Kahn SR, Morrison DR, Cohen JM *et al.* (2013) Interventions for implementation of thromboprophylaxis in hospitalized medical and surgical patients at risk for venous thromboembolism. *Cochrane Database System Rev* (7) CD008201.

Kumpel BM (2002). On the mechanism of tolerance to the Rh D antigen mediated by passive anti-D (Rh D prophylaxis). *Immunol Lett* 82: 67–73.

Lee YS, Kim H, Brahim JS *et al.* (2007). Acetaminophen selectively suppresses peripheral prostaglandin E2 release and increases COX-2 gene expression in a clinical model of acute inflammation. *Pain* 129: 279–86.

Medicines and Healthcare products Regulatory Agency (MHRA) (2012). *Direct Healthcare Professional Communication on ondansetron (Zofran and generics) and dose-dependent QT interval prolongation – new dose restriction for intravenous (IV) use.* Available at: www.mhra.gov.uk/home/groups/comms-ic/documents/websiteresources/con183919.pdf (accessed Dec. 2015).

Metz A, Hebbard G (2007). Nausea and vomiting in adults–a diagnostic approach. *Aust Fam Physician* 36: 688–92.

Mueller-Lissner S, Kamm MA, Wald A *et al.* (2010). Multicenter, 4-week, double-blind, randomized, placebo-controlled trial of sodium picosulfate in patients with chronic constipation. *Am J Gastroenterol* 105: 897–903.

National Institute for Health and Clinical Excellence (NICE) (2013). Intravenous fluid therapy in over 16s in hospital, CG174. Available at: www.nice.org.uk/guidance/cg174 (accessed 30 Jan. 2015).

National Patient Safety Agency (2007). *Reducing the Risk of Hyponatraemia when Administering Intravenous Infusions to Children, Alert 22.* National Patient Safety Agency.

Nijkeuter M, Huisman MV (2004). Pentasaccharides in the prophylaxis and treatment of venous thromboembolism: a systematic review. *Curr Opin Pulm Med* 10: 338–44.

Owen H, Plummer JL, Armstrong I *et al.* (1989). Variables of patient-controlled analgesia. 1. Bolus size. *Anaesthesia* 44: 7–10.

Paice B, Gray JM, McBride D *et al.* (1983). Hyperkalaemia in patients in hospital. *Br Med J (Clin Res Ed)* 286: 1189–92.

Patrignani P, Patrono C (2014). Cyclooxygenase inhibitors: From pharmacology to clinical read-outs. *Biochim Biophys Acta* 1851: 422–32.

Perel P, Roberts I (2013). Colloids versus crystalloids for fluid resuscitation in critically ill patients. *Cochrane Database Syst Rev* (6): CD000567.

Ramkumar D, Rao SS (2005). Efficacy and safety of traditional medical therapies for chronic constipation: systematic review. *Am J Gastroenterol* 100: 936–71.

Roback JD, Grossman BJ, Harris T *et al.* (2011). *AABB Technical Manual*, 17th edn. American Association of Blood Banks Press: Bethesda, MD.

Rose BD, Post TW (2001). *Clinical Physiology of Acid-Base and Electrolyte Disorders*, 5th edn, McGraw-Hill: New York: 285.

Sachdeva A, Dalton M, Amaragiri SV *et al.* (2010). Elastic compression stockings for the prevention of deep venous thrombosis. *Cochrane Database of Systematic Reviews* (7): CD001484a.

Schein JR, Hicks RW, Nelson WW *et al.* (2009). Patient-controlled analgesia-related medication errors in the postoperative period: causes and prevention. *Drug Safety* 32: 549–59.

Scorza K, Williams A, Phillips JD *et al.* (2007). Evaluation of nausea and vomiting. *Am Fam Physician* 76: 76–84.

Shojania KG, Duncan BW, McDonald KM *et al.* (2001). Making health care safer: a critical analysis of patient safety practices. *Evid Rep Technol Assess (Summ).* (43): i–x, 1–668.

Silvergleid AJ (2015). Clinical use of plasma components. In: KleinmanS (ed). *UpToDate.* Wolters Kluwer: Waltham, MA.

Simon GE, Bove JR (1971). The potassium load from blood transfusion. *Postgrad Med* 49: 61.

Slichter SJ (2007). Platelet transfusion therapy. *Hematol Oncol Clin North Am* 21: 697.

Stainsby D, Russell J, Cohen H *et al.* (2005). Reducing adverse events in blood transfusion. *Br J Haematol* 131: 8–12.

Stamer UM, Lehnen K, Höthker F *et al.* (2003). Impact of CYP2D6 genotype on postoperative tramadol analgesia. *Pain* 105: 231–8.

Sterns RH (2014). Maintenance and replacement fluid therapy in adults. In: Emmett M (ed). *UpToDate.* Wolters Kluwer: Waltham, MA.

Tramonte SM, Brand MB, Mulrow CD *et al.* (1997). The treatment of chronic constipation in adults. A systematic review. *J Gen Intern Med* 12: 15.

Tzortzopoulou A, McNicol ED, Cepeda MS *et al.* (2011). Single dose intravenous propacetamol or intravenous paracetamol for postoperative pain. *Cochrane Database Syst Rev* (10): CD007126.

Wofford SA, Verne GN (2000). Approach to patients with refractory constipation. *Curr Gastroenterol Rep* 2: 389.

Zhan C, Miller MR (2003). Excess length of stay, charges, and mortality attributable to medical injuries during hospitalization. *JAMA* 290: 1868–74.

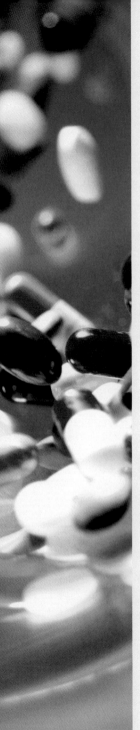

CHAPTER 8

Care of the Elderly

Amy Hawkins

Key topics:

Learning objectives

By the end of this chapter, you should be able to…

- …write prescriptions for elderly patients with osteoporosis, delirium, falls and hyponatraemia, taking into account relevant cautions, contraindications and side effects.

- …discuss the implications of polypharmacy amongst the elderly, and carry out medicines reconciliation.

- …evaluate the key drugs used in the management of the above conditions.

- …discuss the mechanisms of action of the drugs used to treat these conditions.

Essential Practical Prescribing, First Edition. Georgia Woodfield, Benedict Lyle Phillips, Victoria Taylor, Amy Hawkins and Andrew Stanton. © 2016 by John Wiley & Sons, Ltd. Published 2016 by John Wiley & Sons, Ltd.

Bone protection

> **Elizabeth Rowley**
>
> **Age: 80**
>
> **Hospital number: 123456**

🔍 Case study

Presenting complaint: *An 80-year-old woman is admitted with a left-sided fractured neck of femur following a low-impact fall. She has a dynamic hip screw and recovers well postoperatively. She is awaiting a package of care on the ward prior to discharge.*

Background: *She lives with her elderly husband but is normally independent in her activities of daily living. She is an ex-smoker with a 20 pack year smoking history.*

PMH: *Hypertension; hypothyroidism; no previous fractures*

Allergies: *Penicillin – rash*

Examination: *Pulse 80, Sats 97% on air, RR 12*

CVS: *Capillary refill time <2 seconds, pulse regular, no pitting oedema, HS I + II + 0*

RS: *Equal expansion with air entry to both bases and no added sounds*

Abdo: *Soft and non-tender, no masses, bowel sounds present*

MSK: *Well-healing scar left hip*

Diagnosis

Osteoporotic fracture. This patient has sustained a fracture following a low-impact fall.

Initial measures

In women aged 75 years and over, NICE guidelines suggest that a dual energy X-ray absorptiometry (DEXA) scan may not be required. Treatment in this case can be commenced on the presumption of an osteoporotic fracture.

PHARMACY STAMP	AGE 80	FORENAME, SURNAME Elizabeth Rowley
	D.O.B. xx/xx/xxxx	ADDRESS 56 Blythwood Road NHS NUMBER

LEVOTHYROXINE 125 micrograms once daily.

RAMIPRIL 5 mg once daily.

SIGNATURE OF PRESCRIBER   DATE

SP21000

Prescribing for osteoporosis

REGULAR PRESCRIPTIONS

	Circle/enter times below ↓	Day 1	Day 2	Day 3	Day 4
DRUG CALCICHEW-D3 FORTE ®	06				
	⑧				
Dose 1 tablet / Route PO / Freq BD / Start date xx/xx/xx	12				
Signature A. Doctor / Bleep / Review	16				
	⑱				
Additional instructions	22				
DRUG ALENDRONIC ACID	06				
	08				
Dose 70 mg / Route PO / Freq Once weekly (Tuesdays) / Start date xx/xx/xx	12				
Signature A. Doctor / Bleep / Review	16				
	18				
Additional instructions	22				

Calcium and vitamin D: rationale and evidence

The initial priority for all patients with osteoporotic fractures is commencement of calcium and vitamin D supplements. Calcium and vitamin D supplements have been shown to prevent hip fractures in elderly, housebound patients (Moyer, 2013; Prentice *et al.*, 2013).

🔍 Evidence

Calcium and vitamin D supplements and cardiovascular risk

A 7-year randomised, placebo-controlled study investigated the association between calcium and vitamin D supplementation and cardiovascular events. In meta-analyses of three randomised controlled trials, calcium and vitamin D supplementation increased the risk of myocardial infarction (relative risk 1.21) and stroke (relative risk 1.20) (Bolland *et al.*, 2011).

✓ DRUGS checklist for CALCICHEW-D3 FORTE®

Dose	One tablet
Route	Oral
Units	Tablets
Given	Twice daily
Special situations	There are a number of calcium and cholecalciferol preparations available.

Calcium and vitamin D: essential pharmacology

Vitamin D is a fat-soluble vitamin which undergoes hydroxylation twice within the body in order to be converted to activated vitamin D. 1,15-dihydroxyvitamin D_3 is the activated form which binds to vitamin D receptors in the body. Dietary vitamin D is first absorbed in the GI tract. It undergoes hydroxylation in the liver to 25-hydroxycholecalciferol and is then hydroxylated once more in the kidneys to form 1,25-dihydroxyvitamin D.

Bisphosphonates: rationale and evidence

Patients started on a bisphosphonate must be calcium and vitamin D replete; these therapies should be used alongside calcium and vitamin D supplementation. Alendronic acid is the first-line bisphosphonate used; the usual dose is 70 mg given *once weekly*. Patients should be advised to take alendronic acid 30 minutes before breakfast with a full glass of water, and to remain upright for 30 minutes after it has been taken. This helps to prevent development of oesophagitis. Alendronic acid has been shown to reduce the incidence of hip, forearm and spinal fractures.

Other bisphosphonates include risedronate (dosage 35 mg once weekly) and ibandronate (150 mg once a month; can be given orally or intravenously). Zoledronic acid is another bisphosphonate, which is given once yearly as an infusion.

🔍 Evidence

Long-term use of bisphosphonates

Bisphosphonates have been associated with oesophagitis in the short term. There have been reports of long-term use leading to osteonecrosis of the jaw and atypical femoral fractures (Park-Wyllie *et al.*, 2011). As a result, bisphosphonate therapy should be reviewed after 5 years, and bone density can be reassessed with a DEXA scan (Boonen *et al.*, 2012).

ⓘ Guidelines

NICE recommendations: alendronate, etidronate, risedronate, raloxifene, strontium ranelate and teriparatide for the secondary prevention of osteoporotic fragility fractures in postmenopausal women (NICE, 2008):

- Alendronate should be the treatment of choice for secondary prevention of osteoporotic fragility fractures in postmenopausal women.
- Risedronate or etidronate are alternatives in women who do not tolerate alendronate, or in those whose clinical risk fulfils defined criteria.
- Strontium ranelate and raloxifene should be used as third-line agents.

✓ DRUGS checklist for ALENDRONIC ACID

Dose	70 mg
Route	Oral
Units	mg
Given	Once weekly
Special situations	Alendronic acid may cause dyspepsia and oesophagitis. As a result, it should be taken early in the morning (before breakfast) with a whole glass of water, and the patient should sit upright for 30 minutes once the medication has been taken.

Bisphosphonates: essential pharmacology

Bisphosphonates have a number of mechanisms of action. First, they act by inhibiting osteoclastic resorption of bone. They attach to hydroxyapatite binding sites on the surface of bone. Bisphosphonates also act by decreasing osteoclast progenitor development and by promoting apoptosis of osteoclasts. Of note, bisphosphonates also reduce osteoblast apoptosis, thereby reducing bony destruction. Their osteoclastic activity is, however, their primary mechanism of action.

Other treatments used in osteoporosis

- Raloxifene has been shown to reduce the risk of spinal fractures. However, it may increase the risk of deep vein thrombosis (DVT).
- Denosumab is a monoclonal antibody which is given every 6 months by subcutaneous injection. There is a risk of a rebound increase in bone turnover when treatment is stopped, so an alternative agent should be started as soon as it is withdrawn. This is a second-line therapy for most patients.
- Strontium ranelate reduces the risk of fractures and is recommended as a third-line agent.

- Calcitriol may be used in patients with corticosteroid-induced osteoporosis. It works by stimulating calcium absorption.
- Teriparatide is a recombinant fragment of parathyroid hormone (PTH). It is particularly effective in reducing the incidence of spinal fractures. It is given by daily subcutaneous injection.
- Hormone replacement therapy (HRT) has been shown to reduce the risk of osteoporosis in postmenopausal women. However, association with increased risk of stroke, ischaemic heart disease and breast cancer have led to cessation of its use in the management of osteoporosis.

Case outcome and discharge

Mrs Rowley recovered well postoperatively. She undertook daily physiotherapy, and was reviewed by the occupational therapy team. She was discharged home with a twice-daily package of care.

DISCHARGE MEDICATION

Date	Medication	Dose	Route	Frequency	Supply	GP to continue?
xx/xx/xx	CALCICHEW-D3 FORTE	One tablet	PO	Twice daily	14 days	Y
xx/xx/xx	ALENDRONIC ACID	70 mg	PO	Once weekly (Tuesdays)	14 days	Y
xx/xx/xx	PARACETAMOL	1 g	PO	Four times a day	14 days	Y
xx/xx/xx	LEVOTHYROXINE	125 micrograms	PO	Once daily	14 days	Y
xx/xx/xx	RAMIPRIL	5 mg	PO	Once daily	14 days	Y

Notes to patient/GP:

Common pitfalls

- Remember to consider bone protection in all those aged over 75 presenting with a fracture.
- Patients must be calcium and vitamin D replete before a bisphosphonate is commenced.
- Alendronic acid is taken once weekly, and must be taken according to the prescribed instructions in order to prevent oesophagitis.
- Treatment with bisphosphonates should not be continued indefinitely without review, due to the risk of atypical femoral fractures and, rarely, osteonecrosis of the jaw.

SUMMARY

Osteoporosis is a common problem, particularly amongst postmenopausal women. In women aged over 75, a DEXA scan may not be necessary and the fracture can be considered to be secondary to osteoporosis. Prompt management with an appropriate agent is crucial to prevent further fractures.

🔑 Key learning points

- Calcium and vitamin D supplementation should be started in all patients following or at risk of an osteoporotic fracture.
- Bisphosphonates are the first-line therapy for secondary prevention of osteoporotic fractures in those aged over 75 years.
- Bisphosphonate therapy should be reviewed after 5 years, due to a small increase in the risk of atypical femoral fractures in long-term use.
- Other options include raloxifene, strontium ranelate, calcitriol, teriparatide and denosumab.

FURTHER READING

- The National Institute for Health and Care Excellence (NICE) provide clear guidance on secondary prevention of osteoporotic fragility fractures (NICE, 2008).
- A useful review of recent evidence for the management of osteoporotic fractures is: Murad MH, Drake MT, Mullan RJ *et al.* (2012). Clinical review. Comparative effectiveness of drug treatments to prevent fragility fractures: a systematic review and network meta-analysis. *J Clin Endocrinol Metab* 97: 1871–80.

Delirium

Mary Smith

Age: 90

Hospital number: 123456

👤🔍 Case study

Presenting complaint: *A 90-year-old woman is admitted from a residential home with a 2-day history of increasing confusion. She has no diagnosis of dementia and her carers report that she is not normally confused. She denies chest pain, shortness of breath, cough or urinary symptoms. Her carers report that she has been passing urine more frequently than usual and that it is strong smelling.*

Background: *She lives in a residential care home and mobilises with a Zimmer frame. She is a lifelong non-smoker and drinks no alcohol. Her husband died 5 years ago, and she participates fully in the social activities within the nursing home.*

PMH: *Hypertension*

Allergies: *None known*

Examination: *Pulse 88, BP 133/70, Sats 98% on air, RR 14, Temp 38.5*

CVS: *Capillary refill time <2 seconds, pulse regular, no pitting oedema, HS I + II + 0*

RS: *Equal expansion with air entry to both bases and no added sounds*

Abdo: *Soft and non-tender, no masses, bowel sounds present; no palpable bladder*

AMTS: *3/10*

Neurology: *No focal neurological deficit*

Urine dip: *Nitrites +++, protein +, blood ++, leukocytes +++*

Bloods: *White cell count 15.2 (neutrophilia), CRP 167, eGFR 48*

| PHARMACY STAMP | AGE 90 | FORENAME, SURNAME Mary Smith |
| | D.O.B. xx/xx/xxxx | ADDRESS Roseland House NHS NUMBER |

AMLODIPINE 5 mg once daily.

| SIGNATURE OF PRESCRIBER | DATE |

SP21000

Diagnosis

Delirium secondary to urinary tract infection (UTI).

Initial measures

A midstream urine sample (MSU) is sent and a chest X-ray is normal. She is started on intravenous antibiotics (Tazocin 4.5 g TDS) according to the trust protocol for UTIs. Despite this treatment, 48 hours later she remains agitated, is shouting out intermittently and pulling at her IV lines. Her temperature has settled and her inflammatory markers improving.

Prescribing for delirium

Delirium is defined (DSM IV) as a disturbance of consciousness with reduced ability to focus, sustain or shift attention. The disturbance develops over a short period and fluctuates during the day. There should be evidence from the history, examination or investigations that the disturbance is caused by the direct physiological consequence of a general medical condition (Anand and Maclullich, 2013). Following an episode of delirium, elderly patients are at increased risk of death compared with hospital inpatients without delirium (Witlox *et al.*, 2010).

The most commonly used diagnostic scale is the Confusion Assessment Method (CAM):

1. Acute onset and fluctuating course
2. Inattention
3. Disorganised thinking
4. Altered level of consciousness.

A diagnosis of delirium requires 1 and 2 + (3 or 4) (sensitivity 94–100%, specificity 90–95%).

The range of causes include:

1. **Drugs**: a wide range of drugs may be implicated, including opiodes, benzodiazepines and other sedatives
2. **Infection**: chest and urinary tract infections are the most common, but may also be due to cellulitis, thrombophlebitis secondary to IV cannula insertion, infectious gastroenteritis, meningitis or encephalitis
3. **Constipation**
4. **Pain**
5. **Metabolic**: including hypoglycaemia, uraemia, hepatic failure, hyponatraemia and hypercalcaemia

6. **Postoperative** (Zhang *et al.*, 2013)
7. **Alcohol or drug withdrawal**
8. **Cardiac**: including myocardial infarction
9. **Intracranial**: stroke, head injury, tumour and non-convulsive status epilepticus, cerebral vasculitis
10. **Nutritional**: including vitamin B_{12} and thiamine deficiency
11. **Endocrine**: including hypothyroidism
12. **Toxins**: including lead poisoning.

Alongside treating the cause of the patient's delirium (in this case a UTI), initial management of delirium includes orientation of the patient to their surroundings, providing a calm environment, and as much continuity of care as possible (NICE, 2010). First steps include reorientation, minimising disruption to the patient's environment and de-escalation techniques to calm distressed patients.

Historically, there have been concerns regarding use of antipsychotic medications in the elderly and those with dementia. It is now recognised that delirium is associated with longer length of hospital stay, increased admission to long-term care and cognitive impairment can last up to a year. There is increasing recognition that low doses of haloperidol may be appropriate in patients with significant agitation secondary to delirium.

AS REQUIRED MEDICATION					
DRUG HALOPERIDOL				Date	
				Time	
Dose 0.5–1.5 mg	Route PO	Max freq PRN; adjust according to intial response	Start date xx/xx/xx	Dose	
				Route	
Signature/Bleep A. Doctor		Max dose in 24 hrs	Review	Given	
				Check	
Additional instructions					

Haloperidol: rationale and evidence

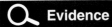 **Evidence**

Haloperidol as prophylaxis in delirium?

In recent years, a number of studies have investigated the potential use of haloperidol in elderly patients at high risk of developing delirium. One randomized controlled trial of intensive care patients found that those who received haloperidol 'prophylaxis' had reduced risk of developing delirium, reduced duration of delirium and improved mortality compared with the control group (Page *et al.*, 2013). However, currently there is no clear, reproducible method of stratifying patients according to risk of developing delirium.

 Guidelines

NICE recommendations: *Delirium: Diagnosis, Prevention and Management* (NICE, 2010):

- Patients should undergo risk assessment for delirium on admission. Those at increased risk include those aged >65, cognitive impairment, current hip fracture and severe illness.
- Prevention is the most crucial intervention, and includes holistic assessment of cognitive impairment, pain, dehydration, constipation, hypoxia and infection.
- Effective communication is crucial with regular reorientation for patients and reassurance for patients and carers.
- Initial management should focus on reorientation and maintaining a calm environment for the patient. De-escalation techniques may be required.
- Only if these non-pharmacological interventions have failed should patients be started on an oral antipsychotic such as haloperidol or olanzapine. Use of these treatments should ideally be limited to less than 1 week and started at the lowest appropriate dose.

✓ DRUGS checklist for HALOPERIDOL

Dose	0.5–1.5 mg
Route	PO
Units	mg
Given	As required; max 2–3 times daily; dose adjusted according to response
Special situations	Contraindicated in Parkinson's disease and Lewy body dementia as haloperidol may worsen symptoms. Baseline ECG should be carried out before haloperidol is started due to risk of long QT syndrome.

Haloperidol: essential pharmacology

Haloperidol is a butyrophenone antipsychotic which acts as an antagonist at D_2 dopaminergic receptors, and also has weak central anticholinergic activity. It has both sedative and antiemetic properties (see Chapter 9). The exact mechanism of action is unclear, but haloperidol is thought to act through inhibition of the reticular activating system of the brainstem. It has actions within the extrapyramidal system, thought to be through inhibition of glutamic acid, and also acts through inhibition of catecholamine receptors.

Case outcome and discharge

Mrs Smith's temperature settled, her inflammatory markers fell and she improved clinically. After 48 hours she was switched to oral antibiotics. However, her delirium persisted for several more days. She required three 0.5 mg doses of haloperidol to settle her agitation. She was discharged home 10 days after admission, with an outpatient appointment for follow up in 2 weeks time.

DISCHARGE MEDICATION						
Date	Medication	Dose	Route	Frequency	Supply	GP to continue?
xx/xx/xx	AMLODIPINE	5 mg	PO	Once daily	14 days	Y

Notes to patient/GP:

Common pitfalls

- Remember that there are multiple causes of delirium and that these may co-exist.
- Don't forget to identify and treat the underlying cause of delirium, and to address environmental and other non-pharmacological factors initially.
- The dose of antipsychotic required in the elderly will be lower; as a guide a starting dose of oral haloperidol should be 0.5 mg. A commonly used alternative is olanzapine 2.5 mg.
- Haloperidol is contraindicated in patients with Parkinson's disease and Lewy body dementia.

SUMMARY

Delirium is extremely common amongst elderly patients but up to one-third of cases are preventable. It is important to recognise risk factors for delirium and carefully investigate for the cause of delirium, and to remember that several causes may coexist. Although urinary tract infections are common in the elderly, a positive urine dipstick only has 30–40% specificity for UTI. Therefore it is important to assess for all possible causes of delirium. There are a number of important steps in managing patients with delirium, including maintaining a calm, quiet environment with as much continuity of care as possible. In patients with marked agitation, low-dose haloperidol may be required.

🔑 Key learning points

- Delirium is a common condition in the elderly, with a multitude of causes.
- Those with existing cognitive impairment are particularly susceptible.
- Initial management of delirium involves identification and treatment of the underlying cause, as well as providing a calm non-threatening environment for patients.
- In patients with marked agitation, a low-dose antipsychotic such as haloperidol may be required.
- It is important to remember, and to counsel patients and relatives, that delirium may continue for many weeks or months after the precipitant has stopped. In some cases, cognitive function may never return to the premorbid level.

FURTHER READING

- National Institute for Health and Care Excellence (NICE) guidelines provide useful information on the management of delirium (NICE, 2010).
- A useful review of management of UTI in the elderly is: Beveridge LA, Davey PG, Phillips G *et al.* (2011). Optimal management of urinary tract infections in older people. *Clin Interv Aging* 6: 173–80.

Polypharmacy

Maureen Phillips

Age: 95

Hospital number: 123456

🔍 Case study

Presenting complaint: *A 95-year-old woman is referred by her GP following a fall. On further questioning she reports that she has had 3–4 falls over the last 4 weeks. There have been no recent changes to her medications. She reports that the falls occur when she gets up to stand from a chair. She feels 'giddy' and falls to the ground. On this occasion, she was unable to get up from the floor, until she was found by her daughter 2 hours later. She denies chest pain, palpitations, shortness of breath or loss of consciousness. There is no evidence of urinary or faecal incontinence, or seizures.*

Background: *She lives alone at home and mobilises with a stick. She has 'meals on wheels' delivered, but has no regular carers.*

PMH: *Hypertension, hypercholesterolaemia, type 2 diabetes, gout, mild cognitive impairment*

Allergies: *None known*

Examination: *Pulse 48, regular, Sats 97% on air, RR 15, temp 37.0. Lying BP 134/82, standing BP 92/70*

CVS: *Capillary refill time <2 seconds, pulse regular, HS I + II + 0, mild pitting oedema to ankles*

RS: *Equal chest expansion with good air entry throughout and no added sounds. No wheeze*

Abdo: *Abdomen soft and non-tender, bowel sounds present*

Neuro: *No focal neurology*

MSK: *No hip tenderness, no head injury*

Diagnosis

Syncopal episodes secondary to iatrogenic postural hypotension.

Initial measures

Thorough assessment of the patient is essential. There is a clear, symptomatic postural drop in blood pressure observed here, so medicines reconciliation is the first priority.

PHARMACY STAMP	AGE 95	FORENAME, SURNAME
		Maureen Phillips
	D.O.B.	ADDRESS
	xx/xx/xxxx	1 Holland Court
		NHS NUMBER

ATENOLOL 50 mg once daily.

RAMIPRIL 5 mg once daily.

AMLODIPINE 5 mg once daily.

ASPIRIN 75 mg once daily.

SIMVASTATIN 40 mg once at night.

METFORMIN 500 mg twice daily.

ALLOPURINOL 100 mg once daily.

SIGNATURE OF PRESCRIBER	DATE

SP21000

REGULAR PRESCRIPTIONS

	Circle/enter times below ↓	Enter dates below			
		Day 1	Day 2	Day 3	Day 4
DRUG AMLODIPINE	06				
	⑧				
Dose 5 mg / Route PO / Freq OD / Start date xx/xx/xx	12				
Signature A. Doctor / Bleep / Review	16				
	18				
Additional instructions	22				
DRUG ASPIRIN	06				
	⑧				
Dose 75 mg / Route PO / Freq OD / Start date xx/xx/xx	12				
Signature A. Doctor / Bleep / Review	16				
	18				
Additional instructions	22				
DRUG SIMVASTATIN	06				
	08				
Dose 40 mg / Route PO / Freq OD / Start date xx/xx/xx	12				
Signature A. Doctor / Bleep / Review	16				
	18				
Additional instructions	㉒				
DRUG METFORMIN	06				
	⑧				
Dose 500 mg / Route PO / Freq BD / Start date xx/xx/xx	12				
Signature A. Doctor / Bleep / Review	16				
Additional instructions	⑱				
	22				
DRUG ALLOPURINOL	06				
	⑧				
Dose 100 mg / Route PO / Freq OD / Start date xx/xx/xx	12				
Signature A. Doctor / Bleep / Review	16				
	18				
Additional instructions	22				

Beta-blockers: rationale and evidence

 Guidelines

NICE recommendations: Hypertension: clinical management of primary hypertension in adults (NICE, 2011):
- Beta-blockers are no longer recommended as first-line treatment for the management of hypertension.
- Current NICE guidelines state that they should only be used in resistant cases (stage 4).
- For those aged under 55 years, the first-line therapy is an angiotensin-converting enzyme (ACE) inhibitor or angiotensin II receptor blocker.
- For those aged over 55 years or those of African Caribbean origin, a calcium channel blocker is the first-line agent.

Prescribing in polypharmacy

This patient has been taking this collection of medications for a number of years, and may have had significant hypertension at one stage. According to current guidelines, the first-line drug for management of hypertension in those aged over 55 is a calcium channel blocker. The target blood pressure in patients over 80 years old is <150/90 mmHg. Atenolol, ramipril and amlodipine could all be contributing to the significant postural drop (significant systolic drop >20 mmHg). It therefore seems unlikely that more than one agent will be needed at present, so atenolol and ramipril would be the most appropriate agents to stop first.

✓ DRUGS checklist for ATENOLOL

Dose	25–100 mg daily
	The starting dose in hypertension is 25 mg; for angina, the maximum dose is 100 mg once daily
Route	Oral
Units	mg
Given	Once or twice daily
Special situations	Beta-blockers can cause bradycardia and are contraindicated in second and third-degree heart block. They are one of the key medical therapies in the management of chronic heart failure, but should be used with caution in acute or unstable cardiac failure. Beta-blockers can cause bronchospasm and should be avoided in patients with a history of asthma. They can cause fatigue, sleep disturbance and cold extremities. Beta-blockers can affect carbohydrate metabolism, causing hypo- or hyperglycaemia. They should therefore be used with caution in patients with diabetes.

Beta-blockers: essential pharmacology

Beta-blockers block the beta-adrenoceptors in the heart, peripheral vasculature, bronchi, pancreas and liver. This inhibits the binding of adrenaline and noradrenaline to these receptors. First-generation beta-blockers act via beta$_1$ and beta$_2$ receptors, and are therefore classified as non-selective. In recent years, a range of cardioselective beta-blockers

have been developed that primarily act upon beta$_1$ receptors.

In the heart, beta-blockers bind to beta-adrenoceptors in the atrioventricular (AV) node, conducting system and cardiac myocytes. The majority of beta-adrenoceptors in the heart are beta$_1$ receptors. Beta-adrenoceptors are G-protein coupled receptors, which activate adenylyl cyclase to form cyclic AMP (cAMP). This activates a cAMP dependent protein kinase, which phosphorylates L-type calcium channels. This causes increased calcium entry into cells, resulting in a positive inotropic effect.

Case outcome and discharge

Mrs Phillips' blood pressure remained 100–125 systolic once atenolol and ramipril were stopped. Amlodipine was subsequently stopped, and her systolic blood pressure remained 130–140 mmHg for the remainder of her admission. All antihypertensives were therefore stopped, and she was discharged to her GP for ongoing blood pressure monitoring. She was assessed by the physiotherapy and occupational therapy teams and a once-daily package of care was arranged on discharge.

DISCHARGE MEDICATION						
Date	Medication	Dose	Route	Frequency	Supply	GP to continue?
xx/xx/xx	ASPIRIN	75 mg	PO	Once daily	14 days	Y
xx/xx/xx	SIMVASTATIN	40 mg	PO	Once at night	14 days	Y
xx/xx/xx	METFORMIN	500 mg	PO	Twice daily	14 days	Y
xx/xx/xx	ALLOPURINOL	100 mg	PO	Once daily	14 days	Y
Notes to patient/GP:						

Common pitfalls

- In this case, all three antihypertensives were discontinued as the patient's blood pressure remained stable.
- During an inpatient admission, it is important to review the drug chart regularly and to stop any medications that are not required or which may be causing unwanted side effects and interactions.

SUMMARY

Polypharmacy is a common problem in the elderly. Postural hypotension is a common side effect of multiple antihypertensive therapies. Medicines reconciliation is the primary intervention in this case.

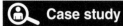 **Key learning points**

- Polypharmacy in the elderly is a common problem and drug charts should be reviewed daily during an inpatient admission.
- A careful drug history, including which drugs have been started or stopped recently, should be obtained.
- Multiple antihypertensives in the elderly can cause significant hypotension.
- If at all unsure of the side effects of any medications, look them up in the BNF (BMA/RPS, 2015).

FURTHER READING

- National Institute for Health and Care Excellence (NICE) guidelines provide useful information on the management of hypertension and postural hypotension (NICE, 2011; NICE, 2013).
- A useful review of treatment options for postural hypotension is: Logan IC, Witham MD (2012). Efficacy of treatments for orthostatic hypotension: a systematic review. *Work Aging Retirement* 41: 587–94.
- For further information on additional therapies that may be required in patients with postural hypotension, see Ziegler MG, Milic M (2012). New therapies for postural hypotension. *Hypertension* 59: 548–9.

Hyponatraemia

Peter Jones

Age: 78

Hospital number: 123456

Case study

Presenting complaint: *A 78-year-old gentleman presents to the emergency department following a* *fall at home. He is found to have sustained a fracture of his right distal radius. A full set of blood tests were sent, and the patient was found to have a sodium of 125. There were no previous blood results available on the system. Urea, creatinine, potassium and all other blood tests were within normal limits.*

Background: *Lives at home with his wife. Mobilises short distances with a stick. Ex-smoker (50 pack year smoking history).*

PMH and family history: *Chronic lymphocytic leukaemia (CLL) – under surveillance, COPD, hypertension, osteoarthritis.*

Allergies: *None known*

Examination: *BP 135/80, Pulse 77, Sats 93% on air, RR 16, Temp 36.7*

CVS: *Capillary refill time <2 seconds, pulse regular, HS I + II + 0, JVP not raised*

RS: *Globally reduced chest expansion, mild wheeze.*

Abdo: *Soft and non-tender, no masses and bowel sounds present*

Neuro: *No focal neurology*

MSK: *Fracture left distal radius; no other injuries*

PHARMACY STAMP	AGE 78 D.O.B. xx/xx/xxxx	FORENAME, SURNAME Peter Jones ADDRESS 24 Grosvenor Road NHS NUMBER

SERETIDE 500 ACCUHALER 1 puff twice daily.

TIOTROPIUM 18 micrograms inhaled once daily.

BENDROFLUMETHIAZIDE 2.5 mg once daily.

BISOPROLOL 1.25 mg once daily.

AMLODIPINE 5 mg once daily.

SALBUTAMOL 2 puffs as required.

PARACETAMOL 1 g four times daily as required.

CITALOPRAM 10 mg once daily.

SIGNATURE OF PRESCRIBER   DATE

SP21000

Diagnosis

Hyponatraemia. There are a number of potential causes of hyponatraemia in this case. These include diuretic therapy, selective serotonin reuptake inhibitor (SSRI therapy) or syndrome of inappropriate antidiuretic hormone (SIADH) (secondary to lung malignancy, which needs to be considered as the patient is an ex-smoker).

Initial measures

Initial management will consist of establishing the patient's fluid status as this will help determine the most likely cause and also the appropriate initial treatment. Medications are a common cause of hyponatraemia in the elderly and there are many common culprits (see Box Drugs that May Cause Hyponatraemia) (Clayton *et al.*, 2006). Initial treatment in this case would involve stopping the bendroflumethiazide, particularly as there is no clear indication along with reviewing if the citalopram is still indicated. Urinary sodium and paired plasma and urine osmolality should also be measured to exclude an alternative cause (i.e. SIADH), but only after stopping drugs such as bendroflumethiazide that affect sodium secretion. It is important to bear in mind that in patients with hyperglycaemia, the sodium may be falsely low and therefore it is always important to check the glucose.

Drugs that may cause hyponatraemia

- Selective serotonin reuptake inhibitors (SSRIs)
- Carbamazepine
- Tricyclic antidepressants
- Tramadol
- Lithium
- Haloperidol
- Diuretics

Prescribing for hyponatraemia

Note here that the bendroflumethiazide is being stopped and BP regularly monitored. Regular analgesia with PRN codeine has been prescribed for pain due to the fracture.

REGULAR PRESCRIPTIONS

DRUG				Circle/enter times below ↓	Enter dates below			
					Day 1	Day 2	Day 3	Day 4

DRUG SERETIDE 500 ACCUHALER

Dose 1 puff	Route INH	Freq BD	Start date xx/xx/xx	06
Signature A. Doctor		Bleep	Review	⑧
				12
Additional instructions				16
				⑱
				22

DRUG TIOTROPIUM

Dose 18 micrograms	Route INH	Freq OD	Start date xx/xx/xx	06
Signature A. Doctor		Bleep	Review	⑧
				12
Additional instructions				16
				18
				22

DRUG BISOPROLOL

Dose 1.25 mg	Route PO	Freq OD	Start date xx/xx/xx	06
Signature A. Doctor		Bleep	Review	⑧
				12
Additional instructions				16
				18
				22

DRUG AMLODIPINE

Dose 5 mg	Route PO	Freq OD	Start date xx/xx/xx	06
Signature A. Doctor		Bleep	Review	⑧
				12
Additional instructions				16
				18
				22

DRUG CITALOPRAM

Dose 10 mg	Route PO	Freq OD	Start date xx/xx/xx	06
Signature A. Doctor		Bleep	Review	⑧
				12
Additional instructions				16
				18
				22

DRUG PARACETAMOL

Dose 1 g	Route PO	Freq QDS	Start date xx/xx/xx	06
Signature A. Doctor		Bleep	Review	⑧
				⑫
Additional instructions				⑯
				⑱
				22

AS REQUIRED MEDICATION

DRUG CODEINE

				Date	
				Time	
Dose 30 mg	Route PO	Max freq QDS PRN	Start date xx/xx/xx	Dose	
Signature/Bleep A. Doctor		Max dose in 24 hrs	Review	Route	
Additional instructions				Given	
				Check	

DRUG SALBUTAMOL

				Date	
				Time	
Dose 2 puffs	Route INH	Max freq QDS PRN	Start date xx/xx/xx	Dose	
Signature/Bleep A. Doctor		Max dose in 24 hrs	Review	Route	
Additional instructions				Given	
				Check	

Thiazide diuretics: rationale and evidence

Evidence

Thiazide diuretics and hyponatraemia

There have been a number of studies that have highlighted hyponatraemia associated with use of thiazide diuretics (Wu *et al.*, 2013; Leung *et al.*, 2011). A study has suggested that age and BMI are significant influences upon risk of developing hyponatraemia with administration of a thiazide diuretic (Rodenberg *et al.*, 2013).

ⓘ Guidelines

NICE recommendations: Hypertension: clinical management of primary hypertension in adults (NICE, 2011):

- The above evidence is reflected in current NICE guidelines – thiazide-like diuretics (such as indapamide and chlorthalidone) are recommended only as a step 4 agent.
- These newer thiazide-like diuretics are now recommended in preference to traditional thiazide diuretics such as bendroflumethiazide.

✓ DRUGS checklist for BENDROFLUMETHIAZIDE

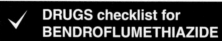

Dose	2.5 mg
Route	Oral
Units	mg
Given	Once daily
Special situations	Thiazide diuretics can exacerbate gout, diabetes and systemic lupus erythematosus (SLE). Electrolyte imbalance including hypokalaemia, hyponatraemia, hypercalcaemia and hyperglycaemia are relatively common side effects.

Thiazide diuretics: essential pharmacology

Thiazide diuretics act by inhibiting the sodium–chloride transporter in the distal convoluted tubule of the nephron. As a consequence, sodium and chloride (and therefore water) reabsorption is inhibited. In contrast, loop diuretics act upon the loop of Henle, and have a greater natriuretic effect than thiazides. Thiazides also increase calcium reabsorption in the distal tubule.

Case outcome and discharge

Mr Jones' hyponatraemia gradually resolved on cessation of bendroflumethiazide. He was reviewed by the orthopaedic team and underwent surgical fixation of his distal radius fracture. He was seen regularly by the physiotherapy and occupational therapy teams and was discharged home with a package of care. Importantly, his GP was asked to follow up the sodium level by repeating the U&Es following discharge.

DISCHARGE MEDICATION

Date	Medication	Dose	Route	Frequency	Supply	GP to continue?
xx/xx/xx	SERETIDE 500 ACCUHALER	1 puff	INH	Twice daily	14 days	Y
xx/xx/xx	TIOTROPIUM	18 micrograms	INH	Once daily	14 days	Y
xx/xx/xx	BISOPROLOL	1.25 mg	PO	Once daily	14 days	Y
xx/xx/xx	AMLODIPINE	5 mg	PO	Once daily	14 days	Y
xx/xx/xx	FUROSEMIDE	40 mg	PO	Once daily	14 days	Y
xx/xx/xx	SALBUTAMOL	2 puffs	INH	As required	14 days	Y
xx/xx/xx	PARACETAMOL	1 g	PO	Four times a day as required	14 days	Y

Notes to patient/GP:

Common pitfalls

- In patients with hyponatraemia, remember to review the drug chart to assess whether there are any drugs that may be contributing.
- Clinical assessment of a patient's fluid status is essential in order to assess the cause of hyponatraemia.

Hyponatraemia is a common clinical problem, which may be asymptomatic or may present with nausea, fatigue, falls and even seizures.

SUMMARY

Key learning points

- Clinical assessment, including a full drug history and thorough examination, are essential in the establishing the differential diagnosis of hyponatraemia.
- Drugs, including thiazide diuretics, are a common cause of hyponatraemia.
- Urinary sodium and paired serum and urine osmolality are crucial to help determine the cause of hyponatraemia.
- Giving 0.9% saline is rarely the most appropriate treatment, unless a patient is clinically dry.
- When replacing losses with 0.9% saline it is critical that sodium is not replaced too quickly, to avoid central pontine myelinosis (maximum rate of correction 8–10 mmol/24 hours).

FURTHER READING

- A useful review of drug-induced hyponatraemia is: Liamis G, Milionis H, Elisaf M (2008). A review of drug-induced hyponatraemia. *Am J Kidney Dis* 52: 144–53.

Now visit **www.wileyessential.com/pharmacology**
to test yourself on this chapter.

References

Anand A, Maclullich AMJ (2013). Delirium in hospitalized older adults. *Medicine* 41: 39–42.

Beveridge LA, Davey PG, Phillips G *et al.* (2011). Optimal management of urinary tract infections in older people. *Clin Interv Aging* 6: 173–80.

Bolland MJ, Grey A, Avenell A *et al.* (2011). Calcium supplements with or without vitamin D and risk of cardiovascular events: reanalysis of the Women's Health Initiative limited access dataset and meta-analysis. *BMJ* 342: d2040.

Boonen S, Ferrari S, Miller PD *et al.* (2012). Post-menopausal osteoporosis treatment with antiresorptives: effects of discontinuation or long-term continuation on bone turnover and fracture risk – a perspective. *J Bone Miner Res* 27: 963–74.

British Medical Association and Royal Pharmaceutical Society of Great Britain (BMA/RPS) (2015). *British National Formulary 69*, 69th edn. BMJ group and Pharmaceutical Press, London.

Clayton JA, Le Jeuine IR, Hall IP (2006). Severe hyponatraemia in medical in-patients: aetiology, assessment and outcome. *Q J Med* 99: 505.

Leung AA, Wright A, Pazo V *et al.* (2011). Risk of thiazide-induced hyponatraemia in patients with hypertension. *Am J Med* 124: 1064–72.

Liamis G, Milionis H, Elisaf M. (2008). A review of drug-induced hyponatraemia. *Am J Kidney Dis* 52: 144–53.

Logan IC, Witham MD (2012). Efficacy of treatments for orthostatic hypotension: a systematic review. *Work, Ageing and Retirement* 41: 587–94.

Moyer VA; U.S. Preventive Services Task Force (2013). Vitamin D and calcium supplementation to prevent fractures in adults: U.S. Preventive Services Task Force recommendation statement. *Ann Intern Med* 158: 691–6.

Murad MH, Drake MT, Mullan RJ *et al.* (2012). Clinical review. Comparative effectiveness of drug treatments to prevent fragility fractures: a systematic review and network meta-analysis. *J Clin Endocrinol Metab* 97: 1871–80.

National Institute for Health and Care Excellence (NICE) (2008). *Alendronate, Etidronate, Risedronate, Raloxifene, Strontium Ranelate and Teriparatide for the Secondary Prevention of Osteoporotic Fragility Fractures in Postmenopausal Women.* Available at: www.nice.org.uk/guidance/ta161 (accessed Dec. 2015).

National Institute for Health and Care Excellence (NICE) (2010). *Delirium: Diagnosis, Prevention and Management.* Available at: www.nice.org.uk/guidance/cg103. (accessed Dec. 2015).

National Institute of Health and Clinical Excellence (NICE) (2011). *Hypertension: Clinical Management of Care Hypertension in Adults.* Available at: www.nice.org.uk/guidance/CG127 (accessed Dec. 2015).

National Institute of Health and Care Excellence (NICE) (2013). *Postural Hypotension in Adults: Fludrocortisone.* Available at: www.nice.org.uk/advice/esuom20/chapter/Key-points-from-the-evidence. (accessed Dec. 2015).

Page VJ, Ely EW, Gates S *et al.* (2013). Effect of intravenous haloperidol on the duration of delirium and coma in critically ill patients (Hope-ICU): a randomised, double-blind, placebo-controlled trial. *Lancet Respir Med* 1: 515–23.

Park-Wyllie L, Mamdani MM, Juurlink DN *et al.* (2011). Bisphosphonate use and the risk of sub-trochanteric or femoral shaft fractures in older women. *JAMA* 305: 783–9.

Prentice RL, Pettinger MB, Jackson RD *et al.* (2013). Health risks and benefits from calcium and vitamin D supplementation: Women's Health Initiative clinical trial and cohort study. *Osteoporos Int* 24: 567–80.

Rodenburg EM, Hoorn EJ, Ruite R *et al.* (2013). Thiazide-associated hyponatraemia: a population- based study. *Am J Kidney Dis* 62: 67–72.

Witlox J, Eurelings LS, de Jonghe JF *et al.* (2010). Delirium in elderly patients and the risk of post-discharge mortality, institutionalization, and dementia. *JAMA* 304: 443–51.

Wu HC, Wemg YL, Wu CJ *et al.* (2013). Fixed-dose combinations containing thiazide as the common cause of severe in-hospital hyponatrae-mia. *Acta Nephrologica* 27: 205–12.

Zhang H, Lu Y, Liu M (2013). Strategies for prevention of postoperative delirium: a systematic review and meta-analysis of randomized trials. *Critical Care* 17: R47.

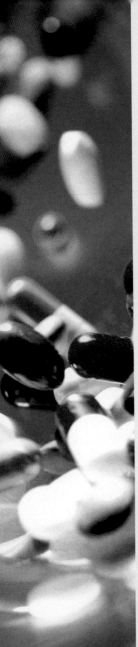

CHAPTER 9

Anticipatory Prescribing at the End of Life

Amy Hawkins

Key topics:

Learning objectives

By the end of this chapter, you should be able to…

- …write prescriptions for patients with symptoms at the end of life, or in anticipation of these symptoms, including:
  - pain
  - breathlessness
  - excess respiratory secretions
  - nausea and vomiting
  - agitation.
- …evaluate the key therapies used in the management of the above symptoms at the end of life.
- …discuss the mechanisms of action of these drugs.

Essential Practical Prescribing, First Edition. Georgia Woodfield, Benedict Lyle Phillips, Victoria Taylor, Amy Hawkins and Andrew Stanton. © 2016 by John Wiley & Sons, Ltd. Published 2016 by John Wiley & Sons, Ltd.

Pain

+-----------------------------------+
| **Sally Green** |
| |
| **Age: 86** |
| |
| **Hospital number: 123456** |
+-----------------------------------+

🔍 Case study

Background: *You are called to review an 86-year-old woman on the care of the elderly ward. She has been diagnosed with metastatic ovarian cancer and is too frail to undergo chemotherapy. In the last week she has deteriorated rapidly and the team feels she is likely to die within hours to days. Until now, she has been comfortable, but her family report that she appears to be in pain. She is struggling to take her oral medications.*

Allergies: *none known*

Examination:

No routine observations are being recorded
Respiratory rate 26
Chest: clear

Abdomen: mildly distended with generalised tenderness
Eyes open to voice
Recent blood tests show eGFR 50

Initial measures

An important first step when assessing a patient in this scenario is to consider the cause of the pain. A full assessment will include taking a history from the patient where possible, seeking a collateral history from her relatives and carrying out a focused examination. The aim of this assessment is to see whether the patient has a reversible cause for her pain, for example a full bladder or rectum or an uncomfortable pressure area. It is also important to review the other medications prescribed on the drug chart. In this case, we are told that the patient is struggling to take her oral medications so these should be reviewed and reconciled as appropriate. It will be important to assess whether the patient is currently receiving any regular analgesia. In this case the patient is no longer able to take her oral paracetamol so an appropriate parenteral drug will need to be given. Mrs Green is 'opioid naïve', that is she doesn't take regular opioid analgesia. As we will see, this has implications for our prescribing choices.

Prescribing for pain at the end of life

It is important to carry out a thorough assessment of the pain. This includes:

- **Nature of the pain:** site, radiation, character and severity should all be included. Remember to assess the impact of the pain on sleep and quality of life.
- **Cause of the pain:** is there evidence of a specific disease causing pain? Is there a reversible or treatable cause? Is pain occurring as a consequence of treatment?
- **Specific type of pain:** for example, is the pain shooting or stabbing in nature, which may suggest neuropathic pain?
- **Psychosocial and spiritual aspects:** is the patient's psychological state impairing their ability to cope with or manage the pain?

REGULAR PRESCRIPTIONS

				Circle/enter times below ↓	↓ Enter dates below			
					Day 1	Day 2	Day 3	Day 4
DRUG RAMIPRIL				06				
				⑧				
Dose 5 mg	Route PO	Freq OD	Start date xx/xx/xx	12				
Signature A. Doctor		Bleep	Review	16				
Additional instructions				18				
				22				
DRUG LEVOTHYROXINE				06				
				⑧				
Dose 100 micrograms	Route PO	Freq OD	Start date xx/xx/xx	12				
Signature A. Doctor		Bleep	Review	16				
Additional instructions				18				
				22				
DRUG LAXIDO				06				
				⑧				
Dose 2	Route PO	Freq BD	Start date xx/xx/xx	12				
Signature A. Doctor		Bleep	Review	16				
Additional instructions				⑱				
				22				
DRUG PARACETAMOL				06				
				⑧				
Dose 1 g	Route PO/IV	Freq QDS PRN	Start date xx/xx/xx	⑫				
Signature A. Doctor		Bleep	Review	⑯				
Additional instructions				⑱				
				22				

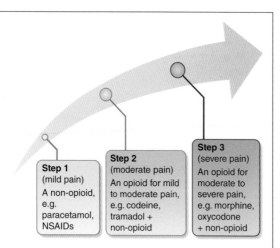

Figure 9.1 The WHO analgesic ladder. Source: Reproduced with permission of WHO.

It is important to consider the WHO 'analgesic ladder' when managing pain (available at: www.who.int/cancer/palliative/painladder/en/). The aim of this model is to start at step one, and gradually add in analgesics at other two steps of the 'ladder' as needed (Figure 9.1).

In this scenario, where oral preparations are not appropriate because the patient is nearing the end of their life and is unlikely to manage to take oral drugs, a subcutaneous opioid is usually the first-choice analgesic. In an elderly opioid-naïve patient with normal renal function, the starting dose of subcutaneous morphine is 1.5–2.5 mg when required, which can be given hourly if needed. This is equivalent to 2.5–5 mg of oral morphine. The dose can be titrated up and a regular dose prescribed based upon how many 'as required' doses have been needed.

AS REQUIRED MEDICATION						
DRUG				Date		
MORPHINE SULPHATE IMMEDIATE RELEASE (IR)				Time		
Dose	Route	Max freq	Start date	Dose		
1.25 mg (ONE POINT TWO FIVE MILLIGRAMS) – 2.5 mg (TWO POINT FIVE MILLIGRAMS) when required	SC	1 - 2 hourly	xx/xx/xx	Route		
Signature/Bleep		Max dose in 24 hrs	Review	Given		
A. Doctor				Check		
Additional instructions						

When prescribing for pain at the end of life in this way, it is important to consider that the patient may also develop other symptoms such as breathlessness, agitation and respiratory secretions. 'Anticipatory' prescribing with medications to counteract these symptoms will help to reduce distress for the patient and family. Aspects of prescribing for these symptoms will be covered later in this chapter.

Morphine: rationale and evidence

Morphine is the first-line strong opioid of choice in patients without significant renal impairment or proven allergy (Bennett *et al.*, 2012; Care, 2001).

⊘ Guidelines

NICE recommendations on opioids in palliative care – safe and effective prescribing of strong opioids for pain in palliative care of adults (NICE, 2012):
- Use of opioids should be tailored to the individual patient and potential side effects of treatment should be communicated clearly.
- The dose of opioid should be carefully titrated, regardless of whether the oral, transdermal or subcutaneous route is most appropriate.
- Important side effects, including constipation, nausea and drowsiness, should be considered.

⌕ Evidence

Morphine for cancer pain
Extensive research has suggested that when used appropriately, opioids are a safe, effective choice of analgesia for patients with cancer pain (McQuay, 1999). Morphine is widely recommended as the first-choice opioid for patients with moderate to severe cancer pain (Hanks *et al.*, 2001). A systematic review has suggested that in patients with moderate to severe cancer pain and renal impairment, fentanyl, alfentanil and methadone are the least likely to cause harm (King *et al.*, 2011).

✓	**DRUGS checklist for MORPHINE**
Dose	Initial starting dose of immediate-release oral morphine in an opioid naïve patient is 2.5–5 mg This is equivalent to 1.25–2.5 mg SC
Route	Oral/subcutaneous (intravenous and intramuscular preparations also available but less comfortable and convenient)
Units	mg
Given	The initial oral dose is usually given 4-hourly, with the PRN dose equal to the 4-hourly dose For anticipatory prescribing, the dose is when required, at a maximum of 1-hourly
Special situations	Constipation and nausea are common side effects. Signs of toxicity include increasing drowsiness, vivid dreams and hallucinations, pinpoint pupils and jerking (myoclonus). Dose reduction or alternative opioids should be used in renal impairment.

Morphine: essential pharmacology

When administered orally, peak plasma concentrations of morphine occur within an hour, with an analgesic effect lasting approximately 4 hours. This is the rationale for 4-hourly dosing you will see on inpatient drug charts. The 'PRN' dose should equal the 4-hourly dose, and the usual frequency for the PRN dose is a maximum of once hourly.

Modified-release oral preparations are taken usually 12-hourly and have a peak concentration within 2–6 hours. The analgesic effect lasts 12–24 hours. Therefore, when dose requirements are uncertain or unstable, it may be more appropriate to use immediate-release formulations. This dose can be switched to a modified-release preparation once analgesic requirements have been established and are at a steady state.

Drugs administered via parenteral routes do not undergo first-pass metabolism. As a result, the relative potency of different formulations varies. Doses must be adjusted accordingly when switching from one dose formulation to another, and from one opioid to another (Mercadante, 2011). When converting from oral to subcutaneous morphine, the dose should be divided by 2 (so for example 10 mg oral morphine is equivalent to 5 mg SC morphine). Table 9.1 provides approximate relative potencies for different opioid analgesics.

Other treatments used for pain management at the end of life

■ **Modified-release morphine preparations** are widely used, including Zomorph and morphine

Table 9.1 Approximate relative potencies of different opioid analgesics.		
Drug and route of administration	**Dose ratio to oral morphine**	**Examples of dose equivalents (in milligrams)**
Oral morphine	1	30
Subcutaneous morphine	1/2	15
Subcutaneous diamorphine	1/3	10
Oral oxycodone	1/2	15
Subcutaneous oxycodone	1/4	7.5
Oral codeine	10	300
Oral tramadol	10	300
Subcutaneous alfentanil	1/30	1

sulphate slow release (MST$_{SR}$). The dose of these preparations is calculated according to the patient's total 24-hour morphine requirement.

- **Diamorphine** may be used in situations where high doses of morphine are required as it is more soluble than morphine and can therefore be delivered in a smaller volume.
- **Oxycodone** may be used as an alternative in patients who tolerate morphine poorly as there is interindividual variability in side effects (Dale, 2011). It is also used in renal impairment. It is available in oral and injectable forms. OxyNorm is the 4-hourly immediate-release formulation, and OxyContin is the 12-hourly modified-release preparation.
- **Fentanyl** may be used as a transdermal patch, but is also available subcutaneously. It is useful in patients with severe renal impairment (eGFR <30 mL/min) as it has no renally excreted metabolites.
- **Alfentanil** is used as an injectable medication for use in a syringe driver in patients with severe renal impairment.
- **Methadone** can be used in cases where pain is poorly responsive to other opioids or where there are unacceptable side effects. However, dose titration is complex and metabolism is variable so it should be used only by specialists.
- **Hydromorphone** is available for oral use in patients who tolerate morphine poorly as there is interindividual variability in side effects. It is available in 4-hourly immediate and 12-hourly modified-release forms. It is not widely used in the UK.

Important point: When prescribing any regular modified-release opioid preparation, remember to prescribe a breakthrough (PRN) dose of the relevant immediate-release preparation at one-sixth of the total daily dose of the regular opioid. If the regular dose is increased the PRN/breakthrough dose is likely to need to be increased accordingly.

Q Evidence

Choice of opioid analgesia

A systematic review found that oral morphine, oxycodone and hydromorphone have similar efficacy and toxicity in patients with cancer pain (Caraceni et al., 2011). Despite this, there are differences between individuals in terms of responses to given opioids, several of which are likely to be genetically mediated (Branford et al., 2012).

Case outcome

Mrs Green had been given 2 × 1.25 mg doses and 6 × 2.5 mg doses of SC morphine during a 24-hour period (equivalent to a total of 17.5 mg SC morphine). A decision was made to add 15 mg of SC morphine to a syringe driver, with a PRN dose of one-sixth of the total 24-hourly requirement (15 mg divided by 6 = 2.5 mg). The patient remained comfortable on this dose and died 2 days later.

Common pitfalls

- A holistic, individualised pain assessment is the key to good pain management at the end of life.
- Remember to consider whether a patient has renal impairment when prescribing opioid analgesics.
- Observe carefully for signs suggestive of opioid toxicity.
- Specialist referral will be required for patients not responding to initial management, or those with severe renal impairment or complex pain needs.

AS REQUIRED MEDICATION													
DRUG MORPHINE SULPHATE IMMEDIATE RELEASE (IR)				Date	xx/xx/xx	xx/xx/xx	xx/xx/xx	xx/xx/xx	xx/xx/xx	xx/xx/xx	xx/xx/xx	xx/xx/xx	
				Time	08.00	10.00	12.00	14.00	16.00	18.00	20.00	22.00	
Dose 2.5 mg (TWO POINT FIVE MILLIGRAMS) - 5 mg (FIVE MILLIGRAMS) when required	Route SC	Max freq 1 - 2 hourly	Start date xx/xx/xx	Dose	1.25 mg	1.25 mg	2.5 mg	2.5 mg	2.5 mg	2.5 mg	2.5 mg	2.5 mg	
				Route	SC	SC	SC	SC	SC	SC	SC	SC	
Signature/Bleep A. Doctor		Max dose in 24 hrs	Review	Given	A. Doctor	A. Doctor	A. Doctor	A. Doctor	A. Doctor	A. Doctor	A. Doctor	A. Doctor	
				Check	A. Doctor	A. Doctor	A. Doctor	A. Doctor	A. Doctor	A. Doctor	A. Doctor	A. Doctor	
Additional instructions For pain													

DRUG MORPHINE SULPHATE				Date									
				Time									
Dose 15 mg (FIFTEEN MILLIGRAMS)	Route SC over 24 hours via syringe driver	Max freq	Start date xx/xx/xx	Dose									
				Route									
Signature/Bleep A. Doctor		Max dose in 24 hrs	Review	Given									
				Check									
Additional instructions Via syringe driver													

Pain is a common symptom amongst patients at the end of life. The WHO Analgesic Ladder provides a useful framework when considering which analgesic to prescribe. Anticipatory prescribing is crucial in order to maintain patient comfort and dignity at the end of life.

SUMMARY

🔑 Key learning points

- Morphine is the first-line opioid for patients with moderate to severe pain at the end of life.
- Alternative opioids may be required for patients who are unable to tolerate morphine, and those with renal impairment.
- Dose conversion is required depending upon the type of opioid and route of administration.
- The breakthrough dose of morphine will be one-sixth of the total 24-hour dose.
- Converting back to oral morphine is a useful way to calculate the dose when changing from one opioid analgesic to another.

FURTHER READING

■ The National Institute for Health and Clinical Excellence (NICE) has issued a guideline for prescribing of opioids in palliative care (NICE, 2012). This gives useful information and is regularly updated.

■ A useful review of the evidence is: Caraceni A, Pigni A, Brunelli C (2011). Is oral morphine still the first choice opioid for moderate to severe cancer pain? A systematic review within the European Palliative Care Research Collaborative guidelines project. *Palliat Med* 25: 402–9.

■ For a comprehensive review of pain management in palliative medicine see Twycross R, Wilcock A, Howard P (eds) (2014). *Palliative Care Formulary* (PCF 5). Available at: www.palliativedrugs.com.

Breathlessness and excess secretions

Henry Martin

Age: 77

Hospital number: 123456

🔍 Case study

Presenting complaint: During a busy on-call shift you go to see a 77-year-old gentleman who is admitted via the emergency department with shortness of breath. He has end-stage metastatic small cell lung cancer which is not suitable for anticancer therapy.

Background: After detailed assessment it is apparent that Mr Martin's disease has progressed rapidly and he is dying. Your consultant discusses this with the family, and they agree that they wish for him to be 'kept comfortable'.

(Continued)

Case study (*Continued*)

Family and social history: *He lives with his wife and has two children living nearby.*

Allergies: *None known*

Examination:
BP 110/70, HR 85, oxygen sats 92% on air, respiratory rate 28, temperature 36.5
Chest: noisy breathing with secretions ++, widespread coarse upper airway secretions
Abdomen: soft and non-tender
Opens eyes transiently to voice – managing only a few mumbled words
eGFR >60

PHARMACY STAMP	AGE 77 D.O.B. xx/xx/xxxx	FORENAME, SURNAME Henry Martin ADDRESS Park Lane NHS NUMBER

METFORMIN: 1 g twice daily (morning and evening).

SIMVASTATIN 20 mg once at night.

ASPIRIN 75 mg once daily.

ORAMORPH 5 mg when required
Max hourly for pain or breathlessness.

SIGNATURE OF PRESCRIBER	DATE

SP21000

Initial measures
As with the case of Mrs Green, it is important to review each medication before it is prescribed on the drug chart. Mr Martin is now minimally responsive and unable to take oral medications, so it is no longer appropriate to prescribe any of his regular medications. Currently, he is prescribed PRN Oramorph for pain and breathlessness, and his family tell you he has been requiring 5 mg once or twice a day. In addition to prescribing specific medications it is worth considering non-pharmacological strategies that can help, for example simple interventions such as a fan are often very helpful.

Prescribing for breathlessness and excess secretions

In this scenario, subcutaneous preparations are appropriate as the patient is no longer able to take oral medications. Morphine is useful for both pain and breathlessness in this context (see Section Pain) (Booth and Dudgeon, 2006). In this case, Mr Martin has only required 5 mg Oramorph once or twice in a 24-hour period, and each dose is equivalent to 2.5 mg of subcutaneous morphine. Therefore, a starting dose of 2.5–5 mg morphine SC when required (up to 1 hourly) is appropriate. We are told that Mr Martin has normal renal function.

In this case, the patient has excess respiratory secretions. There are a number of antimuscarinic drugs that are widely used to manage respiratory secretions in palliative care, but are unlicensed for this purpose. Hyoscine butylbromide is usually the first-line option, although this depends upon local guidelines. Glycopyrronium bromide can be added if symptoms are not adequately controlled with hyoscine butylbromide.

AS REQUIRED MEDICATION					
DRUG MORPHINE SULPHATE IMMEDIATE RELEASE (IR)				Date	
				Time	
Dose 2.5 mg (TWO POINT FIVE MILLIGRAMS) - 5 mg (FIVE MILLIGRAMS) when required	Route SC	Max freq 1 - 2 hourly	Start date xx/xx/xx	Dose	
				Route	
Signature/Bleep A. Doctor		Max dose in 24 hrs	Review	Given	
				Check	
Additional instructions For pain or breathlessness					
DRUG HYOSCINE BUTYLBROMIDE				Date	
				Time	
Dose 20 mg when required	Route SC	Max freq TDS	Start date xx/xx/xx	Dose	
				Route	
Signature/Bleep A. Doctor		Max dose in 24 hrs	Review	Given	
				Check	
Additional instructions For respiratory secretions					

Hyoscine butylbromide: rationale and evidence

Hyoscine butylbromide is a useful drug to reduce respiratory secretions at the end of life, as it is widely available and does not cause unwanted sedation (it does not cross the blood–brain barrier) (Twycross *et al.*, 2014). It is usually given as an initial stat dose of 20 mg, and if it is effective, it can be given at a dose of 60–180 mg over 24 hours via a syringe driver.

🔍 Evidence

Use of antimuscarinic drugs for respiratory secretions at the end of life
A 2008 Cochrane review found no evidence to suggest that any intervention was better than placebo for the treatment of 'death rattle' at the end of life (Wee and Hillier, 2008). However, some studies have suggested that these drugs improve symptoms in up to 80% of patients (Bennett *et al.*, 2002). It is important to review the treatment used regularly, as there are a number of potential adverse effects including dry mouth and urinary retention (Wee and Hillier, 2008).

✓ DRUGS checklist for HYOSCINE BUTYLBROMIDE

Dose	20 mg
Route	Subcutaneous
Units	mg
Given	When required; if effective can be given at a dose of 60–180 mg over 24 hours via a syringe driver
Special situations	As with all antimuscarinic drugs, hyoscine butylbromide can cause dry mouth, urinary retention and constipation.

Hyoscine butylbromide: essential pharmacology

Hyoscine butylbromide is a peripherally acting antimuscarinic agent. As well as its use for respiratory secretions at the end of life, it is also used to treat pain and discomfort caused by abdominal colic, by reducing muscle spasms in the GI tract.

The onset of action of hyoscine butylbromide is from 15 to 30 minutes after administration. It does not cross the blood–brain barrier (unlike hyoscine hydrobromide) so does not cause central effects such as sedation or agitation.

Glycopyrronium: rationale and evidence

Another option for the management of respiratory secretions is glycopyrronium bromide.

AS REQUIRED MEDICATION						
DRUG					Date	
GLYCOPYRRONIUM BROMIDE					Time	
Dose 400 micrograms when required	Route SC	Max freq TDS		Start date xx/xx/xx	Dose	
Signature/Bleep A. Doctor		Max dose in 24 hrs		Review	Route	
					Given	
Additional instructions					Check	
For excess respiratory secretions						

🔍 Evidence

Which antimuscarinic is best?
There is a lack of evidence as to which antimuscarinic drug is most effective for treating respiratory secretions at the end of life (Spiller and Fallon, 2000; Lawry, 2005; Hugel *et al.*, 2006). Indeed, a review of the literature and a Cochrane review found no evidence that any of the commonly used agents (hyoscine butylbromide, hyoscine hydrobromide or glycopyrronium bromide) was more effective than the others (Wee and Hillier, 2008; Bennett *et al.*, 2002). There is some evidence to suggest that glycopyrronium has greater cardiovascular stability. Hyoscine hydrobromide crosses the blood–brain barrier and can cause confusion or even paradoxical agitation (Bennett *et al.*, 2002). These factors must be taken into account when choosing an appropriate antimuscarinic agent.

Initially, glycopyrronium bromide can be used as a subcutaneous injection. If the patient is requiring regular doses and the medication is having a clinical effect, then a syringe driver can be set up with a continuous administration of glycopyrronium.

✓ DRUGS checklist for GLYCOPYRRONIUM BROMIDE

Dose	200–400 micrograms
Route	Subcutaneous
Units	micrograms
Given	When required, maximum dose 1.2 mg in 24 hours
Special situations	Side effects may include dry mouth and urinary retention. Higher doses may result in bradycardia postdose.

Glycopyrronium: essential pharmacology

Glycopyrronium bromide acts by blocking muscarinic receptors, thereby inhibiting cholinergic transmission. It does not cross the blood–brain barrier, so has no central effects. At low doses, glycopyrronium reduces salivary secretions. Bronchial secretions are regulated by muscarinic and non-muscarinic pathways; therefore the clinical impact will be less than is seen with salivary secretions. Moreover, higher doses of glycopyrronium are required to reduce respiratory secretions compared with saliva.

The peak action of glycopyrronium when given subcutaneously occurs after 1–2 hours, in contrast to hyoscine butylbromide and hyoscine hydrobromide (15–30 minutes). However, glycopyrronium has a longer duration of action than these other two agents (the effect of hyoscine butylbromide lasts less than an hour, hyoscine hydrobromide lasts 2–3 hours and glycopyrronium up to 8 hours).

Other treatments used for breathlessness and increased secretions

Hyoscine hydrobromide crosses the blood–brain barrier and can cause sedation or paradoxical agitation. It is therefore used less frequently than hyoscine butylbromide or glycopyrronium.

Case outcome

Mr Martin required three PRN doses of 2.5 mg SC morphine and three PRN doses of 5 mg SC morphine over the next 24 hours (a total of 22.5 mg SC morphine). He had 20 mg hyoscine butylbromide

SC as an initial dose, and then a further dose 8 hours later. This improved his breathlessness and chest secretions. A syringe driver was set up containing 20 mg morphine and 60 mg hyoscine butylbromide. He died comfortably the next day.

REGULAR PRESCRIPTIONS						
DRUG HYOSCINE BUTYLBROMIDE					Date	
					Time	
Dose 60 mg over 24 hours	Route SC syringe driver	Max freq	Start date xx/xx/xx		Dose	
					Route	
Signature/Bleep A. Doctor		Max dose in 24 hrs	Review		Given	
					Check	
Additional instructions WITH						
DRUG MORPHINE SULPHATE					Date	
					Time	
Dose 20 mg (TWENTY MILLIGRAMS) over 24 hours	Route SC syringe driver	Max freq	Start date xx/xx/xx		Dose	
					Route	
Signature/Bleep A. Doctor		Max dose in 24 hrs	Review		Given	
					Check	
Additional instructions						

AS REQUIRED MEDICATION						
DRUG MORPHINE SULPHATE					Date	
					Time	
Dose 2.5 mg (TWO POINT FIVE MILLIGRAMS) - 5 mg (FIVE MILLIGRAMS) when required	Route SC	Max freq 1 - 2 hourly	Start date xx/xx/xx		Dose	
					Route	
Signature/Bleep A. Doctor		Max dose in 24 hrs	Review		Given	
					Check	
Additional instructions For pain or breathlessness						
DRUG HYOSCINE BUTYLBROMIDE					Date	
					Time	
Dose 20 mg	Route SC	Max freq	Start date xx/xx/xx		Dose	
					Route	
Signature/Bleep A. Doctor		Max dose in 24 hrs 180 mg (including syringe driver dose)	Review		Given	
					Check	
Additional instructions As required first line for excess respiratory secretions						

Common pitfalls

- It is important to remember that opioids have a key role to play in the management of breathlessness at the end of life.
- The choice of antimuscarinic for use to reduce respiratory secretions at the end of life will depend upon your local trust protocol.
- There is no definitive evidence to suggest that any antimuscarinic agent should is more efficacious than any other; in practice, hyoscine butylbromide is often chosen first line due to cost and availability.
- Always seek advice from your local palliative care team if you are unsure what to prescribe or if the patient's symptoms fail to improve with initial drug management.

Breathlessness and excess respiratory secretions are common problems amongst patients at the end of life, particularly amongst those with lung malignancy, chronic obstructive pulmonary disease (COPD) and heart failure. There are a number of pharmacological interventions that can be helpful. Options for the management of excess respiratory secretions include hyoscine butylbromide, glycopyrronium and hyoscine hydrobromide. Guidance from your local guidelines and palliative care team will help you decide which agent to use.

SUMMARY

🔑 Key learning points

- In patients with normal renal function and no other contraindications, morphine is the first-line drug of choice for the management of breathlessness.
- In opioid-naïve patients, the initial anticipatory dose of morphine is the same as that used for pain (1.25–2.5 mg SC when required, up to 1–2 hourly).
- Hyoscine butylbromide is a widely used first-choice antimuscarinic.
- Glycopyrronium bromide is often used second line if symptoms do not improve with hyoscine butylbromide.
- Hyoscine hydrobromide is less widely used as it can cross the blood–brain barrier and thus may cause sedation or, more worryingly, paradoxical agitation.

FURTHER READING

- A useful review of evidence and guideline for the use of antimuscarinic drugs at the end of life is: Bennett M, Lucas V, Brennan M *et al.* (2002). Using anti-muscarinic drugs in the management of death rattle: evidence-based guidelines for palliative care. *Palliat Med* 16: 369–74.
- For further information on the management of breathlessness and respiratory secretions at the end of life, see Twycross R, Wilcock A, Howard P (eds) (2014). *Palliative Care Formulary (PCF 5).* Available at: www.palliativedrugs.com.

Nausea and vomiting

Mary Jones

Age: 88

Hospital number: 123456

🔍 Case study

Presenting complaint: During an on-call ward cover shift you are asked to see Mary Jones, an

88-year-old woman with end-stage COPD, admitted with an infective exacerbation. She developed type 2 respiratory failure and had a trial of Bilevel Positive Airway Pressure (BIPAP), but continued to deteriorate despite optimal treatment. The decision has been made with the patient and family that BIPAP and antibiotics should be stopped, and she is to be kept comfortable. You are asked to review her as she is reporting nausea.

Allergies: *None known*

(Continued)

Case study (*Continued*)

Examination:

No routine observations being performed.
Bowels opened yesterday

RS: *Chest clear but reduced air entry bibasally*

Abdomen: *Soft and non-tender, bowel sounds present*
Alert but confused, GCS 14
Two × 1.25 mg and 5 × 2.5 mg PRN doses of SC
morphine were given in the last 24 hours (a total of
15 mg SC morphine, which is equivalent to 30 mg of
oral morphine).

REGULAR PRESCRIPTIONS

				Circle/enter times below ↓	⌐ Enter dates below			
					Day 1	Day 2	Day 3	Day 4
DRUG LAXIDO				06				
Dose 2	Route PO	Freq BD	Start date xx/xx/xx	⑧				
				12				
Signature A. Doctor		Bleep	Review	16				
Additional instructions				⑱				
				22				

AS REQUIRED MEDICATION

DRUG MORPHINE SULPHATE IMMEDIATE RELEASE (IR)				Date	xx/xx	xx/xx	xx/xx	xx/xx	xx/xx	xx/xx	xx/xx
				Time	08.00	10.00	12.00	14.00	16.00	18.00	20.00
Dose 1.25 mg (ONE POINT TWO FIVE MILLIGRAMS) - 2.5 mg (TWO POINT FIVE MILLIGRAMS) when required	Route SC	Max freq Hourly	Start date xx/xx/xx	Dose	1.25mg	1.25mg	2.5mg	2.5mg	2.5mg	2.5mg	2.5mg
				Route	SC	SC	SC	SC	SC	SC	SC
Signature/Bleep A. Doctor		Max dose in 24 hrs	Review	Given	A.D.	A.D.	A.D.	A.D.	A.D.	A.D.	A.D.
Additional instructions For pain or breathlessness				Check							

Initial measures

It is important to consider whether any current medications may be causing nausea and vomiting. Patients with underlying constipation can also suffer from nausea.

Prescribing for nausea and vomiting at the end of life

There are a number of possible mechanisms for nausea and vomiting amongst patients at the end of life. It is important to consider these, as the different antiemetics target different sites (Ang *et al.*, 2010). Therefore some antiemetics will be more appropriate for use in certain types of nausea and vomiting than others. For example, for nausea and vomiting secondary to an intra-abdominal cause resulting in gastric stasis, a prokinetic such as metoclopramide may be most appropriate. However, for a central cause, cyclizine or levomepromazine may be most appropriate. Ondansetron is useful for chemotherapy-induced nausea and vomiting (Hamling, 2011).

The antiemetic you prescribe will depend upon the above factors and also your local guidelines.

Initially, the drug can be given on an 'as required' basis, and if it is of benefit and is being required on a regular basis if can be given via a syringe driver over 24 hours.

In this case, assessment of the patient has suggested that the patient's nausea is opioid induced, and therefore you have chosen haloperidol as the first-line antiemetic of choice. It will be important to check the patient's eGFR as renal impairment can contribute to opioid-induced nausea (in this case the patient has normal renal function, with an eGFR >60). If her nausea does not settle with a regular antiemetic, it may be appropriate to switch to an alternative opioid.

AS REQUIRED MEDICATION

DRUG HALOPERIDOL				Date	
				Time	
Dose 1.5 mg when required	Route PO/SC	Max freq BD	Start date xx/xx/xx	Dose	
				Route	
Signature/Bleep A. Doctor		Max dose in 24 hrs	Review	Given	
Additional instructions For nausea and vomiting				Check	

Haloperidol: rationale and evidence

Haloperidol is the drug of choice for opioid-induced nausea. However, it may cause extrapyramidal side effects, particularly at higher doses, and should be avoided in patients with Parkinsonism.

Evidence

Which antiemetic to use at the end of life?
There is evidence to suggest that nausea is an extremely common symptom at the end of life, particularly amongst patients taking opioids; nausea and vomiting affects up to 30% of patients in this group (Mannix, 2006). There is insufficient evidence in the literature to advocate use of one particular antiemetic over another, and the choice of antiemetic will depend upon the cause of nausea and vomiting (Laugsand *et al.*, 2011; Glare *et al.*, 2011).

Guidelines

Management of opioid-induced nausea and vomiting in cancer patients: systematic review and evidence-based recommendations (Laugsand et al., 2011).

- This study reviewed the literature in an attempt to develop guidelines for the use of antiemetics in this population. However, the evidence reviewed was too weak to enable recommendation of one antiemetic in preference to another.
- The guideline does suggest that changing the opioid or route of administration can be helpful.

✓ DRUGS checklist for HALOPERIDOL

Dose	1.5 mg
Route	Subcutaneous or oral
Units	mg
Given	Up to twice daily as required initially. May also be used in a syringe driver over 24 hours, in this case the dose is 2.5 to 7.5 mg over 24 hours
Special situations	May cause extrapyramidal side effects, although this is rare at low doses. Should be avoided in patients with parkinsonism as it may worsen symptoms.

Haloperidol: essential pharmacology

Haloperidol is a pure dopamine D_2 antagonist, which has a profound inhibitory effect at the chemoreceptor trigger zone. At higher doses it has antipsychotic properties. It is therefore useful in the management of delirium in patients at the end of life. It is heavily protein bound and is metabolised via the liver.

Other treatments used for nausea and vomiting at the end of life

There are a number of other drugs used in the management of nausea and vomiting at the end of life. Here are some of the most common of those:

- Cyclizine acts at H_1 antihistamine receptors, and also has some anticholinergic action. It may be given orally, intravenously or subcutaneously at a dose of 50 mg 8-hourly/PRN where the cause of the nausea and vomiting is felt to be centrally mediated.
- Metoclopramide is a dopamine D_2 antagonist and prokinetic. It is therefore useful in gastric stasis but should be avoided in patients with intestinal obstruction. At higher doses (40–80 mg daily) it has activity at serotonergic receptors.
- Levomepromazine is a first-generation antipsychotic, which is used in palliative medicine for its antiemetic and/or antipsychotic properties. It can cause sedation, particularly at higher doses.
- Ondansetron is a $5HT_3$ antagonist. It is used to control postchemotherapy nausea and vomiting. However, prolonged use should be avoided as it causes significant constipation.

Case outcome

Mrs Jones required two 1.5-mg doses of haloperidol during a 24-hour period, which she was given SC as she was too drowsy to take oral medications. So a syringe driver was started with 3 mg haloperidol over 24 hours. Her nausea settled. Morphine was also added to the syringe driver for pain, at a dose of 10 mg over 24 hours. She was discharged home under a 'fast-track' process within 48 hours.

Remember that doses for controlled drugs must be written in words and figures, and the quantity to be supplied must be stated. In addition to the TTA, injectable medication charts were sent with the patient on discharge, with a dose range for morphine and haloperidol so the dose could be increased by the district nurses in the community as needed in consultation with the community palliative care team.

DISCHARGE MEDICATION

Date	Medication	Dose	Route	Frequency	Supply	GP to continue?
xx/xx/xx	HALOPERIDOL	3 mg	Subcutaneous	Over 24 hours via syringe driver	14 days	Y
xx/xx/xx	MORPHINE SULPHATE 10 mg/mL (TEN MILLIGRAMS PER MILLILITRE)	10 mg (TEN MILLIGRAMS)	Subcutaneous	Over 24 hours via syringe driver	Please supply 14 (FOURTEEN) x 1 mL (ONE MILLILITRE) ampoules	Y
xx/xx/xx	HALOPERIDOL (1st line antiemetic)	1.5 mg	Subcutaneous	As required up to a total dose of 7.5 mg in 24 hours, including CSCI dose	14 days	Y
xx/xx/xx	LEVOMEPROMAZINE (2nd line antiemetic)	6.25–12.5 mg	Subcutaneous	As required up to a total dose of 50 mg in 24 hours	14 days	Y
xx/xx/xx	MORPHINE SULPHATE 10 mg/mL (TEN MILLIGRAMS PER MILLILITRE)	1.25 mg (ONE POINT TWO FIVE MILLIGRAMS) to 2.5 mg (TWO POINT FIVE MILLIGRAMS)	Subcutaneous	As required up to 1–2 hourly for pain or breathlessness	Please supply 5 (FIVE) x 1 mL (ONE MILLILITRE) ampoules	Y

Notes to patient/GP:

Common pitfalls

- It is important to consider the cause of the nausea and vomiting, as the appropriate antiemetic will vary depending on the cause.
- Remember that nausea is a common side effect of opioids, so consider whether switching opioids or reducing the dose may be appropriate.
- Patients taking opioids should be prescribed PRN laxatives and antiemetics.
- Haloperidol, levomepromazine and metoclopramide all have central antidopaminergic side effects. Therefore, they should **not routinely be used in combination**. Moreover, these drugs may enhance the extrapyramidal side effects of other drugs, including selective serotonin reuptake inhibitors (SSRIs) and tricyclic antidepressants. They should be avoided in Parkinson's disease.
- The prokinetic mechanism of metoclopramide is partly cholinergic. Cyclizine has anticholinergic properties. Therefore best practice suggests that they should not be used in combination.

SUMMARY

Nausea and vomiting are common symptoms at the end of life, and the causation is often multifactorial. A range of antiemetics is available depending upon the cause. Your local guidelines and palliative care team will help you decide which agent to use.

Key learning points

- A careful assessment is required to establish the cause of nausea.
- Remember that opioids cause nausea in 30–50% of patients so a PRN antiemetic is required.
- The choice of antiemetic will depend upon the likely cause of the nausea and vomiting. Therefore careful assessment of the patient is crucial.
- Local guidelines vary according to which antiemetics are recommended.
- In some patients, more than one agent may be required.

FURTHER READING

- A useful review of evidence regarding management of opioid induced nausea and vomiting is: Laugsand EA, Kaasa S, Klepstad P (2011). Management of opioid-induced nausea and vomiting in cancer patients: systematic review and evidence-based recommendations. *Palliat Med* **25**: 442–53.
- For detailed information regarding the management of nausea and vomiting at the end of life, see Twycross R, Wilcock A, Howard P (eds) (2014). *Palliative Care Formulary* (PCF 5). Available at: www.palliativedrugs.com.

Agitation

Betty Baker

Age: 75

Hospital number: 123456

🔍 Case study

Presenting complaint: *You are asked to review a 75-year-old woman by nursing staff on an acute medical ward. The nursing staff tell you that she has metastatic breast cancer and is dying. You are told that she appears agitated.*

Allergies: *None known*

Examination:
RS: *Reduced air entry bibasally, but otherwise clear*
Abdomen: *Soft and non-tender, no palpable bladder, bowel sounds present*
GCS: *14*

No evidence of bony tenderness, calves soft and non-tender, pressure areas intact. Appears restless. No evidence of visual hallucinations or 'plucking' at objects.

AS REQUIRED MEDICATION									
DRUG MORPHINE SULPHATE				Date	xx/xx/xx	xx/xx/xx	xx/xx/xx	xx/xx/xx	
				Time	08.00	10.00	12.00	14.00	
Dose 1.25 mg (ONE POINT TWO FIVE MILLIGRAMS) - 2.5 mg (TWO POINT FIVE MILLIGRAMS) when required	Route SC	Max freq 1 - 2 hourly	Start date xx/xx/xx	Dose	1.25mg	1.25mg	2.5mg	2.5mg	
				Route	SC	SC	SC	SC	
Signature/Bleep A. Doctor		Max dose in 24 hrs	Review	Given	A.D.	A.D.	A.D.	A.D.	
				Check					
Additional instructions Two breakthrough doses of 1.25 mg SC and 2 doses of 2.5 mg SC given over the last 6 hours, with no effect on agitation									

Initial measures

It is important to perform a thorough assessment of the patient to ascertain if there is a specific reason why the patient is agitated. For example, the agitation may be related to pain or discomfort from bony metastases, or from urinary retention or a pressure ulcer. In this case, there do not seem to be any signs that the patient is in pain, and her agitation has persisted despite PRN morphine. The patient may have symptoms of nausea, vomiting or constipation that are causing distress. The symptoms may be side effects of medication or may be due to delirium secondary to sepsis, for example (Breitbart and Alici, 2008). In this case, the patient does not appear to be delirious (the pharmacological management of terminal agitation and delirium differ, see Section Other Treatments Used for Agitation at the End of Life).

It is important to note that for many patients, terminal agitation may to some extent be caused by emotional distress related to psychosocial factors or existential distress.

Once any treatable causes of agitation have been excluded, if the patient remains agitated, she is likely to require a sedative medication as her agitation is clearly causing distress to the patient and her family. This should be discussed with her family, and it is important to pay attention to environmental factors. In this case it would be appropriate to try and move the patient into a side-room if possible.

Prescribing for agitation at the end of life

Midazolam is the first-line treatment of choice for managing terminal agitation. In an elderly patient it can be given at an initial dose of 1.25–2.5 mg SC, and uptitrated according to the patient's response.

AS REQUIRED MEDICATION					
DRUG MIDAZOLAM				Date	
				Time	
Dose	Route	Max freq	Start date	Dose	
1.25 mg (ONE POINT TWO FIVE MILLIGRAMS) - 2.5 mg (TWO POINT FIVE MILLIGRAMS) when required	SC	1 -2 hourly	xx/xx/xx	Route	
Signature/Bleep A. Doctor		Max dose in 24 hrs	Review	Given	
				Check	
Additional instructions For agitation					

Midazolam: rationale and evidence

Midazolam is a benzodiazepine, which is widely used as the drug of choice for patients with agitation at the end of life.

 Guidelines

Terminal agitation

Guidelines from the European Association of Palliative Care (EAPC) set standards for the management of agitation at the end of life (Cherny *et al.*, 2009).

These guidelines describe a 10-item framework, which highlights the importance of discussion with patients and families, and careful assessment to exclude reversible causes of agitation.

✓ DRUGS checklist for MIDAZOLAM

Dose	1.25–2.5 mg
Route	Subcutaneous
Units	mg
Given	When required, maximum hourly. Depending on the patient's requirements, a syringe driver may be started with 5–30 mg midazolam over 24 hours

Special situations For some patients, midazolam may be insufficient to treat their symptoms of agitation. In this case, specialist input should be sought.

Midazolam: essential pharmacology

Midazolam is a short-acting benzodiazepine, which acts through enhancing the effect of the neurotransmitter GABA on GABA-A receptors. It is metabolised through cytochrome P-450 enzymes and glucuronide conjugation and is poorly absorbed orally. In addition to sedative properties, midazolam also has activity as an anticonvulsant.

Other treatments used for agitation at the end of life

- For patients with signs of delirium (including visual hallucinations, and 'plucking' at sheets or other objects), an antipsychotic agent such as haloperidol or levomepromazine should be used first line (Twycross *et al.*, 2014).
- If agitation persists despite appropriate doses of Midazolam, and Haloperidol or Levomepromazine given via continuous subcutaneous injection in a syringe driver, occasionally additional agents such as Phenobarbitone may be required. Specialist advice should be sought before such agents are used, and in cases of terminal agitation or delirium which do not respond to low doses of appropriate medication (De Graeff and Dean, 2007).

Case outcome

Mrs Baker required 2 × 1.25 mg SC midazolam and 3 × 2.5 mg doses of SC midazolam during a 24-hour period (a total dose of 10 mg SC midazolam). She also required 3 × 2.5 mg doses of SC morphine (a total of 7.5 mg SC morphine). She was commenced on a syringe driver with 7.5 mg midazolam and 5 mg SC morphine over 24 hours.

DISCHARGE MEDICATION

Date	Medication	Dose	Route	Frequency	Supply	GP to continue?
xx/xx/xx	MIDOLAZAM 5 mg/mL (FIVE MILLIGRAMS PER MILLILITRE)	20 mg (TWENTY MILLIGRAMS)	Subcutaneous	Over 24 hours via syringe driver	Please supply 28 (TWENTY-EIGHT) x 2 mL (TWO MILLILITRE) ampoules	Y
xx/xx/xx	MORPHINE SULPHATE 10 mg/mL (TEN MILLIGRAMS PER MILLILITRE)	10 mg (TEN MILLIGRAMS)	Subcutaneous	Over 24 hours via syringe driver	Please supply 14 (FOURTEEN) x 1 mL (ONE MILLILITRE) ampoules	Y
xx/xx/xx	MIDOLAZAM 1 mg/mL (ONE MILLIGRAM PER MILLILITRE)	2.5 mg (TWO POINT FIVE MILLIGRAMS) to 5 mg (FIVE MILLIGRAMS)	Subcutaneous	As required, up to 1–2 hourly for agitation	Please supply 15 (FIFTEEN) x 2 mL (TWO MILLILITRE) ampoules	Y
xx/xx/xx	MORPHINE SULPHATE 10 mg/mL (TEN MILLIGRAMS PER MILLILITRE)	1.25 mg (ONE POINT TWO FIVE MILLIGRAMS) to 2.5 mg (TWO POINT FIVE MILLIGRAMS)	Subcutaneous	As required, up to 1–2 hourly for pain or breathlessness	Please supply 5 (FIVE) x 1 mL (ONE MILLILITRE) ampoules	Y

Notes to patient/GP:

Over the next 72 hours, the doses were up-titrated according to symptoms and her use of PRN medications to 20 mg midazolam and 10 mg morphine via a syringe driver over 24 hours. She remained comfortable and was discharged home 2 days later. Remember that doses for controlled drugs must be written in words and figures, and the quantity to be supplied must be stated. In addition to the TTA, injectable medication charts were sent with the patient on discharge, with a dose range for morphine and midazolam so the dose could be increased as appropriate by community teams.

Common pitfalls

- A detailed, comprehensive assessment of the possible causes for agitation is crucial, including physical examination.
- Important causes of agitation include pain, urinary retention, constipation, nausea and vomiting, and existential distress. These causes should be considered and managed individually.
- An 'as required' dose of midazolam is often sufficient to reduce symptoms of agitation at the end of life. The dose can be uptitrated as required and given over 24 hours via a syringe driver.

SUMMARY

Terminal agitation is a common symptom at the end of life, which may have specific remediable causes.

🔑 Key learning points

- Agitation is a relatively common symptom at the end of life, which may have a range of causes including pain, urinary retention, constipation and existential distress.
- A holistic approach that assesses and takes account of psychosocial factors is key.
- Midazolam is the first-line drug of choice for the management of terminal agitation at the end of life.

(Continued)

> ### 🔑 Key learning points (*Continued*)
>
> - An antipsychotic (haloperidol or levomepromazine) should be used first line for patients with delirium at the end of life.
> - For patients who experience ongoing symptoms despite doses of haloperidol, levomepromazine or midazolam, specialist help should be sought and the patient should be reassessed to identify any additional causes of unresolved or worsening agitation.

FURTHER READING

- A useful review of evidence regarding terminal agitation is: Cherny NI, Radbruch L (2009). European Association for Palliative Care (EAPC) recommended framework for the use of sedation in palliative care. *Palliat Med* 23: 581–93.
- For up-to-date information regarding the management of terminal agitation and delirium at the end of life, please see Twycross R, Wilcock A, Howard P (eds) (2014). *Palliative Care Formulary* (PCF 5). Available at: www.palliativedrugs.com.

Now visit **www.wileyessential.com/pharmacology** to test yourself on this chapter.

References

Ang SK, Shoemaker LK, Davis MP (2010). Nausea and vomiting in advanced cancer. *Am J Hosp Palliat Care* 27: 219–25.

Bennett MI, Graham J, Schmidt-Hansen M *et al.* (2012). Prescribing strong opioids for pain in adult palliative care: summary of the NICE guidance. *BMJ* 344: e2806.

Bennett M, Lucas V, Brennan M *et al.* (2002). Using anti-muscarinic drugs in the management of death rattle: evidence-based guidelines for palliative care. *Palliat Med* 16: 369–74.

Booth S, Dudgeon D (eds) (2006). *Dyspnoea in Advanced Disease: a Guide to Clinical Management.* Oxford: Oxford University Press: 189–202.

Branford R, Droney J, Ross JR (2012). Opioid genetics: the key to personalized pain control? *Clin Genet* 82: 301–10.

Breitbart W, Alici Y (2008). Agitation and delirium at the end of life: 'we couldn't manage him'. *JAMA* 300: 2898–910.

Caraceni A, Pigni A, Brunelli C (2011). Is oral morphine still the first choice opioid for moderate to severe cancer pain? A systematic review within the European Palliative Care Research Collaborative guidelines project. *Palliat Med* 25: 402–9.

Care P (2001). Morphine and alternative opioids in cancer pain: the EAPC recommendations. *Br J Cancer* 84: 587–93.

Cherny NI, Radbruch L; Board of the European Association for Palliative Care (2009). European Association for Palliative Care (EAPC) recommended framework for the use of sedation in palliative care. *Palliat Med* 23: 581–93.

Dale O (2011). European palliative care research collaborative pain guidelines: opioid switching to improve analgesia or reduce side effects: a systematic review. *Palliat Med* 25: 494–503.

De Graeff A, Dean M (2007). Palliative sedation therapy in the last weeks of life: a literature review and recommendations for standards. *J Palliat Med* 10: 67–85.

Glare P, Miller J, Nikolova T *et al.* (2011). Treating nausea and vomiting in palliative care: a review. *Clin Interv Aging* 6: 243–59.

Hamling K (2011). The management of nausea and vomiting in advanced cancer. *Int J Palliat Nurs* 17: 321–7.

Hanks GW, de Conno F, Cherny N *et al.* (2001). Morphine and alternative opioids in cancer pain: the EAPC recommendations. *Br J Cancer* 84: 587–93.

Hugel H, Ellershaw J, Gambles M (2006). Respiratory tract secretions in the dying patient: a comparison between glycopyrronium and hyoscine hydrobromide. *J Palliat Med* 9: 279–84.

King S, Forbes K, Hanks GW *et al.* (2011). A systematic review of the use of opioid medication in those with moderate to severe cancer pain and renal impairment: a European Palliative Care Research Collaborative opioid guidelines project. *Palliat Med* 25: 525–52.

Laugsand EA, Kaasa S, Klepstad P (2011). Management of opioid-induced nausea and vomiting in cancer patients: systematic review and evidence-based recommendations. *Palliat Med* 25: 442–53.

Lawrey H (2005). Hyoscine vs glycopyrronium for drying respiratory secretions in dying patients. *Br J Community Nurs* 10: 421–6.

Mannix K (2006). Palliation of nausea and vomiting in malignancy. *Clin Med* 6: 144–7.

McQuay H (1999) Opioids in pain management. *Lancet* 353: 2229–32.

Mercadante S (2011). Conversion ratios for opioid switching in the treatment of cancer pain: a systematic review. *Palliat Med* 25: 504–15.

National Institute for Health and Care Excellence (NICE) (2012). *Palliative Care for Adults: Strong Opioids for Pain Relief*, CG140. Available at: www.nice.org.uk/guidance/cg140 (accessed Dec. 2015).

Spiller JA, Fallon M (2000). The use of Scopoderm in palliative care. *Hosp Med* 61: 782–4.

Twycross R, Wilcock A, Howard P (eds) (2014). *Palliative Care Formulary* (PCF 5). Available at: www.palliativedrugs.com.

Wee B, Hillier R (2008). Interventions for noisy breathing in patients near to death. *Cochrane Database Syst Rev* (1): CD005177.

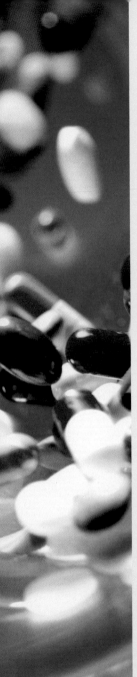

CHAPTER 10
Renal
Benedict Lyle Phillips

Key topics:

Learning objectives

By the end of this chapter you should…

- …understand that there are multiple mechanisms of acute kidney injury in an unwell patient.

- …be able to recognise common nephrotoxic drugs so that these can be withheld.

- …understand that investigations with intravenous contrast can be nephrotoxic, and how to minimise insult to the kidney.

- …be able to talk about the mechanisms of action of the key drugs that cause acute kidney injury.

- …be able to recognise and prescribe medications to treat hyperkalaemia.

Essential Practical Prescribing, First Edition. Georgia Woodfield, Benedict Lyle Phillips, Victoria Taylor, Amy Hawkins and Andrew Stanton. © 2016 by John Wiley & Sons, Ltd. Published 2016 by John Wiley & Sons, Ltd.

Acute kidney injury

Jeremy Sykes
Age: 79
Hospital number: 123456

 Case study

Presenting complaint: A 79-year-old man presents to accident and emergency with fever and rigors.

Background: This patient has had a 1-week history of dysuria and urinary frequency for which he first presented to his general practitioner. He was treated with a 5-day course of trimethoprim for a urinary tract infection. However, the patient continued to have fevers and rigors following completion of the antibiotics, and has presented to A&E. He has multiple comorbidities but is not known to have kidney disease.

PMH: Ischaemic heart disease – coronary artery stenting with drug-eluding stents 4 months ago.
Chronic obstructive pulmonary disease
Giant cell arteritis
Osteoarthritis
Hypertension
Hypercholesterolaemia

Regular medications: see FP10 form

Allergies: None

FH: Nil relevant

Social history: Ex-smoker 20 pack years

Examination, observations and investigations:
Weight 80 kg
CVS: Capillary refill time 3 seconds, pulse regular, HS I + II + 0
RS: Equal expansion with air entry to both bases and no added sounds
Abdo: Soft and non-tender. No masses or organomegaly
Dry mucosal surfaces, low JVP
Observations: Temp 38.0, BP 95/65, HR 90, Sats 90% room air

Blood tests: Hb 127 g/dL, WCC 20 $\times 10^9$/L, Neut 19 $\times 10^9$/L

| PHARMACY STAMP | AGE 79 | FORENAME, SURNAME Jeremy Sykes |
| | D.O.B. xx/xx/xxxx | ADDRESS Kingston Street NHS NUMBER |

TRIMETHOPRIM 200 mg twice daily
(5 day course recently finished).

ASPIRIN 75 mg once daily.

CLOPIDOGREL 75 mg once daily.

SALBUTAMOL INHALER 400 microgram as required, max four times daily.

BUDESONIDE INHALER 1 puff twice daily.

PREDNISOLONE 5 mg once daily.

IBUPROFEN 400 mg three times daily.

RAMIPRIL 10 mg once daily.

SIMVASTATIN 40 mg once nightly.

TRAMADOL 100 mg four times daily.

SIGNATURE OF PRESCRIBER   DATE

SP21000

Creatinine 210 micromole/L (baseline renal function dated 2 months earlier: creatinine 67 micromole/L)
Urea 20 mmol/L, eGFR 29 mL/min/1.73m^2, CRP 150 mg/L, K 4.5 mmol/L, Na 137 mmol/L

Diagnosis
Acute kidney injury (KDIGO Stage 3); sepsis of unknown origin.

Initial measures
Recognition of acute kidney injury (AKI) is an important first step. Failure to recognise AKI will prolong and potentially worsen the injury. In particular, identifying and reversing the cause of AKI is of utmost importance. Life-threatening complications of AKI include hyperkalaemia, pulmonary oedema and uraemia, and should be treated immediately.

Prescribing in acute kidney injury

Acute kidney injury (AKI) is a reversible decline in glomerular filtration rate (GFR), which results in an increase in serum creatinine, urea, potassium and other waste products that are normally excreted by the kidney. The Kidney Disease Improving Global Outcomes (KDIGO) group defines AKI as any of the following:

- Increase in serum creatinine by ≥26.5 micromole/L or more within 48 hours **or**
- Increase in serum creatinine to 1.5 times baseline or more within the last 7 days **or**
- Urine output less than 0.5 mL/kg/h for 6 hours.

The term AKI is preferentially being used instead of acute renal failure, as it is believed that the injury does not result in 'failure'. The term 'acute renal failure' should no longer be used.

In 2012, KDIGO published clinical guidance on AKI (Acute Kidney Injury Work Group, 2012). Within these guidelines, it was recommended that clinicians should use a staging system to quantify the severity of AKI (Table 10.1).

Initial measures in AKI are:

1. Management of life-threatening electrolyte and metabolic derangements. Life-threatening hyperkalaemia (>6.5 mmol/L but problems can occur >6.0 mmol/L) and severe metabolic acidosis (pH <7.1) are complications of AKI and should be treated immediately. Patients who do not respond to medical treatment of these complications may need urgent haemodialysis. For the treatment of hyperkalaemia see Section Hyperkalaemia.
2. Management of life-threatening pulmonary oedema.
3. Management of life-threatening uraemia, such as uraemic pericarditis or encephalopathy.

4. Assessment of fluid status:
   (a) Hypervolaemia: in AKI, the kidneys have an impaired ability to excrete water and sodium. This predisposes patients to fluid overload. This can be exacerbated confounded by overzealous IV fluid therapy.
   (b) Hypovolaemia: this can be a cause of prerenal AKI. IV fluid is used to normalise reduced intravascular circulating volume.
5. Nephrotoxicity: stop non-essential nephrotoxic medications, replacing these with non-nephrotoxic alternatives. Some medications may require drug level monitoring with dose adjustment accordingly.
6. Renal excretion: identify medications that are excreted by the kidney, and reduce the dose/stop them according to the degree of renal dysfunction.
7. Reversal of the cause of AKI (the list is not exhaustive but states the most common causes):
   (a) Acute prerenal disease
       i. Volume depletion from diarrhoea or unreplenished insensible losses
       ii. Circulatory shock (including sepsis)
       iii. Haemorrhage
       iv. Decompensated systolic heart failure
   (b) Acute intrinsic renal disease
       i. Acute interstitial nephritis (induced by nephrotoxic medications)
       ii. Acute tubular necrosis (ATN)
       iii. Acute nephrotic or nephritic syndrome (including glomerulonephritis, vasculitis and others)
   (c) Acute postrenal disease
       i. Obstructive nephropathy: obstruction to the flow of urine at any point from the renal pelvis to the urethra.

Table 10.1 KDIGO staging for AKI severity.

Stage	Serum creatinine	Urine output
1	1.5–1.9 times baseline in 48 hours or ≥26.5 micromol/L increase in 48 hours	<0.5 mL/kg/hour for 6 hours
2	2–2.9 times baseline in 48 hours	<0.5 mL/kg/hour for 6 hours
3	3 times baseline in 48 hours or Increase in serum creatinine to ≥354 micromol/L in 48 hours or Initiation of renal replacement therapy	<0.3mL/kg/hour for 24 hours or Anuria for >12 hours

Sepsis and hypoperfusion:
- Severe sepsis
- Haemorrhage
- Dehydration
- Cardiac failure
- Liver failure
- Renovascular insult

Toxicity:
- Nephrotoxic drugs
- Iodinated radiological contrast

Obstruction:
- Bladder outflow
- Stones
- Tumour
- Surgical ligation of ureters
- Extrinsic compression
- Retroperitoneal fibrosis

Parenchymal kidney disease:
- Glomerulonephritis
- Tubulointerstitial nephritis
- Rhabdomyolysis
- Haemolytic uraemic syndrome
- Myeloma kidney
- Malignant hypertension

Figure 10.1 STOP' AKI checklist of the important causes of AKI. The checklist acts as an aide memoire to junior doctors. Source: London AKI Network, 2015.

The traditional way of viewing the causes of AKI has been in the format of prerenal, renal and postrenal disease. A comprehensive checklist of the important causes of AKI is shown in Figure 10.1.

This patient has signs of sepsis, which may have caused AKI. In addition to investigating and treating AKI, the initial treatment should also include management of sepsis (see Box The Sepsis Six and Chapter 11).

The Sepsis Six

The surviving sepsis campaign has highlighted six key intervention in patients with sepsis:
1. Administration of high flow oxygen
2. Take blood cultures
3. Give broad-spectrum antibiotics
4. Give intravenous fluid challenges
5. Measure serum lactate and haemoglobin
6. Measure accurate hourly urine output

Nephrotoxicity: evidence and rationale

Nephrotoxicity is the poisonous effect of substances to the kidneys. In the context of AKI, this is commonly iatrogenic from the patient's own medications or new drug therapies initiated in hospital.

Acute kidney injury may occur due to a number of causes. Nephrotoxic drugs may be implicated as the primary insult, or may have acted as an exacerbating factor to another primary insult. Nevertheless, nephrotoxic drugs should be stopped in AKI. Some medications may require drug level monitoring with dose adjustment accordingly (see Box). In the context of AKI, drugs known to be nephrotoxic should be used only if absolutely essential, and only once a nephrologist has been consulted.

Drugs whose serum blood levels can be measured, and their dose adjusted in the context of renal dysfunction

(Ashley Currie, 2014)

Aciclovir	Dalteparin (antifactor Xa levels)	Phenytoin
Amikacin	Digoxin	Rifampicin
Aminophylline	Ethambutol	Sirolimus
Amiodarone	Everolimus	Streptomycin
ATG	Gentamicin	Tacrolimus
Bromocriptine	Lithium	Tobramycin
Ciclosporin	Methotrexate	Zidovudine

Drug-induced nephrotoxicity is an increasing problem, with medication being implicated as a primary cause in 20% of cases of AKI (Bellomo, 2006). This figure is even higher in the elderly population (Kohli *et al.*, 2000). This is due to the rising age of patients and the increasing number of comorbidities, resulting in rising problem of polypharmacy (Hoste and Kellum, 2006).

The most important strategy to prevent drug-induced renal injury is prevention(Schetz *et al.*, 2005). By identifying risk factors for AKI, nephrotoxicity may be prevented (see Box Patient-related Risk Factors for AKI.

Patient-related risk factors for AKI

- Intravascular volume depletion (diarrhoea, vomiting, increased insensible losses)
- Age >60 years
- Diabetes mellitus
- Reduced intravascular circulating volume (heart failure, nephrotic syndrome, liver failure)
- Sepsis
- Severe hypercalcaemia (which causes direct toxicity, renal arteriole vasoconstriction and volume depletion)
- Underlying chronic kidney disease (eGFR <60, stage 3 or more)
- Proteinuria (with otherwise normal eGFR)

Contrast-induced nephropathy (CIN) is defined as the impairment of renal function following IV contrast. CIN is measured as either a 25% increase in serum creatinine from baseline or 44.2 micromol/L increase in absolute value within 48–72 hours of the introduction of IV contrast. CIN has been reported to be the third most common cause of AKI in patients who are admitted into hospital (Hou *et al.*, 1983). This is mainly in the context of intra-arterial contrast media, used in percutaneous angiography (such as coronary angiography), or intravenous contrast, used in computed tomography (CT) scans (Clec'h *et al.*, 2013). This risk of CIN is higher when using iodine contrast of high osmolarity.

The most important risk factors for contrast-induced nephropathy are:

- Estimated glomerular filtration rate (eGFR) <60 mL/min/1.73m^2
- Concomitant AKI
- Diabetes mellitus, metformin use
- Volume depletion
- Use of diuretics

When ordering a CT scan it is important to consider whether IV contrast is required. The purpose of IV contrast is to enhance the visibility of bleeding, blood vessels and intravisceral pathology. You must ask yourself whether the pathology that you are most concerned about will be detected without the need for contrast. The radiology department should also advise you on the need for contrast in detecting suspected pathology. Common examples of CT scans which do **not** require IV contrast are:

- CT kidney ureter bladder (CT KUB)
- CT brain, in the context of head injury, stroke or intracerebral haemorrhage
- CT spine.

There is no specific treatment for contrast-induced nephropathy once AKI has developed. First and foremost, avoid the use of iodine-based contrast (Briguori *et al.*, 2011). Magnetic resonance imaging (MRI) does not use iodised-contrast. Instead it uses gadolinium-contrast which is significantly less nephrotoxic. Alternatively, CT scans can sometimes be performed with carbon dioxide contrast (either alone, or with a small amount of IV contrast), mainly in vascular imaging in the form of digital subtraction angiography (which is used in the investigation of peripheral vascular disease). However, if IV iodine-based contrast is required, there is a strategy to reduce the risk of AKI:

- IV sodium chloride infusion (to keep the patient euvolaemic); 1 mL/kg/h of 0.9% saline is given 12 hours before and after the IV contrast is administered (depending on volume status). Maintaining good intravascular filling is fundamentally important (Trivedi *et al.*, 2003).
- Stop non-essential nephrotoxic medications temporarily, such as diuretics. Also consider stopping angiotensin-converting inhibitors and angiotensin-receptor blockers.
- Stop metformin due to the risk of lactic acidosis (though there is weak evidence supporting this).
- Consider *N*-acetylcysteine (NAC) before and after the scan, though there is no evidence supporting this practice.
- Consider IV sodium bicarbonate infusion (discuss with nephrology doctor).
- Monitor creatinine and urea 72 hours following IV contrast, and alter doses of renally excreted medications accordingly.
- If IV contrast is given in the context of an outpatient CT scan, the general practitioner should be asked to check renal function blood tests 72 hours after IV contrast administration.

IV fluid therapy with isotonic saline (0.9% sodium chlorine) has been shown to reduce the incidence of contrast-induced nephropathy, especially in diabetic patients (Mueller *et al.*, 2002). Most patients who undergo CT scans with IV contrast are outpatients, and do not get IV fluid replacement. These patient's should maximise their oral fluid intake before and after the scan.

N-acetylcysteine (NAC) is a thiol compound with vasodilatory and antioxidant effects. Anecdotally, NAC may help to reduce the intraglomerular vasoconstriction and oxygen free-radical generation caused by IV iodised contrast. However, there is heterogeneity in the result from individual studies, and contradictions between meta-analyses (Kshirsagar *et al.*, 2004; Fishbane, 2008). Never the less, given that NAC does not show any significant adverse effects, and is inexpensive, the KDIGO guidelines 2012 support its use in the prevention of contrast-induced nephropathy(Acute Kidney Injury Work Group, 2012).

There are some instances where the nephrotoxic medication is deemed essential to the patient's survival, and that renal dysfunction is a predictable complication. In these rare instances, the necessary supportive measures should be put in place support the patient's renal function. A common example of this is in the intensive care setting. In severe life-threatening sepsis, nephrotoxic antimicrobial agents may be continued despite their insult on the kidneys, at adjusted doses. However, in most contexts outside the intensive care unit, nephrotoxic medications should be stopped, and replaced with a non-nephrotoxic alternative if possible. A multidisciplinary team approach in this setting is strongly advised.

 Guidelines

The London AKI network has published a useful guideline on avoiding contrast-induced nephropathy (CIN). The guideline supports the use of CIN prophylaxis in patients who:

- Require high volume (>100 mL) iodine-based contrast
- Have chronic kidney disease with eGFR <60 mL/min/1.73m^2 (especially those with diabetes or AKI)

The London AKI network advices the use of 0.9% saline 1 mL/kg/h for 12 hours before and after contrast administration.

IV sodium bicarbonate 1.26% is also used, but should be discussed with a nephrologist.

The London AKI network does not find sufficient evidence to support the stopping of metformin or ACE inhibitors.

The full guideline is available at: www.londonaki.net/downloads/LondonAKInetwork-ContrastInducedNephropathyProphylaxis.pdf

---

[TOP TIP] Preventing drug-induced nephrotoxicity

1. Check the patient's renal function before prescribing any nephrotoxic drugs.
2. When ordering investigations, consider whether you need IV contrast or not.
3. If patients have risk factors for contrast-induced nephropathy, consider alternative imaging such as MRI (gadolinium contrast is much less nephrotoxic than iodine contrast) or ultrasound.
4. If nephrotoxic medications are essential, ensure that patients remain euvolaemic with IV fluid and *N*-acetylcysteine (though the latter is lacking in evidence).
5. Consult the *British National Formulary* (BNF) (BMA/RPS, 2015) or ask a nephrologist for advice.

A nephrologist must be consulted prior to giving nephrotoxic or renally excreted medications to patients in end-stage renal disease (ESRD), even if they have already been established on renal replacement therapy. Likewise, a nephrologist must be consulted prior to considering IV iodine-based contrast in ESRD. Patients in ESRD should be given gadolinium contrast with extreme caution, as they may develop a rare condition called nephrogenic systemic fibrosis (NSF).

 Guidelines

Management of AKI –The Four Ms
AKI is often predictable and preventable. However, AKI continues to be recognised late. The Four M's, devised by the London AKI network, may be used as a way of remembering key steps in the management of AKI.

Monitor patient: Observations and EWS, regular blood tests, pathology alerts, fluid charts, urine volumes)

(Continued)

Guidelines (*Continued*)

Maintain circulation: Hydration, resuscitation, oxygenation)

Minimise kidney insults: Nephrotoxic medications, surgery or high risk interventions, iodinated contrast and prophylaxis, hospital acquired infection)

Manage the acute illness: Sepsis, heart failure, liver failure

(London AKI network, 2015. *London AKI Network Manual*. Available at: http://londonaki. net/downloads/LondonAKInetwork-Manual.pdf (accessed May 2015)).

 Evidence

Gadolinium contrast in patients with end stage renal disease

Contrast medium used in magnetic resonance imaging (MRI) is associated with a rare condition called nephrogenic systemic fibrosis (NSF), in patients in ESRD. A case–control study involving 565 participants showed that exposure of gadolinium to patients in ESRD is associated with NSF. The risk of NSF is highest among patients already on dialysis. NSF is a rare condition, so if MRI with gadolinium is indicated, discuss with a nephrologist (Elmholdt *et al.*, 2011).

Guidelines

- NICE has published a useful guideline on Acute Kidney Injury: Prevention, detection and management of acute kidney injury up to the point of renal replacement therapy, CG169, 2013. Available at:www. nice.org.uk/guidance/cg169 (accessed Dec. 2015).
- The Renal Association has published a useful guideline on acute kidney injury (Lewington and Kanagasundaram, 2011). Available at: www.renal.org/guidelines/ modules/acute-kidney-injury (accessed Dec. 2015).

Nephrotoxicity: essential pharmacology

In order to avoid inadvertent drug-induced nephrotoxicity, the prescriber must be aware of the pathogenic mechanisms of renal injury, as well as patient and medication-related risk factors for renal injury.

There are a number of pathways by which the medications that we prescribe can cause renal injury. Furthermore, medications can cause this nephrotoxicity through one or multiple modes.

1. **Interstitial nephritis**: this is inflammatory infiltration of the renal interstitium. This can be acute or chronic. Acute interstitial nephritis (AIN) is most commonly caused by drugs, and can be seen as a type of allergic reaction. Aside from drugs, AIN may also be caused by autoimmune or infective conditions.
   Examples: penicillins, cephalosporins, sulfonamides, thiazide diuretics, furosemide, NSAIDs and rifampicin.

2. **Glomerulonephritis**: this is inflammatory infiltration affecting the glomerulus. Whilst glomerulonephritis is usually associated with primary nephrotic and nephritic syndromes, certain medications may cause a secondary glomerulonephritis as well.
   Examples: penicillamine, gold, captopril, phenytoin, penicillins, sulphonamides, rifampicin.

3. **Altered intraglomerular haemodynamics**: this mechanism of action results in loss of vasodilatation of either the afferent arterioles, prior to entering the glomerulus, or the efferent arterioles, after leaving the glomerulus. Altered blood flow through the glomerulus causes ischaemia.
   Examples: angiotensin-converting enzyme inhibitors and NSAIDs.

4. **Direct tubular cell toxicity**: this is a subtype of acute tubular necrosis that causes proximal tubular epithelium necrosis. Other parts of the tubule may also be injured.
   Examples: aminoglycosides (like gentamicin), ciclosporin, amphotericin tenofovir (proximal tubular injury) and cisplatin (diffuse tubular injury).

5. **Rhabdomyolysis**: this is the destruction of skeletal muscle cells, resulting in a toxic release of muscle cell-containing substances, including creatine kinase, myoglobin and electrolytes. Myoglobin is directly toxic to the kidney (Bosch *et al.*, 2009).
   Examples: statins, selective serotonin reuptake inhibitors, zidovudine, colchicine, lithium, methadone. Also illicit drugs such as heroin, cocaine, amphetamines and D-lysergic acid diethylamide (LSD).

6. **Crystal nephropathy**: certain medications can precipitate within the renal tubules to form crystals which cause damage to the tubules (Yarlagadda and Perazella, 2008).
   Examples: aciclovir, sulphonamide antibiotics, methotrexate, protease inhibitors.

7. **Thrombotic microangiopathy**: this microvascular injury due to arteriolar and capillary thrombosis (George and Nester, 2014).
   Examples: mitomycin-C, ciclosporin, quinine, and ticlopidine.

There are a large number of medications that are nephrotoxic. This chapter will focus on those nephrotoxic medications that junior doctors are likely to encounter. For a complete list of nephrotoxic medications with clinical advice, look at the Further Reading section.

Renally excreted medications: rationale and evidence

Renal dysfunction results in the reduced excretion of waste products into urine. This explains why urea, creatinine and potassium excretion falls in renal dysfunction. Renally excreted medications also accumulate in systemic circulation in the presence of renal failure. It is for this reason that drugs that are renally excreted should either be reduced in dose or stopped completely. This is because medications may be toxic if allowed to accumulate. Many renally excreted drugs are nephrotoxic, others may be hepatotoxic or ototoxic.

Renally excreted drugs should be dosed according to the glomerular filtration rate. This is so that the reduced excretion of drugs is matched with a reduced dosage. In basic terms, if the plug hole of a bath is draining slower, then the amount of water entering the bath should be reduced in order to avoid the bath overflowing.

For advice regarding specific renally excreted medications, consult the *Renal Drug Handbook* (Ashley, and Currie, 2014).

Commonly prescribed renally excreted medications

- Antibiotics:
  - Penicillins
  - Cephalosporins
  - Aminoglycosides
  - Tetracycline
- Beta-blockers
- Diuretics
- ACEIs
- ARBs
- Metformin
- NSAIDs
- Lithium
- Digoxin
- Opioids
- Procainamide
- Ranitidine, cimetidine

Medications that should not be started in AKI are listed in Table 10.2.

Renally excreted medications: essential pharmacology

The kidneys excrete a number of water-soluble substances to produce urine. They kidneys also act as the principle organs in the excretion of medications.

Plasma, from blood, reaching the glomerulus in the nephron is filtered through pores in the glomerular epithelium. Water and electrolytes are actively and passively absorbed from the renal tubules back into circulation. However, many drug metabolites are ionised molecules. These cannot diffuse through the renal tubules back into circulation. Instead they remain within the tubules and are excreted in urine.

Table 10.2 Medications that should NOT be started in AKI.

Drug	Problem	Replace it with...
ACE Inhibitors	Antagonises ACE action, vasodilating the efferent arterioles of the glomeruli and thereby decreasing GFR	Depends on situation and indication- could give another antihypertensive without renal effects e.g. beta blocker (but be aware that these can also accumulate)
Metformin	Causes lactic acidosis in AKI	Consider insulin sliding scale, if BMs are high
Gentamicin	Well known to cause renal toxicity, will worsen AKI of any cause	Consider different antibiotic, seek micro advice, reduce dose, check levels if already given
Antihypertensives- if the AKI is pre- renal in origin	If dehydration and hypotension have caused AKI, do not give drugs that will further lower BP	Withhold all antihypertensives until BP and renal function recover
Digoxin	Digoxin is renally excreted and has a narrow therapeutic margin = risk of digoxin toxicity in AKI	Check digoxin levels. Omit or reduce dose until AKI recovered.
NSAIDs	NSAIDS inhibit the enzyme cyclooxygenase (COX) and therefore reduce the production of prostaglandins to decrease pain. However, prostaglandins also act in the glomerulus by causing vasodilatation of the afferent arteriole. NSAIDS therefore inhibit afferent arteriole vasodilatation, causing renal ischaemia	Another form of analgesia such as paracetamol, codeine, opioids (low dose as will accumulate in renal failure) or a topical opioids such as fentanyl patch which is not renally excreted.

However, not all drug metabolites are renally excreted. There are three ways in which drug metabolites may evade being excreted by the kidneys:

1. Drug metabolites that bind to plasma proteins are not filtered through the glomerular epithelium and remain in circulation.
2. Unionised drug metabolites are filtered by the glomerulus into the renal tubules, but may passively diffuse back into circulation.
3. Certain drug metabolites have transportation systems within the renal tubules that actively reabsorb these molecules back into circulation, such as dextrose, vitamin C and B vitamins.

Urine pH has an important influence on drug reabsorption and excretion. Urine pH, which varies from 4.5 to 8.0, determines the ionised state of weak acids and bases:

- Acidic urine: increases reabsorption and decreases excretion
- Alkaline urine: decreases reabsorption and increases excretion.

Case outcome and discharge

Jeremy Sykes was rapidly identified as a patient with two life-threatening conditions: acute kidney injury and sepsis.

The patient was treated for sepsis:

- High-flow oxygen was started: 15 L/min via non-rebreathe mask. This was changed within 30 minutes to controlled oxygen delivery due to the patient's chronic obstructive pulmonary disease (COPD). Oxygen was delivered via a Venturi mask 24%.
- Blood cultures were taken.
- IV antibiotics were started.
- Serum lactate was checked and found to be 3.0 mmol/L. This reduced to 2.0 mmol/L following IV fluid therapy.
- Urine output was monitored accurately and documented in the bedside notes.

Antibiotic therapy was determined by local microbiology guidelines.

Acute kidney injury was initially treated by gaining IV access and starting IV fluids. His urine output was monitored with a urinary catheter. He was clinically found to be volume deplete – IV fluid therapy was titrated to a urine output of 0.5 mL/kg/h.

The IV fluid was administered according to the NICE guidelines (NICE, 2013). The fluid of choice should be any crystalloid with a sodium concentration of 130–154 mmol/L. This means that either Hartmann's solution or 0.9% sodium chloride could be used. Colloids are no longer recommended as resuscitation fluids (Perel and Roberts, 2013).

 Evidence

Choice of IV fluid in resuscitation
In 2013, the Cochrane Library performed a meta-analysis of 74 trials comparing crystalloid and colloid fluids in critically unwell patients requiring fluid resuscitation. The authors state that 'there is no evidence from randomised controlled trials that resuscitation with colloids reduces the risk of death, compared to resuscitation with crystalloids, in patients with trauma, burns or following surgery' (Perel and Roberts, 2013).

The patient was on a number of regular medications, some of which were identified as nephrotoxic or renally excreted. The admitting medical team informed the on-call nephrology registrar of the patient's admission into hospital. The nephrology team provided advice regarding the management of AKI over the phone, and saw the patient on their ward round. Management of the patient's medications is summarised in Table 10.3.

Table 10.3 Management of medications for the example acute kidney injury case.

Patient's regular medication	Action taken by admitting medical team
Trimethoprim 200mg BD	This is not nephrotoxic. However, it has an interesting effect on the renal tubules. It causes inhibition of the tubular secretion of creatinine. This increases serum creatinine, but not as a result of renal injury. A recent course of trimethoprim may have increased the patient's serum creatinine but has not caused renal injury. Nonetheless, trimethoprim may increase serum potassium levels by acting as a potassium sparing diuretic, and should therefore be stopped.
Clopidogrel 75mg OD	Drug continued, as drug eluding stent inserted <6 months ago
Budesonide inhaler 1 puff BD	Drug continued
Ibuprofen 400mg TDS	Nephrotoxic: drug stopped
Simvastatin 40mg ON	Nephrotoxic: drug stopped
Aspirin 75mg OD	Drug continued, as drug eluding stent inserted <6 months ago
Salbutamol inhaler 400microgram PRN, max QDS	Drug continued
Prednisolone 5mg OD	Dose doubled in the context of acute illness, to avoid Addisonian Crisis
Ramipril 10mg OD	Nephrotoxic: drug stopped. Blood pressure monitored.
Tramadol 100mg QDS	Renally excreted: dose reduced to 50mg TDS

DISCHARGE MEDICATION

Date	Medication	Dose	Route	Frequency	Supply	GP to continue?
xx/xx/xx	ASPIRIN	75 mg	PO	Once daily	14 days	Y
xx/xx/xx	CLOPIDOGREL	75 mg	PO	Once daily	14 days	Y
xx/xx/xx	SALBUTAMOL INHALER 400 micrograms	2 puffs	INH	As required, maximum four times daily	14 days	Y
xx/xx/xx	BUDESONIDE INHALER	1 puff	INH	Twice daily	14 days	Y
xx/xx/xx	PREDNISOLONE	10 mg	PO	Once daily	For one week then reduce back to 5 mg once daily	Y
xx/xx/xx	TRAMADOL	50 mg	INH	As required, maximum four times daily	14 days	Y

Notes to patient/GP:

Common pitfalls

- Inadvertent prescription of nephrogenic or renally excreted medications without checking patients' renal function first.
- Failure to withhold nephrotoxic medications that the patient was already taking.
- Inappropriate use of IV contrast in CT scans.
- Failure to identify alternatives to CT scans with IV contrast, such as alternative contrast (CO_2) or alternative imaging (MRI, ultrasound).
- Failure to gain advice from nephrologist prior to giving patients nephrotoxic drugs in the context on AKI or chronic renal impairment.

SUMMARY

Nephrotoxic and renally excreted drugs should be used with caution. It is important to check patients' renal function prior to delivering these medications. The list of nephrotoxic and renally excreted medications is long, and the specific advice of stopping or altering dosage can be sought in the *Renal Drug Handbook* (Ashley and Currie, 2014). The 'STOP' AKI checklist helps doctors to consider the important causes of AKI. However, the best treatment remains prevention. Consider the four Ms in preventing AKI in patients (Monitor patient, Maintain circulation, Minimise kidney insult, Manage the acute illness).

IV contrast is an important cause of AKI. However, junior doctors should understand that not all IV contrast is nephrotoxic. Iodine-based contrast, which is mainly used for CT scans, is the main nephrotoxic contrast medium. Gadolinium-based contrast is much less nephrotoxic and is used in MRI. This can be used as an alternative imaging modality to CT in patients who required contrast-enhanced imaging. Ultrasound is another alternative that does not require a contrast medium.

🔑 Key learning points

Acute kidney injury (AKI)
- KDIGO defines AKI as
  - Increase in serum creatinine by ≥26.5 micro mol/L or more within 48 hours **or**
  - Increase in serum creatinine to 1.5 times baseline or more within the last 7 days **or**
  - Urine output less than 0.5 mL/kg/h for 6 hours.
- AKI is caused by numerous factors (easily remembered as the 'STOP' AKI checklist)
  - Sepsis and hypoperfusion
  - Toxicity
  - Obstruction
  - Parenchymal kidney disease.

Use the 'STOP' AKI checklist as an aide memoire of the important causes of AKI that should be urgently reversed.
- Prevention is the best treatment. Consider the four Ms.
- AKI causing hyperkaemia or acidosis may require resolution using haemofiltration/ dialysis if not responding to fluid challenges and other medical measures.
- Always assess the risk of contrast-induced nephropathy when using IV iodine-based contrast.

FURTHER READING

- Acute Kidney Injury Work Group (2012). Kidney Disease: Improving Global Outcomes (KDIGO) - Clinical Practice Guideline for Acute Kidney Injury. *Kidney Int* 2: 1–138.
- London AKI Network (2015). *'STOP AKI' and Checklist.* Available at: www.londonaki.net/downloads/LondonAKInetwork-STOPAKIchecklist.pdf (accessed May 2015).
- London AKI Network (2015). *London AKI Network Manual.* Available at: londonaki.net/downloads/LondonAKInetwork-Manual.pdf (accessed May 2015).
- NICE (2013). *Acute Kidney Injury: Prevention, Detection and Management of Acute Kidney Injury up to the Point of Renal Replacement Therapy*, CG169. Available at: www.nice.org.uk/guidance/cg169 (accessed May 2015).
- Ashley C, Currie A (2014). *Renal Drug Handbook: The Ultimate Prescribing Guide for Renal Practitioners*, 4th edn. Radcliffe Publishing, London.

Hyperkalaemia

Jane Tenette

Age: 61

Hospital number: 123456

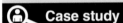 **Case study**

Presenting complaint: *A 61-year-old woman presents to accident and emergency with haematuria*

Background: *This woman, who is under investigation for hypertension by her GP, presents to the hospital with a 1-week history of macroscopic haematuria. She has also noted oedema of her legs.*

PMH: *Recent throat infection 3 weeks ago*

Regular medications: *None*

Allergies: *None*

FH: *Nil relevant*

Social history: *Smoker 4/day*

Examination, observations and tests:
Weight 66 kg

CVS: Capillary refill time 3 seconds, pulse regular, HS I + II + 0 .
RS: Bibasal crepitations
Abdo: Soft and non-tender. No masses or organomegaly

Observations: *Temp 37.0, BP 180/90, HR 80, Sats 99% room air*

ECG *(Figure 10.2) Tall tented T waves leads I, II, V_2–V_5*

Blood tests: *Hb 127 g/dL, WCC 4.0 × 10^9/L, Neut 4.0 × 10^9/L, Na 137 mmol/L, K^+ 7.0 mmol/L Creatinine 250 micromol/L (baseline renal function dated 2 months earlier: creatinine 71 micromol/L) Urea 31 mmol/L, eGFR 17 mL/min/1.73m^2 , CRP 15 mg/L*

Diagnosis
Hyperkalaemia; acute kidney injury (KDIGO stage 3); possible poststreptococcal glomerulonephritis.

Initial measures
Hyperkalaemia is defined as a serum potassium of greater than 5.5 mmol/L (Chapagain and Ashman, 2012). However, the threshold for urgent inpatient treatment is:

- Potassium >6.0 mmol/L with ECG changes

(Continued)

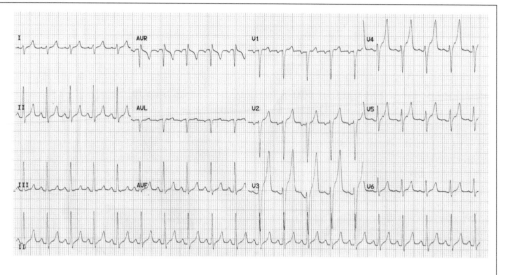

Figure 10.2 Electrocardiogram showing tall tented T waves in leads I, II, V₂–V₅. This is suggestive of dangerous hyperkalaemia.

Case study (*Continued*)

- Potassium >6.5 mmol/L with or without ECG changes (Mount, 2015).

  Hyperkalaemia is a life-threatening emergency. Therefore the initial measure in this case is to treat the hyperkalaemia. The specific treatment and investigation of AKI should wait until after serum potassium is corrected, although general resuscitation of the patient will of course be ongoing.

  The patient should be moved to an area with cardiac monitoring, such as the resuscitation room or acute medical unit. A 12-lead ECG should be urgently arranged to establish whether there is cardiac destabilisation.

  The patient also has AKI, which should also be urgently managed (see Section Acute Kidney Injury).

Prescribing for hyperkalaemia

The complications of hyperkalaemia are ascending muscle weakness, paralysis, cardiac arrhythmias and death. Prior to these life-threatening complications, patients may remain entirely asymptomatic. Hyperkalaemia therefore remains silent, but soon manifests as a periarrest situation. Prevention is the most important treatment. However, patients with hyperkalaemia may be treated acutely with a combination of drugs.

ECG changes consistent with hyperkalaemia are tall tented T waves. P waves flatten and then disappear altogether. There may be progressive lengthening of the PR interval. Some patients also develop a bundle branch block or advanced atrioventricular block. Any brady- or tachyarrhythmia may be caused by underlying hyperkalaemia. These changes indicate cardiac instability, and warrant immediate attention.

The treatment of hyperkalaemia should be initiated in the following order.

1. Patient moved to an area with cardiac monitoring (resuscitation room, acute medical unit)
2. 12-lead ECG:
   (a) ECG changes consistent with hyperkalaemia: urgent treatment with intravenous 10% calcium gluconate. This should be delivered as 1–10 ml, in 1-ml aliquots until there is 'cardiac stabilisation' (ECG changes normalise).
   (b) Normal ECG: continue treatment below. Calcium gluconate should not be given to patients who do not show evidence of ECG changes consistent with hyperkalaemia.

3. Intravenous insulin and 50% dextrose infusion. Following insulin/dextrose, a 5% dextrose infusion is recommended in order to avoid hypoglycaemia.
4. Nebulised salbutamol 5 mg.
5. Stop drugs that cause hyperkalaemia.
6. Reverse any medical conditions that cause hyperkalaemia.
7. Repeat serum potassium within 4 hours to ensure resolution. Repeat the above if potassium remains raised.
8. Haemodialysis is indicated if patients are:
   (a) Already established on haemodialysis
   (b) In ESRD and do not produce urine
   (c) In refractory hyperkalaemia that does not respond to the medical treatment detailed above.
9. Long-term: low potassium diet (0–2 g daily).

ONCE ONLY PRESCRIPTIONS							
Date	Time to be given	DRUG	Dose	Route	Time	Prescriber	
						Signature	Bleep
xx/xx/xx	xx:xx	CALCIUM GLUCONATE 10%	10 ml	IV	Over 10 minutes	A. Doctor	
xx/xx/xx	xx:xx	SALBUTAMOL	5 mg	NEB	STAT	A. Doctor	

FLUID CHART							
Date	Infusion fluid			Drug to be added		Signature	Print name
	Name and strength	Volume	Rate	Approved name	Dose		
xx/xx/xx	50% DEXTROSE	50 ml	Over 30 minutes	ACTRAPID INSULIN	10 units	A. Doctor	A. Doctor

Although acute and chronic renal dysfunction are common causes of hyperkalaemia, as excretion of potassium is impaired in these conditions, disorders and medications affecting the renin-angiotensin system may also cause hyperkalaemia.

Potassium (K^+) is an intracellular anion. An increase in extracellular potassium makes the resting potential across cell membranes less electronegative, and partly depolarises the cell membrane. A less-negative cell membrane requires a smaller depolarising stimulus to generate an action potential. In simpler terms, the cell membrane becomes temporarily more excitable (Kalra et al., 1999). However, persistent depolarisation causes sodium channels in the cell membrane to deactivate, which decreases cell membrane excitability.

It is cardiac and skeletal muscle that is most sensitive to an increase in extracellular potassium. In the heart, decreased cell membrane excitability results in impaired cardiac conduction. This may cause cardiac arrhythmias which are life-threatening. The more rapid the increase in serum potassium, the greater the cardiac toxicity (Paice et al., 1983). This explains why patients with chronically high potassium may be more tolerant of hyperkalaemia, whilst others develop ECG changes sooner.

The rational of the treatment regimen in hyperkalaemia is threefold:
1. Stabilise the myocardium
2. Encourage extracellular potassium to enter the intracellular space
3. Encourage excretion of excess potassium from the body.

> **(!) Guidelines**
>
> The Renal Association has published a guideline on the treatment of hyperkalaemia: Alfonzo et al. (2014). *Treatment of Acute Hyperkalaemia in Adults*. Available at: www.renal.org/guidelines/joint-guidelines/treatment-of-acute-hyperkalaemia-in-adults (accessed Dec. 2015).

Calcium gluconate: rationale and evidence

The Renal Association recommends intravenous calcium gluconate in hyperkalaemia in the presence of ECG evidence of hyperkalaemia (1A evidence) (Renal Association, 2014; see Box Guidelines).

Calcium (Ca^{2+}) acts as a direct antagonist to the membrane actions of hyperkalaemia (Winkler *et al.*, 1939). IV calcium therefore acts to stabilise the myocardium from the effects of hyperkalaemia. This stabilisation is therefore required if there is demonstrated ECG changes.

The Renal Association, in its guidelines on the treatment of hyperkalaemia in adults, highlighted a common pitfall in the use of calcium gluconate in this setting. In clinical practice, calcium gluconate is often used inappropriately in patients with no ECG changes. IV calcium is not without risk, including bradycardia, therefore calcium should only be reserved for patients with ECG changes of hyperkalaemia.

The correct dose of calcium gluconate in the treatment of hyperkalaemia is 1000 mg. When using a solution with a strength of 10% calcium gluconate, this equates to 10 mL.

The actions of IV calcium are rapid – the effect of calcium begins within minutes, but only lasts for 30–60 minutes. Intravenous calcium gluconate (10%) should be administered, by the prescribing doctor, in 1-mL aliquots, whist the patient is on cardiac monitoring, until ECG changes normalise. Up to 10 ml may be given. If the ECG fails to resolve, a further doses can be given, though a senior doctor should be involved at this point.

An exception to the use of calcium gluconate is hyperkalaemia caused by digoxin toxicity. This is because acute hypercalcaemia exacerbates the toxic effects of digoxin. In this situation, calcium gluconate can be made into a more dilute solution, and given slowly (>30 minutes) (Mount, 2015). Advice should be gained from your pharmacist. An alternative is to give the patient antidigoxin antibodies prior to treatment.

Calcium should never be given with solutions containing bicarbonate, because this will lead to precipitations of solid calcium carbonate (chalk).

Given	Once only over 10 minutes in 1-mL aliquots
Special situations	Patients should be on cardiac monitoring whilst this is being administered as arrhythmias may occur.
	This concentrated preparation of calcium gluconate is contraindicated if hyperkalaemia is caused by digoxin toxicity (dilute solution of calcium gluconate, given over 30 minute infusion should be considered).
	Calcium carbonate is an alternative to calcium gluconate.
	Do not give with solutions containing bicarbonate.

Calcium gluconate: essential pharmacology

The active ingredient of calcium gluconate is calcium anions (Ca^{2+}). When delivered as an IV solution, calcium ions act on myocardial and skeletal muscle cells. Calcium directly antagonises the dangerous effect of a high serum potassium concentration. Raised extracellular potassium initially causes the resting potential across muscle cell membranes to be less electronegative, causing cells to depolarise more easily. When this occurs persistently, sodium channels become less active, causing cardiac and skeletal muscle cells to become less excitable. In the heart, this causes conduction problems. Calcium gluconate therefore competes with the excess of potassium ions and helps to restore the normal electrical activity of cells. Calcium gluconate therefore corrects conduction abnormalities caused by hyperkalaemia.

However, calcium will neither encourage potassium into cells, nor excrete potassium out of the body. It therefore will not cause a fall in serum potassium.

✓	**DRUGS checklist for CALCIUM GLUCONATE 10%**
Dose	10 ml
Route	IV
Units	ml

Insulin–dextrose infusion: rationale and evidence

Insulin acts by encouraging extracellular potassium into cells. Total body potassium therefore remains unchanged, but intracellular potassium is not in the circulation and therefore not dangerous.

Clearly, if insulin were given alone, the patient would soon suffer from life-threatening hypoglycaemia. Insulin in this setting is therefore given with an infusion of 50% dextrose (50 mL) in order to keep glycaemia stable. After the insulin/dextrose mix, a further 5% dextrose infusion is recommended to avoid hypoglycaemia. Blood glucose should be monitored during and after this infusion.

Actrapid 10 units, which is a short-acting insulin, is added to 50 mL of 50% dextrose, and delivered IV over 30 minutes. The effect of Actrapid begins in 10 minutes and lasts for 4–6 hours. This should be prescribed on the IV drug infusion part of the drug chart.

✓	**DRUGS checklist for INSULIN and DEXTROSE INFUSION**
Dose	10 units Actrapid insulin in 50 mL of 50% dextrose
Route	IV
Units	Actrapid: International units
	Dextrose: mL of fluid
Given	Infusion over 30 minutes
	Can be repeated as required according to potassium level
Special situations	Ensure that the insulin is in the same syringe as the 50% dextrose, as on no account do you want the insulin to be given alone. This would cause a life-threatening drop in blood glucose level and precipitate coma.

The insulin–dextrose infusion results in a fall in serum potassium by 0.5–1.2 mmol/L (Emmett, 2000), and this lasts for 4–6 hours (Ahmed and Weisberb, 2001).

Insulin–dextrose infusion: essential pharmacology

Insulin has many action in homeostasis. In the context of potassium balance, insulin acts on Na-K-ATPase pumps, mainly in skeletal muscle, to exchange extracellular potassium with intracellular sodium (Halperin and Kamel, 1998). This effect is independent of insulin's action on glucose.

Insulin is considered to be the most reliable drug in encouraging extracellular potassium into cells (Weisberg, 2008). Insulin's effect on potassium transport is potentiated if given with B_2 agonists, such as nebulised salbutamol (Allon and Copkney, 1990). Insulin–dextrose infusion and salbutamol are given via different routes, making their combined use easy and effective.

The main risk of insulin–dextrose infusion is hypoglycaemia. Therefore close monitoring of patient glycaemia is mandatory. Patients with acute or chronic renal dysfunction may experience delayed hypoglycaemia (up to 6 hours later) (Williams *et al.*, 1988).

Other medications used in hyperkalaemia

- **Nebulised salbutamol**: Salbutamol is a B_2 adrenergic agonist, which also acts by stimulating Na-K-ATPase to encourage extracellular potassium into cells. Insulin and salbutamol therefore act in the same way in this regard (Mount and Zandi-Nejad, 2008). The route of administration is inhalation through a nebuliser, which rapidly acts to reduce extracellular potassium. Salbutamol 5 mg may reduce serum potassium by 0.5–1.5 mmol/L (Liou *et al.*, 1994). B_2 adrenergic agonists do have unwanted effects, such as tachycardia and angina, in susceptible patients. B_2 adrenergic agonists are therefore contraindicated in patients with acute coronary syndrome.
- **Loop diuretics,** e.g. furosemide: This acts by increasing the excretion of potassium into urine. This is not generally used as acute hyperkalaemia management but may be used as an adjunct in refractory cases. However, loop diuretics are not effective if renal function is markedly impaired.
- **Sodium bicarbonate**: This acts by increasing the pH of blood, which encourages extracellular potassium to move into cells. Sodium bicarbonate is generally only used in acidotic patients (pH <7.2) in this setting. However, there is little evidence supporting its efficacy in reducing serum potassium and should not be used without the advice of a nephrologist.

- **Cation exchange resins,** e.g. Calcium Resonium: These are used in the prevention of hyperkalaemia, and not in the acute setting as they do not act rapidly. However, Calcium Resonium is a chalky powder, which has to be swallowed or inserted per rectally. Both these routes of administration are poorly tolerated by patients and therefore this is not commonly used anymore.
- Nephrology doctors may also use **laxatives** or **fludrocortisone** to reduce serum potassium in the long-term management of recurrent or chronic hyperkalaemia, depending on patients' volume status.

Further aspects of hyperkalaemia management – dialysis

Dialysis is indicated in the treatment of hyperkalaemia (Ahmed and Weisberg, 2001) if patients are:
- Already established on dialysis
- In refractory hyperkalaemia which does not respond to aggressive or optimum medical treatment.

  There are three main forms of dialysis:
- **Haemodialysis**: This occurs via a non-tunnelled line (temporary), a tunnelled internal jugular line (such as a permacath or tesiocath), an arteriovenous fistula or graft.
- **Haemofiltration**: This occurs via a central venous catheter and is used in the intensive care setting. Haemofiltration occurs over a longer period (hours to days) and is haemodynamically better tolerated by patients. It can therefore be used in patients with hypotension.
- **Peritoneal dialysis**: This occurs via a peritoneal dialysis (PD) catheter. The peritoneum is used as a membrane for exchange of fluid, electrolytes and waste products. Insertion of a peritoneal dialysis catheter requires an invasive procedure. Although hyperkalaemia is not a contraindication to PD catheter insertion, peritoneal dialysis is less commonly used in the acute setting.

  Haemodialysis is the most commonly used renal replacement therapy in the treatment of hyperkalaemia. This is because access via a catheter is quickly and easily established. It is therefore used in patients who have not got access to dialysis via an arteriovenous fistula/graft or peritoneal catheter.

Haemodialysis also removes serum potassium faster than peritoneal dialysis (Nolph *et al.*, 1978). Haemofiltration is another option, particularly in centres without a dialysis unit, but it removes potassium much more slowly. However, haemofiltration does have the added advantage of being used in haemodynamically unstable patients. In end-stage renal patients who have already been established on peritoneal dialysis, a nephrologist may expedite their dialysis session to treat hyperkalaemia.

Case outcome and discharge

Jane Tenette was treated urgently for hyperkalaemia. Her ECG showed Tall tented T waves leads I, II, V_2–V_5. She was therefore moved to the resuscitation room and placed on a cardiac monitor. The emergency department registrar treated her with 10% calcium gluconate (7 mL were required to demonstrate normalisation of her ECG, therefore the remaining 3 mL calcium gluconate were discarded.)

An infusion of 50 mL 50% dextrose containing 10 units of Actrapid was given over 30 minutes. Her blood glucose levels were monitored and did not fall below 5.0 mmol/L. She also received a nebulised of 5 mg salbutamol.

She was then referred to the nephrology team for investigation and treatment of her AKI. Blood tests were taken to investigate acute intrinsic renal disease, and an ultrasound kidney/ureter/bladder was arranged to rule out obstructive causes.

During her inpatient stay, nephrotoxic medications were avoided. Venous thromboembolism (VTE) prophylaxis was started in the form of unfractionated heparin 5000 units SC BD. She was given a no-potassium diet.

She was discharged to outpatient renal follow up without any medications, as her renal function returned to acceptable levels and needs ongoing monitoring postdischarge.

Common pitfalls

- The most common error is delivering calcium gluconate in patients with no cardiac or skeletal muscle abnormalities. If indicated, this should be given with the patient on cardiac monitoring. Patients may receive 1–10 mL of 10% calcium gluconate until ECG changes resolve.

- Ensure patient's blood glucose is monitored, to avoid hypoglycaemia.
- Hyperkalaemia may return within 4–6 hours of treatment. Therefore recheck serum potassium 2–4 hours after treatment.

- Early referral to nephrologist if the patient is in ESRD, established on dialysis or has refractory hyperkalaemia.
- Remember that it is not always about what to prescribe for hyperkalaemia, it is equally important to know what **not** to prescribe. Medications that should not be started in patients with hyperkalaemia are listed in Table 10.4.

Table 10.4 Medications that should NOT be started in patients with hyperkalaemia.

Drug	Problem	Replace it with...
ACE Inhibitors eg. Ramipril ARBs eg. Losartan	Decreased angiotensin leads to decreased aldosterone. Aldosterone is key in increasing sodium uptake and excreting potassium in the nephron.	A different antihypertensive eg. Ca channel blockers, beta blockers, diuretic
K+ sparing diuretics eg. Spironolactone, Amiloride	Spironolactone is an aldosterone antagonist. Amiloride inhibits epithelial sodium channels in the distal nephron, reducing K excretion	A loop or thiazide diuretic
Any medication causing AKI see above table	If a patient has hyperkalaemia secondary to AKI, look at the cause of AKI and correct it as well as treating hyperkalaemia	See above table for drugs causing AKI
Blood Transfusions	RBC trauma and lysis causes release of intracellular potassium into the plasma	Blood is not contraindicated in hyperkalaemia, however hyperkalaemia should be treated concurrently. Monitor serum potassium, consider slowing blood, and treat hyperkalaemia.
Trimethoprim	Same mechanism as amiloride (Perazella, 2000)	Discuss with microbiologist regarding other antibiotics
Sando-K	This is a potassium supplement. This seems obvious, but can be easily missed	Stop medication

Hyperkalaemia is defined as a serum potassium of greater than 5.0 mmol/L. However, the threshold for urgent inpatient treatment is if there are ECG changes and/or a serum potassium of >6.5 mmol/L (Mount, 2015). The complications of hyperkalaemia are ascending muscle weakness, paralysis, cardiac arrhythmias and death. Prior to these life-threatening complications, patients may remain entirely asymptomatic. The rationale of the treatment regimen in hyperkalaemia is to stabilise the myocardium, encourage extracellular potassium to enter the intracellular space and to increase excretion of potassium from the body. The underlying cause can then be investigated once the patient is stable.

SUMMARY

Key learning points

Hyperkalaemia

- Patients with ECG changes require urgent calcium gluconate to stabilise the myocardium and prevent life-threatening arrhythmias.
- Insulin and dextrose acts by encouraging potassium into cells, thereby decreasing circulating K levels.
- Salbutamol acts in a similar way to insulin and is generally well tolerated.
- For patients with refractory hyperkalaemia, haemofiltration or haemodialysis may be required.
- Urgent consideration and correction of the cause should be a priority, as soon as the patient has received the hyperkalaemia correction medications, as otherwise hyperkalaemia may reoccur.
- Fluid resuscitation is often required simultaneously, as hyperkalaemia often goes with AKI.
- Common culprit drugs include ACEIs, ARBs and spironolactone.
- Repeat K levels must be taken 2–4 hours after treatment, as a repeat of treatment may be necessary.

FURTHER READING

- Mahoney BA, Smith WAD, Lo D *et al.* (2005). Emergency interventions for hyperkalaemia. *Cochrane Database Syst Rev* (2): CD003235.
- Maxwell A, Linden K, O'Donnell S *et al.* (2013). Management of hyperkalaemia. *J R Coll Physicians Edinb* 43: 246–51.

Now visit **www.wileyessential.com/pharmacology** to test yourself on this chapter.

References

Acute Kidney Injury Work Group (2012). Kidney disease: improving global outcomes (KDIGO) – clinical practice guideline for acute kidney injury. *Kidney Inter* 2: 1–138.

Bellomo R (2006). The epidemiology of acute renal failure: 1975 versus 2005. *Curr Opin Crit Care* 12: 557–60.

Ahmed J, Weisberg LS (2001). Hyperkalemia in dialysis patients. *Semin Dial* 14: 348–56.

Emmett M (2000). Non-dialytic treatment of acute hyperkalemia in the dialysis patient. *Semin Dial* 13: 279–80.

Alfonzo A, Soar J, MacTier R *et al.* (2014). *Treatment of Acute Hyperkalaemia in Adults*. Renal Association. Available at: www.renal.org/guidelines/joint-guidelines/treatment-of-acute-hyperkalaemia-in-adults (accessed Dec. 2015).

Allon M, Copkney C (1990). Albuterol and insulin for treatment of hyperkalaemia in haemodialysis patients. *Kidney Int* 38: 869–72.

Ashley C, Currie A (2014). *Renal Drug Handbook: The Ultimate Prescribing Guide for Renal Practitioners*, 4th edn. Radcliffe Publishing, London.

Bosch X, Poch E, Grau JM (2009). Rhabdomyolysis and acute kidney injury. *N Engl J Med* 361: 62–72.

Briguori C, Visconti G, Ricciardelli B *et al.* (2011). Renal insufficiency following contrast media administration trial II (REMEDIAL II): RenalGuard system in high-risk patients for contrast-induced acute kidney injury: rationale and design. *EuroIntervention* 6: 1117.

British Medical Association and Royal Pharmaceutical Society of Great Britain (2015). *British National Formulary 69*. 69th edn. BMJ group and Pharmaceutical Press, London.

Chapagain A, Ashman N (2012). Hyperkalaemia in the age of aldosterone antagonism. *QJM* 105: 1049–57.

Clec'h C, Razafimandimby D, Laouisset M *et al.* (2013). Incidence and outcome of contrast-associated acute kidney injury in a mixed medical-surgical ICU population: a retrospective study. *BMC Nephrol* 14: 31.

Elmholdt TR, Pedersen M, Jørgensen B *et al.* (2011). Nephrogenic systemic fibrosis is found only among gadolinium-exposed patients with renal insufficiency: a case-control study from Denmark. *Br J Dermatol* 165: 828–36.

Fishbane S (2008). N-acetylcysteine in the prevention of contrast-induced nephropathy. *Clin J Am Soc Nephrol* 3: 281.

George JN, Nester CM (2014). Syndromes of thrombotic microangiopathy. *N Engl J Med* 371: 654–66.

Halperin ML, Kamel KS (1998). Potassium. *Lancet* 352: 135–40.

Hou SH, Bushinsky DA, Wish JB *et al.* (1983). Hospital-acquired renal insufficiency: a prospective study. *Am J Med* 74: 243–8.

Hoste EA, Kellum JA (2006). Acute kidney injury: epidemiology and diagnostic criteria. *Curr Opin Crit Care* 12: 531–7.

Kalra PA, Kumwenda M, MacDowall P *et al.* (1999). Questionnaire study and audit of use of angiotensin converting enzyme inhibitor and monitoring in general practice: the need for guidelines to prevent failure. *BMJ* 318: 234–7.

Kohli HS, Bhaskaran MC, Muthukumar T *et al.* (2000). Treatment-related acute renal failure in the elderly: a hospital-based prospective study. *Nephrol Dial Transplant* 15: 212–7.

Kshirsagar AV, Poole C, Mottl A *et al.* (2004). N-acetylcysteine for the prevention of radiocontrast induced nephropathy: a meta-analysis of prospective controlled trials. *J Am Soc Nephrol* 15: 761–9.

Lewington A, Kanagasundaram S (2011). *Acute Kidney Injury Guidelines.* Renal Association, March 2011. Available at: www.renal.org/guidelines/modules/acute-kidney-injury (accessed Dec. 2015).

Liou HH, Chiang SS, Wu SC *et al.* (1994). Hypokalemic effects of intravenous infusion or nebulization of salbutamol in patients with chronic renal failure: comparative study. *Am J Kidney Dis* 23: 266–71.

Mount DB (2015). Treatment and prevention of hyperkalaemia in Adults. In: Sterns RH (ed), UpToDate. Waltham, MA.

Mount DB, Zandi-Nejad K (2008). Disorders of potassium balance. In: Brenner BM (ed). *Brenner and Rector's The Kidney,* 8th edn. WB Saunders Co, Philadelphia: 547.

Mueller C, Buerkle G, Buettner HJ *et al.* (2002). Prevention of contrast media-associated nephropathy: randomized comparison of 2 hydration regimens in 1620 patients undergoing coronary angioplasty. *Arch Intern Med* 162: 329–36.

National Institute for Health and Care Excellence (NICE) (2013). *Intravenous Fluid Therapy in Adults in Hospital.* Available at: www.nice.org.uk/guidance/cg174 (accessed Dec. 2015).

Nolph KD, Popovich RP, Ghods AJ *et al.* (1978). Determinants of low clearances of small solutes during peritoneal dialysis. *Kidney Int* 13: 117–23.

Paice B, Gray JM, McBride D *et al.* (1983). Hyperkalaemia in patients in hospital. *Br Med J (Clin Res Ed)* 286: 1189–92.

Perazella M (2000). Trimethoprim-induced hyperkalaemia: clinical data, mechanism, prevention and management. *Drug Saf* 22: 227–36.

Perel P, Roberts I (2013). Colloids versus crystalloids for fluid resuscitation in critically ill patients. *Cochrane Database Systematic Review* (6): CD000567.

Schetz M, Dasta J, Goldstein S *et al.* (2005). Drug-induced acute kidney injury. *Curr Opin Crit Care* 11: 555–65.

Trivedi HS, Moore H, Nasr S *et al.* (2003). A randomized prospective trial to assess the role of saline hydration on the development of contrast nephrotoxicity. *Nephron Clin Pract* 93: C29.

Weisberg LS (2008). Management of severe hyperkalaemia. *Crit Care Med* 36: 3246–51.

Williams PS, Davenport A, Bone JM (1988). Hypoglycaemia following treatment of hyperkalaemia with insulin and dextrose. *Postgrad Med J* 64: 30–2.

Winkler AW, Hoff HE, Smith PK (1939). Factors affecting the toxicity of potassium. *Am J Physiol* 127: 430.

Yarlagadda SG, Perazella MA (2008). Drug-induced crystal nephropathy: an update. *Expert Opin Drug Saf* 7: 147–58.

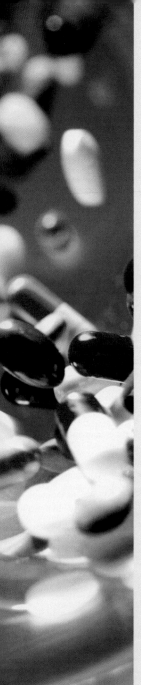

CHAPTER 11
Microbiology
Victoria Taylor

Key topics:

Learning objectives

By the end of this chapter you should…

- …be able to write a safe prescription for patients with sepsis and infections.

- …be able to talk about the mechanisms of action of the main groups of antibiotics.

- …be able to describe the measures you can take to ensure good antibiotic stewardship.

- …be aware of some of the specific aspects of prescribing for neutropenic sepsis.

Essential Practical Prescribing, First Edition. Georgia Woodfield, Benedict Lyle Phillips, Victoria Taylor, Amy Hawkins and Andrew Stanton. © 2016 by John Wiley & Sons, Ltd. Published 2016 by John Wiley & Sons, Ltd.

Sepsis and antibiotics

Mrs Oluremi Lawal

Age: 80 years

Hospital number: 123456

🔍 Case study

Mrs Lawal has been admitted from her residential home where her carers have noticed that she has become more drowsy and withdrawn over the last few days. She has been off her food and not joining in with group activities as she normally does, spending most of her time in her room, sleeping. When they checked her temperature, she was found to be febrile at 39° so the carers called an ambulance.

PMH: *Hypertension, type 2 diabetes (diet controlled), atrial fibrillation, hysterectomy 25 years ago.*

DH: *See FP10*

Allergies: *None known*

Salient examination findings:
T 38.8°C, HR 85, BP 90/50, RR 25, Sats 96% on air
CVS: No murmurs heard
Chest: No crackles heard
Abdomen: Soft, some suprapubic tenderness but no renal angle tenderness, bowel sounds present
Drowsy, AMT 3/10
No hot, swollen joints or rashes

Bedside investigations:
Urine dip: Positive for leukocytes, nitrites and blood
ECG: Atrial fibrillation at 90 bpm, left axis deviation, no ischaemic changes
CXR: Clear lung fields
Point-of-care tests: WCC 17, Hb 11, vBG lactate 3, creatinine 97
Weight: 66 kg

Diagnosis
Sepsis, probably originating in the urinary tract.

Initial management
The most important step in managing sepsis is *recognising* sepsis – a systemic inflammatory

| PHARMACY STAMP | AGE 80 | FORENAME, SURNAME Oluremi Lawal |
| | D.O.B. xx/xx/xxxx | ADDRESS Pinetrees Care Home NHS NUMBER |

RAMIPRIL 2.5 mg, one tablet daily.

BISOPROLOL 2.5 mg, one tablet daily.

ADCAL D3 FORTE, two tablets daily.

ALENDRONIC ACID 70 mg weekly.

FERROUS FUMARATE 210 mg, one tablet daily.

PARACETAMOL 1 g as needed, max four times daily.

WARFARIN variable dose.

SIGNATURE OF PRESCRIBER   DATE

SP21000

response in the presence of an infection. You also need to look out for evidence of severe sepsis (acute organ dysfunction in the presence of sepsis) and septic shock (hypotension despite adequate fluid resuscitation). Key early steps shown to be effective in the management of sepsis include: high flow oxygen, taking blood cultures, IV antibiotics, IV fluid therapy and measuring the Hb, lactate and hourly urine output – the so-called 'sepsis six' (Daniels *et al.*, 2010). If the patient doesn't respond to fluid resuscitation, it may be appropriate to discuss the case with the ICU team.

Don't be fooled: Patients taking beta-blockers or other negatively chronotropic medications may not manifest the tachycardic response you expect when they are septic as the adrenergic supply to their heart is blunted.

Prescribing for sepsis

FLUID CHART

Date	Fluid	Dose	Route	Rate	Signature	Print name
xx/xx/xx	SODIUM CHLORIDE 0.9%	500 ml	IV	STAT	A. Doctor	A. Doctor

ONCE ONLY PRESCRIPTIONS

Date	Time to be given	DRUG	Dose	Route	Prescriber Signature	Bleep
xx/xx/xx	xx:xx	GENTAMICIN	330 mg	IV	A. Doctor	

REGULAR PRESCRIPTIONS

DRUG				Circle/enter times below ↓	Day 1	Day 2	Day 3	Day 4
ADCAL D3 FORTE				06				
Dose 2 tablets	Route PO	Freq OD	Start date xx/xx/xx	⑧				
				12				
Signature A. Doctor		Bleep	Review	16				
				18				
Additional instructions				22				
ALENDRONIC ACID				06				
Dose 70 mg	Route PO	Freq Weekly	Start date xx/xx/xx	⑧	X	X		X
				12				
Signature A. Doctor		Bleep	Review	16				
				18				
Additional instructions				22				
FERROUS FUMARATE				06				
Dose 210 mg	Route PO	Freq BD	Start date xx/xx/xx	⑧				
				12				
Signature A. Doctor		Bleep	Review	16				
				18				
Additional instructions				22				

VARIABLE DOSE ANTICOAGULANT

Anticoagulant WARFARIN	Therapeutic range 2-3	Duration of therapy Ongoing
Indication for anticoagulation AF	Prescriber's signature A. Doctor	Date xx/xx/xx

FOR ADVICE PLEASE CONTACT THE ANTICOAGULATION CLINIC ON EXTENSION ** OR BLEEP ****

New to warfarin? Y/(N)	Previous dose (if known) warfarin patient) 3.5 mg daily	Pre-treatment INR Awaited	Pre-treatment FBC/LFTs checked? Y/N

Date	First dose					
INR		First test				
Warfarin dose (mg)						
Doctor or Practitioner (initials)						
Given by (give @ 6pm)						

AS REQUIRED MEDICATION

DRUG **PARACETAMOL**				Date		
				Time		
Dose 1 g	Route PO	Max freq QDS	Start date xx/xx/xx	Dose		
				Route		
Signature/Bleep A. Doctor		Max dose in 24 hrs 4 g	Review	Given		
				Check		
Additional instructions						

A fluid challenge has been prescribed as well as an initial dose of antibiotics. Hospital guidelines in this case suggested gentamicin as the initial empirical antibiotic. The patient's usual medications have been prescribed except for the angiotensin-converting enzyme (ACE) inhibitor and the beta-blocker, which have been held temporarily due to the patient's low blood pressure and in order to avoid nephrotoxicity.

Gentamicin dosing

Gentamicin dosing is based on (1) the patient's weight and (2) the patient's renal function. In obese patients dosing is based on ideal body weight (see also gentamicin DRUGS checklist).

Calculating creatinine clearance

A patient's renal function is usually based on the estimated glomerular filtration rate (eGFR) or creatinine clearance (CrCl). Many hospitals have their own CrCl calculators for you to use and versions are available online but you can also work out a patient's CrCl yourself. If you're calculating it yourself using the Cockcroft–Gault equation (Cockcroft and Gault, 1976). Be aware that there are two different units used for measuring creatinine: **micromole/L** and **mg/dL**. The original equation used mg/dL so if your hospital uses micromole/L, you need to multiply the creatinine by **0.0113** to make the equation work (i.e. 1 micromole = 0.0113 mg/dL).

$$CrCl = \frac{(140 - age)\,(\text{weight in kg}) \times (0.85 \text{ if female})}{72 \times (\text{serum creatinine})\,(\times 0.113 \text{ if using micromole/L})}$$

In this case:

$$CrCl = \frac{(140 - 80) \times 66 \times 0.85}{72 \times 97 \times 0.0113} = \frac{3366}{78.9} = 42.7 \text{ mL/min}$$

Caveat: The calculation is less accurate at extremes of weight and in these cases ideal body weight should be used, which is why many gentamicin calculators ask for the patient's height.

Working out a gentamicin dose

Many hospitals have a gentamicin dosing calculator for you to use, which automatically takes into account the patient's renal function and weight to provide you with the correct gentamicin dose.

Gentamicin toxicity arises from persistently elevated levels of the drug in the renal tubules. Therapeutic drug monitoring (TDM) should be performed where further doses of gentamicin are required. There are basically two strategies for monitoring gentamicin when using once-daily dosing:

1. The Hartford nomogram: dosing interval is adjusted according to blood levels 6–14 hours after the previous dose.
2. Withholding gentamicin until blood levels fall below a threshold.

Hospitals vary as to which method they use but the Hartford nomogram is supported by better evidence. Ototoxicity may also arise from inappropriately high serum gentamicin levels but is less predictable and may occur with apparently non-toxic concentrations, especially in the elderly. Vestibular toxicity is irreversible. Diuretics (e.g. furosemide) given in combination with gentamicin may further increase the risk of renal and ototoxicity.

There is a balance to be struck between adequately treating a case of sepsis and avoiding further renal impairment. Gentamicin in this case has been prescribed at a dose of 5 mg/kg, that is 330 mg ($5 \times 66 = 330$).

General principles of prescribing antibiotics

- Start antibiotics early in cases of sepsis.
- Always give a review and stop date.
- Document the indication for antibiotics in the medical notes and if possible on the drug chart.
- Aim to rationalise antibiotics when appropriate: narrow the spectrum of cover once the causative pathogen is known and switch to an oral preparation once the patient is improving clinically.
- Review prescriptions daily and in light of culture results.

Antibiotics in sepsis: rationale and evidence

Antibiotics are a group of drugs that take advantage of the differences between bacterial and human cells to selectively damage or destroy bacteria. They have greatly diminished the burden of human disease and allow previously risky procedures such as surgery to proceed safely.

The Surviving Sepsis Campaign (Dellinger *et al.*, 2013) recommends giving antibiotics within 1 hour of recognition of sepsis as part of a care bundle designed to improve outcomes in sepsis. Other antibiotic-related recommendations that have been shown to improve outcomes in sepsis include taking blood cultures prior to giving antibiotics, using broad-spectrum antibiotics in the first instance to cover all the likely organisms and consideration of combination antibiotic therapy in certain circumstances (Levy *et al.*, 2010; Daniels *et al.*, 2010; Ibrahim *et al.*, 2000).

🔍 Evidence

A large multicentre retrospective cohort study looked at a group of adult patients with septic shock. They examined the delay between onset of hypotension and the administration of antibiotics and demonstrated a correlation between this and the chances of a patient surviving to discharge. Patients who received antibiotics within the first hour after the onset of hypotension had a 79.9% chance of survival to discharge with a mean decrease in survival of 7.6% for every hour of delay thereafter (Kumar *et al.*, 2006).

This is reflected elsewhere in the literature (although there is no randomised controlled trial (RCT)-level evidence of this). For example, a large multicenter observational study found that early administration of broad-spectrum antibiotics to adults with severe sepsis or septic shock was associated with increased survival to discharge (Ferrer *et al.*, 2009).

In sepsis especially, antibiotics can be life-saving and there is good evidence that the sooner they are administered, the better the outcome (see Evidence). This does, however, need to be balanced against the injudicious or inappropriate use of antibiotics. When considering the choice of antibiotics, as well as referring to local guidelines, factors you should take into account include: allergies, any recent courses of antibiotics taken by the patient, previous organisms cultured from the patient and their sensitivities, underlying co-morbidities and local sensitivity patterns. You should also take note of other drugs the patient may be taking, which may interact with the antibiotic, for example warfarin, diuretics and statins.

It is again highlighted that once the causative pathogen has been identified, the antibiotic regimen should be rationalised and refined to avoid complications and the development of antibiotic resistance.

Antibiotics: essential pharmacology

Below, we cover the main groups of antibiotics in use today, with a summary of how they work and their main characteristics. As a general rule, if you are not sure which antibiotic to use, are treating an unusual infection or just aren't sure about some aspect of antibiotic prescribing, you should consult your hospital microbiologist.

Antibiotics that inhibit bacterial cell wall synthesis

Penicillins, cephalosporins and carbapenems

Mechanism of action: The penicillins, cephalosporins and carbapenems all work by interfering with the production of peptidoglycan bacterial cell walls (there are a few bacteria that lack a cell wall – clearly these antibiotics won't work here!). This action is selectively harmful to bacteria as human cells do not have cell walls.

Penicillins

Penicillins are beta-lactam antibiotics. Beta-lactam refers to a particular chemical structure, which interferes with the synthesis of bacterial cell walls.

Activity: Penicillins are broad-spectrum antibiotics, active against many Gram-positive and Gram-negative bacteria.

Side effects: These include nausea, vomiting, diarrhoea and rash. Less common side effects include: hypersensitivity, transiently deranged LFTs, haematological abnormalities (usually cytopenias) and candidal superinfection.

Pharmacokinetics: The penicillins distribute widely into body fluids including the joints and pleural space. They are lipid insoluble and as such have low penetrance across the blood–brain barrier unless the meninges are inflamed. Their excretion is mainly renal and it is suggested their dose be decreased in renal impairment. They are also secreted into bile (Datapharm, 2015).

✓ DRUGS checklist for AMOXICILLIN/ AMPICILLIN and FLUCLOXACILLIN		
	AMOXICILLIN/ AMPICILLIN	**FLUCLOXACILLIN**
Dose	500 mg–1 g	500 mg–2 g
Route	PO (amoxicillin) IV (ampicillin)	PO IV
Units	Milligrams (mg)	Milligrams (mg)
Given	TDS	Typically QDS
Special situations	In patients with Epstein–Barr virus infection (glandular fever), amoxicillin may cause a non-allergic rash and is usually avoided.	Especially good activity against staphylococci and therefore useful in skin infections; flucloxacillin is also active against beta-haemolytic streptococci which cause skin infections.

Other examples: Other examples of penicillins are benzylpenicillin and piperacillin (a component of Pip-Taz: see Section Neutropenic Sepsis).

[TOP TIP] When a patient informs you they are 'allergic' to penicillin, or any other medication, always ask if they can remember what the 'allergy' consists of and be sure to document this. Side effects are not uncommon with antibiotics, for example many people develop nausea whilst taking antibiotics but this can be managed with suitable antiemetics and should not preclude them from receiving these life-saving medications in the future. If however, they inform you of a rash or of symptoms consistent with anaphylaxis (facial swelling or breathing difficulties) during previous treatment with penicillin, it would be extremely dangerous to administer the drug again. For a fuller discussion of anaphylaxis and its treatment, see Chapter 1.

Add-ons: Beta-lactamase inhibitors. Beta-lactamase is an enzyme possessed by many bacteria which enables them to lyse the active component of a beta-lactam antibiotic. There are many types of beta-lactamase enzymes. By adding an agent that disables this enzyme, the antibiotic can get on and do its job.

Examples include **clavulanic acid** and **tazobactam**:
- clavulanic acid + amoxicillin = co-amoxiclav
- tazobactam + piperacillin = Pip-Taz

Don't forget that despite their deceptive names, Pip-Taz (Tazocin) and co-amoxiclav contain penicillin and must not be given to patients who are allergic to penicillin!

Cephalosporins

Cephalosporins are another group of beta-lactam antibiotics.

Activity: Cephalosporins are broad-spectrum antibiotics, active against many Gram-positive and Gram-negative bacteria. Subsequent generations of cephalosporins have increasing activity against Gram-negative bacteria but decreasing activity against staphylococcal bacteria. They are not active against *Listeria monocytogenes* (hence the addition of ampicillin in patients at risk of *Listeria* meningitis) or enterococci, and are not effective in cases of methicillin-resistant *Staphylococcus aureus* (MRSA).

Side effects: These include loose stool and diarrhoea (beware *Clostridium difficile*), nausea, vomiting, hypersensitivity, risk of superinfection, haematological reactions and transiently deranged LFTs. The injectable solutions also contain a significant amount of sodium.

Pharmacokinetics: Cephalosporins are mainly given as intravenous preparations and distribute widely in the body. Several can cross the blood–brain barrier (cefotaxime, ceftriaxone, cefuroxime). Most cephalosporins are excreted via the kidneys and require dose adjustment in renal impairment (Datapharm, 2015).

✓ DRUGS checklist for CEFUROXIME and CEFTAZIDIME		
	CEFUROXIME	**CEFTAZIDIME**
Dose	750 mg–1.5 g	1–2 g
Route	IV	IV/ IVI/ IM
Units	Milligrams (mg)/ grams (g)	Grams (g)
Given	TDS–QDS	TDS

(Continued)

✓ DRUGS checklist for CEFUROXIME and CEFTAZIDIME (*Continued*)

Special situations	In meningitis a higher dose regimen of up to 3 mg TDS can be used. Dose adjustments: CrCl 10–20 mL/min: 750 mg BD CrCl <10 mL/min: 750 mg OD.	Active against Pseudomonas aeruginosa; should not be used for staphylococcal infections. Dose adjustments: CrCl 31–51 mL/min: 1 g BD CrCl 16–30 mL/min: 1 g OD CrCl 6–15 mL/min: 500 mg OD CrCl <mL/min: 500 mg alternate days.

Other examples:

- First generation: cefalexin (PO), cefadroxil
- Second generation: cefuroxime, cefaclor, cefoxitin
- Third generation: ceftazidime, cefotaxime, ceftriaxone, cefixime
- Fourth generation: cefepime.

Cephalosporin allergy and cross-reactivity:
Because of similarities in their structures, there are concerns that patients who are allergic to penicillins may also be allergic to cephalosporins. However, it has been suggested that the commonly cited rate of cross-reactivity of 10% is an over-estimate, determined in the 1970s when cephalosporins were often contaminated with penicillin due to the manufacturing processes used (Pegler and Healy, 2007). Rates of cross-reactivity may well be much lower than this (see Evidence). Many hospitals allow cephalosporins to be given to patients who are penicillin allergic in a monitored environment, after discussion with a senior team member or microbiologist. That said, most manufacturers of cephalosporins recommend that cephalosporins should not be given to patients with a history of immediate anaphylaxis to penicillin (as opposed to rash).

🔍 Evidence

A meta-analysis (Pichichero and Casey, 2007) found that there was an increased odds ratio of allergy in penicillin-allergic patients receiving a first-generation cephalosporin, whereas cross-reactivity was 'negligible' with second or third-generation cephalosporins. They suggest that most cross-reactivity is due to similarities in their side chains rather than the central beta-lactam ring. A later literature review (Campagna *et al.*, 2012) came to similar conclusions, giving a cross-reactivity rate of 1% between penicillin and first-generation cephalosporins or second-generation cephalosporins with a similar R1 side chain, but finding negligible cross-reactivity between penicillins and third or fourth-generation cephalosporins or those with dissimilar side chains.

Carbapenems

Carbapenem antibiotics consist of a beta-lactam ring attached to a penem ring.

Activity: The carbapenems are very broad-spectrum beta-lactam antibiotics and are not lysed by most bacterial beta-lactamase enzymes. They are active against a wide range of Gram-positive and Gram-negative bacteria, including *Pseudomonas aeruginosa*. They are not active against bacteria that lack a cell wall (*Chlamydia* spp., *Mycoplasma* spp.), nor reliably against *Listeria monocytogenes;* they are not active against MRSA.

Side effects: These include nausea and vomiting, diarrhoea, rash, injection site reactions, hypersensitivity, thrombocytosis, deranged LFTs and superinfection.

Pharmacokinetics: The carbapenems distribute into many body tissues and fluids. They are mainly excreted unchanged via the renal tract, with about 30% metabolised to an inactive metabolite (Datapharm, 2015).

✓ DRUGS checklist for MEROPENEM

Dose	500 mg–2 g
Route	IV
Units	Milligrams (mg) or grams (g)
Given	TDS
Special situations	Meropenem may decrease serum valproate levels. Dose adjustment in renal dysfunction: CrCl 26–50 mL/min: maximum 2 g BD CrCl 10–25 mL/min: maximum 1 g BD CrCl <10 mL/min: maximum 1 g OD.

Other examples: ertapenem, imipenem.

Can carbapenems be used safely in patients with penicillin or cephalosporin allergy? Because they share the beta-lactam ring structure, there is concern that patients who are allergic to penicillin or cephalosporins may demonstrate cross-reactivity to carbapenem antibiotics. There are very limited data in this area. What evidence there is may suggest that the incidence of IgE-mediated allergic cross-reactivity between the carbapenems and other beta-lactam antibiotics is low (see Evidence). It is not possible to predict anaphylaxis to meropenem from penicillin allergy and vice versa. However, as with the cephalosporins, manufacturers still list anaphylaxis to another beta-lactam antibiotic as a contraindication to administration of carbapenems.

🔍 Evidence

A systematic review (Kula *et al.*, 2014) looked at a mixture of prospective studies, retrospective studies and case reports regarding patients with a history of IgE-mediated penicillin or cephalosporin allergy (either proven, suspected or possible) who were subsequently treated with systemic carbapenems. Of the 838 patients with previous allergy, 4.3% had some type of reaction to a subsequent carbapenem. Of the 221 *proven* cases, one patient (0.5%) went on to have a *proven* IgE-mediated reaction to a carbapenem. Caveats include that the data was drawn from heterogeneous patients groups, with variability in the way the reactions were reported.

Glycopeptides

Mechanism of action: Glycopeptides bind to peptidoglycan in bacterial cell walls (at a different site to the beta-lactams) and prevent cross-linkage of these structures, thereby inhibiting bacterial cell wall synthesis.

Activity: Glycopeptides are active against many Gram-positive bacteria and are used primarily for severe staphylococcal infections where penicillins or cephalosporins cannot be used due to previous treatment failure, resistance (e.g. MRSA) or allergy. They can also be used to treat *C. difficile* infection when given by the oral route. The glycopeptides have a narrow spectrum of activity (Gram-positive organisms only) and caution is therefore advised in their use as a monotherapy unless the causative pathogen is already known.

Side effects: These include nausea, rashes and cutaneous reactions, fever, hypersensitivity, allergy, superinfection, cytopenias and deranged LFTs. The glycopeptides are potentially ototoxic and nephrotoxic. Infusion reactions can occur if vancomycin is administered too quickly.

Pharmacokinetics: Glycopeptides distribute into pleural, pericardial, ascitic and synovial compartments but have poor penetration of the CNS (although vancomycin has reasonable penetration of the CSF if the meninges are inflamed). They aren't absorbed from the GI tract and are only effective orally in cases of *C. difficile*-associated pseudomembranous colitis. They are mostly eliminated via the renal tract and are not metabolised to any large extent (Rybak, 2006; Datapharm, 2015).

Therapeutic drug monitoring (TDM): TDM needs to be performed to ensure that vancomycin particularly is administered within a therapeutic window without toxicity. Teicoplanin is less likely to be toxic but TDM may need to be performed in prolonged treatment of severe infections to ensure adequate dosing.

✓ DRUGS checklist for VANCOMYCIN and TEICOPLANIN

	VANCOMYCIN	TEICOPLANIN
Dose	500 mg–1 g (125 mg PO)	6–12 mg/ kg 400 mg–800 mg (100 mg–200 mg PO)
Route	IV slow infusion (PO in *C. difficile* infection)	IV (PO in *C. difficile* infection)
Units	Milligrams (mg)	Milligrams (mg)
Given	BD (1 g) or QDS (500 mg) (125 mg QDS if PO)	Every 12 hours for the first 3 doses (loading); once daily thereafter (maintenance) (100 mg–200 mg BD if PO)
Special situations	Vancomycin is an irritant and extravasation can lead to tissue necrosis. Red man syndrome is a rare rate-dependent reaction which may occur when given IV. The dose should be decreased in renal impairment. Requires therapeutic drug monitoring.	May require therapeutic drug monitoring. The maintenance dose (but not loading doses) should be adjusted in renal impairment. On the fourth day of treatment: CrCl 30–80 mL/min: halve the dose or give a dose alternate days CrCl <30 mL/min: give a third of the dose or give a dose every third day.

Antibiotics that inhibit bacterial protein synthesis

There are several antibiotic groups that act to disrupt bacterial protein synthesis. These include the macrolide, tetracycline and aminoglycoside antibiotics. As they act on bacterial protein synthesis rather than the bacterial cell wall, they are effective against organisms that lack a cell wall (unlike the beta-lactams and glycopeptides).

Macrolides

Mechanism of action: The macrolides bind the 50S subunit of bacterial ribosomes to inhibit protein synthesis.

Activity: The macrolides have activity against a range of Gram-positive and Gram-negative bacteria, both aerobic and anaerobic. They are also active against atypical organisms that lack a cell wall, such as *Mycoplasma* and *Chlamydia* species.

Side effects: These include rashes, hypersensitivity, nausea and GI disturbance, deranged LFTs, superinfection and cardiac dysrhythmias, especially in the elderly and those with pre-existing heart disease. The effect is caused by prolongation of the QT interval and may be fatal. Caution should be used where patients are taking other drugs that have this effect, for example antidepressants. The macrolides may worsen weakness in patients with myasthenia gravis.

Pharmacokinetics: Macrolides are well absorbed from the gastrointestinal tract and this is unaffected by administration alongside food. They are primarily excreted by the liver, in bile (Datapharm, 2015).

✓ DRUGS checklist for ERYTHROMYCIN and CLARITHROMYCIN

	ERYTHROMYCIN	CLARITHROMYCIN
Dose	250 mg–1 g	250 mg–500 mg
Route	PO Suspension available	PO or IV Suspension available
Units	Milligrams (mg)	Milligrams (mg)
Given	BD–QDS	BD
Special situations	May cause ototoxicity at high doses. Active against *Treponema pallidum* (syphilis).	Clarithromycin has excellent bioavailability when taken orally and therefore only needs to be given IV if the patient is nil by mouth.

Other example: azithromycin.

Enzyme inhibitors: interaction alert!

Clarithromycin and erythromycin are cytochrome P450 enzyme inhibitors acting on the enzyme CYP3A (Datapharm, 2015). This leads to interactions with a number of other medications. By inhibiting this enzyme they can potentially slow the breakdown of other medications including:

- **Warfarin:** This may lead to an increase in the INR and an increased risk of bleeding. The INR should be checked more frequently during macrolide therapy and the warfarin dose may need to be temporarily decreased.
- **Simvastatin:** This is associated with an increased risk of myopathy. Simvastatin should be temporarily held during treatment with a macrolide antibiotic.
- **Carbamazepine:** Levels may be increased, leading to an increased risk of toxicity. You should monitor for side effects.

Other enzyme inhibitors: Metronidazole is another notable enzyme inhibitor. The antifungal agents fluconazole, itraconazole and ketoconazole are also enzyme inhibitors.

Tetracyclines

Mechanism of action: Tetracycline antibiotics bind reversibly to the 30S subunit of bacterial ribosomes to prevent the binding of tRNA and inhibit bacterial protein synthesis.

Activity: Tetracyclines are active against a range of Gram-positive and Gram-negative organisms as well intracellular bacteria such as *Chlamydia*, *Mycoplasma* and *Rickettsia*. They are used in Lyme disease (caused by the spirochete *Borrelia burgdorferi*) and syphilis (caused by the spirochete *Treponema pallidum*) and are also active against a number of protozoan parasites, for example *Plasmodium* spp., which cause malaria.

Side effects: These include nausea, vomiting, diarrhoea, superinfection, hypersensitivity reactions and photosensitivity.

Cautions and contraindications: Systemic lupus erythematosus and myasthenia gravis may both be exacerbated by the use of tetracyclines. Tetracyclines may impair bone growth and cause permanent tooth discolouration and are therefore contraindicated in children and women who are pregnant or breast feeding.

Pharmacokinetics: Apart from doxycycline, tetracyclines administered enterally are incompletely absorbed and this is further impaired in the presence of food, milk, iron tablets or antacids. They should therefore be taken 1 hour before or 2 hours after food. They are widely distributed and undergo both renal and hepatic excretion. It is important to give an initial loading dose with doxycycline, to prevent initial subtherapeutic concentrations, which may permit resistance to emerge early in treatment (Roberts, 2003; Datapharm, 2015).

Pharmacokinetics: Gentamicin is not metabolised and is excreted unchanged via the renal tract; its dose should therefore be adjusted in renal impairment (Datapharm, 2015).

✓ DRUGS checklist for DOXYCYCLINE	
Dose	100 mg–200 mg
	For example, in exacerbations of chronic obstructive pulmonary disease (COPD), give a loading dose of 200 mg on day 1, then 100 mg daily thereafter.
Route	PO
Units	Milligrams (mg)
Given	OD or BD depending on indication
Special situations	The absorption of doxycycline, unlike other tetracyclines, is not impaired by food or milk.

Other examples: tetracycline, minocycline and oxytetracycline. Tetracyclines have anti-inflammatory properties and are also used in the treatment of non-infectious conditions such as acne (see Chapter 13), but usually at a lower dose.

Aminoglycosides

Mechanism of action: Aminoglycosides irreversibly bind the 30S subunit of the bacterial ribosomal, inhibiting protein synthesis.

Activity: Aminoglycosides are active against many Gram-negative organisms (including *Pseudomonas*) and some Gram-positive organisms, as well as many organisms resistant to other antibiotics. They are often used in severe Gram-negative infections.

Side effects: These include nausea and vomiting, hypersensitivity, rash, deranged LFTs and blood dyscrasias. Aminoglycosides may be nephrotoxic and ototoxic at high concentrations; vestibular toxicity may arise idiosyncratically and there may be an hereditary predisposition.

✓ DRUGS checklist for GENTAMICIN	
Dose	Check hospital protocol; however, the usual initial dose with normal renal function is 5–7 mg/kg
Route	IV (slow injection or infusion)
Units	Milligrams (mg)
Given	Various regimens depending on the infection, usually once daily
Special situations	Dose reduction is usually recommended in the elderly (e.g. 4 mg/kg) and sometimes in renal impairment. Requires therapeutic drug monitoring (see Box Monitoring Gentamicin).
	Potentially nephrotoxic and ototoxic (especially with repeated doses, giving cumulative toxicity – a problem in cystic fibrosis).
	Contraindicated in myasthenia gravis.

Other examples: amikacin, tobramycin and streptomycin.

Monitoring gentamicin

NB. Recommendations may differ slightly between hospitals.

Therapeutic drug monitoring (TDM) should be performed where more than one dose of gentamicin is required. There are basically two strategies for monitoring gentamicin when using once daily dosing:

1. The Hartford Nomogram (Figure 11.1)
   - Take a gentamicin level 6–14 hours after the dose has been given.

- Specify the time the last dose was given and the time the sample was taken on the blood form. Random levels cannot be interpreted.
- The result should be available to be reviewed before prescribing the next dose.
- The concentration of gentamicin and the time since the dose was given are plotted on the Hartford Nomogram to determine when the next dose should be given, i.e. 24, 36 or 48 hours after the previous dose. An electronic gentamicin calculator is often available and calculates this for you.
- Repeat levels twice weekly if stable.

2. Withholding gentamicin until blood levels fall below a threshold
   - Take the initial predose level 18–24 hours after the first dose, i.e. just before the second dose.
   - The predose level of gentamicin in the blood should be less than 1.0 mg/L, i.e. the blood concentration should have fallen sufficiently to show that the patient is clearing gentamicin well.
   - For patients >65 years, those with renal impairment or those who have had high levels reported previously, **wait** for the result before giving the next dose. For other patients the second dose can be given without waiting for the results although do not give more than one further dose to any patient without reviewing the reported level result.
   - Postdose levels are not required with once-daily dosing.
   - Repeat levels twice weekly if stable.

Dosing regimens

Some conditions are not suitable for once daily gentamicin dosing because the volume of distribution of the drug is affected. These include pregnancy and burns. Other conditions such as endocarditis and listeriosis will have multiple daily dosing regimens if gentamicin is required.

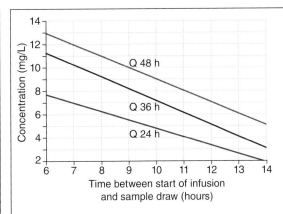

Figure 11.1 The Hartford nomogram. Source: Ross S (2014) Prescribing at a Glance. Reproduced with permission of Wiley.

Antibiotics that inhibit bacterial DNA repair and replication

Fluoroquinolones

Mechanism of action: The fluoroquinolones inhibit bacterial DNA gyrase, preventing one of the initial steps in DNA replication.

Activity: Fluoroquinolones are used primarily to treat infections with Gram-negative organisms. One of the main advantages of the quinolones is their activity against *Pseudomonas aeruginosa*. However, the use of ciprofloxacin is limited by its potential to predispose patients to developing *C. difficile* infection. Levofloxacin is increasingly used in the treatment of pneumonia in penicillin-allergic patients.

Side effects: These include nausea, diarrhoea, headaches, dizziness, photosensitivity reactions, superinfection (especially *C. difficile* infection), lowering of seizure threshold in patients with epilepsy and deranged LFTs (cases of hepatic failure have been reported). The quinolones can cause QT prolongation and should be used in caution in patients at risk of ventricular arrhythmias, with a known prolonged QT interval or when used in combination with other medications which cause QT prolongation. Systemic quinolones may cause tendonitis and tendon rupture.

Pharmacokinetics: The fluoroquinolones are absorbed extensively from the GI tract (i.e. have excellent oral bioavailability) and reach high concentrations in the lungs and urogenital tract. Intravenous ciprofloxacin is expensive and is rarely needed, unless the oral route is unavailable. They are excreted largely unchanged, mostly via the renal tract (apart from moxifloxacin which is mainly cleared via the liver with some contribution from the kidneys) (Wolfson and Hooper, 1989; Datapharm, 2015).

✓	**DRUGS checklist for CIPROFLOXACIN**
Dose	250 mg–750 mg (PO)
	400 mg (IV)
Route	PO (rarely IV)
Units	Milligrams (mg)
Given	BD
	Not with milk
Special situations	There is very little difference in bioavailability between oral and IV formulations.
	Inhibits the enzyme CYP1A2 and may increase levels of other drugs, including theophylline and warfarin.
	Dose adjustments: CrCl 30–60 mL/min: maximum 500 mg BD CrCl <30 mL/min: maximum 500 mg OD.

Other examples: levofloxacin and moxifloxacin.

Miscellaneous antibiotics

Key points on other miscellaneous antibiotics are as follows (Rang *et al.*, 2003; Datapharm, 2015).

Metronidazole: Metronidazole inhibits nucleic acid synthesis. It is a prodrug and becomes active only when reduced to its active form by certain bacteria. It is therefore *only* active against anaerobes and certain protozoa and has no activity against aerobic bacteria of any species (see also Section Infections Related to Antibiotic Use).

Nitrofurantoin: Bacterial reductases activate nitrofurantoin by converting it into reactive metabolites, which then go on to damage the bacteria. Nitrofurantoin is active against the majority of bacteria causing urinary tract infections. Caution is advised in the elderly and those with renal failure. It is concentrated in the urine of patients with normal renal function and is thus only effective for cystitis, not for frank urosepsis or pyelonephritis; it will not work in patients with a low GFR.

Trimethoprim: Trimethoprim is a dihydrofolate reductase inhibitor, which antagonises folate synthesis and prevents synthesis of some amino acids. It is used in urinary tract infections, although increasing resistance is reducing its utility. Because is depletes folate, it is contraindicated in pregnancy.

Co-trimoxazole (trimethoprim+sulfmethoxazole): Sulfamethoxazole (a sulfonamide) inhibits folate synthesis via inhibition of dihydropteroate synthetase and has a synergistic effect when combined with trimethoprim. Co-trimoxazole is used in treatment of, and prophylaxis against, *Pneumocystis jiroveci* pneumonia, as well as for exacerbations of COPD. It is an antibiotic that is being revisited for some infections, for example hospital-acquired pneumonia, because of emerging resistance to other agents and because it has a relatively low risk of causing *C. difficile*-associated disease. Because is depletes folate, it is contraindicated in pregnancy.

Clindamycin: Clindamycin inhibits protein synthesis by reversibly binding the 50S subunit of bacterial ribosomes. It is useful for infections caused by staphylococci, streptococci and anaerobes. It may be active against MRSA, but has a high risk of causing *C. difficile* and where there is sensitivity to other agents (e.g. doxycycline), these should be used instead for mild MRSA infections.

Linezolid: Linezolid inhibits bacterial protein synthesis. It is active against most aerobic

Gram-positive cocci, including vancomycin-resistant enterococci (VRE) (see Section Infections Related to Antibiotic Use). It is very expensive and has a long list of interactions and side effects, some irreversible. It should only be used on the advice of a clinical microbiologist.

Rifampicin: The rifamycins inhibit bacterial RNA synthesis. Rifampicin is used in the treatment of tuberculosis, prophylaxis of bacterial meningitis and in serious staphylococcal infections. A potent enzyme inducer, rifampicin may increase the metabolism of other drugs. It can be hepatotoxic.

Other aspects of sepsis management

Guidance regarding fluid resuscitation is covered in Chapter 7.

Vasopressors and inotropic drugs

These are medications used to support the circulatory system in seriously unwell patients. They are used predominantly in an ICU setting. Examples include: noradrenaline (norepinephrine), adrenaline (epinephrine), dobutamine (especially for cardiac support) and vasopressin. Dopamine has largely fallen out of favour.

Venous thromboembolism (VTE) prophylaxis

Infection is a risk factor for the development of venous thromboembolism and therefore consideration of VTE prophylaxis is an important part of the management of a septic patient, provided no contraindications are present.

Case outcome and discharge

After 24 hours, Mrs Lawal was feeling better and her fevers had settled. Within 48 hours she was looking brighter with her pulse and blood pressure back within the normal range. Her urine culture grew an *Escherichia coli* sensitive to co-amoxiclav and gentamicin but resistant to trimethoprim. *E. coli* was also isolated from blood culture bottles. In view of the sensitivity results and the fact that

she had not spiked a temperature for 48 hours, it was decided that her antibiotics could be safely switched to oral co-amoxiclav to complete a 7-day course. Her INR was checked on alternate days to ensure that her warfarin levels weren't being adversely affected by the antibiotic therapy she was receiving. She was observed on the ward to ensure she was responding to the co-amoxiclav and her ramipril and bisoprolol were restarted. She finally went back to her care home 5 days after admission, following physiotherapy assessments to ensure that her mobility was back at a baseline level. Her GP was asked to recheck her INR in the community.

DISCHARGE MEDICATION						
Date	Medication	Dose	Route	Frequency	Supply	GP to continue?
xx/xx/xx	CO-AMOXICLAV	625 mg	PO	Three times daily	To complete a 7 day course, i.e. until xx/xx/xx	N
xx/xx/xx	RAMIPRIL	2.5 mg	PO	Once daily	14 days	Y
xx/xx/xx	BISOPROLOL	2.5 mg	PO	Once daily	14 days	Y
xx/xx/xx	ADCAL D3	TT	PO	Once daily	14 days	Y
xx/xx/xx	ALENDRONIC ACID	70 mg	PO	Once weekly	14 days	Y
xx/xx/xx	FERROUS FUMARATE	210 mg	PO	Once daily	14 days	Y
xx/xx/xx	WARFARIN	Variable	PO	Once daily	14 days	Y
xx/xx/xx	PARACETAMOL	1 g	PO	As needed, maximum four times daily	14 days	Y

Notes to patient/GP:

No changes to regular medications. Would you be able to re-check Mrs Lawal's INR on xx/xx/xx, in view of her ongoing course of co-amoxiclav. Many thanks.

Common pitfalls

- **Antibiotics that require therapeutic drug monitoring:** Therapeutic drug monitoring is a tricky subject. Each hospital tends to have its own guidelines as to when and how medications should be monitored but there are some general principles.
  - **Peak level:**
    When? One hour after a dose is given.
    Why? To establish whether the patient is receiving a sufficient dose to achieve a therapeutic effect.
  - **Trough level:**
    When? Just before the next dose is given.
    Why? To establish whether the patient is at risk of toxicity (Garner, 2013).

- **Drugs that require monitoring:**

  Aminoglycosides: Gentamicin trough levels can be monitored twice weekly in a stable patient but a change in renal function should trigger a reassessment of levels as well as considering a change in dose. Where multiple daily dosing is required (e.g. for endocarditis), peak and trough levels will be required.

  Glycopeptides: Teicoplanin requires therapeutic monitoring if high doses are used or with prolonged courses. Check a trough level before the fourth dose and weekly thereafter to determine the timing of subsequent doses.

- **Antibiotics in renal failure:** Many antibiotics require dose adjustments in patients with renal impairment. If you are unsure, you can check online (www.medicines.org.uk/emc/), in the BNF (BMA/RPS, 2015) or ask your local pharmacist.

- **Antibiotics and warfarin:** Don't forget to check the INR regularly whilst a patient is taking antibiotics, especially clarithromycin, erythromycin and metronidazole.

- **What is in a name?** Don't forget that despite their deceptive name, co-amoxiclav and Pip-Taz both **contain penicillin** and must **not** be given to patients who are penicillin allergic!

SUMMARY

Sepsis is a life-threatening condition, which is potentially curable with antibiotics and supportive measures. However, the clinical syndrome must be promptly recognised and treated to ensure a good outcome for the patient. Prescribing antibiotics is a complicated business, both in terms of selecting an effective antibiotic for the patient and also in preserving antibiotic utility for future generations. In addition to this, there are constantly changing patterns of bacterial sensitivity and resistance to be aware of.

☞ Key learning points

Key points when prescribing antibiotics:

- Do not delay the administration of antibiotics in a case of suspected sepsis.
- Think carefully about your choice of antibiotic, referring to local guidelines and expertise: most hospitals have 24/7 on-call microbiology advice service.
- Basic knowledge about your antibiotic of choice will make prescriptions safer for patients.

Antibiotics stewardship:

- Always give a review date or a stop date and document the indications for antibiotics in the notes and on the drug chart if possible.
- Review microbial culture and sensitivity results regularly and aim to step down to a narrower-spectrum antibiotic as soon as it is clinically indicated.
- Aim to switch from the IV to the oral route of administration as soon as it is clinically indicated.

FURTHER READING

- A good review article is: MacGowan A, Macnaughton E (2013). Antimicrobial therapy: principles of use. *Medicine* 41: 635–41.
- It is also worthwhile looking at the website of the Surviving Sepsis Campaign. Available at: www.survivingsepsis.org (accessed Dec. 2015).

Infections related to antibiotic use

Mr Burt Bickerstaff

Age: 71 years

Hopital number: 123456

🔍 Case study

Three weeks ago, Mr Bickerstaff developed cellulitis of his right leg, with a small area of ulceration. His GP noted a green exudate, which he thought was indicative of Pseudomonas infection and treated with oral ciprofloxacin 500 mg BD. Subsequently Staphylococcus aureus, resistant to ciprofloxacin but sensitive to flucloxacillin was grown from the ulcer swab and treatment was changed to oral flucloxacillin 250 mg QDS and amoxicillin 500 mg TDS. When this didn't work, he was referred to the acute medical unit for intravenous antibiotics. On the advice of a microbiology consultant, his treatment was intensified. The dose of flucloxacillin was increased to 1 g QDS and the amoxicillin was discontinued. The cellulitis has now almost completely resolved but for the last 3 days he has suffered with increased abdominal pains, anorexia and smelly green diarrhoea. There is no history of recent travel or unwell contacts and he is not taking laxatives.

PMH: Type 2 diabetes, hypertension

DH: See FP10

Allergies: Peanuts

Salient examination findings:
T 37.5°C, HR 96 bpm, BP 100/60, Sats 97% on air, RR 20
He has dry mucous membranes and decreased skin turgor
Abdomen: mild generalised tenderness, no guarding
Right leg: area of healing cellulitis

Bedside investigations:
ECG: Sinus rhythm at 92 bpm.
Point-of-care tests: WCC 13.2, Hb 12, Plt 285

| PHARMACY STAMP | AGE 71 | FORENAME, SURNAME Burt Bickerstaff |
| | D.O.B. xx/xx/xxxx | ADDRESS 7 Hazel Close NHS NUMBER |

GLICLAZIDE 80 mg twice daily.

OMEPRAZOLE 20 mg once daily.

ASPIRIN 75 mg.

AMLOPIDINE 5 mg.

SIGNATURE OF PRESCRIBER   DATE

SP21000

Diagnosis
Likely to be *Clostridium difficile* infection.

Initial management
It is important to recognise the significance of recent courses of antibiotics in diagnosing this condition.

An urgent stool sample should be sent promptly and if the abdominal pain worsens, an abdominal radiograph should be performed and a surgical review considered. The dehydration will need to be addressed with fluids and you should consider withholding any drugs that may compromise renal function further, for example ACE inhibitors, NSAIDs etc. You should inform the infection control team and nurse the patient in isolation with advice to staff to wash their hands with soap and water before and after each contact with the patient.

A note on prescribing in cellulitis

Common causes of treatment failure in cellulitis are misdiagnosis (deep vein thrombosis, venous eczema, gout) and inadequate treatment or poor antibiotic selection. You will occasionally hear colleagues talking about characteristic colours and odours associated with particular infections, for example a 'pseudomonasy' green exudate or an 'anaerobic' smell.

This is not a scientific method of selecting antibiotics, with no evidence to support it. In this case, the initial antibiotic, ciprofloxacin, was inappropriate; the green exudate was the patient's own pus cells. The subsequent dose of flucloxacillin (250 mg) was inadequate. Flucloxacillin may be given orally in doses of up to 1 g QDS, although the dose may need to be reduced due to nausea. Where flucloxacillin is given in adequate doses, there is no need to add in amoxicillin or benzylpenicillin as almost all organisms causing cellulitis, for example *Staphylococcus aureus* (apart from MRSA) and beta-haemolytic streptococci, are susceptible to flucloxacillin alone. This patient's *C. difficile* infection could probably have been avoided with better prescribing practice.

Evidence

A Cochrane review (Kilburn *et al.*, 2010) has suggested that intravenous antibiotics are of no benefit over oral agents for the treatment of simple cellulitis. There is even weak evidence that oral treatment may be superior and this also has the advantage of protecting patients from the complications associated with admissions for IV antibiotics.

Prescribing for *Clostridium difficile* infection

FLUID CHART

Date	Fluid	Dose	Route	Rate	Signature	Print name
xx/xx/xx	SODIUM CHLORIDE 0.9%	500 ml	IV	STAT	A. Doctor	A. Doctor

REGULAR PRESCRIPTIONS

Circle/enter times below ↓ / Enter dates below / Day 1 / Day 2 / Day 3 / Day 4

DRUG METRONIDAZOLE
Dose 400 mg / Route PO / Freq TDS / Start date xx/xx/xx
Signature A. Doctor / Bleep / Review xx/xx/xx
Additional instructions
(06) 08 12 (14) 18 (22)

DRUG GLICLAZIDE
Dose 80 mg / Route PO / Freq BD / Start date xx/xx/xx
Signature A. Doctor / Bleep / Review
Additional instructions
06 (08) 12 16 (18) 22

DRUG OMEPRAZOLE
Dose 20 mg / Route PO / Freq OD / Start date xx/xx/xx
Signature A. Doctor / Bleep / Review
Additional instructions
06 (08) 12 16 18 22

DRUG ASPIRIN
Dose 75 mg / Route PO / Freq OD / Start date xx/xx/xx
Signature A. Doctor / Bleep / Review
Additional instructions
06 (08) 12 16 18 22

DRUG AMLODIPINE
Dose 5 mg / Route PO / Freq OD / Start date xx/xx/xx
Signature A. Doctor / Bleep / Review
Additional instructions
06 (08) 12 16 18 22

AS REQUIRED MEDICATION

DRUG PARACETAMOL
Dose 1 g / Route PO / Max freq QDS / Start date xx/xx/xx
Signature/Bleep A. Doctor / Max dose in 24 hrs 4 g / Review
Additional instructions
Date / Time / Dose / Route / Given / Check

Metronidazole is the current first-line treatment for mild to moderate cases of *C. difficile* infection requiring treatment.

You should stop antibiotics that are not required and review the need for any proton pump inhibitor

(PPI) currently prescribed; there is emerging evidence that PPIs may predispose to *C. difficile* infection (Janarthan *et al.*, 2012) (see Chapter 5).

Antibiotics in *Clostridium difficile* infection: rationale and evidence

C. difficile is an anaerobic, Gram-positive, spore-forming bacteria, which can produce toxins leading to inflammation of the gut and diarrhoea. In more severe cases it can result in pseudomembranous colitis and toxic megacolon, which can be life-threatening. Metronidazole is active against anaerobic organisms including *Clostridia* and is relatively inexpensive. It is the antibiotic of choice in mild and moderate cases of *C. difficile* infection requiring treatment. Vancomycin (125 mg QDS, orally, for 10–14 days) is widely used in more severe cases. This is a more expensive treatment.

As always, it is recommended that you refer to local guidelines prior to starting antibiotic treatment.

 Guidance

Public Health England (PHE, 2013) guidance suggests that, in severe cases, vancomycin should be used preferentially as there is some evidence it evokes a more rapid clinical response and there are recent reports of high failure rates with metronidazole.

PHE guidance also suggests that any case satisfying one of the following criteria be treated as 'severe':
- WCC >15×10^9/L
- Creatinine >50% above baseline
- Temperature >38.5°C
- Evidence of severe colitis.

Evidence

Systematic reviews investigating antibiotic therapy for *C. difficile*-associated diarrhoea or 'CDAD' (Nelson *et al.*, 2011; Drekonja *et al.*, 2011) have failed to demonstrate superiority of any one antibiotic over another, except to say that fidaxomicin may result in a lower recurrence rate. Few studies so far have stratified patients by the severity of their condition, although one

such study (Zar *et al.*, 2007) does suggest superiority of vancomycin in severe C. difficile associated diarrhoea. However, concerns regarding the methodology used in this study means its results may not be generalisable.

Other treatments for *C. difficile* infection that you may come across are:

- **Fidaxomicin:** Dose 200 mg BD for 10–14 days. Fidaxomicin is a newer treatment, which may be superior in terms of a sustained response and is sometimes used for patients suffering recurrent episodes of *C. difficile* infection but is considerably more expensive than the other treatments available (about £1600 per course!).
- **Faecal transplant:** This is a newer treatment where faeces from a healthy donor are administered via enema/ nasogastric tube/ at colonoscopy into the recipient with the intention of restoring the normal bowel flora. It has the highest success rate of any treatment but is not widely available and may not be acceptable to everyone!
- **Surgery:** Some patients with severe disease who develop toxic megacolon may require a partial or total colectomy.

Metronidazole: essential pharmacology

Mechanism of action: Metronidazole is administered as a prodrug, which is selectively converted to its active form inside anaerobic bacteria, where it inhibits DNA synthesis and degrades existing DNA.

Activity: Metronidazole is active against anaerobic bacteria and protozoa.

Common side effects: GI disturbance and anorexia, taste disturbance, oral mucositis, disulfiram reactions when taken with alcohol (severe nausea and vomiting); prolonged courses can cause neurotoxicity and psychiatric disturbance.

Pharmacokinetics: Metronidazole is metabolised by hepatic oxidation and caution is advised in patients with severe hepatic insufficiency. No dose reduction is needed in patients with renal impairment (Datapharm, 2015).

✓ DRUGS checklist for METRONIDAZOLE

Dose	400 mg (PO)/ 500 mg (IV)
Route	PO or IV
	Can also be given PR
Units	Milligrams (mg)
Given	TDS
Special situations	Alcohol should be avoided during and for 48 hours following treatment; concomitant use may lead to disulfiram-like reaction.
	Metronidazole is an enzyme inhibitor and may therefore interact with other medications, notably warfarin.
	Dose reduction in severe hepatic impairment:
	Give 400 mg (PO) or 500 mg (IV) TDS.

Common pitfalls

- The clinical effects of *C. difficile* range from asymptomatic colonisation to mild diarrhoea to pseudomembranous colitis to toxic megacolon. Treatment is not necessarily required unless there is a significant symptom burden.
- Colonisation may be distinguished from infection based on a toxin test; however, the test is not 100% sensitive and sometimes patients with toxin-negative results have symptomatic *C. difficile* diarrhoea requiring treatment.
- Patients should be monitored on a daily basis while on treatment for *C. difficile*. Worsening abdominal pain and distension associated with sudden decrease in stool frequency are features to look out for; a plain abdominal radiograph and serum lactate should be performed.
- Do not use antiperistaltic agents in acute diarrhoeal infection as this may delay clearance of the toxin.
- Recurrence of *C. difficile* infection is common; patients and staff should be vigilant for this.

Case outcome and discharge

Mr Bickerstaff was treated with metronidazole. He suffered some worsening of his symptoms over the first 24 hours but an abdominal radiograph did not show any worrying features. He suffered with nausea, probably as a complication of the metronidazole, which was managed with oral antiemetics and he was encouraged to continue with treatment. The diarrhoea settled over the next 7 days and he was discharged to complete a 10-day course of metronidazole in total. His GP was asked to review the ongoing need for omeprazole over the next few months.

DISCHARGE MEDICATION

Date	Medication	Dose	Route	Frequency	Supply	GP to continue?
xx/xx/xx	METRONIDAZOLE	400 mg	PO	Three times daily	To complete a 10 day course, i.e. until xx/xx/xx	N
xx/xx/xx	GLICLAZIDE	80 mg	PO	Twice daily, with meals	14 days	Y
xx/xx/xx	ASPIRIN	75 mg	PO	Once daily	14 days	Y
xx/xx/xx	AMLODIPINE	5 mg	PO	Once daily	14 days	Y

Notes to patient/GP:
Omeprazole stopped due to possible link to C. difficile infection. Please review the ongoing need for antireflux medications in due course. Many thanks.

Discussion of infections related to antibiotic use

Whilst antibiotics are often life-saving medications, their widespread use can lead to problems:

- At an individual level, antibiotics risk depleting the body's normal flora and may leave patients susceptible to secondary infections.
- At a population level, bacterial resistance is a growing concern, with the emergence of so-called 'superbugs'.

Secondary infections

Antibiotic therapy acts not only against the intended pathological bacteria but also some of the body's normal flora. This normal commensal flora usually has a protective effect, out-competing invading organisms. Without the normal flora, the body is susceptible to colonisation by other, sometimes pathogenic organisms.

C. difficile: One of the side effects of treatment with broad-spectrum antibiotics is the unintended disruption of normal gut flora. This allows certain species of bacteria, such as *C. difficile*, to multiply and potentially overwhelm the GI tract, causing diarrhoea and, in severe cases, pseudomembranous colitis. Complications of pseudomembranous colitis include toxic megacolon, dehydration and acute kidney injury, all of which can be potentially fatal, especially in older patients (Bouza *et al.*, 2005). *Clostridia* can be part of normal gut flora and some people are colonised by *C. difficile* without any symptoms; these patients do not require treatment. It is the presence of *C. difficile* in the context of significant illness that necessitates treatment.

The *Clostridium* culprits:

- Co-amoxiclav
- Cephalosporins
- Clindamycin
- Ciprofloxacin
- Carbapenems

Candida: It is very common for patients to develop secondary *Candida* infections (colloquially known as 'thrush') during or soon after receiving a course of antibiotics. The treatment for this is usually with topical or systemic antifungal agents, such as nystatin drops, clotrimazole cream or fluconazole tablets.

Resistant organisms

The widespread use of antibiotics favours the growth of resistant organisms, via natural selection. Some organisms are intrinsically resistant to certain antibiotics, for example enterococci and cephalosporins, aerobic bacteria and metronidazole. However, resistance can also develop in bacterial populations either via enzymes that inhibit the actions of the antibiotic, by alteration of the antibiotic binding site or by preventing the antibiotic gaining access to its binding site (Shales *et al.*, 1997), or by efflux pumps which extrude the antibiotic. Resistant organisms cause infection in a similar way to non-resistant organisms but are harder to treat. Patients colonised or infected with these organisms may be subject to infection control procedures to prevent their spread within a hospital.

Methicillin-resistant *Staphylococcus aureus* (MRSA): This is a strain of *Staphylococcus aureus* that is not sensitive to the usual beta-lactam antibiotics such as flucloxacillin. Antibiotic resistance here is primarily due to an alteration in the organism's 'penicillin-binding protein' (Shales *et al.*, 1997), which prevents the antibiotic binding to the organism. Many people carry MRSA as part of their normal flora but when it causes an infection, it usually requires treatment with a glycopeptide antibiotic such as vancomycin or teicoplanin. Mild infections may be treated with doxycycline or a macrolide; however, susceptibility is unpredictable. It is routinely screened for and eradicated in inpatients. Eradication therapy usually consists of topical mupirocin with or without chlorhexidine. Note, you may come across the term MSSA for methicillin-sensitive *Staphylococcus aureus*.

Resistant Gram-negative bacteria: There has been a recent rise in the number of infections caused by resistant Gram-negative bacteria. Extended spectrum beta-lactamases (ESBLs), AmpC beta-lactamases and carbapenamases are types of *enzyme* that are produced by bacteria and confer a degree of antibiotic resistance to the organisms that produce them (Hawkey and Jones, 2009). The term 'multiply resistant gram-negative organisms' (MRGNO) is sometimes used because ESBLs are not the only mechanism of Gram-negative resistance.

Vancomycin-resistant enterococci (VRE) also known as glycopeptide-resistant enterococci (GRE): Enterococci usually occupy the gastrointestinal tract and female genital tract. Although they can cause infections such as endocarditis, they are often not pathogenic. However, they have become a not infrequent cause of hospital-acquired infections and many strains are intrinsically resistant to commonly used antibiotics. The emergence of enterococci carrying genes for vancomycin resistance is of great concern as infections with these organisms can be extremely difficult to treat. Even if not causing an infection themselves, there is concern they could transfer some of their vancomycin-resistance genes to other pathogenic bacteria, causing serious problems (Cetinkaya *et al.*, 2000). Patients carrying VRE may need to be isolated or special infection control measures taken.

Addressing the problem: antibiotic stewardship

Antibiotic stewardship comprises the mechanisms by which we (as individuals and as organisations) conserve the effectiveness of antimicrobial agents and at the same time minimise antimicrobial side effects.

Each hospital should have evidence-based antimicrobial guidelines, which take into account local resistance patterns to guide antibiotic prescribing. Hospitals are encouraged to audit the mechanisms they have in place to ensure good antibiotic stewardship (DoH, 2011). On an individual level, doctors and nurses who prescribe antibiotics should be aware of the measures they can take to minimise both (1) the occurrence of secondary infections and (2) the emergence of resistant bacteria.

Whilst clinicians are encouraged to provide broad-spectrum antibiotic cover early in the treatment of severe infections, it should also be highlighted that in low-risk scenarios, antibiotics with narrower antimicrobial cover, chosen based on the expected causative organism, should be used preferentially. Likewise, intravenous preparations should be reserved for the most severe cases, with oral administration preferred wherever feasible.

When the intravenous route of administration is deemed necessary, this should be reviewed daily and switched to the oral route once the patient is clinically improving and able to manage enteral preparations (DoH, 2011).

Evidence

In 2011, antimicrobial resistance was a focus of the Chief Medical Officer's annual report (Davies, 2013). It gives the goals of antibiotic stewardship as follows:
- Optimise therapy for individual patients
- Prevent overuse, misuse and abuse
- Minimise development of resistance at patient and community levels.

Clinicians are encouraged to obtain specimens for microscopy, culture and sensitivity ('M, C & S') before initiating antimicrobial treatment wherever possible, with the caveat that this should not delay antibiotic treatment in cases of fulminant sepsis. The results of specimens sent for analysis should be reviewed daily and acted upon promptly (DoH, 2011), in conjunction with the local microbiology team where necessary.

Good documentation of antibiotic choices and the rationale behind their choice is an important part of antibiotic stewardship, as is documenting the expected duration of treatment or a review date (DoH, 2011).

Complementary to good prescribing practice are infection control measures, which are designed to lessen the burden of infection in the hospital environment by preventing the spread of organisms (especially the resistant ones!).

The use of antibiotics prior to surgical procedures is discussed in Chapter 7.

SUMMARY

Whilst antibiotics are important life-saving medications, doctors should be aware of the consequences of their widespread or injudicious use. Anyone prescribing antibiotics should be aware of the concept of 'antibiotic stewardship'. It is important both to be vigilant for *secondary infections*, in patients who have previously received antibiotics as well as being aware of the implications of *drug-resistant organisms*.

🔑 Key learning points

Prescribing for *C. difficile* infection:
- Simple colonisation with *C. difficile* does not require treatment.
- In symptomatic *C. difficile* infection, use either metronidazole or vancomycin in the first instance, depending on the severity of the condition.

Antibiotic stewardship:
- Think carefully about your choice of antibiotic, referring to local guidelines and expertise.
- Always give a review date or a stop date.
- Review microbial culture and sensitivity results regularly and aim to step down to a narrower-spectrum antibiotic as soon as it is clinically indicated.
- Aim to switch from the IV to the oral route of administration as soon as it is clinically indicated.
- Ask your local microbiologist if you are unsure about which antibiotic to prescribe or the duration of treatment.
- Be alert for symptoms of antibiotic-related infections.

FURTHER READING

- Public Health England guidance *Clostridium difficile: Guidance, Data and Analysis* is a readable document providing guidance on the treatment of *C. difficile*. Available at: www.gov.uk/government/collections/clostridium-difficile-guidance-data-and-analysis (accessed Dec. 2015).
- The Royal College of Physicians provides advice for antibiotic prescribing as part of their 'Top Ten Tips' series. Available at: www.rcplondon.ac.uk/resources/top-ten-tips-series (accessed Dec. 2015).

Neutropenic sepsis

> **Mr Hari Ranasinghe**
> **Age: 35 years**
> **Hospital number: 123456**

🔍 Case study

Mr Ranasinghe was diagnosed with Hodgkin's lymphoma 8 months ago and has been started on a course of chemotherapy (ABVD) for this. He has been doing well so far and received his third cycle of treatment 7 days ago. He developed a fever of 38.5°C last night with rigors and, as advised by his haematology team, has come straight into hospital.

PMH: *Hodgkin's lymphoma*

DH: *See FP10*

Allergies: None known

Salient examination findings:
T 40.2°C, HR 115, BP 87/50, RR 25, Sats 96% on air
Weight: 73 kg
He is sitting up and talking, although he reports feeling 'rubbish'
CVS: He has warm peripheries and looks flushed and vasodilated. His pulse is fast but regular. HS I+II+0; JVP not seen
Chest: Air entry to both bases, no added sounds
Abdomen: soft and non-tender
No neurological deficit is noted
There are no indwelling lines and no rashes or swollen joints

Bedside investigations:
Point-of-care tests: WCC 1.0, neutrophils 0.2, Hb 97, Plt 78
vBG: lactate 4

Urine dip: Awaited
ECG: Sinus tachycardia at 112 bpm without isch-
aemic changes

PHARMACY STAMP	AGE 35	FORENAME, SURNAME Hari Ranasinghe
	D.O.B. xx/xx/xxxx	ADDRESS 15 Courtlands Avenue
		NHS NUMBER

ALLOPURINOL 300 mg, once daily, 21 days.

METOCLOPRAMIDE, 10 mg, as needed (max three times daily).

L

SIGNATURE OF PRESCRIBER	DATE

SP21000

Diagnosis

Neutropenic sepsis.

Initial management

This is a potentially very sick patient. Important early interventions and investigations are the same as for sepsis and include: high-flow oxygen, blood cultures, IV antibiotics, IV fluid therapy and measuring hourly urine output (using bottles; catheters can introduce further infection in patients with neutropenia) along with checking the Hb and lactate (Daniels *et al.*, 2010). It is important to try and identify a source, performing a careful examination (don't forget to examine any vascular access sites as well as looking for oral mucositis) and taking relevant investigations, including blood cultures, urine samples, sputum samples, skin swabs and stool samples where relevant. It can be trickier to pin down a source for neutropenic sepsis as localising signs are usually caused by the immune response, which may be blunted in immunosuppressed states (Sickles *et al.*, 1975). It is important to inform the oncology or haematology team when a patient who is receiving chemotherapy develops neutropenic sepsis. If the patient doesn't respond to initial fluid resuscitation, it is sensible to discuss the case with the ICU team.

Prescribing for neutropenic sepsis

FLUID CHART

Date	Fluid	Dose	Route	Rate	Signature	Print name
xx/xx/xx	SODIUM CHLORIDE 0.9%	500 ml	IV	STAT	A. Doctor	A. Doctor
xx/xx/xx	SODIUM CHLORIDE 0.9%	500 ml	IV	STAT	A. Doctor	A. Doctor
xx/xx/xx	SODIUM CHLORIDE 0.9%	500 ml	IV	STAT	A. Doctor	A. Doctor

REGULAR PRESCRIPTIONS

		Circle/enter times below	Day 1	Day 2	Day 3	Day 4
DRUG PIP-TAZ		(06) 08				
Dose 4.5 g	Route IV	Freq QDS	Start date xx/xx/xx	(12)		
Signature A. Doctor	Bleep	Review xx/xx/xx	16			
Additional instructions		(18)				
		(22)				

As there was no clear source of infection and the patient's renal function was normal, he was empirically prescribed a standard dose of a broad-spectrum beta-lactam with pseudomonal cover: Pip-Taz (Tazocin). Some units are still using empirical combination therapy (e.g. Pip-Taz plus gentamicin), although recent evidence has shown monotherapy with a broad-spectrum beta-lactam to be superior (see Evidence).

Fluid challenges were given with good response, titrated to his blood pressure, urine output and serum lactate concentration.

Fluid resuscitation is discussed in Chapter 7.

Antibiotics in neutropenic sepsis: rationale and evidence

Neutropenic sepsis is a medical emergency where prompt treatment can be life-saving. It can rapidly escalate and untreated has a reported mortality rate of between 2% and 21% (NICE, 2012). Patients often present with a fever in the context of being neutropenic, without evidence of full-blown sepsis, so-called 'febrile neutropenia'. This is usually initially treated as neutropenic sepsis, even in the absence of other markers of sepsis, partly because the inflammatory response may be attenuated and partly because it may be detrimental to the patient to wait until the other signs are manifest before providing treatment.

The treatment provided is often empirical as these patients often lack localising signs of infection to help guide antibiotic choices. Other agents *may* be required empirically, depending on the clinical features of the infection. For example, if the patient is thought to have a pneumonia as the source of their infection, adding an agent to cover atypical causes of pneumonia such as a macrolide (e.g. clarithromycin) may be wise (de Naurois *et al.*, 2010); equally, if there is persistent hypotension, this may indicate a Gram-negative sepsis and at this point an aminoglycoside (e.g. gentamicin) may be added to the regimen. As in any other case of sepsis, the antibiotic regimen should be rationalised once culture results and microbiological sensitivities are available, in conjunction with the microbiology team.

The duration of antibiotic treatment depends on a number of factors. Where there is evidence of a particular site of infection or where an organism is identified, this will guide the duration of treatment, although treatment should continue at least until the neutrophil count has recovered (Freifeld *et al.*, 2011). For an unexplained fever in the context of neutropenia, it has been suggested that antibiotic treatment could be stopped once the neutrophil count has recovered (Freifeld *et al.*, 2011).

Piperacillin-tazobactam: essential pharmacology

Pip-Taz (Tazocin) is a broad-spectrum beta-lactam antibiotic (piperacillin) with a built-in beta-lactamase inhibitor (tazobactam). It is active against many aerobic and anaerobic Gram-positive and Gram-negative bacteria, including *Pseudomonas* species. It is not active against bacteria that lack a cell wall (e.g. *Chlamydia* spp., *Mycoplasma* spp.) and species that have acquired resistance to it (e.g. MRSA) (Datapharm, 2015).

Pip-Taz should not be given to patients with anaphylactic reactions to penicillin. Treatment of neutropenic sepsis in penicillin-allergic patients varies between hospitals and local guidelines should be followed.

For further antibiotic pharmacology, see Section Sepsis and Antibiotics.

Evidence

A systematic review of 71 trials (Paul *et al.*, 2013) compared empirical beta-lactam monotherapy with empirical combination therapy (beta-lactam plus aminoglycoside) for febrile neutropenia. The review found that not only did patients who received monotherapy have a lower all-cause mortality but also have a lower risk of fungal superinfection and lower rate of adverse events, notably, nephrotoxicity.

✓ DRUGS checklist for PIPERACILLIN/ TAZOBACTAM (TAZOCIN)	
Dose	4.5 g (4 g piperacillin + 0.5 g tazobactam)
Route	IV infusion (over 30 minutes)
Units	Grams (g)
Given	QDS in neutropenia (usually TDS)
Special situations	Contains penicillin; relatively high sodium content.
	In renal impairment (CrCl <40 mL/min): CrCl 20–40 mL/min: 4.5 g TDS CrCl <20 mL/min: 4.5 g BD.

Other medications used in neutropenic sepsis

Granulocyte-colony stimulating factor (G-CSF) stimulates the bone marrow to make granulocytes (white blood cells). It is sometimes recommended by oncology or haematology teams in cases of neutropenia.

✓	DRUGS checklist for GRANULOCYTE-COLONY STIMULATING FACTOR
Dose	Filgrastim: 30 or 48 megaunits
	Lenograstim: 13 or 34 megaunits
Route	SC
Units	Megaunits (million international units)
Given	OD
Special situations	Side effects include bone and muscle pains, headache, nausea and hypersensitivity reactions.
	Dose is weight dependent.
	Not used in myeloid malignancy as it can promote the growth of myeloid cells.

Further aspects of managing neutropenic sepsis

ⓘ Guidelines

NICE (NICE, 2012) defines neutropenic sepsis as:

- Neutrophil count of ≤0.5 × 10^9/L

plus

- Temperature >38°C or other clinical evidence of sepsis.

NICE provides the following guidance for patients with neutropenic sepsis, where the neutropenia is due to anticancer treatment:

- Prioritise neutropenic sepsis as a medical emergency.

- Provide immediate empiric antibiotic therapy. Current guidance recommends beta-lactam monotherapy and piperacillin-tazobactam is suggested.
- A healthcare professional experienced in the management of complications of anticancer therapy should assess the risk of septic complications within 24 hours of presentation.

Case outcome and discharge

Mr Ranasinghe was admitted to the haematology ward, to an isolation room, and was treated with Pip-Taz until he was clinically better and his neutrophil count had recovered. He was also prescribed G-CSF by the haematology team until his neutrophil count had recovered. Despite cultures being sent, no organism or source of infection was isolated, as is often the case in neutropenic sepsis. He recovered well and was discharged with advice to come straight back if he noticed any deterioration.

DISCHARGE MEDICATION						
Date	Medication	Dose	Route	Frequency	Supply	GP to continue?
xx/xx/xx	ALLOPURINOL	300 mg	PO	Once daily	To complete a 21 day course (as per chemotherapy regimen)	N
xx/xx/xx	METOCLOPRAMIDE	10 mg	PO	As needed, max three times daily	As per chemotherapy regimen	N
Notes to patient/GP: No changes to regular medications.						

Common pitfalls

Culture leucocyte-negative urine: Urine should be cultured even if there are no leucocytes on urine dip as the neutropenic patient is leucocyte deplete by definition. The urine may still grow organisms on culture, which can be vital to treating the underlying infection. You should highlight to the laboratory on the request form that the patient is neutropenic and that you would still like the urine to be cultured whether or not there is a high leucocyte count.

Don't be fooled by a clear chest X-ray if there are clinical signs: Similarly, a chest X-ray may not show consolidation in neutropenic patients as there are no white cells or leucocytes to create the 'pus' which causes consolidation (Sickles *et al.*, 1975). You should rely on clinical signs and observations and add in antibiotics to cover 'chest organisms' where there is a clinical suspicion of a chest source (low oxygen saturations, raised respiratory rate, pleuritic chest pains etc.).

Think about unusual organisms: If there is no response to the usual antibiotics, think outside the box: could this be a resistant organism, a fungal infection or a viral infection, requiring a different type of treatment?

SUMMARY

Neutropenic sepsis is a medical emergency and should be treated promptly with antibiotics as well as other supportive measures such as fluid resuscitation. Physicians working in emergency departments and acute medical units should be familiar with the initial treatment of this life-threatening condition.

Key learning points

Neutropenic sepsis management:
- Prompt recognition and treatment of neutropenic sepsis can be life-saving and antibiotics must be given within 1 hour.
- Empiric therapy is with a broad-spectrum beta-lactam antibiotic (or as directed by local guidelines in penicillin allergy).
- Fluid resuscitation is important and should proceed as for any other patient with sepsis.
- Neutropenic patients should be nursed in isolation.
- The oncology or haematology team should be contacted for advice.

FURTHER READING

- A succinct summary article regarding infections in immunosuppressed patients, including those with neutropenia, is: Barnes R (2012). Infection in cancer and transplantation. *Medicine* 41: 624–7.

Now visit **www.wileyessential.com/pharmacology** to test yourself on this chapter.

References

Bouza E, Muñoz P, Alonso R (2005). Clinical manifestations, treatment and control of infections caused by Clostridium difficile. *Clinical Microbiol Infect* 11 (Suppl. 4): 57–64.

British Medical Association and Royal Pharmaceutical Society of Great Britain (BMA/RPS) (2015). *British National Formulary 69*, 69th edn. BMJ group and Pharmaceutical Press, London.

Campagna JD, Bond MC, Schabelman E *et al.* (2012). The use of cephalosporins in penicillin-allergic patients: a literature review. *J Emerg Med* 42: 612–20.

Cetinkaya Y, Falk P, Mayhall CG (2000). Vancomycin-resistant enterococci. *Clin Microbiol Rev* 13: 686–707.

Cockcroft DW, Gault MH (1976). Prediction of creatinine clearance from serum creatinine. *Nephron* 16: 31–41.

Daniels R, Nutbeam T, McNamara G *et al.* (2010). The sepsis six and the severe sepsis resuscitation bundle: a prospective observational cohort study. *Emerg Med J* 28: 507–12.

Datapharm (2015). *Electronic Medicines Compendium (eMC) Summaries of Product Characteristics (SPC)*. Available at: www.medicines.org.uk (accessed Dec. 2015).

Davies SC (2013). *Annual Report of the Chief Medical Officer,* Vol. 2, 2011. *Infections and the Rise of Antimicrobial Resistance*. Department of Health: London. Available at: www.gov.uk/government/uploads/system/uploads/attachment_data/file/138331/CMO_Annual_Report_Volume_2_2011.pdf (accessed Dec. 2015).

Dellinger RP, Levy MM, Rhodes A *et al.* (2013). Surviving sepsis campaign: international guidelines for management of severe sepsis and septic shock: 2012. *Crit Care Med* 41: 580–637.

de Naurois J, Novitzky-Basso I, Gill MJ *et al.*, on behalf of the ESMO Guidelines Working Group. (2010). Management of febrile neutropenia: ESMO clinical practice guidelines. *Ann Oncol* 21 (Suppl. 5): v252–6.

Department of Health (DoH) Advisory Committee on Antimicrobial Resistance and Healthcare Associated Infections (2011). *Antimicrobial Stewardship Guidance for Secondary Care, England;* *Start Smart – Then Focus*. Department of Health. Available at: www.gov.uk/government/publications/antimicrobial-stewardship-start-smart-then-focus (accessed Dec. 2015).

Drekonja DM, Butler M, MacDonald R *et al.* (2011). Comparative effectiveness of *Clostridium difficile* treatments: a systematic review. *Ann Intern Med* 155: 839–47.

Ferrer R, Artigas A, Suarez D *et al.* for the Edusepsis Study Group (2009). Effectiveness of treatments for severe sepsis: a prospective, multicenter, observational study. *Am J Respir Crit Care Med* 180: 861–6.

Freifeld AG, Bow EJ, Sepkowitz KA *et al.*, Infectious Diseases Society of America (2011). Clinical practice guideline for the use of antimicrobial agents in neutropenic patients with cancer: 2010 update by the Infectious Diseases Society of America. *Clin Infect Dis* 52: e56–93.

Garner DP (2013). *Microbiology Nuts and Bolts*. Available at: www.microbiologynutsandbolts. co.uk (accessed Dec. 2015).

Hawkey PM, Jones AM (2009). The changing epidemiology of resistance. *J Antimicrob Chemother* 64 (Suppl. 1): i3–i10.

Ibrahim EH, Sherman G, Ward S *et al.* (2000). The influence of inadequate antimicrobial treatment of bloodstream infections on patient outcomes in the ICU setting. *Chest* 118: 146–55.

Janarthanan S, Ditah I, Adler DG *et al.* (2012). Clostridium difficile-associated diarrhea and proton pump inhibitor therapy: a meta-analysis. *Am J Gastroenterol* 107: 1001–10.

Kilburn SA, Featherstone P, Higgins B *et al.* (2010). Interventions for cellulitis and erysipelas. *Cochrane Database Syst Rev* (6): CD004299.

Kula B, Djordjevic G, Robinson JL (2014). A systematic review: can one prescribe carbapenems to patients with IgE-mediated allergy to penicillins or cephalosporins? *Clin Infect Dis* 59: 1113–22.

Kumar A, Roberts D, Wood KE *et al.* (2006). Duration of hypotension before initiation of effective antimicrobial therapy is the critical determinant of survival in human septic shock. *Crit Care Med* 34: 1589–96.

Levy MM, Dellinger RP, Townsend SR *et al.* (2010). The Surviving Sepsis Campaign: results of an international guideline-based performance improvement program targeting severe sepsis. *Crit Care Med* 38: 367–74.

Nelson RL, Kelsey P, Leeman H *et al.* (2011). Antibiotic treatment for *Clostridium difficile*-associated diarrhea in adults. *Cochrane Database Syst Rev* (9): CD004610.

National Institute for Health and Care Excellence (NICE) (2012). Neutropenic sepsis: prevention and management in people with cancer, CG151. Available at: www.nice.org.uk/guidance/cg151 (accessed Dec. 2015).

Paul M, Dickstein Y, Schlesinger A, *et al.* (2013). Beta-lactam versus beta-lactam-aminoglycoside combination therapy in cancer patients with neutropenia. *Cochrane Database Syst Rev* (6): CD003038.

Pegler S, Healy B (2007). In patients allergic to penicillin, consider second and third generation cephalosporins for life threatening infections *BMJ* 335: 991.

Pichichero ME, Casey JR (2007). Safe use of selected cephalosporins in penicillin-allergic patients: A meta-analysis. *Otolaryngol Head Neck Surg* 136: 340–7.

Public Health England (PHE) (2014). *The characteristics, diagnosis, management, surveillance and epidemiology of Clostridium difficile (C. difficile)*. Available at: www.gov.uk/government/collections/clostridium-difficile-guidance-data-and-analysis (accessed Dec. 2015).

Rang HP, Dale MM, Ritter JM *et al.* (2003). *Pharmacology*, 5th edn. Churchill Livingstone.

Roberts MC (2003). Tetracycline therapy: update. *Clin Infect Dis* 36: 462–7.

Rybak MJ (2006). The pharmacokinetic and pharmacodynamic properties of vancomycin. *Clin Infect Dis* 42 (Suppl. 1): S35–9.

Shales DM, Gerding DN, John JF *et al.*: Society for Healthcare Epidemiology of America and Infectious Diseases Society of America Joint Committee on the Prevention of Antimicrobial Resistance (1997). Guidelines for the prevention of antimicrobial resistance in hospitals. *Infect Control Hosp Epidemiol* 18: 275–91.

Sickles EA, Greene WH, Wiernik PH (1975). Clinical presentation of infection in granulocytopenic patients. *Arch Intern Med* 135(5): 715–9.

Wolfson JS, Hooper DC (1989). Fluoroquinolone antimicrobial agents. *Clin Microbiol Rev* 2: 378–424.

Zar FA, Bakkanagari SR, Moorthi KM *et al.* (2007). A comparison of vancomycin and metronidazole for the treatment of *Clostridium difficile*-associated diarrhea, stratified by disease severity. *Clin Infect Dis* 45: 302–7.

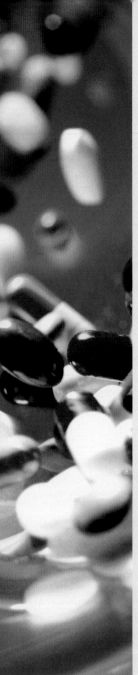

CHAPTER 12

Rheumatology

Victoria Taylor

Key topics:

Learning objectives

By the end of this chapter, you should be able to…

- …safely prescribe a range of commonly used analgesic preparations.

- …prescribe safely for patients with some of the commonly encountered rheumatological and musculoskeletal conditions.

- …determine when it is safer not to prescribe for patients with these conditions and when to seek help.

- …discuss the roles and implications of using some of the disease-modifying antirheumatic drugs (DMARDs) and newer biological therapies used in the treatment of rheumatoid arthritis.

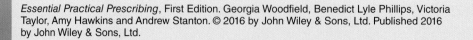

Essential Practical Prescribing, First Edition. Georgia Woodfield, Benedict Lyle Phillips, Victoria Taylor, Amy Hawkins and Andrew Stanton. © 2016 by John Wiley & Sons, Ltd. Published 2016 by John Wiley & Sons, Ltd.

Osteoarthritis

> **Mr Arthur Cartwright**
>
> **Age: 62**
>
> **Hospital number: 123456**

PC: Mr Cartwright was admitted to hospital a week ago with an ischaemic stroke affecting his right arm and leg. The physiotherapists have started to work with him on his mobility but ask if you would review him as he is suffering with a lot of pain in his left knee. When you speak to him, he says the pain has been getting gradually worse over the last 6 months and describes the pain as occurring mainly on and after mobilising. He describes only 15 minutes of morning stiffness. When you ask about other joints, he says they are mostly ok, although some of the joints in his hands get a little sore in the winter.

PMH: *IHD (MI 6 years ago), hypercholesterolaemia, hypothyroidism*

Allergies: None

Examination:
HR 75, BP 165/87, Sats 98% on air, RR 16, T 36.7°C
The knee is not red, hot or swollen and there is no apparent effusion, although he reports his knee does sometimes become swollen and it is a little tender to touch. There is a slightly limited range of active and passive movement with marked crepitus on knee flexion. The hip joint gives a little pain on internal rotation; no abnormality is found in the ankle joint. You note the presence of Heberden's nodes in his fingers.

Investigations:
A left knee X-ray shows no fracture but does shows evidence of joint-space narrowing, with an osteophyte visible on the medial aspect of the tibial plateau.

Weight: *82 kg*

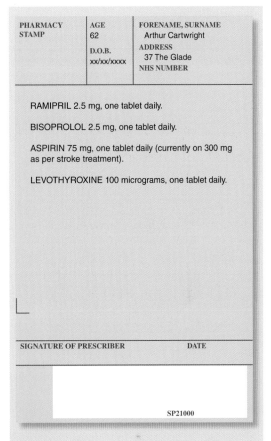

| PHARMACY STAMP | AGE 62 | FORENAME, SURNAME Arthur Cartwright |
| | D.O.B. xx/xx/xxxx | ADDRESS 37 The Glade NHS NUMBER |

RAMIPRIL 2.5 mg, one tablet daily.

BISOPROLOL 2.5 mg, one tablet daily.

ASPIRIN 75 mg, one tablet daily (currently on 300 mg as per stroke treatment).

LEVOTHYROXINE 100 micrograms, one tablet daily.

SIGNATURE OF PRESCRIBER   DATE

SP21000

Diagnosis

Mr Cartwright has features of osteoarthritis of his left knee without features of an inflammatory arthritis.

Initial management

This is a chronic condition for which there are conservative, medical and surgical options. The most important interventions are non-pharmacological (e.g. weight loss, physiotherapy) and must be instituted before any regular medication, especially opiates.

Prescribing for osteoarthritis

When prescribing for osteoarthritis (OA), it is recommended that you use a stepwise approach, starting with simple analgesia, such as paracetamol or non-steroidal anti-inflammatory drugs (NSAIDs), and only escalating to stronger medications (such

REGULAR PRESCRIPTIONS

DRUG RAMIPRIL				Circle/enter times below ↓	Enter dates below			
					Day 1	Day 2	Day 3	Day 4
				06				
				(08)				
Dose 5 mg	Route PO	Freq OD	Start date xx/xx/xx	12				
Signature A. Doctor		Bleep	Review	16				
				18				
Additional instructions				22				

DRUG BISOPROLOL					06				
				(08)				
Dose 2.5 mg	Route PO	Freq OD	Start date xx/xx/xx	12				
Signature A. Doctor		Bleep	Review	16				
				18				
Additional instructions				22				

DRUG LEVOTHYROXINE					06				
				(08)				
Dose 100 micrograms	Route PO	Freq OD	Start date xx/xx/xx	12				
Signature A. Doctor		Bleep	Review	16				
				18				
Additional instructions				22				

DRUG ASPIRIN					06				
				(08)				
Dose 300 mg	Route PO	Freq OD	Start date xx/xx/xx	12				
Signature A. Doctor		Bleep	Review	16				
				18				
Additional instructions				22				

DRUG PARACETAMOL					(06)				
				08				
Dose 1 g	Route PO	Freq QDS	Start date xx/xx/xx	(12)				
Signature A. Doctor		Bleep	Review	16				
				(18)				
Additional instructions				(22)				

AS REQUIRED MEDICATION

DRUG CODEINE PHOSPHATE				Date			
				Time			
Dose 30 mg	Route PO	Max freq QDS	Start date xx/xx/xx	Dose			
				Route			
Signature/Bleep A. Doctor		Max dose in 24 hrs	Review	Given			
				Check			
Additional instructions							

In this section, we cover paracetamol and the weak opioids. NSAIDs are discussed in the Gout section of this chapter.

Paracetamol: rationale and evidence

Paracetamol (or acetaminophen if you're American) is an effective and safe analgesic at the recommended doses, with few side effects. Its efficacy should not be underestimated even in severe pain. There is evidence that NSAIDs are more effective in OA but these medications also come with a number of cautions and side effects and most would agree that paracetamol should be the first-line treatment in OA (see Evidence and Guidelines).

⊙ Guidelines:

At the time of writing, NICE is awaiting the outcome of an MRHA report on the safety of over-the-counter analgesics before issuing new guidance on the pharmacological management of OA. At present the guidance recommends paracetamol or topical NSAIDs as first-line treatment for OA (NICE, 2014).

🔍 Evidence

A number of systematic reviews have looked at the efficacy of paracetamol in OA. One such review (Towheed et al., 2006) looked at 15 RCTs, seven of which compare paracetamol to placebo and 12 of which compare paracetamol to an NSAID. Outcomes included measures of pain, function and global assessment. A meta-analysis of the data showed paracetamol to have a small but significant advantage over placebo in terms of reducing pain with no differences in toxicity. NSAIDs appeared to be more effective than paracetamol although there was an increased number of withdrawals due to GI side effects from NSAIDs. The longer-term safety of using paracetamol or NSAIDs in OA was difficult to assess as the trials tended to be of short duration (median 6 weeks).

as the weak opioids) if this along with non-drug interventions (weight loss, physiotherapy etc.) fail. In mild or intermittent pain states is usual to start with analgesics on an 'as needed' basis, although for pain that is present most of the time, regular analgesia is helpful to provide background analgesia and prevent distressing 'spikes' in pain. It was decided to treat Mr Cartwright with regular paracetamol and codeine as needed, to achieve a good level of analgesia during his daily physiotherapy sessions.

✓ DRUGS checklist for PARACETAMOL

Dose	500 mg–1 g
	Decreased doses are advised for patients weighing <50 kg (see Special Situations)
Route	PO (also available as an IV preparation, requiring no dose adjustment)
Units	Grams (g) or milligrams (mg)
Given	Maximum QDS
Special situations	Paracetamol is also an effective antipyretic agent.
	Side effects are rare but hypersensitivity can occur.
	Toxicity can occur with doses only a little higher than the therapeutic dose and patients with low body weight are especially at risk. The BNF advises that daily doses of paracetamol should not exceed 60 mg/kg when prescribed for adults weighing <50 kg (BMA/RPS, 2015). The maximum daily dose should be reduced to 3 g for adult patients with hepatocellular insufficiency, chronic alcoholism, chronic malnutrition or dehydration. Be aware of the possibility of patients having taken paracetamol-containing cold and flu remedies.

Paracetamol: essential pharmacology

The mechanism of action of paracetamol, despite being one of the most widely used analgesic medications, remains to be fully elucidated. It has been shown to have a weak anti-inflammatory effect, seemingly mediated via inhibition of prostaglandin synthesis (i.e. similar to the NSAIDs). There are studies suggesting that under conditions of mild but not severe inflammation, paracetamol inhibits the actions of cyclo-oxygenase-2 (COX-2), raising concerns by some about the co-administration of paracetamol and NSAIDs (Hinz and Brune, 2012). Other studies have suggested that the antinociceptive effects of paracetamol are dependent on the serotonergic and/or cannabinoid systems (Mallet *et al.*, 2008; Ottani *et al.*, 2006).

Paracetamol is well absorbed orally, reaching peak plasma concentrations in 30 minutes–2 hours. It is metabolised in the liver and its metabolites are excreted in urine (Datapharm, 2015).

The weak opioid analgesics: rationale and evidence

Codeine and tramadol are commonly used analgesic medications, which appear to be effective in pain caused by OA (see Evidence). As with all opioids, prominent side effects include nausea and constipation. Patients with a tendency towards constipation may require concomitant treatment with laxatives.

Dihydrocodeine is very similar to codeine and used interchangeably in clinical practice.

🔍 Evidence

A systematic review (Cepeda *et al.*, 2006) looked at the efficacy of tramadol in OA. Eleven placebo-controlled RCTs were reviewed, although only two studies used tramadol in addition to paracetamol (as is perhaps more common in clinical practice). The results suggest that tramadol is effective in controlling pain and improving global assessment scores in OA, with a number needed to treat to benefit (NNTB) of 6. However, it was associated with significantly more adverse events than placebo with an overall number needed to treat to harm (NNTH) of 8, which may limit its usefulness. The authors note that 10 out of the 11 studies were industry funded.

One RCT (Wilder-Smith *et al.*, 2001) compared tramadol and dihydrocodeine (both slow-release preparations), showing both to be effective in controlling OA-related pain when used in addition to NSAIDs, with tramadol seemingly better at controlling rest pain. Overall adverse effects were more common in the tramadol group although dihydrocodeine seemed slightly more constipating.

✓ **DRUGS checklist for CODEINE PHOSPHATE**

Dose	30–60 mg (maximum 240 mg daily); lower doses are available in over-the counter-preparations
Route	PO
Units	Milligrams (mg)
Given	As needed, up to four times per day (QDS)
Special situations	Codeine also has some antitussive (anticough) effects.
	Side effects include: constipation, nausea, vomiting, headache, rash or pruritis, blurred vision and biliary spasm. Although rarely seen, codeine can be addictive.
	Codeine can cause respiratory depression, especially in patients with underlying predisposition towards type 2 respiratory failure and caution is advised in renal impairment. In patients with hepatic impairment, it may precipitate coma.
	Patients mustn't drive or operate heavy machinery whilst taking codeine and it is contraindicated in breastfeeding women.

✓ **DRUGS checklist for TRAMADOL**

Dose	50–100 mg
Route	PO (also available as an IV preparation, requiring no dose adjustment)
Units	Milligrams (mg)
Given	As needed, up to four times per day (QDS)
Special situations	A modified-release version also exists which should only be given BD. Be sure you know what you're prescribing when transcribing a patient's usual medications onto a hospital drug chart.
	Side effects include: nausea, dizziness, constipation vomiting, headache, dry mouth, fatigue and sweating. It can also cause psychiatric reactions, including hallucinations. Tramadol is felt to have low dependence potential.
	Patients mustn't drive or operate heavy machinery whilst taking tramadol.
	In renal impairment (CrCl <30 mL/min) or hepatic impairment, 12-hourly dosing is recommended and it is contraindicated once CrCl <10 mL/min.
	It may be better tolerated with a slow up-titration of dose (Ruoff, 1999).

The weak opioid analgesics: essential pharmacology

Pain is a subjective experience comprising (often but not always) a noxious stimulus and an affective component. The opioid analgesics are effective in reducing both aspects of the experience of pain. They work by interacting with the μ-opioid receptor, which mediates the antinociceptive effects of the drugs as well as many of their side effects (Rang *et al.*, 2003).

Codeine is a weak agonist at the μ-opioid receptor and is metabolised to morphine, an active metabolite, by the cytochrome P450 enzyme, CYP2D6. Interestingly, the presence and activity of the CYP2D6 enzyme varies between populations with 7% of Caucasians being deficient, meaning the drug is ineffective and 29% of Ethiopian Africans being ultrametabolisers, potentially putting them at risk of toxicity (see Box Pharmacogenetics) (Datapharm, 2015). Codeine is metabolised in the liver and excreted by the kidney.

Pharmacogenetics

Pharmacogenetics is the study of how genetic variability can be used to predict individual patient responses to a drug, both in terms of efficacy as well as toxicity. This field has the potential to help select out patients for whom a drug would be ineffective or even dangerous. One example of pharmacogenetics in current use is the practice of screening for thiopurine-*S*-methyltransferase (TPMT) polymorphisms prior to using azathioprine in inflammatory bowel disease (IBD) to avoid the profound bone marrow suppression that can be associated with low enzyme activity (Weinshilboum and Wang, 2004).

Tramadol is a weak agonist at the μ-opioid receptor and also acts as a weak noradrenaline reuptake inhibitor. It may also enhance serotonin release and, in combination with other serotonergic drugs, can potentially contribute to the development of serotonin syndrome. It too has an active metabolite, *O*-desmethyl tramadol, which has a higher affinity for the μ-opioid receptor than tramadol itself, although it is not known which of

these primarily contributes to its analgesic effect. Tramadol is excreted via the kidneys (Datapharm, 2015).

Further aspects of osteoarthritis management

Other pharmacological treatments used in OA include topical NSAIDs, capsaicin cream and glucocorticoid joint injections. Glucosamine and chondroitin (the so-called 'nutraceuticals') are not recommended by NICE.

The allied health professions including physiotherapists and occupational therapists often have an important role to play in managing OA. Non-pharmacological strategies include:

- Weight loss
- Strengthening and aerobic exercise
- Supports and braces
- Assistive devices, e.g. walking sticks.

Case outcome

Mr Cartwright found that regular paracetamol allowed him to continue his physiotherapy and a topical NSAID (ibuprofen gel) was added in, which helped settle any additional pain after a session of physiotherapy. He only required codeine on a couple of occasions. When he was discharged, a week later, his GP was advised of this new diagnosis.

DISCHARGE MEDICATION						
Date	Medication	Dose	Route	Frequency	Supply	GP to continue?
xx/xx/xx	RAMIPRIL	5 mg	PO	Once daily	14 days	Y
xx/xx/xx	BISOPROLOL	2.5 mg	PO	Once daily	14 days	Y
xx/xx/xx	CLOPIDOGREL	75 mg	PO	Once daily	14 days	Y
xx/xx/xx	LEVOTHYROXINE	100 micrograms	PO	Once daily	14 days	Y
xx/xx/xx	PARACETAMOL	1 g	PO	Four times daily	14 days	Review in 2 weeks
xx/xx/xx	IBUPROFEN GEL (IBUGEL FORTE®, IBUPROFEN 10%)	⊤	Topical (left knee)	As needed, max three times daily	14 days	Review in 2 weeks

Notes to patient/GP:
Aspirin switched to clopidogrel following an ischaemic stroke. Paracetamol and ibuprofen gel started for knee osteoarthritis. Please would you review Mr Cartwright's symptoms and analgesic medications in 2 weeks' time? Many thanks.

Common pitfalls

- Watch out for the many over-the-counter and prescribed paracetamol-containing preparations, such as co-codamol, co-dydramol, Anadin Extra®, Beechams All-In-One®, Codipar®, Lemsip Cold & Flu®, Migraleve®, Night Nurse®, Panadol®, Zapain®. Type 'paracetamol' into the search bar at www.medicines.org.uk/ to see a full list of paracetamol-containing products. It is important to advise patients of this phenomenon and of the maximum recommended daily dosage. See Chapter 1 for details of how to treat paracetamol overdose.
- Don't forget that paracetamol should be prescribed at a lower dose for those with low body weight. If the patient looks like they might weigh <50 kg, prescribe a lower dose until their weight has been checked.
- Don't forget that codeine is a weak opioid and may be associated with some of the side effects of the stronger opioids such as respiratory depression.

SUMMARY

Osteoarthritis is a commonly seen chronic musculoskeletal condition resulting in joint pain and often associated with some level of functional disability. Pain has a huge impact on a patient's quality of life and providing good analgesia is one of the most important things you can do as a doctor, but keep in mind that no drug is without side effects or potential adverse consequences. Think about these when you are prescribing and how they might relate to the individual patient you are prescribing for.

🔑 Key learning points

Management of osteoarthritis:
- Use analgesia, following a step-wise approach, alongside non-pharmacological measures to achieve pain control.
- It is important to be aware of relevant side effects and cautions when prescribing analgesic medications.

FURTHER READING

- A good review article is available in the *BMJ*: Bennell KL, Hunter DJ, Hinman RA (2012). Management of osteoarthritis of the knee. *BMJ* 345: e4934.
- An interesting article covering the evolution of pharmacogenetics is freely available from the journal *Nature*: Meyer UA (2004). Pharmacogenetics – five decades of therapeutic lessons from genetic diversity. *Nat Rev Genetics* 5: 669–76.

Gout

> **Mr Giles McKenzie**
>
> **Age: 58 years**
>
> **Hospital number: 123456**

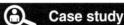 Case study

Mr McKenzie has been admitted to hospital with an acute kidney injury secondary to a prolonged bout of diarrhoea and vomiting. He is feeling a little better but you are asked to see him as his left knee has become swollen and tender. He has had two similar episodes in the last year, previously in his right big toe, although he thinks this is by far the worst.

PMH: *Gout, hypertension, diabetes*

DH: *See FP10*

Allergies: *None*

Salient examination findings:
HR 93, BP148/89, Sats 98% on air, RR 16, T 37.7°C
Left knee: red, hot, swollen and tender to touch
Other joints: No swelling or tenderness

Investigations:
Stool culture: negative
Urine culture: negative
Latest renal function results:
Na: 136, K: 4.6, urea: 9, creatinine: 147 (baseline creatinine: 90)

PHARMACY STAMP	AGE 58	FORENAME, SURNAME Giles McKenzie
	D.O.B. xx/xx/xxxx	ADDRESS Cliplet Close NHS NUMBER

BENDROFLUMETHIAZIDE 5 mg, one tablet daily.

RAMIPRIL 2.5 mg, one tablet daily.

METFORMIN 500 mg twice daily.

ALLOPURINOL 100 mg, one tablet daily.

SIGNATURE OF PRESCRIBER	DATE

SP21000

Latest glucose: 5.7
Aspiration of the joint reveals straw-coloured fluid which has no organisms seen on microscopy but numerous needle-shaped negatively birefringent crystals.

Diagnosis
Acute gout, with acute kidney injury.

Initial measures
In acute gout, the patient should be advised to rest the affected joint and adequate analgesia should be provided. If there is a suspicion of septic arthritis, IV antibiotics should be started as per local guidelines once urgent joint aspiration has been performed, and should be continued until aspirate results exclude septic arthritis.

Prescribing for acute gout

Gout is a crystal arthropathy with deposition of monosodium urate crystals within articular and periarticular tissues, causing acute pain. The treatment of acute gout therefore consists of measures to control the pain. Commonly used medications include:

- NSAIDs
- Colchicine
- Intra-articular steroids (only if joint is non-septic).

However, consideration of any co-existing conditions requires some thought before prescribing. Neither NSAIDs nor colchicine are ideal medications in the above situation because of the acute kidney injury (Mr McKenzie's bendroflumethiazide, ramipril and metformin have also been stopped here for this reason). Opiate analgesics can be used as adjunct although they have their own limitations in renal failure. Ice-packs can also be a helpful adjunct.

Allopurinol should not be started during an acute flare of gout but should be continued at a previously established dose.

ONCE ONLY PRESCRIPTIONS

Date	Time to be given	DRUG	Dose	Route	Prescriber Signature	Bleep
xx/xx/xx	15:00	PARACETAMOL	1 g	PO	A. Doctor	

REGULAR PRESCRIPTIONS

	Circle/enter times below ↓	Enter dates below			
		Day 1	Day 2	Day 3	Day 4
DRUG DALTEPARIN	06				
	(08)				
Dose 5000 units / Route SC / Freq OD / Start date xx/xx/xx	12				
Signature A. Doctor / Bleep / Review	16				
	18				
Additional instructions	22				
DRUG ~~BENDROFLUMETHIAZIDE~~	06				
	(08)				
Dose ~~2.5 mg~~ / Route ~~PO~~ / Freq ~~OD~~ / Start date xx/xx/xx	12				
Signature A. Doctor / Bleep / Review	16				
	18				
Additional instructions	22				
DRUG ~~RAMIPRIL~~	06				
	(08)				
Dose ~~5 mg~~ / Route ~~PO~~ / Freq ~~OD~~ / Start date xx/xx/xx	12				
Signature A. Doctor / Bleep / Review	16				
	18				
Additional instructions	22				
DRUG ALLOPURINOL	06				
	(08)				
Dose 100 mg / Route PO / Freq OD / Start date xx/xx/xx	12				
Signature A. Doctor / Bleep / Review	16				
	18				
Additional instructions	22				
DRUG ~~METFORMIN~~	06				
	(08)				
Dose ~~500 mg~~ / Route ~~PO~~ / Freq ~~BD~~ / Start date xx/xx/xx	12				
Signature A. Doctor / Bleep / Review	16				
	(20)				
Additional instructions	22				
DRUG PARACETAMOL	(06)				
	08				
Dose 1 g / Route PO / Freq Max QDS / Start date xx/xx/xx	(12)				
Signature A. Doctor / Bleep / Review	16				
	(18)				
Additional instructions	(22)				

AS REQUIRED MEDICATION

DRUG CODEINE PHOSPHATE	Date		
	Time		
Dose 60 mg / Route PO / Max freq QDS / Start date xx/xx/xx	Dose		
	Route		
Signature/Bleep A. Doctor / Max dose in 24 hrs / Review	Given		
	Check		
Additional instructions			

Non-steroidal anti-inflammatory medications: rationale and evidence

Gout is an acute inflammatory condition and therefore responds to treatment with medications that counter the inflammatory response. There are a wide range of NSAIDs available, including ibuprofen, naproxen, diclofenac and indomethacin. They have anti-inflammatory and antipyretic effects. There is no good evidence for choosing one over another NSAID in terms of efficacy (see Evidence) but naproxen is thought to have a milder side-effect profile.

🔍 Evidence

Comparative studies have not demonstrated that there is any one superior NSAID in gout. One randomised, double-blind study (Schumacher et al., 2002) compared indomethacin with etoricoxib (a selective COX-2 inhibitor) in acute gout and showed that both had similar efficacy in reducing patients' symptoms as well as physician-assessed measures of joint inflammation.

Whilst NSAIDs are good anti-inflammatories, they have a number of side effects (see Section Non-steroidal Anti-inflammatory Medications: Essential Pharmacology) and caution is advised, especially in patients with renal failure. Concurrent treatment with gastroprotective agents (e.g. with a PPI or H2-antgonist) may be advisable.

✓ DRUGS checklist for NAPROXEN

Dose	250 mg–500 mg
Route	PO
Units	Milligrams (mg)
Given	BD or TDS (max 1 g per day) In gout, an initial dose of 750 mg has been suggested, followed by 250 mg TDS for 1–2 weeks

Special situations	Side effects: acute kidney injury, gastric irritation and ulcers, bleeding (platelet dysfunction), elevations in liver function tests.
	Caution is advised in patients with asthma, elderly patients with multiple co-morbidities and NSAIDs are not recommended in IBD.
	NSAIDs are contraindicated in the last trimester of pregnancy, people with previous GI bleeding due to NSAIDs or active peptic ulcers, hypersensitivity (allergy or asthma) and in severe hepatic, renal or cardiac disease.

Non-steroidal anti-inflammatory medications: essential pharmacology

How do they work?

NSAIDs work by inhibiting the enzyme cyclo-oxygenase (COX, otherwise known as prostaglandin G/H synthetase), which is present in nearly all tissues. COX converts arachidonic acid to prostanoids, which go on to act in a number of physiological and potentially pathological processes. There are two isoenzymes: COX-1, which is constitutively active (i.e. active all the time) and COX-2, which is inducible in response to inflammation (although largely true, the actual situation is more complex than this). The traditional NSAIDs are non-selective and inhibit both isoforms to some extent, decreasing prostanoid production and preventing its down-stream effects. The desired clinical end-point is a decrease in the pain caused by localised inflammation, although depletion of prostanoids, as discussed in Section Unwanted Effects, also accounts for the undesired effects of the NSAIDs.

A note on aspirin: Although aspirin has many similarities to the NSAIDs, when used in analgesic doses (>600 mg), uric acid excretion may be impaired, worsening gout (Jordan *et al.*, 2007).

Selective COX-2 inhibitors

In the 1990s, a second generation of COX-inhibitors, which acted selectively on the COX-2 isoenzyme, was produced, with the idea that the analgesic effects of COX-inhibition could be separated from the gastrointestinal side effects. However, in the 2000s, data emerged suggesting that these medications increased the risk of cardiovascular events and rofecoxib (Vioxx) was taken off the market following a trial which showed a fivefold increased risk of MI compared to naproxen. Subsequent meta-analyses showed that all non-naproxen NSAIDs carried an approximately twofold increased risk of MI and that this risk was comparable amongst the various agents studied (Kearney *et al.*, 2006).

COX-2 inhibitors include: celecoxib, etoricoxib and rofecoxib (no longer available).

Unwanted effects

The side effects of NSAIDs are related to their ability to deplete prostanoids. Certain prostanoids, namely prostaglandin E2 (PGE2) and prostacyclin (PGI2), inhibit gastric acid production and promote gastric mucus production, both of which protect the mucosa from erosions and ulcers (Rang *et al.*, 2003). The depletion of these prostanoids may lead to an increased risk of gastric erosions and ulcers, although it is also possible that inhibition of platelet-derived COX-1 predisposes to bleeding complications from gastric erosions whether secondary to NSAID use or not. In the renal glomeruli, prostanoids are responsible for dilating the afferent arterioles and thereby maintaining glomerular flow, in conditions of decreased renal perfusion. The depletion of prostanoids by NSAID medications may therefore lead to renal impairment in susceptible individuals (i.e. those already at risk of renal dysfunction due to heart failure, liver cirrhosis, dehydration etc.), by impairing their ability to deal with renal compromise (Whelton, 1999). As with aspirin, NSAIDs can cause a hypersensitivity syndrome and can trigger asthma attacks in some people with asthma.

Pharmacokinetics

NSAIDs are eliminated via the kidneys by glomerular filtration and may accumulate in renal failure or where renal blood flow is impaired (e.g. heart failure, liver cirrhosis) (Datapharm, 2015).

Colchicine: rationale and evidence

Colchicine is an alkaloid derivative of the autumn crocus plant (*Colchicum autumnale*, a member of the lily family) and has been used in gout for over 2000 years (Terkeltaub, 2009). However, in modern medicine, it is usually used as a second-choice agent in patients who are unable to take NSAIDs. It is recommended at low doses (see Evidence and British Society of Rheumatology (BSR) guidelines, available at: www.rheumatology.org.uk), larger doses being limited by its side effects.

✓ DRUGS checklist for COLCHICINE

Dose	500 micrograms (BSR recommended dosing regimen)
Route	PO
Units	Micrograms (do not abbreviate)
Given	BD–QDS (BSR recommended dosing regimen) No more frequently than QDS. The authors suggest avoiding the aggressive uptitration described in the BNF (BMA/RPS, 2015).
Special situations	Higher doses are poorly tolerated, causing diarrhoea, nausea and vomiting. Other less frequent side effects include: rash, hepatic and renal impairment, peripheral neuropathy, myopathy, alopecia and with prolonged use may cause bone marrow suppression.
	Dose reductions are suggested if CrCl <50 mL/min.
	It is contraindicated in severe renal impairment (CrCl <10 mL/min) and in pregnancy.

🔍 Evidence

A systematic review (van Echteld *et al.*, 2014) looked at the efficacy of colchicine in acute gout. It found that there was a lack of high-quality evidence, with only two placebo-controlled RCTs found and no trials comparing colchicine to other treatments. From these trials the authors concluded that there is low-quality evidence that low-dose colchicine is effective in acute gout (high-dose colchicine was associated with very high frequency of side effects, namely diarrhoea, vomiting or nausea).

It should be borne in mind that a lack of good evidence does not necessarily equate to a lack of efficacy; it is simply that the evidence we have cannot prove the efficacy of this drug at the current time.

Colchicine: essential pharmacology

It is not known exactly how colchicine works in acute gout. It is known to bind tubulin, a component of microtubules. Microtubules form the cytoskeleton, a structure with multiple roles in the cell including cell division, cell migration and cellular secretion, to name but a few. Colchicine's main pharmacological actions in gout are thought to lie in its ability to disrupt the function of cellular microtubules. It is thought that colchicine inhibits the migration of leucocytes to areas of inflammation, and may also inhibit their phagocytic and secretory functions, with an associated reduction in the leucocyte-mediated inflammatory response (phagocytosis of sodium monourate crystals by leucocytes is thought to contribute to the inflammatory reaction that occurs in acute gout) (Terkeltaub, 2009).

Interactions: Colchicine is metabolised by the CYP3A4 enzyme. As such its serum levels may be affected by CYP3A4 inhibitors such as the macrolide antibiotics (clarithromycin, erythromycin etc.) and azoles (ketoconazole etc.). Other interactions are due to effects on the multidrug transporter ABCB1, which is modulated by ciclosporin as well as the macrolides and statins, leading to potential interactions with colchicine (Datapharm, 2015).

Pharmacokinetics: Colchicine is well absorbed from the GI tract. It is eliminated by kidneys and liver (Datapharm, 2015).

Glucocorticoids in gout

For patients who cannot tolerate NSAIDs or colchicine, glucocorticoids are effective treatment for acute gout (see Evidence). In monoarticular gout, intra-articular (IA) glucocorticoid injections can be used, whereas in polyarticular gout, oral (PO) or intramuscular (IM) steroid can be used. Joint infection should be excluded prior to their use. See the Section Rheumatoid Arthritis for further information about glucocorticoids.

🔍 Evidence

A double-blind, randomised trial (Janssens *et al.*, 2008) showed oral prednisolone (35 mg, OD) to be as effective as naproxen (500 mg, BD) in terms of pain reduction during the first 4 days of an acute flare of gout.

A systematic review (Wechalekar *et al.*, 2013) found no randomised controlled trial-level evidence to support the use of intra-articular corticosteroids in acute gout, although they are commonly used in clinical practice and are shown to be effective and safe in other rheumatological conditions.

Further aspects of managing acute gout

Non-pharmacological interventions: It is suggested that the affected joint be rested during a flare of gout. Ice-packs may be of symptomatic value (Jordan *et al.*, 2007).

Precipitating factors: It is important to look for the precipitating factors:
- Excessive intake of purine-rich foods:
  - Ask about diet; foods that commonly precipitate gout include beer, red meat and shellfish
- Impaired uric acid excretion:
  - Diuretics
  - Renal impairment
  - Ciclosporin
- Excessive cell breakdown and uric acid release:
  - Myeloproliferative disease
  - Chemotherapy.

Pharmacological management of chronic gout

Chronic gout is usually managed in general practice or in a rheumatology clinic. The aim of treatment is to keep blood uric acid levels <300 micromole/L, which should prevent acute flares. The BSR has excellent guidelines to guide treatment (available at: www.rheumatology.org.uk/resources/guidelines/default.aspx).

Allopurinol: rationale and evidence

Allopurinol is a first-line medication used in prevention of gout attacks and has been shown to be effective in lowering serum uric acid concentrations (see Evidence). It is not commenced until 1–2 weeks after the acute inflammation has settled as a decrease in serum uric acid can precipitate an acute attack of gout. That said, for patients already taking allopurinol, it does not need to be held during an acute attack.

⚠ Guidelines

The British Society of Rheumatology (BSR) produces guidelines on starting prophylactic treatment (Jordon *et al.*, 2007). Uric acid lowering therapy is usually commenced if:
- There are multiple attacks within 1 year
- Tophi are present

(Continued)

ⓘ Guidelines (*Continued*)

- There is concurrent renal failure
- The patient suffers with gout in conjunction uric acid-renal stones
- The patient suffers with gout but needs to take diuretics

Initial treatment should be covered with NSAIDs, colchicine or corticosteroids.

⌕ Evidence

Two studies were identified in the course of a systematic review (Seth *et al.*, 2014) which compared allopurinol to placebo in the treatment of chronic gout. These studies (Schumacher *et al.*, 2008; Taylor *et al.*, 2012) found that whilst allopurinol was effective in lowering serum urate concentration, there was no significant decrease in the incidence of gout attacks. However, the doses of allopurinol used in these trials only went up to a maximum of 300 mg and for a maximum of 28 weeks. The data was felt to be of moderate quality.

✓ DRUGS checklist for ALLOPURINOL

Dose	100 mg–900 mg
Route	PO
Units	Milligrams (mg)
Given	Once daily up to a dose of 300 mg
	In divided doses once taking >300 mg
	Wait until 1–2 weeks after the inflammation of acute gout has settled before commencing treatment with allopurinol

Special situations	Allopurinol should be titrated to uric acid levels: aim to increase the dose by 50–100 mg every 2–4 weeks until the uric acid levels is <300 micromole/L.
	Dose reduction is advised if CrCl <20 mL/min.
	Side effects include: rash, elevations in liver function tests, nausea, vomiting and diarrhoea and hypersensitivity.

Allopurinol: essential pharmacology

Hyperuricaemia (excessive serum uric acid concentrations) can lead to deposition of uric acid in body tissues; gout is a clinical manifestation of this. Purines, which are taken in as part of a normal diet, are broken down and metabolised to uric acid, before being excreted in the urine. The final stage of this process is catalysed by xanthine oxidase. Allopurinol is a xanthine oxidase inhibitor, which inhibits the conversion of xanthine to uric acid, lowering the serum uric acid concentration.

Interactions: Xanthine oxidase is responsible for metabolism of 6-mercaptopurine and its prodrug azathioprine. Therefore, concurrent administration of allopurinol with azathioprine may result in elevated concentrations of azathioprine and toxicity.

Pharmacokinetics: Allopurinol is itself metabolised to oxipurinol, which is also inhibits xanthine oxidase, prolonging the duration of action. Both allopurinol and oxipurinol are excreted by the kidneys (Datapharm, 2015).

Other medications used to prevent gout

Other xanthine oxidase inhibitors: These inhibit the conversion of purine metabolites into uric acid.

- Febuxostat (may be more effective than allopurinol in lowering serum urate levels).

Uricosuric agents: These accelerate the excretion of uric acid.

- Benzbromarone (can be used in renal failure)
- Sulfinpyrazone
- Probenecid.

Recombinant urate oxidase: This converts uric acid into 'allantoin' which is readily excreted in urine.

- Rasburicase (very expensive; rarely used in gout)

Cancer, chemotherapy and hyperuricaemia

Chemotherapy treatment of certain haematological malignancies can lead to accelerated cell breakdown, releasing large amounts of uric acid into the systemic circulation, which can cause renal damage, as well as gout.

Rasburicase is an intravenous, recombinant urate oxidase enzyme, usually used in patients at high risk of tumour lysis syndrome, in the context of chemotherapy for leukaemia or lymphoma. It is very expensive and is rarely used in gout.

A note on pseudogout

Pseudogout has a similar aetiology to gout except that the crystals are formed of calcium pyrophosphate dehydrate (CPPD). The attacks are similar but tend to be less severe. Treatment is also similar, with NSAIDs or corticosteroids (there is some evidence for colchicine), although no long-term prophylactic option has been established (Marinayagam *et al.*, 2014).

Case outcome and discharge

Intra-articular injection of methylprednisolone provided a good analgesic effect, supplemented occasionally with simple analgesics. Mr McKenzie's renal function continued to improve and he was discharged 3 days later with advice to continue to rest the left knee at home. An information leaflet on gout was provided with dietary advice and instructions for how to manage an acute flare.

DISCHARGE MEDICATION

Date	Medication	Dose	Route	Frequency	Supply	GP to continue?
xx/xx/xx	RAMIPRIL	2.5 mg	PO	Once daily	14 days	Y
xx/xx/xx	AMLODIPINE	5 mg	PO	Once daily	14 days	Y
xx/xx/xx	ALLOPURINOL	100 mg	PO	Once daily	14 days	Y
xx/xx/xx	METFORMIN	500 mg	PO	Twice daily, with meals	14 days	Y
xx/xx/xx	PARACETAMOL	1 g	PO	As needed, max four times daily	7 days	N
xx/xx/xx	CODEINE PHOSPHATE	60 mg	PO	As needed, max four times daily	7 days	N

Notes to patient/GP:
Bendroflumethiazide stopped (as may contribute to gout) and amlodipine started instead. A corticosteroid joint injection was administered on xx/xx/xx and analgesic medications are supplied to cover the acute episode of gout. Please would you up-titrate Mr McKenzie's allopurinol until the uric acid level is <300 micromole/L, to a maximum of 900 mg per day, starting 1–2 weeks after the inflammation has settled. Many thanks.

Common pitfalls

- A single, red, hot, swollen joint should be treated as septic arthritis until proven otherwise.
- Take care when treating gout in patients with renal impairment.
- Do not stop a pre-existing allopurinol prescription during acute attacks of gout.
- Do not up-titrate colchicine until diarrhoea occurs.

Gout is a common medical condition caused by hyperuricaemia (elevated serum uric acid levels). Acute attacks can be severely painful and may mimic septic arthritis. The inpatient population is at especially high risk of gouty attacks due to the high prevalence of co-morbidities, often requiring medications that can predispose to acute gouty attacks, as well as their age profile. Most doctors will have treated a patient who has developed gout during an acute admission at some point. This population is especially challenging to treat, as the above case illustrates, as they often have complicating factors such as concurrent renal impairment.

SUMMARY

⚷ Key learning points

Management of acute gout:
- Exclude septic arthritis where appropriate.
- Use NSAIDs, colchicine or corticosteroids to provide pain relief.
- Other analgesic agents can be used but may be less effective.
- Do not up-titrate colchicine to the 'maximum dose tolerated'– your patient won't thank you for it!

Management of chronic gout:
- Aim to keep uric acid levels <300 micromole/L.
- Start a xanthine oxidase inhibitor as per BSR guidelines, but not during an acute episode; wait until 1–2 weeks after the inflammation has settled.

FURTHER READING:

- A shortened version of the BSR guidelines is available and gives a more detailed review of the management of gout: Jordan KM, Cameron JS, Snaith M *et al.* (2007). British Society for Rheumatology and British Health Professionals in Rheumatology guideline for the management of gout. *Rheumatology* 46: 1372–4.

Rheumatoid arthritis

Mrs Helen Parker

Age: 43 years

Hospital number: 123456

 Case study

A 43-year-old woman is admitted on the acute medical take with a week-long history of fevers, shortness of breath and a cough.

PMH: *Rheumatoid arthritis*

DH: *See FP10*

Allergies: *None*

Salient examination findings:
HR 95, BP 120/65, Sats 93% on air, RR 25, T 37.8 °C
CRT <2 seconds, warm peripheries.
Crackles heard at right lung base.
No signs of heart failure detected.

PHARMACY STAMP	AGE 43	FORENAME, SURNAME Helen Parker
	D.O.B. xx/xx/xxxx	ADDRESS 32 Hatfield Close NHS NUMBER

METHOTREXATE 15 mg weekly.

FOLIC ACID 5 mg weekly.

HYDROXYCHLOROQUINE 200 mg once daily.

SIMVASTATIN 20 mg once at night.

SIGNATURE OF PRESCRIBER	DATE

SP21000

Investigations:
CXR: Consolidation with air-bronchograms at the right lung base
WCC 12.4, CRP 132

Diagnosis
Community-acquired pneumonia on a background of immunosuppression.

Initial management
A: Patent
B: Provide oxygen, aiming for oxygen saturations of 94 – 98%.
C: Gain IV access, take blood cultures, give fluids and antibiotics.
Immunosuppressant medications should be stopped when patients are admitted to hospital with evidence of infection.

Prescribing in rheumatoid arthritis

What is wrong with the drug chart?
1. This patient's immunosuppressant medications have been continued in the presence of an active infection.
2. It is recommended that simvastatin be held when administering clarithromycin.

Although not a severe pneumonia on CURB-65 criteria, given the immunosuppression and her clinical appearance, a more aggressive approach with antibiotics is not unreasonable.

Medications used in rheumatoid arthritis

The treatment of rheumatoid arthritis (RA) is usually managed by a specialist rheumatology team. Whilst a GP might initiate treatment of a flare with steroid therapy, more potent immunosuppressant medications require careful specialist monitoring and follow up. However, a good understanding of the various medications used in the treatment of RA, as well as their possible side effects, is important as it is a common condition and misprescription of immunosuppressants can have serious side effects.

RA is a chronic immune-mediated inflammatory arthropathy which predominantly affects the small joints of the hands and feet. Prolonged inflammation over time can lead to destructive changes in the joints as well as damage to the tendons and wasting of the muscles, impairing patients' functional abilities. The aim of treatment in RA is therefore both to reduce symptoms as well as preventing these destructive changes from

REGULAR PRESCRIPTIONS

					Circle/enter times below ↓	Day 1	Day 2	Day 3	Day 4
DRUG AMOXICILLIN					⑥				
					08				
Dose 1 g	Route IV	Freq TDS for 5 days		Start date xx/xx/xx	⑫				
Signature A. Doctor		Bleep		Review xx/xx/xx	16				
					18				
Additional instructions					㉒				
DRUG CLARITHROMYCIN					⑥				
					08				
Dose 500 mg	Route PO	Freq BD for 5 days		Start date xx/xx/xx	12				
Signature A. Doctor		Bleep		Review xx/xx/xx	16				
					⑱				
Additional instructions					22				
DRUG METHOTREXATE					06				
					⑧	X		X	X
Dose 15 mg	Route PO	Freq Weekly: Fridays		Start date xx/xx/xx	12				
Signature A. Doctor		Bleep		Review	16				
					18				
Additional instructions					22				
DRUG FOLIC ACID					06				
					⑧	X	X		X
Dose 5 mg	Route PO	Freq Weekly: Saturdays		Start date xx/xx/xx	12				
Signature A. Doctor		Bleep		Review	16				
					18				
Additional instructions					22				
DRUG HYDROXYCHLOROQUINE					06				
					⑧				
Dose 200 mg	Route PO	Freq OD		Start date xx/xx/xx	12				
Signature A. Doctor		Bleep		Review	16				
					18				
Additional instructions					22				
DRUG SIMVASTATIN					06				
					08				
Dose 40 mg	Route PO	Freq ON		Start date xx/xx/xx	12				
Signature A. Doctor		Bleep		Review	16				
					18				
Additional instructions					㉒				

FLUID CHART

Date	Fluid	Dose	Route	Rate	Signature	Print name
xx/xx/xx	SALINE 0.9%	1 L	IV	Over 6 hours	A. Doctor	A. Doctor

occurring. Whilst NSAIDs alleviate symptoms, they do not prevent the long-term destructive changes that lead to deformity and disability and it is important to start one of the so-called disease-modifying antirheumatic drugs (DMARDs) early on in the disease course. Steroids work well in rheumatoid arthritis but have many side effects, which limit their long-term use in this chronic condition. More recently a new generation of disease-modifying agents, the biologics, have come into use.

Medications used in the management of RA are:

- NSAIDs
- Glucocorticoid steroids: tablets or injections
- Traditional (synthetic) DMARDs:
  - Methotrexate
  - Sulfasalazine
  - Leflunomide
  - Hydroxychloroquine
  - Others include: azathioprine, ciclosporin, D-penicillamine, auranofin (oral gold), myco-phenolate mofetil (MMF)

These are commonly used in combination where monotherapy has proved insufficient to adequately control symptoms.

- Biological therapies (sometimes termed bDMARDs):
  - TNF-α inhibitors: adalimumab (Humira), etanercept (Enbrel), infliximab (Remicade)
  - Anti-B cell therapy: rituximab
  - IL6 inhibitor: tocilizumab
  - Abatacept

Usually given in addition to rather than instead of the traditional DMARDs.

Response to treatment is monitored using specially designed assessment tools. One such tool in common use is called DAS-28 (Disease Activity Score in 28 joints). It takes into account how many joints are painful, how many are swollen, the CRP or ESR and also includes a subjective patient score of how bad their disease is currently on a 0–100 scale. The aim of treatment is to achieve remission, which equates to a DAS-28 score of <2.6.

Here we discuss the use of glucocorticoids in RA as well as the most commonly used DMARD, methotrexate. We also cover some general rules regarding immunosuppressant drugs and also briefly touch on the newer biological therapies. An in-depth discussion of each of the DMARDs and biological therapies is beyond the scope of this book.

Glucocorticoids in rheumatoid arthritis: rationale and evidence

Glucocorticoid steroids are indicated in RA for achieving rapid relief of symptoms whilst waiting for DMARDs to take effect ('bridging'), and for rapid control of flares ('rescue'). Some patients remain on low-dose glucocorticoids in the longer term if their symptoms are very difficult to control. Systemic glucocorticoids can either be given as an oral preparation, usually prednisolone, or as an intramuscular injection, usually methylprednisolone (you may come across Depo-Medrone, which is a trade name). They are also useful in the form of a joint injection for a single painful joint, although obviously this approach is not helpful in active polyarthritis. The use of steroids in the longer term is limited by their side effects.

Evidence

A systematic review (Gorter *et al.*, 2010) looked at the efficacy of glucocorticoids in RA. The paper reviews 11 publications including three Cochrane reviews. It concludes that:

- Glucocorticoids are effective 'bridging therapy', that is they prevent radiological progression and lessen the clinical symptom-burden in the time between starting a DMARD and the DMARD taking full clinical effect.
- The addition of glucocorticoids to either DMARD monotherapy or combination therapy has benefits in terms of symptom-burden and radiological progression.
- Glucocorticoids are effective both in early RA (mainly in terms of slowing radiological progression) and in established RA (mainly in terms of controlling disease activity).

✓ DRUGS checklist for PREDNISOLONE

Dose	2.5 mg–60 mg
Route	PO
Units	Milligrams (mg)
Given	Once daily
	Usually in the morning as steroids tend to cause wakefulness; however, there is some evidence that the symptom of 'morning stiffness' can be controlled more effectively by taking prednisolone at night (Arvidson *et al.*, 1997).
Special situations	Side effects include: dyspepsia and peptic ulceration, hyperglycaemia, psychiatric disturbances, proximal myopathy, immunosuppression, salt and water retention, hypertension, skin atrophy and osteoporosis.
	Patients receiving more than 7.5 mg for more than 3 weeks need a tapering dose before stopping treatment (see Section Glucocorticoids in Rheumatoid Arthritis: Essential Pharmacology).

✓ DRUGS checklist for IM/IA METHYLPREDNISOLONE

Dose	IM: 80–120 mg
	IA: Depends on joint size; up to 80 mg for large joints
Route	Intramuscular (IM), intra-articular (IA)
Units	Milligrams (mg)
Given	As a one-off dose, with sterile technique.
	IA methylprednisolone is sometimes combined with lidocaine for added anaesthetic effect.
	After administration of IA methylprednisolone, the joint should be rested for the remainder of the day.
Special situations	Injecting methylprednisolone through the skin can cause subcutaneous or cutaneous atrophy. IM administration via the deltoid muscle is not recommended.
	IM methylprednisolone: the usual steroid-induced side effects are applicable to systemically administered methylprednisolone.
	IA methylprednisolone: there is a risk of septic arthritis and injections should not be given into previously infected or unstable joints. Some systemic absorption can be expected with IA methylprednisolone.

Glucocorticoids in rheumatoid arthritis: essential pharmacology

How do they work?

As discussed elsewhere (see Chapters 2 and 6), glucocorticoids are lipophilic and diffuse through cell membranes to act on the intracellular glucocorticoid receptor to modulate gene transcription although other, less well-defined, shorter-term effects are also produced via interaction with cell surface receptors. Downstream effects of glucocorticoid therapy include inhibition of prostaglandin production via several mechanisms including suppressing transcription of cyclo-oxygenase 2 (COX2) and inducing transcription of annexin-1 and MAPK phosphatase 1. The glucocorticoid–receptor complex also blocks the transcriptional activity of another transcription factor (NF-κB) which would otherwise promote transcription of cytokines, chemokines, cell adhesion molecules and complement factors, all of which are involved in the inflammatory or immune response (Rhen and Cidlowski, 2005). Prednisolone is mainly metabolised in the liver and a mixture of unchanged prednisolone and its metabolites are excreted in the urine. Methylprednisolone is metabolised in the liver to inactive metabolites by the CYP34A enzyme.

Steroid tapering

A steroid-reducing regimen is required where patients have taken supraphysiological steroid doses for more than 3 weeks or very high steroid doses for a shorter period. In these situations, the hypo-thalamo–pituitary–adrenal (HPA) axis may have become suppressed and to withdraw the exoge-nous steroid abruptly may trigger potentially fatal acute adrenal insufficiency with severe hypoten-sion. Manufacturers of steroid preparations recom-mend that a reducing regimen be employed where patients have received a dose of more than 1 mg dexamethasone equivalent (i.e. 7.5 mg prednisolone or 30 mg hydrocortisone) for more than 3 weeks. Factors that make HPA suppression more likely and therefore may necessitate a reducing regimen even if the steroid course was less than 3 weeks include: repeated courses of steroid treatment, previous long-term steroid use, doses higher than 6 mg dexameth-asone equivalent, the presence of other risk factors for adrenocortical insufficiency or evening dosing. The speed of reduction also depends on the likeli-hood of disease relapse with steroid withdrawal.

Patients on long-term steroid therapy may need their steroid dose increased during acute illness as their own ability to produce extra steroid in response to stress may be impaired.

Methotrexate: rationale and evidence

Methotrexate (MTX) is the most commonly used DMARD in RA and has been used in the treatment of this condition for over 40 years. It is effective in controlling symptoms as well as halting the progression of destructive changes in RA (see Evidence). Other indications for methotrexate include certain neoplastic diseases as well as psoriasis, psoriatic arthritis, Crohn's disease and some of the connective tissue diseases.

🔍 Evidence

A systematic review (Suarex-Almazoor et al., 1998) looked at the evidence for the efficacy and toxicity of methotrexate in established RA. It reviewed five placebo-controlled trials looking at outcome measures including number of swollen joints, number of tender joints, pain, function, ESR, radiological damage and global assessment. The trials used doses of 7.5–25 mg, for a period of between 12 and 18 weeks and found that methotrexate was superior to placebo in all the above areas except for reduction in ESR. There was, however, a significant dropout rate for methotrexate due to adverse effects. There was a similar overall dropout rate for placebo, although mainly due to lack of response rather than adverse effects.

Methotrexate is always taken alongside folic acid, which has been shown to reduce the elevation in hepatic transaminases and may reduce gastroin-testinal side effects without a significant effect on methotrexate efficacy, perhaps in keeping with the idea that methotrexate's intended effect in RA and its side effects are medicated by different pathways (Whittle and Hughes, 2004). A dose regimen of 5–10 mg folic acid per week is suggested. It is sug-gested that this is taken the day after methotrexate is given, although there is little evidence to support any particular regimen. Folinic acid also seems to be effective in preventing adverse effects due to methotrexate but it is significantly more costly and there is a suggestion from one study that it decreases methotrexate efficacy. As a consequence, folic acid is generally preferred. When it is first introduced, prednisolone is often given alongside the metho-trexate until it takes clinical effect and then grad-ually weaned.

✓ DRUGS checklist for METHOTREXATE

Dose	5–25 mg (increments of 2.5 mg)
Route	PO (can also be given IM, SC or IV with 1:1 equivalent dosing)
Units	Milligrams (mg)
Given	Once weekly.
	This must be explicitly stated on drug charts for inpatients remaining on maintenance methotrexate. It is important to cross through the days when methotrexate is not to be given on the drug chart. Inappropriate daily administration of methotrexate is a 'never event' that must be avoided.
Special situations	Side effects include: GI side effects, mucositis, bone marrow suppression, liver dysfunction, renal failure, pulmonary fibrosis and a range of rashes. It may also impair fertility although this appears to be reversible upon stopping methotrexate therapy.
	It is contraindicated in pregnancy and breast feeding, in bone marrow failure and in the presence of infection. Conception should be avoided during treatment and for 3 months after stopping methotrexate. Patients taking methotrexate should not receive live vaccines.
	Methotrexate requires monitoring for potential toxicity.
	A reduced dose is suggested in renal impairment.
	Methotrexate may take 6 weeks–3 months to exert its full effect (Chakravarty *et al.*, 2008).

Methotrexate: essential pharmacology

How does it work?

Methotrexate (sometimes written as 'MTX') is a dihydrofolate reductase inhibitor, and therefore a folate antagonist which inhibits DNA synthesis. It is not known whether this mechanism accounts for its efficacy in RA. Hypotheses include an effect on other folate-dependent enzymes, a reduction in toxic oxygen species or modulation of the cytokine response, all of which may exhibit a down-stream anti-inflammatory effect. Nevertheless, as explained above, it seems to be clinically effective in lessening both the symptoms and destructive changes which occur in untreated RA. That said, methotrexate has a relatively high discontinuation rate, mainly due to adverse effects and much of this can be explained by its antifolate properties. Inhibition of DNA synthesis impairs cell division and more rapidly dividing cells are disproportionately affected. This includes cells that are present in mucosal surfaces, as well as the cells of the bone marrow, which explains some of the adverse effects associated with methotrexate including mucositis, which can occur anywhere along the GI tract (aphthous ulcers, intestinal ulceration) or urogenital tracts (rarely: cystitis, haematuria, vaginitis, vaginal ulcers) and bone marrow suppression, which can cause leucopenia, thrombocytopenia or anaemia. Rapidly dividing cells are also, of course, present in the growing fetus, which is why methotrexate is strictly contraindicated in pregnancy: it causes congenital malformations as well as fetal death.

 Guidelines

Monitoring methotrexate
British Society of Rheumatology (BSR) guidelines suggest the following with regards to methotrexate monitoring (Chakravarty *et al.*, 2008):
Prior to starting treatment, check: FBC, U&E, LFT and baseline CXR.
Signs of potential toxicity are:
- WCC <3.5 × 10^9/ L neutrophils <2 × 10^9/ L or recurrent infections

(*Continued*)

Guidelines (*Continued*)

- Platelet count <150 × 10⁹/L or easy bruising
- AST or ALT more than 2 times the upper limit of normal or an unexpected drop in albumin
- New cough or dyspnoea
- Rash, oral ulcers, vomiting and diarrhoea. According to BSR guidelines, FBC and LFTs should be reviewed every 2 weeks for at least 6 weeks or until the dose is stable, then monthly until the disease and dose has been stable 1 year. Thereafter the frequency of monitoring is at the discretion of the clinician. Abnormal findings should prompt omission of methotrexate and a specialist review.

Methotrexate elimination is mainly by renal excretion (Datapharm, 2015). Therefore in cases of acute kidney injury, methotrexate should be withheld and folinic acid rescue considered (see Section Folinic acid rescue). There are a number of medications which impair methotrexate excretion in the kidneys, thereby increasing the likelihood of toxicity for a given dose of methotrexate. These include NSAIDs and aspirin, oral hypoglycaemics, thiazide diuretics, phenytoin and a number of antibiotics including the penicillins, tetracyclines and ciprofloxacin (which arguably shouldn't be used concurrently anyway if their indication is infection!).

Folate

Folate is important in DNA synthesis as it is converted, via dihydrofolate reductase (DHFR) into tetrahydrofolate, a precursor of purines which make up the building blocks of DNA. Folinic acid is readily converted to tetrahydrofolate in the absence of DHFR and, as such, has been used in situations where toxicity results from DHFR inhibition, so-called 'folinic acid rescue'. Other folate antagonists you may come across include trimethoprim and sulfmethoxazole (called co-trimoxazole when used in combination).

Folinic acid rescue

In cases of methotrexate overdose, severe haematological toxicity or acute renal failure, treatment with folinic acid can be considered. BSR guidelines suggest an intravenous dose of at least 20 mg followed by oral doses of 15 mg, 6 hourly until the abnormalities are resolved (Chakravarty *et al.*, 2008). This should be discussed with relevant specialists.

Newer therapies in rheumatoid arthritis: a brief guide

Thanks to advances in molecular biology, newer more-targeted treatments (the biologics) have been developed against specific parts of the immune response, including tumour necrosis factor-α (TNF-α), interleukin-6 (IL-6), B cells and T cells (Table 12.1). These are generally either monoclonal antibodies or receptor blocking agents. These treatments offer good options for patients who fail to achieve adequate disease control with the conventional DMARDs.

Monoclonal antibodies

Monoclonal antibodies are immunoglobulins targeted against a specific epitope or antigen ('monoclonal' refers to the fact that all the antibodies are identical). They are commonly used in autoimmune and malignant conditions.

Tip: **m**onoclonal **a**nti**b**odies end in the suffix '-mab'.

Side effects and cautions

The most common side effect of these targeted therapies is an infusion-related reaction. There are also some rare but potentially serious side effects to take into consideration. These treatments all target the immune system and as such patients are at risk of acquiring infections. In addition to this, the biologics have been associated with reactivation of underlying infections such as latent tuberculosis or HBV infection. It is recommended that patients

Table 12.1 Biologics for treatment of rheumatoid arthritis (Bukhari *et al.*, 2011; Ding *et al.*, 2010; NICE, 2012).

Biologics	Specific features
TNF-α inhibitors: Adalimumab Etanercept Infliximab	These treatments target TNF-α, a cytokine which is involved in multiple inflammatory pathways as well as regulation of the immune response
	Adalimumab and etanercept are given as SC injections (alternate weeks and twice weekly, respectively), whereas infliximab is given as IV infusions at 0, 2 and 6 weeks and every 8 weeks thereafter.
Anti-B cell therapy: Rituximab	Rituximab targets the CD20 surface marker on B cells, depleting the B-cell population. Patients who are negative for rheumatoid factor or ACPA[a] are less likely to have a good response.
	Given as an IV infusion. This can be repeated if there is a good response but no more frequently than every 6 months.
IL-6 inhibitor: Tocilizumab	Tocilizumab targets the IL-6 receptor. IL-6 is a cytokine involved in many inflammatory and immune regulatory pathways, including B-cell differentiation, thereby inducing antibody production.
	Can cause elevated lipid levels. Given as a SC injection on a weekly basis or as an IV infusion over 1 hour, every 4 weeks.
T-cell co-stimulatory module inhibitor: Abatacept	Abatacept blocks the co-stimulatory signal required for full T-cell activation.
	Given as a SC injection on a weekly basis ± an initial IV infusion.

[a] ACPA, anticitrullinated protein antibodies, a relatively specific marker of RA.

undergoing treatment with biologics be screened for tuberculosis as well as hepatitis B and C and HIV, although recommendations vary slightly with each treatment. Live vaccines are not recommended during treatment with biologics and non-live vaccines may not be as effective, as they work by stimulating an immune response. Immunomodulatory agents such as these have also been associated with an increased risk of malignancy. Although no increased risk has yet been identified for many of the agents in use, an association with latent cancers may well emerge with time (see Section Biologics register). Caution is advised in heart failure and with demyelinating conditions with the TNF-α inhibitors and with rituximab (Bukhari *et al.*, 2011; Ding *et al.*, 2010; NICE, 2012).

[TOP TIP] As with other immunosuppressant medications, healthcare professionals must be vigilant for signs of infection during treatment. In the case of medications such as these, given by intermittent injection, it may not be apparent from a repeat prescription or drug chart that a patient is taking them and, as such, if you come across a patient who has an autoimmune or malignant condition it is important to document the therapies they have received in the last 6–12 months that could impact upon their current situation.

Biologics register

The BSR collects information about these newer drug treatments on the BSR Biologics Register (BSRBR). There is one register for RA and one for ankylosing spondylitis. Here, data is collected about patients receiving these newer treatments, specifically with regard to any adverse effects or long-term effects that might emerge. Further details can be found online on the BSR website.

Guidelines

NICE and the BSR regularly update their guidance on the criteria for when and how to use these newer biological treatments. Up-to-date details can be found on their websites.

In general, to qualify for biologic treatment, a patient must have moderate to severely active RA (DAS-28 score >3.2) and have an inadequate response or intolerance to at least two DMARD therapies, usually given concurrently and for a reasonable time period. The newer biologics are given in combination with methotrexate where possible. Usually, the TNF inhibitors are tried first, followed by rituximab or tocilizumab.

Other aspects of management of rheumatoid arthritis

Non-pharmacological management

As with any chronic disease, pharmacological therapy is only one aspect of management. Management involves patient education and input from members of the multidisciplinary team, which may include specialist nurses, physiotherapists and occupational therapists.

Cardiovascular risk prophylaxis

Research has suggested that patients with chronic inflammatory conditions such as RA have an above-average risk of cardiovascular events such as strokes and myocardial infarctions (Lindhardsen *et al.*, 2011). Therefore, part of the management of RA involves managing this risk by assessing possible co-existing risk factors and starting medications such as statins at an appropriate time.

Case outcome and discharge

The rheumatology specialist nurse and consultant rheumatologist reviewed Mrs Parker and high-lighted the importance of stopping immunosuppressant medications during an acute infection or illness. They arranged for the specialist nurse to see Mrs Parker in clinic a week after her discharge with a plan to restart her RA medications if she remained well. The sputum culture was awaited but as she had not had a fever for 48 hours, her antibiotics were switched to an oral preparation with a plan to let her go home if she remained well over the next 24 hours. Follow-up was booked with rheumatology as above and with the acute physicians for 6 weeks' time with a repeat CXR to ensure that the pneumonia had cleared completely and that there were no underlying pulmonary abnormalities.

DISCHARGE MEDICATION						
Date	Medication	Dose	Route	Frequency	Supply	GP to continue?
xx/xx/xx	AMOXICILLIN	500 mg	PO	Three times daily	To complete a 7 day course, i.e. until xx/xx/xx	N
xx/xx/xx	CLARITHROMYCIN	500 mg	PO	Twice daily	To complete a 7 day course, i.e. until xx/xx/xx	N

Notes to patient/GP:
Methotrexate, folic acid and hydroxychloroquine have been held until review in rheumatology clinic in 1 week's time. Simvastatin should be held until the course of antibiotics is complete due to a potential interaction between clarithromycin and simvastatin.

Common pitfalls

- Immunosuppressant medications such as the DMARDs and biological therapies used in RA and other rheumatological conditions should be stopped immediately if a patient develops evidence of an active infection, and advice sought from local specialist teams.
- Methotrexate is given as a **once weekly** regimen. Severe adverse reactions may occur if it is given more frequently.

Think carefully about patients receiving immunosuppressant medications. Many trusts do not allow these medications to be prescribed by anyone less senior than a registrar.

 Key learning points

Prescribing in rheumatoid arthritis
- Treatment is usually managed by a specialist.
- It is of the utmost importance that patients do not continue their immunosuppressant medication(s) whilst they are unwell.
- Advice should be sought from the rheumatology specialist nurse or a specialist physician as well as from your ward pharmacist if you are unsure about any of these medications.
- Methotrexate must be prescribed and administered weekly. Accidental daily administration is a 'never event'.

FURTHER READING

- A good and up-to-date summary of the drug treatment of rheumatoid arthritis is as follows (two of the authors were also involved in creating the BSR guidelines): Garner R, Ding T, Deighton C (2014). Management of rheumatoid arthritis. *Medicine* 42: 237–42.

Giant cell arteritis and polymyalgia rheumatica

Mrs Vivian Redwood

Age: 70 years

Hospital number: 123456

 Case study

Mrs Redwood has suffered with increasingly severe headaches over the last week, to the point where she can't even brush her hair anymore. She feels tired and lethargic. Doctors in the emergency department have referred her on to the medical team as they are concerned this might be giant cell arteritis. When you ask specifically, she does admit to jaw pain on chewing, but has not noticed any change in her vision or pain in her arms.

PMH: *Hypertension*

DH: *See FP10*

Allergies: *None*

Salient examination findings:
HR 78, BP (R) 145/78, (L)152/80
Sats 98% on air, RR 16, T 37.7 °C

Case study *(Continued)*

Her scalp is tender to touch.
There are no signs of meningism.
No abnormal neurology is detected; importantly, the visual fields appear normal with no RAPD.
Upper limb pulses are present and equal.

Investigations:
Hb 124, Plt 478, WCC 8.2
Renal and liver function: normal
ESR: 98 mm/h
Urine dip: negative
CXR: normal heart size, narrow mediastinum, clear lung fields
Weight: 62 kg

PHARMACY STAMP	AGE 70	FORENAME, SURNAME Vivian Redwood
	D.O.B. xx/xx/xxxx	ADDRESS South Street
		NHS NUMBER

BENDROFLUMETHIAZIDE 5 mg.

SIGNATURE OF PRESCRIBER   DATE

SP21000

Diagnosis
Probable giant cell arteritis (sometimes called temporal arteritis)

Initial management
Giant cell arteritis (GCA) is a sight-threatening diagnosis and therefore is a medical emergency. Mrs Redwood should be started on high-dose steroids and referred for a temporal artery biopsy, which is usually performed by either ENT or vascular surgeons. Some centres are now using temporal artery ultrasound as an alternative/ adjunct to temporal artery biopsy; the presence of a 'halo' around blood flow identified by Doppler is said to be extremely specific for GCA. If there were to be visual symptoms, an ophthalmology opinion would be valuable. The patient is usually followed up by a rheumatology specialist, who will also be able to give advice in the acute setting.

Prescribing for suspected giant cell arteritis

| ONCE ONLY PRESCRIPTIONS | | | | | Prescriber | |
Date	Time to be given	DRUG	Dose	Route	Signature	Bleep
xx/xx/xx	10:30	PREDNISOLONE	60 mg	PO	A. Doctor	

The treatment of suspected GCA usually requires high-dose oral prednisolone, although if there are visual symptoms, pulsed methylprednisolone may be indicated (see Guidelines).

(!) **Guidelines**

The British Society of Rheumatology (BSR) guidelines (Dasgupta *et al.*, 2010) suggest the following:
- Uncomplicated GCA: 40–60 mg prednisolone per day, but not less than 0.75 mg/kg/day
- Evolving visual symptoms: 500 mg–1 g methylprednisolone IV for 3 days
- Established visual symptoms: at least 60 mg prednisolone per day.

Prednisolone: rationale and evidence

GCA is a granulomatous vasculitis of the medium and large arteries. It is an inflammatory condition and therefore responds to treatment with medications that counter the inflammatory response.

The aim of treatment is to control the symptoms but more importantly to prevent the ophthalmic complications, including permanent visual loss, which occurred in 14.6% of cases in one study (Gonzalez-Gay *et al.*, 2000). It is possible that starting treatment with steroids will affect the results of a subsequent temporal artery biopsy but treatment should not be delayed due to the risk of irreversible visual loss which can occur without treatment.

Evidence

High-dose steroid treatment has been used in GCA for many years. For obvious reasons, placebo-controlled trials have not been performed.

✓ DRUGS checklist for PREDNISOLONE in uncomplicated GCA	
Dose	40–60 mg/day (but not <0.75 mg/kg/day, as per BSR guidelines)
	Many physicians give 1 mg/kg/day (usually rounded to the nearest 5 mg)
	Dose continued until resolution of symptoms and inflammatory markers and should be gradually tapered thereafter (see Special Situations).
Route	PO
Units	Milligrams (mg)
Given	Once daily, usually in the morning
Special situations	Side effects include: dyspepsia and peptic ulceration, hyperglycaemia, psychiatric disturbances, proximal myopathy, immunosuppression, salt and water retention, hypertension, skin atrophy, cataracts and osteoporosis.

Whilst any patient receiving more than 7.5 mg prednisolone for more than 3 weeks will need a tapering dose, this needs to be done particularly slowly and carefully in GCA due to the risk of relapse if steroids are withdrawn too quickly.

Guidelines

The following tapering regimen is suggested by the BSR (Dasgupta *et al*, 2010):
40–60 mg (but not <0.75 mg/kg) daily until resolution of symptoms and normalization of inflammatory markers then:
- decrease prednisolone by 10 mg every 2 weeks until a dose of 20 mg daily is reached, then
- decrease prednisolone by 2.5 mg every 2–4 weeks until a dose of 10 mg daily is reached, then
- decrease prednisolone by 1 mg every 1–2 months, providing there is no evidence of relapse.

The full guideline along with updates can be found on the BSR website (available at: www.rheumatology.org.uk).

Prednisolone: essential pharmacology

Prednisolone is a glucocorticoid. The essential pharmacology of the glucocorticoids is discussed in the Rheumatoid Arthritis section of this chapter.

Further aspects treating giant cell arteritis

Implications of long-term steroid treatment: Patients with GCA are likely to need treatment with prednisolone for 1–2 years and, as such, it is recommended, once the diagnosis is confirmed that concomitant bone protection (calcium supplements and a bisphosphonate) as well as a gastroprotective agent (such as a proton-pump inhibitor or H2 receptor antagonist) be prescribed (see Chapters 5 and Chapter 8).

Steroid-sparing agents: A rheumatologist may recommend methotrexate or azathioprine as steroid-sparing treatments in the longer-term management of GCA.

Low-dose aspirin: There is some evidence (see Evidence) that long-term low-dose aspirin reduces cranial ischaemic complications (strokes and visual loss) in GCA and it is recommended in most guidelines that low-dose aspirin be started, provided there are no contraindications.

🔍 Evidence

A retrospective observational study (Nesher et al., 2004) found that significantly fewer patients who were already on low-dose aspirin developed cranial ischaemic complications from GCA (8% vs. 29%). However, there is no RCT-level evidence available to support this possibility (Mollan et al., 2014).

A note on polymyalgia rheumatic

One of the most common indications for long-term steroid treatment, polymyalgia rheumatic is an inflammatory condition of the muscles, which leads to proximal myopathy as well as systemic symptoms such as lethargy and weight loss. There is a significant association between polymyalgia rheumatic and GCA (Smeeth et al., 2006).

Treatment of polymyalgia rheumatic (without evidence of GCA) is with lower-dose prednisolone, usually starting around 15 mg/ day, which is gradually tapered (see Guidelines), with the aim of withdrawing steroids altogether, although this often takes months or years. As with GCA, it is recommended that bone protection and gastroprotection be considered during long-term steroid treatment.

⚠ Guidelines:

The following tapering regimen is suggested by the BSR (Dasgupta et al., 2009):
- 15 mg for 3 weeks, then
- 12.5 mg for 3 weeks, then
- 10 mg for 4–6 weeks, then
- decrease prednisolone by 1 mg every 4–8 weeks, or consider alternate-day reductions.

The full guideline along with updates can be found on the BSR website (available at: www.rheumatology.org.uk).

Case outcome and discharge

Mrs Redwood was reviewed by the ENT team and booked in for a temporal artery biopsy the following day. She was counselled about the implications of long-term steroid use and follow-up was organised with one of the local rheumatologists.

DISCHARGE MEDICATION						
Date	Medication	Dose	Route	Frequency	Supply	GP to continue?
xx/xx/xx	BENDROFLUMETHIAZIDE	5 mg	PO	Once daily	14 days	Y
xx/xx/xx	PREDNISOLONE	60 mg	PO	Once daily	14 days	For review in rheumatology clinic
xx/xx/xx	OMEPRAZOLE	20 mg	PO	Once daily	14 days	Y; whilst on steroids
xx/xx/xx	ADCAL D3	2 tablets	PO	Twice daily	14 days	Y; whilst on steroids
xx/xx/xx	ALENDRONIC ACID	70 mg	PO	Once weekly	14 days	Y; whilst on steroids

Notes to patient/GP:
Please seek urgent medical help should you notice any change in your vision. Please note, alendronic acid should be taken in the morning, whilst seated upright, or standing, 30 minutes prior to food.

SUMMARY

Giant cell arteritis is the most common of the vasculitides and prompt recognition and management can be sight saving. That said, it is a diagnosis that commits a patient to long-term steroid treatment with their accompanying risks and side effects and, as such, the diagnosis should not be taken lightly and should be confirmed with a temporal artery biopsy as soon as possible.

🔑 Key learning points

Management of GCA:
- Prednisolone dose depends on the presence of visual symptoms.
- Prednisolone is continued until symptoms and inflammatory markers have normalised.
- Prompt referral for temporal artery biopsy is recommended.
- Once the diagnosis is confirmed, consider bone protection and gastroprotection and discuss the implications of being on long-term steroids.

FURTHER READING

- A good review of GCA and polymyalgia rheumatic is available in the *Lancet*: Salvarani C, Cantini F, Hunder GG (2008). Polymyalgia rheumatica and giant-cell arteritis. *Lancet* 372: 234–45.

Now visit **www.wileyessential.com/pharmacology** to test yourself on this chapter.

References

Arvidson NG, Gudbjörnsson B, Larsson A *et al.* (1997). The timing of glucocorticoid administration in rheumatoid arthritis. *Ann Rheum Dis* 56: 27–31.

British Medical Association and Royal Pharmaceutical Society of Great Britain (BMA/RPS) (2015). *British National Formulary 69*, 69th edn. BMJ group and Pharmaceutical Press, London.

Bukhari M, Abernethy R, Deighton C *et al.*, on behalf of the BSR and BHPR Standards, Guidelines and Audit Working Group (2011). BSR and BHPR guidelines on the use of rituximab in rheumatoid arthritis. *Rheumatology* 50: 2311–3. Full guideline available at: www.rheumatology.org.uk/resources/guidelines/default.aspx (accessed Dec. 2015).

Cepeda MS, Camargo F, Zea C *et al.* (2006). Tramadol for osteoarthritis. *Cochrane Database Syst Rev* (3): CD005522.

Chakravarty K, McDonald H, Pullar T *et al.*, on behalf of the British Society for Rheumatology, British Health Professionals in Rheumatology Standards, Guidelines and Audit Working Group in consultation with the British Association of Dermatologists (2008). BSR/BHPR guideline for disease-modifying anti-rheumatic drug (DMARD) therapy in consultation with the British Association of Dermatologists. *Rheumatology* 49: 1197–9. Full guideline available at: www.rheumatology.org.uk/resources/guidelines/default.aspx (accessed Dec. 2015).

Dasgupta B, Borg FA, Hassan N *et al.* on behalf of the BSR and BHPR Standards, Guidelines and Audit Working Group (2009). *BSR and BHPR Guidelines for the Management of Polymyalgia Rheumatic*. Available at: http://www.rheumatology.org.uk/resources/guidelines/bsr_guidelines.aspxwww.rheumatology.org.uk/resources/guidelines/default.aspx (accessed Dec. 2015).

Dasgupta B, Borg FA, Hassan N *et al.* on behalf of the BSR and BHPR Standards, Guidelines and Audit Working Group (2010). BSR and BHPR guidelines for the management of giant cell arteritis. *Rheumatology* 49: 1594–7. Full guideline available at: www.rheumatology.org.uk/resources/guidelines/default.aspx (accessed Dec. 2015).

Datapharm (2015). *Electronic Medicines Compendium (eMC) Summaries of Product Characteristics (SPC)*. Available at: www.medicines.org.uk (accessed Dec. 2015).

Ding T, Ledingham J, Luqmani R *et al.* on behalf of the Standards, Audit and Guidelines Working Group of BSR Clinical Affairs Committee and BHPR (2010). BSR and BHPR rheumatoid arthritis guidelines on safety of anti-TNF therapies. *Rheumatology* 49: 2217–9. Full guideline available at: www.rheumatology.org.uk/resources/guidelines/default.aspx (accessed Dec. 2015).

Gonzalez-Gay MA, Garcia-Porrua C, Llorca J *et al.* (2000). Visual manifestations of giant cell arteritis: trends and clinical spectrum in 161 patients. *Medicine (Baltimore)* 79: 283–92.

Gorter SL, Bijlsma JW, Cutolo M *et al.* (2010). Current evidence for the management of rheumatoid arthritis with glucocorticoids: a systematic literature review informing the EULAR recommendations for the management of rheumatoid arthritis. *Ann Rheum Dis* 69: 1010–14.

Hinz B, Brune K (2012). Paracetamol and cyclooxygenase inhibition: is there a cause for concern? *Ann Rheum Dis* 71: 20–5.

Janssens HJ, Janssen M, van de Lisdonk EH *et al.* (2008). Use of oral prednisolone or naproxen for the treatment of gout arthritis: a double-blind, randomised equivalence trial. *Lancet* 371: 1854–60.

Jordan KM, Cameron JS, Snaith M *et al.* British Society for Rheumatology and British Health Professionals in Rheumatology Standards, Guidelines and Audit Working Group (SGAWG) (2007). British Society for Rheumatology and British Health Professionals in Rheumatology guideline for the management of gout. *Rheumatology* 46: 1372–4.

Kearney PM, Baigent C, Godwin J *et al.* (2006). Do selective cyclo-oxygenase-2 inhibitors and traditional non-steroidal anti-inflammatory drugs increase the risk of atherothrombosis? Meta-analysis of randomised trials. *BMJ* 332: 1302–8.

Lindhardsen J, Ahlehoff O, Gislason GH *et al.* (2011). The risk of myocardial infarction in rheumatoid arthritis and diabetes mellitus: a Danish nationwide cohort study. *Ann Rheum Dis* 70: 929–34.

Mallet C, Daulhac L, Bonnefont J *et al.* (2008). Endocannabinoid and serotonergic systems are needed for acetaminophen-induced analgesia. *Pain* 139: 190–200.

Marianayagam T, Koduri G, Ellis S (2014). Crystal arthropathies. *Medicine* 42: 208–12.

Mollan SP, Sharrack N, Burdon MA *et al.* (2014). Aspirin as adjunctive treatment for giant cell arteritis. *Cochrane Database Syst Rev* (8): CD010453.

National Institute for Health and Care Excellence (NICE) (2012). *Tocilizumab for the Treatment of Rheumatoid Arthritis (Rapid Review of Technology Appraisal Guidance 198)*, TA247. Available at: www.nice.org.uk/guidance/ta247 (accessed Nov. 2014).

National Institute for Health and Care Excellence (NICE) (2014). *Osteoarthritis: Care and Management in Adults*, CG177. Available at: www.nice.org.uk/guidance/CG177 (Accessed Nov. 2014).

Nesher G, Berkun Y, Mates M *et al.* (2004). Low-dose aspirin and prevention of cranial ischemic complications in giant cell arteritis. *Arthritis Rheum* 50: 1332–7.

Ottani A, Leone S, Sandrini M *et al.* (2006). The analgesic activity of paracetamol is prevented by the blockade of cannabinoid CB1 receptors. *Eur J Pharmacol* 531: 280–1.

Rang HP, Dale MM, Ritter JM *et al.* (2003). *Pharmacology*, 5th edn. Churchill Livingstone.

Rhen T, Cidlowski JA (2005). Anti-inflammatory action of glucocorticoids—new mechanisms for old drugs. *N Engl J Med* 353: 1711–23.

Ruoff GE (1999). Slowing the initial titration rate of tramadol improves tolerability. *Pharmacotherapy* 19: 88–93.

Schumacher HR Jr, Boice JA, Daikh DI *et al.* (2002). Randomised double blind trial of etoricoxib and indometacin in treatment of acute gouty arthritis. *BMJ* 324: 1488–92.

Schumacher HR, Becker MA, Wortmann RL *et al.* (2008). Effects of febuxostat versus allopurinol and placebo in reducing serum urate in subjects with hyperuricemia and gout: a 28-week, phase III, randomized, double-blind, parallel-group trial. *Arthritis Rheum* 59: 1540–8.

Seth R, Kydd ASR, Buchbinder R *et al.* (2014). Allopurinol for chronic gout. *Cochrane Database Syst Rev* (10): CD006077.

Smeeth L, Cook C, Hall AJ (2006). Incidence of diagnosed polymyalgia rheumatica and temporal arteritis in the United Kingdom, 1990 to 2001. *Ann Rheum Dis* 65: 1093–8.

Suarez-Almazor ME, Belseck E, Shea B *et al.* (1998). Methotrexate for treating rheumatoid arthritis. *Cochrane Database Syst Rev* (2): CD000957.

Taylor TH, Mecchella JN, Larson RJ *et al.* (2012). Initiation of allopurinol at first medical contact for acute attacks of gout: a randomized clinical trial. *Am J Med* 125: 1126–34.

Terkeltaub RA (2009). Colchicine Update: 2008. *Semin Arthritis Rheum* 38: 411–9.

Towheed T, Maxwell L, Judd M *et al.* (2006). Acetaminophen for osteoarthritis. *Cochrane Database Syst Rev* (1): CD004257.

van Echteld I, Wechalekar MD, Schlesinger N *et al.* (2014). Colchicine for acute gout. *Cochrane Database Syst Rev* (8): CD006190.

Wechalekar MD, Vinik O, Schlesinger N *et al.* (2013). Intra-articular glucocorticoids for acute gout. *Cochrane Database Syst Rev* (4): CD009920.

Weinshilboum R, Wang L (2004). Pharmacogenomics: bench to bedside. *Nat Rev Drug Discov* 3: 739–48.

Whittle SL, Hughes RA (2004). Folate supplementation and methotrexate treatment in rheumatoid arthritis: a review. *Rheumatology* 43: 267–71.

Whelton A (1999). Nephrotoxicity of nonsteroidal anti-inflammatory drugs: physiologic foundations and clinical implications. *Am J Med* 106: 13S.

Wilder-Smith CH, Hill L, Spargo K *et al.* (2001). Treatment of severe pain from osteoarthritis with slow-release tramadol or dihydrocodeine in combination with NSAID's: a randomised study comparing analgesia, antinociception and gastrointestinal effects. *Pain* 91: 23–31.

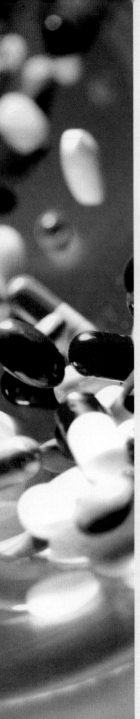

CHAPTER 13
Dermatology
Amy Hawkins

Key topics:

Learning objectives

By the end of this chapter, you should be able to…

- …write prescriptions for patients with eczema, psoriasis, allergic rashes, cellulitis, fungal infections or acne, taking into account relevant cautions, contraindications and side effects.

- …evaluate the key topical and systemic therapies used in the management of the above conditions.

- …discuss the mechanisms of action of the key drugs used to treat these conditions.

Essential Practical Prescribing, First Edition. Georgia Woodfield, Benedict Lyle Phillips, Victoria Taylor, Amy Hawkins and Andrew Stanton. © 2016 by John Wiley & Sons, Ltd. Published 2016 by John Wiley & Sons, Ltd.

Eczema

Finlay Reed

Age: 6

Hospital number: 123456

Case study

Presenting complaint: A 6-year-old boy is brought by his mother to see his GP with an itchy rash affecting his elbows and knees.

Background: He lives with his parents and older sister. There are no developmental concerns and the family do not have pets.

PMH and family history: Finlay has asthma, which is well controlled with his inhalers. He has never been admitted to hospital for his asthma or any other conditions. He is up to date with all his immunisations. His sister Sarah has hay fever and eczema.

Allergies: None known

Examination:
Looks well and is happily playing in the waiting room

Skin: Symmetrical rash affecting the flexural aspects of the elbows and knees. The skin in these areas is erythematous and excoriated with some bleeding points. There is no evidence of blistering or secondary infection. There is a small area of skin affected behind the left ear.

Diagnosis
Atopic eczema. The patient has a history of an itchy rash affecting the flexures. The skin is excoriated from repeated scratching and the skin has begun to bleed in some areas. This can lead to secondary infection so prompt treatment is important. He has a strong personal and family history of atopy, and there is no history to suggest an irritant source.

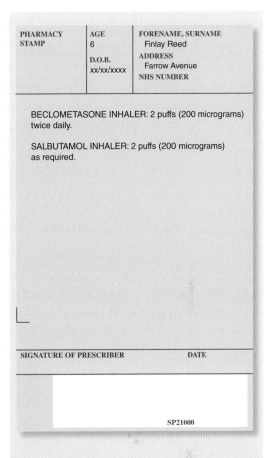

PHARMACY STAMP	AGE 6	FORENAME, SURNAME Finlay Reed
	D.O.B. xx/xx/xxxx	ADDRESS Farrow Avenue NHS NUMBER

BECLOMETASONE INHALER: 2 puffs (200 micrograms) twice daily.

SALBUTAMOL INHALER: 2 puffs (200 micrograms) as required.

SIGNATURE OF PRESCRIBER   DATE

SP21000

Initial measures
A detailed explanation and education for the child and their family are of paramount importance. In this case, the family already have one child with eczema, but it will still be important to give education and lifestyle advice. Useful advice includes wearing loose clothing over affected areas, keeping the child's fingernails short and avoiding potential precipitants, including pets and dust.

Prescribing for eczema

The mainstay of treatment in eczema is topical therapy. Systemic therapies can be added in severe disease under specialist supervision.

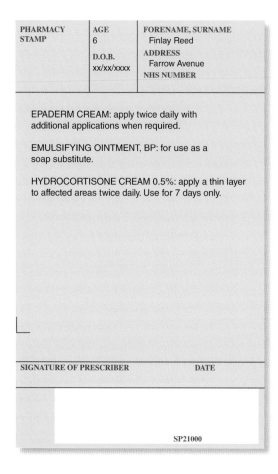

| PHARMACY STAMP | AGE 6 | FORENAME, SURNAME Finlay Reed |
| | D.O.B. xx/xx/xxxx | ADDRESS Farrow Avenue NHS NUMBER |

EPADERM CREAM: apply twice daily with additional applications when required.

EMULSIFYING OINTMENT, BP: for use as a soap substitute.

HYDROCORTISONE CREAM 0.5%: apply a thin layer to affected areas twice daily. Use for 7 days only.

SIGNATURE OF PRESCRIBER   DATE

SP21000

Emollients: rationale and evidence

The first line of treatment is emollients (Baron *et al.*, 2012). These should be applied liberally to the skin as lotions and soap substitutes on a regular basis (at least twice daily) even when eczema is less active. A range of different emollients are available and can be used depending on disease severity (Bieber *et al.*, 2008). For example, Epaderm is useful for more severe eczema, and Diprobase is a less greasy preparation for less-severe disease.

 Guidelines

NICE recommendations on use of emollients in atopic childhood eczema (NICE, 2007):
- Emollients should form the mainstay of management of atopic eczema.

- They should be used at all times, even during periods of less disease activity.
- Additional therapies should be added in a stepwise manner according to symptom severity.

🔍 Evidence

Emollients in eczema

There is currently a lack of evidence regarding which emollients are most effective. There is currently a Cochrane review underway to assess the effectiveness and relative efficacy of different emollients. Interestingly, one study found that there were no studies on the use of bath emollients, nor any studies comparing use of base emollients and directly applied emollients (Tarr and Iheanacho, 2009). More research in this area is needed.

✓ DRUGS checklist for EPADERM

Dose	One application
Route	Topical
Units	N/A
Given	When required, at least twice daily
Special situations	Where a spatula or spoon is provided this should be used to avoid contamination of the emollient. Emollients should be applied in the direction of hair growth to reduce the risk of folliculitis.

Emollients: essential pharmacology

Skin becomes dry due to insufficient water in a layer of the skin called the stratum corneum. In eczema, skin is flaky due to partial detachment of keratinocytes from the skin surface. This also occurs in psoriasis (see Section Psoriasis).

Emollients work by softening and moistening the skin. They provide an occlusive barrier on top of the skin surface. This reduces the rate of water loss from the skin, increasing the moisture content of the stratum corneum. The extent to which this barrier is formed depends on the type of emollient – ointments are the most occlusive, followed by creams, then lotions, and lastly soap substitutes. This explains why the choice of emollient depends upon the severity of the eczema and which area is affected.

Topical steroids: rationale and evidence

The next topical therapy to be considered is topical steroids. These range in potency from hydrocortisone (least potent), to Eumovate, Betnovate and Dermovate (most potent). Choice depends upon severity, site and the patient's age. It is important to remember that topical steroids are absorbed systemically and may also cause thinning of the skin. For this reason, it is important to use the appropriate strength depending on the site and severity of eczema.

Evidence

Topical steroids in eczema
There is evidence to suggest that short-term use of potent topical steroids is equivalent to the use of long-term use of mild steroids (Thomas *et al.*, 2002). One study has suggested that prolonged use of topical steroid can reduce the frequency of disease flare-ups, but this has to be balanced against the risks and side effects described in this section (Berth-Jones *et al.*, 2003).

✓ DRUGS checklist for TOPICAL HYDROCORTISONE

Dose	One application
Route	Topically (to affected areas only)
Units	N/A
Given	Once/twice daily depending on severity
Special situations	Short-term use of mild and moderately potent steroids is associated with few side effects. Particular caution should be taken when using potent steroids. Local side effects include thinning of the skin, contact dermatitis and worsening of underlying infection. Absorption through the skin can rarely cause adrenal suppression.

Topical steroids: essential pharmacology

Topical steroids work by reducing skin inflammation; this is thought to occur through induction of phospholipase A2 inhibitory proteins called lipocortins. These proteins control the synthesis of inflammatory mediators including prostaglandins and leukotrienes by inhibiting the release of arachidonic acid.

It is important to note that the pharmacokinetics of topical steroids is affected by the extent of scaling or flaking of skin so inflammation and flaking are likely to increase the degree of steroid absorption.

Other treatments used in eczema

- Wet wraps and compresses: these are helpful in the acute phase of treatment.
- Antibiotics: for areas of skin that have become secondarily infected, either topical or for more severe cases, systemic, antibiotics may be required.
- Coal tar preparations: may be used for cases with severe lichenification.
- Non-steroidal topical immunosuppressants: tacrolimus ointment (Protopic) may be used as a steroid-sparing agent.
- Sedative antihistamine: may be required at night for cases in which severe itching disturbs sleep.

- Phototherapy: both PUVA and narrow-band UVB therapy are helpful steroid-sparing strategies in chronic eczema.
- Systemic steroids or ciclosporin: only required in the most severe cases under expert supervision.
- Azathioprine and methotrexate: increasingly used under expert supervision as systemic treatments of severe refractory eczema.

Evidence

Topical calcineurin inhibitors versus topical steroids in eczema

A 2005 systematic review and meta-analysis (Ashcroft *et al.*, 2005) found limited evidence that topical tacrolimus was more effective than placebo or mild topical steroids for moderate to severe eczema. Following this analysis, an RCT of almost 500 patients has found improved efficacy for topical tacrolimus compared with moderately potent topical steroids (Reitamo *et al.*, 2005). However, a systematic review of 17 trials comparing tropical steroids with topical tacrolimus (0.1% or 0.03%) found that the efficacy of these drugs was comparable to mild to moderate topical steroids.

Further aspects of eczema management

Remember that atopic eczema is just one type of eczema. Treatments for other forms of the condition may vary:

- Irritant and contact dermatitis: may be caused by chemicals, water, solvents or detergents. Typically this form of eczema affects a specific area that has been in contact with the irritant. Management relies heavily on identification and avoidance of the allergen or irritant in addition to the treatment steps described in this Section.
- Seborrhoeic dermatitis: a chronic, scaly eruption affecting the scalp, face and chest (areas of the skin with more sebaceous glands). Mild topical steroid or antifungal creams and shampoo can be used.

- Discoid eczema: coin-shaped lesions affecting the limbs, which may be vesicular or chronically become lichenified. Secondary infection is more common and antibiotics may be required.
- Pompholyx eczema: this form of eczema characteristically affects hands and feet and involves an intensely itchy vesicular eruption. Potent topical steroids are often required.

Case outcome and discharge

Finlay's parents applied emollients regularly every day, in the morning before school, when he got home from school and in the evenings before bed. The emollients were applied by the school nurse at lunchtime. He used the soap substitute as prescribed, and topical hydrocortisone was applied for 7 days. Regular use of the emollients was required but his skin cleared up after 3–4 weeks.

PHARMACY STAMP	AGE 6	FORENAME, SURNAME Finlay Reed
	D.O.B. xx/xx/xxxx	ADDRESS Farrow Avenue
		NHS NUMBER

EPADERM CREAM: apply twice daily with additional applications when required.

EMULSIFYING OINTMENT, BP: for use as a soap substitute.

HYDROCORTISONE CREAM 0.5%: apply a thin layer to affected areas twice daily. Use for 7 days only.

BECLOMETASONE INHALER: 2 puffs (200 micrograms) twice daily.

SALBUTAMOL INHALER: 2 puffs (200 micrograms) as required.

SIGNATURE OF PRESCRIBER   DATE

SP21000

Common pitfalls

- It is important to emphasise to patients and families that long-term treatment is likely to be required.
- Remember not to prescribe long courses of topical steroid treatment as this can produce systemic side effects. Use the lowest strength steroid possible for the least time possible, on the smallest area required.
- Specialist referral will be required for those patients not responding to first-line therapies.

SUMMARY

Eczema is a common condition, which is controlled using topical therapies in the vast majority of patients. Emollients may be used liberally, but it is important to recognise that topical steroids can have harmful side, effects, which may be systemic. The minimum quantity of the minimum potency for the minimum time period required to treat the skin disease should therefore be used. Education and psychological support are important for the patient and their family. Non-atopic eczema has a range of forms and treatments may vary. Use of systemic immunosuppressive therapy should only be used in severe disease and under supervision from a specialist.

🔑 Key learning points

Atopic eczema
- First-line therapy is an emollient (at least twice daily) such as Epaderm or Diprobase, in addition to soap substitutes.
- Next, a topical steroid can be added. In order of potency these are:
  hydrocortisone < Eumovate < Betnovate < Dermovate.
- A multidisciplinary approach is crucial to the management of eczema.

Other forms of eczema
- In irritant (contact) dermatitis, identification and removal of the causative agent is the key to effective management.
- Pompholyx eczema often requires treatment with a potent topical steroid.

FURTHER READING

- National Institute for Health and Care Excellence (NICE, 2007) and British Association of Dermatologists guidelines (BAD, 2010) give excellent guidance about the treatment of eczema and are regularly updated.
- A useful review of recent evidence for the management of eczema can is: Torley D, Futamura M, Williams HC *et al.* (2013). What's new in atopic eczema? An analysis of systematic reviews published in 2010–11. *Clin Exp Dermatol* 28: 449–56.

Psoriasis

> **Sarah Evans**
>
> **Age: 43**
>
> **Hospital number: 123456**

🔍 Case study

Presenting complaint: *A 43-year-old woman presents to her GP with a 6-month history of a rash affecting her knees, elbows and buttocks. The rash is scaly and slightly itchy; she has been too embarrassed to seek help before now.*

Background: *She lives with her husband and 12-year-old daughter.*

PMH: *She had an appendicectomy aged 12 years. She is obese and has type 2 diabetes.*

Family and social history: *She has no family history of skin conditions. She has a 20 pack year smoking history.*

Allergies: *Elastoplast causes rash*

Skin examination: *Symmetrical rash affecting the extensor aspects of the elbows and knees, as well as the buttocks. There are well demarcated erythematous plaques topped with silvery scale.*

Diagnosis

Plaque psoriasis. The patient has a history of a rash affecting the extensor surfaces. The classic description is of plaques with a 'silvery scale'. Occasionally, the surface of the plaques may become keratinised so that it is hard and thickened.

Initial measures

It is important to assess the impact of the disease on each individual patient – some patients will be relatively undisturbed by extensive psoriasis,

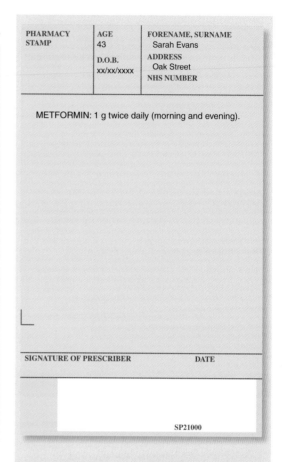

PHARMACY STAMP	AGE 43	FORENAME, SURNAME Sarah Evans
	D.O.B. xx/xx/xxxx	ADDRESS Oak Street
		NHS NUMBER

METFORMIN: 1 g twice daily (morning and evening).

SIGNATURE OF PRESCRIBER DATE

SP21000

whereas others may be distressed by what may appear to be minimal disease. Lifestyle advice including smoking cessation is also important. Most patients are managed successfully on an outpatient basis.

Prescribing for psoriasis

Generally, topical treatments are safest and are used first line. Second-line treatments should only be used when topical treatments are no longer sufficient. Biological therapies are used as third-line agents due to their immunosuppressive effects.

Topical therapies are often supplemented with phototherapy.

PHARMACY STAMP	AGE 43	FORENAME, SURNAME Sarah Evans
	D.O.B. xx/xx/xxxx	ADDRESS Oak Street
		NHS NUMBER

CALCIPOTRIOL OINTMENT: apply twice daily to affected areas.

BECLOMETASONE DIPROPIONATE 0.025% CREAM: apply thinly 1-2 times daily to affected areas.

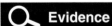

SIGNATURE OF PRESCRIBER   DATE

SP21000

✓ DRUGS checklist for TOPICAL CALCIPOTRIOL

Dose	One application
Route	Topically (to affected areas)
Units	N/A
Given	Once/twice daily (max 100 g weekly for those >12 years)
Special situations	May cause photosensitivity or dry skin; rare side effects include facial or perioral dermatitis.

Topical vitamin D analogues: essential pharmacology

Calcipotriol is a vitamin D3 analogue, which works by inhibiting epidermal cell proliferation and improving cell differentiation. It is thought to act through binding to vitamin D receptors, thereby altering gene transcription.

Generally, treatment with topical vitamin D analogues is well tolerated. However, side effects may include irritant dermatitis.

Topical steroids: rationale and evidence

Topical steroids are an effective and convenient treatment option, although long-term treatment is often required, which can cause skin atrophy and worsening of psoriasis when stopped.

Topical vitamin D analogues: rationale and evidence

Topical vitamin D analogues such as calcipotriol have similar efficacy to topical steroids but have a slower response (Svensson *et al.*, 2011). Combined steroid–calcipotriol preparations are also used.

🔍 Evidence

Topical vitamin D analogues
Vitamin D analogues suppress the activity of proinflammatory cytokines, which drive the disease (Hegyi *et al.*, 2013). A study found that topical vitamin D analogues were more efficacious and better tolerated than coal tar preparations in patients with plaque psoriasis (Singh *et al.*, 2013).

🔍 Evidence

Topical steroids in psoriasis
A systematic review has suggested that, used in combination, topical steroids and vitamin D analogues are more than twice as effective as using vitamin D analogues alone (Devaux *et al.*, 2012). There is also evidence to suggest that potent topical corticosteroids either used alone or in combination with vitamin D analogues are the most cost-effective option for patients with trunk or limb psoriasis (Sawyer *et al.*, 2013).

✓ **DRUGS checklist for BECLOMETASONE**

Dose	One thin application
Route	Topically (to affected areas only)
Units	N/A
Given	Once/twice daily depending on severity
Special situations	Short-term use of mild and moderately potent steroids is associated with few side effects. Particular caution should be taken when using potent steroids. Local side effects include thinning of the skin, contact dermatitis and worsening of underlying infection. Absorption through the skin can rarely cause adrenal suppression.

Topical steroids: essential pharmacology

See Topical Steroids: Essential Pharmacology in Eczema section.

Other treatments used in psoriasis

- Coal tar-based therapies have long been an effective, safe therapy for psoriasis (Slutsky et al., 2010). However, these substances are messy and inconvenient to apply. Tar extracts are less effective but more convenient and pleasant to use.
- Dithranol (anthralin) has a relatively slow onset of action but can lead to prolonged remission. Unlike topical steroids, it has a shorter contact time and does not lead to rebound worsening of disease on withdrawal. However, it stains skin, clothing and towels a yellow-brown colour and can cause local skin irritation.

- Topical retinoids have limited efficacy and are teratogenic.
- Phototherapy using UVB is a commonly used therapy in psoriasis, usually as an adjunct to topical therapies. Psoralen UVA (PUVA) is also used.
- Systemic therapies include methotrexate, acitretin and ciclosporin. Methotrexate is the most widely used. It is important to note that these drugs have significant side-effect profiles and as such are used as second-line therapies. For example, acitretin is teratogenic and ciclosporin is nephrotoxic and can cause immunosuppression.
- Biological agents such as adalimumab and etanercept are costly immunosuppressive agents and have to be given intravenously. They are currently only used in severe cases when other therapies have failed and in patients with psoriatic arthritis (Christophers et al., 2013; Mease et al., 2000).

🔍 **Evidence**

Biological therapies for psoriasis
A study comparing biological therapies with other treatment options found that more patients receiving biological treatments reported symptomatic improvement from severe to mild or moderate compared with topical treatment, phototherapy or conventional systemic treatment.

One study found that 4 weeks after treatment with adalimumab, patients with psoriatic arthropathy had significantly improved quality of life compared to pretreatment scores (Tsuji et al., 2013).

Case outcome and discharge

Sarah used the calcipotriol and beclometasone as prescribed. This resulted in some improvement in her symptoms, but her plaques did not resolve entirely. She was referred to a dermatologist for PUVA treatment.

PHARMACY STAMP	AGE 43	FORENAME, SURNAME Sarah Evans
	D.O.B. xx/xx/xxxx	ADDRESS Oak Street
		NHS NUMBER

CALCIPOTRIOL OINTMENT: apply twice daily to affected areas.

BECLOMETASONE DIPROPIONATE 0.025% CREAM: apply thinly 1-2 times daily to affected areas.

METFORMIN: 1 g oral twice daily.

SIGNATURE OF PRESCRIBER   DATE

SP21000

Common pitfalls

- You may encounter patients with psoriasis who are taking systemic therapies. Remember that these will have immunosuppressive effects, which should be considered when managing acute episodes of illness, especially intercurrent infection (where immunosuppressives should be withheld).
- As with eczema, remember to avoid protracted courses of topical steroid treatment.
- Specialist referral will be required for those patients not responding to first-line therapies.

SUMMARY

Psoriasis is associated with both genetic factors (including HLA associations), as well as environmental factors such as smoking, high alcohol intake and some drugs. It may have a significant psychological impact upon sufferers. Topical therapies are the first line of treatment and include topical steroids and topical vitamin D analogues. Use of systemic immunosuppressive therapy, including novel biological agents, should only be used in severe disease and under supervision from a specialist.

Key learning points

Psoriasis
- Topical treatments are used first line, including topical steroids, topical vitamin D analogues (e.g. calcipotriol) and coal tar preparations.
- There is evidence to suggest that use of a topical steroid and vitamin D analogue in combination may be more effective than each treatment alone.

(Continued)

🔑 Key learning points (*Continued*)

- Phototherapy (PUVA/UVB) is a common adjunctive treatment.
- Systemic therapies are used second line and include acetretin and ciclosporin.
- Biological therapies are used in severe refractory disease and in patients with associated psoriatic arthropathy.

FURTHER READING

- National Institute for Health and Care Excellence (NICE) and British Association of Dermatologists (BAD) guidelines give useful guidance about the treatment of psoriasis and are regularly updated.
- A useful review of recent evidence for the management of psoriasis using topical therapies is: Mason AR, Mason J, Cork M *et al.* (2013). Topical treatments for chronic plaque psoriasis (review). *Cochrane Database Syst Rev* (3): CD005028.

Allergic rashes

> **Ruby Smith**
> **Age: 78**
> **Hospital number: 123456**

Case study

Presenting complaint: *An 78-year-old woman is referred to her local hospital by her GP. She presented with a 2-day history of cough, shortness of breath and fever. She has been given IV co-amoxiclav for community-acquired pneumonia. Since then she has developed a widespread itchy rash.*

Background: *She lives with her husband in a bungalow. She is independent at home.*

PMH and family history: *She has hypothyroidism and hypertension.*

Allergies: *None known*

Examination: *Pulse 102, Sats 95% on air, RR 24*

CVS: *Capillary refill time <2 seconds, BP 126/75*

RS: *Chest clear*

Skin: *Widespread morbilliform maculopapular rash. There are raised wheals varying from a few millimetres to a few centimetres in size. The rash is itchy.*

| PHARMACY STAMP | AGE 78 | FORENAME, SURNAME Ruby Smith |
| | D.O.B. xx/xx/xxxx | ADDRESS Cedar Road NHS NUMBER |

LEVOTHYROXINE 100 micrograms once daily.

RAMIPRIL 5 mg once daily.

SIGNATURE OF PRESCRIBER   DATE

SP21000

Diagnosis

Allergic rash. The patient has developed a rash following administration of a penicillin derivative. Patients may have a documented allergy or this may be a new reaction. It is important to ensure that the patient remains haemodynamically stable and that the rash does not develop into anaphylaxis. There is no evidence here of angioedema or respiratory compromise.

Initial measures

A thorough 'ABC' approach is required in this situation to ensure that the patient is not developing anaphylaxis. Once you are sure that the patient is stable and a rash is the only symptom present, further management can commence.

Prescribing for allergic rashes

The first step in the management of an allergic rash is to remove the precipitant. In the case of a drug allergy, if an IV infusion is the cause, then this should be stopped as soon as possible. If a drug has already been given, it should be crossed off the drug chart and formally documented as an allergy to prevent further doses being given. Drug rashes may occur several weeks after starting a new drug, so a careful drug history is essential.

For symptomatic relief, an antihistamine can be given. This can be given orally, except in the case of anaphylaxis when it is given intravenously or intramuscularly along with intramuscular adrenaline, intravenous hydrocortisone and nebulised salbutamol. Rarely, there can be other severe skin manifestations of drug reactions including erythroderma and Stephen–Johnson syndrome.

Chlorphenamine: rationale and evidence

Chlorphenamine is used to provide symptomatic relief from itch in allergic rashes. It non-selectively antagonises central and peripheral H1 histamine receptors. This leads to a number of effects including suppression of the medullary cough centre, antidyskinetic, antiemetic and sedative effects. It is metabolised in the liver and GI tract and is excreted via the kidneys.

| PHARMACY STAMP | AGE 78 | FORENAME, SURNAME Ruby Smith |
| | D.O.B. xx/xx/xxxx | ADDRESS Cedar Road NHS NUMBER |

CHLORPHENAMINE: 4 mg 3-4 times daily (max dose 24 mg/24 hours).

SIGNATURE OF PRESCRIBER   DATE

SP21000

✔	**DRUGS checklist for CHLORPHENAMINE**	
Dose	4 mg for itch or rash	
	10 mg for anaphylaxis	
Route	Oral for itch or rash	
	IV or IM for anaphylaxis	
Units	mg	
Given	Every 4–6 hours for itch or rash, maximum 24 mg daily	
	For anaphylaxis, can give up to 4 doses of 10 mg in 24 hours	
Special situations	May cause drowsiness; rarely exfoliative dermatitis and tinnitus have been reported.	

Chlorphenamine: essential pharmacology

In an allergic reaction, the allergen cross-links with surface IgE antibodies on mast cells and basophils. Once this complex has formed, this causes histamine release. Histamine then causes itch, vasodilatation, flushing, tachycardia and a rash through its action on H1 receptors. Chlorphenamine is a short-acting alkylamine antihistamine and histamine antagonist. It acts by binding to the H1 histamine receptor to block the action of endogenous histamine.

Case outcome and discharge

Mrs Smith's itchy rash resolved later that day. The rash was documented on her medical records as an allergy to co-amoxiclav.

Common pitfalls

- In this case, the clue to the cause of the rash was in the history – never forget to ask about recent changes in medication.
- When examining a rash, try to describe it as thoroughly as possible, and think through some key differential diagnoses.
- Remember that chlorphenamine may cause drowsiness – it is important to warn patients of this, and it may be appropriate for it to be taken at night for this reason.

PHARMACY STAMP	AGE 78	FORENAME, SURNAME
		Ruby Smith
	D.O.B. xx/xx/xxxx	ADDRESS Cedar Road
		NHS NUMBER

CHLORPHENAMINE: 4 mg 3-4 times daily (max dose 24 mg/24 hours).

LEVOTHYROXINE 100 micrograms once daily.

RAMIPRIL 5 mg once daily.

SIGNATURE OF PRESCRIBER   DATE

SP21000

SUMMARY

Allergic rash is common and has a wide range of causes, including drug reactions. The degree of reaction can vary widely from rash to anaphylaxis, or other cutaneous manifestations including erythroderma. Antihistamines are useful in the management of simple allergic rash.

🔑 Key learning points

Allergic rash
- An initial ABC approach is required in the assessment of a drug reaction.
- The cause of the rash should be removed, and if symptoms and signs of anaphylaxis are present, emergency management with adrenaline and hydrocortisone is required (see Chapter 2).
- An antihistamine such as chlorphenamine is useful in the management of allergic rash.

FURTHER READING

- A useful review of recent evidence of drug-associated rashes is: Stern RS (2012). Exanthematous drug eruptions. *N Engl J Med* 366: 2492–501.

Cellulitis

Marjorie Butler

Age: 72

Hospital number: 123456

Case study

Presenting complaint: *A 72-year-old woman presents to accident and emergency with fever and a red, hot, swollen and tender area on her left lower leg.*

Background: *She is retired and lives at home with her husband.*

PMH and family history: *Hypertension, non-ST-elevation myocardial infarction (NSTEMI) 3 years ago, atrial fibrillation (on warfarin), cholecystectomy 20 years ago.*

Allergies: *none known*

Examination:
Pulse 115, Sats 96% on air, RR 24, temperature 38.5

CVS: *capillary refill time <2 seconds, BP 145/83, HS normal, mild bilateral pitting oedema to mid-shin*

RS: *Chest clear*

Abdo: *Soft and non-tender*

Skin: *Erythematous, warm, tender area of skin over left lower leg and foot. No skin ulceration and no clinical evidence of DVT*

Diagnosis

Cellulitis. This often occurs following a breach to the skin such as an insect bite, eczema, psoriasis or ulcer. The leg is the most commonly affected site.

| PHARMACY STAMP | AGE 72 | FORENAME, SURNAME Marjorie Butler |
| | D.O.B. xx/xx/xxxx | ADDRESS Rose Lane NHS NUMBER |

ASPIRIN 75 mg oral once daily.

AMLODIPINE 5 mg oral once daily.

BENDROFLUMETHIAZIDE 2.5 mg oral once daily.

SIMVASTATIN 20 mg oral once at night.

WARFARIN as per INR oral once daily.

SIGNATURE OF PRESCRIBER   DATE

SP21000

It presents as a red, hot, swollen and tender area. The diagnosis is largely clinical.

Initial measures

Management will depend upon the severity of the cellulitis and the degree of systemic illness. In this case, the patient is febrile and tachycardic, suggestive of more severe infection. Inflammatory markers are also a useful indicator of severity. Here, intravenous antibiotics are the most appropriate option.

Prescribing for cellulitis

REGULAR PRESCRIPTIONS					Circle/enter times below ↓	⅍ Enter dates below			
						Day 1	Day 2	Day 3	Day 4
DRUG BENZYLPENICILLIN					06				
Dose 1.2 g	Route IV	Freq QDS	Start date xx/xx/xx		08				
					12				
Signature A. Doctor		Bleep	Review		16				
					18				
Additional instructions CELLULITIS R/V 48 hours					22				
DRUG FLUCLOXACILLIN					06				
Dose 500 mg	Route IV	Freq QDS	Start date xx/xx/xx		08				
					12				
Signature A. Doctor		Bleep	Review		16				
					18				
Additional instructions CELLULITIS R/V 48 hours					22				

Other measures include elevation of the affected limb and analgesia. The affected area should be marked initially and reviewed daily to assess the efficacy of antibiotic therapy.

Penicillins: rationale and evidence

The choice of antibiotic therapy will vary depending upon local protocols. Patients with mild cellulitis and no systemic symptoms can be treated with oral antibiotics such as flucloxacillin. Clindamycin is an alternative in penicillin-allergic patients. In patients who are known to be colonised with methicillin-resistant *Staphylococcus aureus* (MRSA), intravenous vancomycin should be used. Teicoplanin or linezolid are suitable alternatives. There is a lack of evidence regarding duration of antibiotic therapy; many guidelines now suggest 10–14 days of oral therapy.

🔍 Evidence

Antibiotic choice in cellulitis
There remains a lack of consensus in terms of the most appropriate antibiotic choice in cellulitis. A Cochrane review analysed 25 randomised controlled trials but could not draw any definitive conclusions as a wide range of different antibiotics were

used (Kilburn *et al.*, 2010). Current guidelines suggest that the majority of cases caused by *Streptococcus* and *Staphylococcus aureus* should be treated with flucloxacillin or amoxicillin, making sure to test an individual's MRSA status (CREST, 2005).

✓ DRUGS checklist for FLUCLOXACILLIN

Dose	Oral: 250–500 mg QDS
	Intravenous: 250 mg to 2 g QDS
Route	Oral, intravenous or intramuscular
Units	mg
Given	Four times a day
Special situations	May cause hypersensitivity reactions including rash, fever and joint pains. Rarely angioedema, anaphylaxis, convulsions, gastrointestinal disturbances, and thrombocytopenia.

✓ DRUGS checklist for BENZYLPENICILLIN

Dose	1.2–2.4 g QDS
Route	Intravenous or intramuscular
Units	mg
Given	Four times a day
Special situations	Rarely, can cause hypersensitivity reactions. Even more rare are CNS toxicity, interstitial nephritis and coagulopathy.

Penicillins: essential pharmacology

Penicillins are a group of antibiotics that contain a beta-lactam ring. Benzylpenicillin (penicillin G) has a relatively narrow spectrum, and is used to treat infections caused by Gram-positive organisms, including

Pneumococcus and *Streptococcus*. Most *Staphylococcus aureus* strains produce penicillinase, and are therefore resistant to the action of benzylpenicillin. Benzylpenicillin acts by binding to penicillin-binding proteins in the cell wall, inhibiting cell wall synthesis. It has poor oral absorption and so is given intravenously or intramuscularly. Diffusion to most of the body tissues occurs with peak plasma levels after 15–30 minutes. However, penetration to the brain is poor. The half-life of benzylpenicillin is approximately 30 minutes and it is renally excreted.

Flucloxacillin has activity against Gram-positive organisms, including beta-lactamase-producing staphylococci. It has an isoxazolyl group, and therefore is not inactivated by beta-lactamase. Like benzylpenicillin, it acts by inhibiting cell wall synthesis. Unlike benzylpenicillin, flucloxacillin is not broken down by gastric acid so it can be given orally, intravenously or intramuscularly.

Case outcome and discharge

Mrs Butler completed 48 hours of intravenous antibiotics. The cellulitis responded well to treatment, her inflammatory markers fell and her temperature settled. She was switched to oral antibiotics and discharged home.

DISCHARGE MEDICATION

Date	Medication	Dose	Route	Frequency	Supply	GP to continue?
xx/xx/xx	PENICILLIN V	500 mg	PO	Four times a day	10 days	N
xx/xx/xx	FLUCLOXACILLIN	500 mg	PO	Four times a day	10 days	N
xx/xx/xx	ASPIRIN	75 mg	PO	Once daily	14 days	Y
xx/xx/xx	AMLODIPINE	5 mg	PO	Once daily	14 days	Y
xx/xx/xx	BENDROFLUMETHIAZIDE	2.5 mg	PO	Once daily	14 days	Y
xx/xx/xx	SIMVASTATIN	20 mg	PO	Once at night	14 days	Y
xx/xx/xx	WARFARIN	As per INR	PO	Once daily	14 days	Y

Notes to patient/GP:

Common pitfalls

- Remember to mark the affected area of skin.
- Don't forget to check your local antibiotic guidelines as antibiotic choice will vary between trusts.
- Patients with mild cellulitis without systemic infection can be treated with oral antibiotics and discharged home.
- Approximately 30% of patients will have a recurrence of cellulitis. This can be prevented by improving skin integrity; the most common causes are fungal infections and toe web intertrigo.

SUMMARY

Cellulitis is a relatively common skin infection, particularly in patients with diabetes or pre-existing skin disease. Management includes analgesia, elevation of the affected limb, marking of the area and antibiotic therapy. For mild disease without systemic features, oral antibiotics may be sufficient. For patients with systemic symptoms and severe cellulitis, hospital admission for intravenous antibiotics may be required.

🔑 Key learning points

Cellulitis
- Patients invariably require antibiotic therapy.
- Options include oral and intravenous antibiotics.
- In patients with fever, tachycardia and significantly raised inflammatory markers, those with extensive cellulitis, or treatment failure with oral antibiotics, intravenous therapy is likely to be indicated.

(Continued)

> ### 🔑 Key learning points (*Continued*)
>
> - Optimal antibiotic choice remains contentious and you should be guided by your local protocols.
> - Be sure to check the MRSA status of your patient – this will affect the antibiotic regimen used.

FURTHER READING

- A useful review of recent evidence for the management of cellulitis is: Phoenix G, Das S, Joshi M (2012). Diagnosis and management of cellulitis. *BMJ* 345: e4955.

Fungal infections

> ### Rosie Wroughton
> ### Age: 12
> ### Hospital number: 123456
>
> ### 🔍 Case study
>
> ***Presenting complaint:*** *A 12-year-old girl presents to her GP with an itchy, scaly scalp.*
>
> ***Background:*** *She lives with her mother and younger siblings. Her siblings have had similar symptoms in the last few weeks.*
>
> ***PMH and family history:*** *She has no past medical history of note, has no family history of skin conditions and has never been admitted to hospital.*
>
> ***Allergies:*** *None known*
>
> ***Skin examination:*** *Thickened, scaly scalp with raised red rings. No skin lesions associated and no hair loss.*
>
> ***Diagnosis***
>
> Tinea capitis (scalp ringworm). Tinea capitis is a dermatophyte infection of the scalp occurring mainly in children. Clinical signs are variable, but the scalp is often scaly, there may be the classic

ring lesions, or kerion. There may be alopecia in more severe cases. In this case, we are told that the patient has young siblings with similar symptoms; it will also be important for them to be diagnosed and treated.

Initial measures

Treatment of superficial fungal infections will vary widely depending upon the type and location of infection. Thus it is particularly important to obtain samples through skin scraping or scalp brushing to determine the causative organism.

Tinea can also affect the feet (tinea pedis) or body (tinea corporis). Fungal infections can also affect the nails (onychomycosis). Other superficial fungal infections include candidiasis and malassezia infection, including pityriasis versicolor.

Prescribing for superficial fungal infections

Most superficial fungal skin infections can be treated with topical therapy, but tinea capitis requires systemic treatment. Options include griseofulvin, terbinafine or itraconazole. The use of griseofulvin has been widely superseded by the use of newer antifungals.

PHARMACY STAMP	AGE 12	FORENAME, SURNAME
		Rosie Wroughton
	D.O.B. xx/xx/xxxx	ADDRESS
		Riversdale Close
		NHS NUMBER

TERBINAFINE: 250 mg once daily for 2-4 weeks.

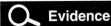

SIGNATURE OF PRESCRIBER	DATE

SP21000

Terbinafine: rationale and evidence

Azole antifungals such as ketoconazole and fluconazole act through inhibition of cytochrome P-450 enzymes. It is important to note that these drugs can therefore interact with the many other medications metabolised through this pathway. Allylamines including terbinafine act in a similar way to azoles.

Q Evidence

Choice of oral antifungal treatment in tinea capitis

A systematic review suggested that newer antifungals such as terbinafine have similar efficacy and safety profiles to griseofulvin, and can be used for shorter time periods (Bell-Syer *et al.*, 2012). In another systematic

review of treatment of children, terbinafine was found to be more effective in the treatment of *Trychophyton* spp., whereas grisofulvin was more effective for *Microsporum* spp. (Gupta and Drummond-Main, 2013). In this study terbinafine treatment was for 4 weeks and grisofulvin was for 8 weeks. This highlights the importance of sending scalp samples for analysis to identify the causative organism.

Q Evidence

Treatment of tinea coporis and tinea pedis

For tinea corporis, topical treatment is used first line; there is no evidence that one agent is superior to another. Terbinafine 1% for 4–6 weeks is usually the treatment of choice (Moriarty *et al.*, 2012).

For tinea pedis, a Cochrane review analysed randomised controlled trials comparing a range of topical antifungal treatments with placebo. The most effective topical therapy in this study was terbinafine (Crawford and Hollis, 2007).

✓ DRUGS checklist for TERBINAFINE

Dose	Orally: 250 mg for 2–4 weeks (can be up to 3 months in nail infections)
	Topically: one application 1–2 times daily for 2 weeks
Route	Oral or topical
Units	mg
Given	Once daily
Special situations	Oral terbinafine should be avoided in hepatic impairment. Dose reduction to 50% is recommended if the eGFR <50 mL/min. Side effects may include nausea, loss of appetite, abdominal discomfort, diarrhoea, headache and urticarial rash.

Terbinafine: essential pharmacology

Terbinafine acts by inhibiting a fungal enzyme called squaline epoxidase. This prevents the synthesis of ergosterol, a key component of the fungal cell wall and causes cell lysis. Terbinafine has good oral absorption and binds to albumin and other plasma proteins, becoming concentrated within fat cells in the skin and nails. As a result, the concentration of the drug in keratinised tissues is considerably higher than in plasma, and therapeutic levels of the drug may persist in these tissues for months after cessation of oral therapy.

Case outcome and discharge

Rosie was reviewed by her GP after 2 weeks of treatment with terbinafine, and she was found to have some residual tinea infection. She therefore continued treatment for a further 2 weeks (4 weeks in total), at which stage the tinea had resolved.

Common pitfalls

- Think carefully about your choice of antifungal – you may wish to contact your local microbiology department for advice.
- Remember that many antifungal therapies can interact with other medications so always refer to the BNF (BMA/RPS, 2015) before prescribing.

PHARMACY STAMP	AGE 12	FORENAME, SURNAME Rosie Wroughton
	D.O.B. xx/xx/xxxx	ADDRESS Riversdale Close
		NHS NUMBER

TERBINAFINE: 250 mg oral once daily for 2-4 weeks.

SIGNATURE OF PRESCRIBER   DATE

SP21000

SUMMARY

Superficial fungal infections, including tinea capitis, pedis and corporis, are relatively common and treatment depends upon the site. Tinea pedis and corporis can usually be managed with topical therapy, whereas tinea capitis requires systemic antifungals. Fungal infections affecting the nails (onychomycosis) are more difficult to treat with topical therapy than tinea pedis and corporis.

🔑 Key learning points

Tinea infections

- First-line therapy for tinea pedis and corporis should be a topical antifungal.
- For tinea pedis, there is evidence to suggest that terbinafine is the most effective treatment.
- For tinea corporis, there is a lack of robust evidence as to which antifungal is the most effective.
- For tinea capitis, oral therapy is required. Terbinafine is generally well tolerated and requires a shorter duration of therapy compared to griseofulvin.

FURTHER READING

■ A useful review of recent evidence for the management of superficial fungal infections is: Salmon N, Fuller C (2013). Fungal skin infections: current approaches to management. *Prescriber* 24: 31–7.

Acne

> **Joseph James**
>
> **Age: 18**
>
> **Hospital number: 123456**

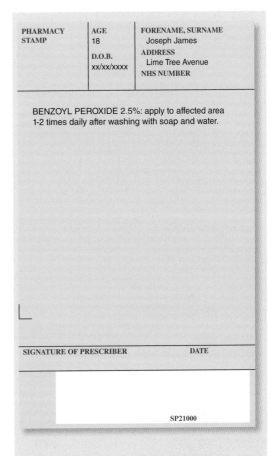

Case study

Presenting complaint: *An 18-year-old man presents to his GP with worsening acne. He initially saw his GP 2 months ago and was prescribed topical benzoyl peroxide. However, his symptoms are continuing to worsen and he is starting to feel low in mood and self-conscious about his skin, and has recently stopped going out with his friends because of this.*

Background: *He works as an apprentice plumber and smokes 20 cigarettes a day.*

PMH and family history: *He has been previously fit and well. No family history of skin conditions.*

Allergies: *Elastoplast – rash*

Skin examination: *Numerous open and closed comedones, inflamed nodules, papules and pustules on the patient's face. No excoriations or scarring.*

Diagnosis

Moderately severe acne. We are told that the patient has numerous comedones, nodules, papules and pustules. He has tried one topical therapy which has not improved his symptoms. We are also told that his mood and social activities are being affected by his acne.

Initial measures

It is important to remember the psychosocial implications of acne, and that the extent of skin disease may not necessarily correlate with the impact of acne upon a patient's life. Initial advice includes smoking cessation, and advice to avoid scratching or squeezing lesions, as this may cause scarring.

Prescribing for acne

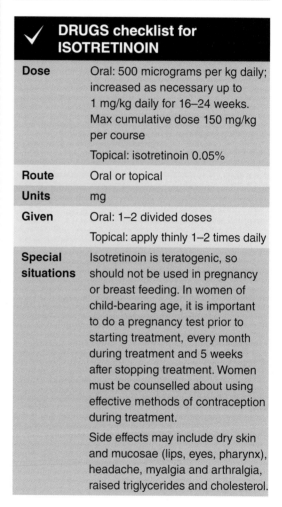

PHARMACY STAMP	AGE 18	FORENAME, SURNAME Joseph James
	D.O.B. xx/xx/xxxx	ADDRESS Lime Tree Avenue NHS NUMBER

TOPICAL ISOTRETINOIN 0.05%: apply thinly 1-2 times daily.

TETRACYCLINE 500 mg twice daily for 12 weeks.

SIGNATURE OF PRESCRIBER   DATE

SP21000

Isotretinoin: rationale and evidence

Topical retinoids such as isotretinoin have become the mainstay of topical therapy are now recommended for all patients with acne, except those taking oral retinoids. These agents may cause skin irritation, and have been reported to cause an initial worsening of symptoms. Like oral retinoids, topical retinoids should be avoided in pregnancy and breastfeeding, and women of child-bearing age should be given contraceptive advice.

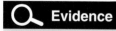

Evidence

Isotretinoin

Both topical and systemic retinoids are used in acne. Several studies have suggested that

benzoyl peroxide should be added alongside topical retinoids when inflammatory lesions are present (Hughes *et al.*, 1992; Gollnick *et al.*, 2003); this has been reflected in European guidelines (Nast *et al.*, 2012). Oral isotretinoin has been shown to be highly efficacious in patients with severe acne (Haider and Shaw, 2004).

✓ DRUGS checklist for ISOTRETINOIN

Dose	Oral: 500 micrograms per kg daily; increased as necessary up to 1 mg/kg daily for 16–24 weeks. Max cumulative dose 150 mg/kg per course
	Topical: isotretinoin 0.05%
Route	Oral or topical
Units	mg
Given	Oral: 1–2 divided doses
	Topical: apply thinly 1–2 times daily
Special situations	Isotretinoin is teratogenic, so should not be used in pregnancy or breast feeding. In women of child-bearing age, it is important to do a pregnancy test prior to starting treatment, every month during treatment and 5 weeks after stopping treatment. Women must be counselled about using effective methods of contraception during treatment.
	Side effects may include dry skin and mucosae (lips, eyes, pharynx), headache, myalgia and arthralgia, raised triglycerides and cholesterol.

Isotretinoin: essential pharmacology

Retinoids act by binding to and activating retinoic acid receptors (RARs). Retinoid receptors are intranuclear and act as transcription factors; they bind to regulatory regions in DNA and activate gene transcription. Release of growth factors causes epidermal hyperplasia, due to proliferation of basal keratinocytes.

Isotretinoin acts by reducing the size of seborrhoeic glands and reducing sebum production, reducing the production of comedones, reducing colonisation with *Propionibacterium acnes*, and reducing the abnormal desquamation involved in the pathogenesis of acne.

Tetracycline: rationale and evidence

Systemic antibiotics can be used and have antimicrobial and anti-inflammatory effects (James, 2005). Options include doxycycline, minocycline, lymecycline, erythromycin and tetracycline. There is a lack of evidence as to which antibiotic is the most efficacious (Simonart *et al.*, 2008). Studies do suggest, however, that as with topical antibiotics, oral antibiotics should be used in conjunction with other therapies. Antibiotic courses should be limited to 12 weeks where possible.

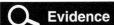

Evidence

Combination therapy in acne: retinoids and antibiotics

A phase IV study investigated the use of a topical retinoid, topical antibiotic or benzoyl peroxide and an oral antibiotic and has suggested that these agents were effective, well tolerated and reduced the need for oral isotretinoin use (Zaenglein *et al.*, 2013).

✓ DRUGS checklist for TETRACYCLINE

Dose	500 mg
Route	Oral
Units	mg
Given	Twice daily
Special situations	Side effects may include nausea, vomiting and diarrhoea. Rarely, hepatotoxicity and photosensitivity may occur.

Tetracycline: essential pharmacology

Tetracycline has bacteriostatic effects, binding to the bacterial ribosomal 30S and 50S subunits, preventing aminoacyl tRNA from binding and preventing translation. Additional effects include altering the bacterial cytoplasmic membrane causing leakage of intracellular contents.

In addition to use in acne, tetracyclines are used in *Rickettsia*, *Coxiella* and *Borrelia burgdorferi* (Lyme disease) infections.

Other treatments used in acne

Topical agents:

- Topical benzoyl peroxide is an antimicrobial agent with bactericidal and anti-inflammatory properties. Skin irritation may occur, although this often resolves with prolonged treatment. The strength of treatment varies from 2.5 to 10%; skin irritation is worse at higher concentrations. Benzoyl peroxide can also bleach clothing, bedding and hair.
- Topical antibiotics such as erythromycin and clindamycin are useful when inflammatory lesions are present.
- A number of antibiotic–retinoid and antibiotic–benzoyl peroxide combination treatments are available; these are more expensive but may improve treatment compliance.
- Azelaic acid is an alternative to topical retinoids. It has comedolytic, anti-inflammatory and antimicrobial properties, but may cause skin hypopigmentation.
- Topical salicylic acid may be used as an alternative topical agent when other treatments are not tolerated. There is limited evidence as to the efficacy of topical salicylic acid in acne, although some studies suggest that it may be better tolerated than the other agents.

Systemic agents: There are a number of systemic agents available for patients with moderate to severe acne:

- In women, the combined oral contraceptive pill (COCP) can be effective; a Cochrane review found that the COCP was effective for patients with inflammatory and non-inflammatory acne. Some formulations contain cyproterone acetate; however, use of these drugs has a higher risk of venous thromboembolism and there is no clear evidence that they are more effective (Arowojolu *et al.*, 2009).
- Oral isotretinoin is used in the treatment of severe acne, and moderate acne that is resistant to other therapies. It is recommended to be used first line

and as monotherapy in such cases. Treatment takes 4–8 weeks to take effect, and patients usually complete a 16 to 24-week course. Meta-analyses have highlighted the effectiveness of oral isotretinoin; approximately 80% of patients will not require further treatment (Chivot , 2005; Newman *et al.*, 2011). However, there are a number of important side effects – see DRUGS checklist for isotretinoin.

Evidence

Resistance to topical antibiotic treatment

There is increasing evidence to suggest that resistance to topical antibiotic treatment may occur in *P. acnes* infection. A systematic review suggested that efficacy of topical antibiotic therapy with erythromycin and clarithromycin in acne decreases with time (Gamble *et al.*, 2012). There is also some resistance to *Staphylococcus* and *Streptococcus* infections (Leyden *et al.*, 2009). Therefore, current guidelines recommend that topical antibiotics should not be used as monotherapy, and should be used for a maximum of 12 weeks where possible (Ozolins *et al.*, 2004).

Case outcome and discharge

After 3 months, Joseph returned to his GP. His acne had improved, but he still experienced troubling symptoms. He was referred to a dermatologist for consideration of oral isotretinoin therapy.

Common pitfalls

- Remember to assess the clinical severity of acne as this will guide treatment.

| PHARMACY STAMP | AGE 18 | FORENAME, SURNAME Joseph James |
| | D.O.B. xx/xx/xxxx | ADDRESS Lime Tree Avenue NHS NUMBER |

TOPICAL ISOTRETINOIN 0.05%: apply thinly 1-2 times daily.

BENZOYL PEROXIDE 2.5%: apply to affected areas 1-2 times daily after washing with soap and water.

TETRACYCLINE 500 mg twice daily for 12 weeks.

SIGNATURE OF PRESCRIBER   DATE

SP21000

- Combination therapy using a topical retinoid and topical or systemic antibiotic is particularly effective.
- Each of the drugs used in acne have important side-effect profiles – it is important to consider this, particularly for patients prescribed oral or topical isotretinoin.

SUMMARY

Acne can have significant psychosocial morbidity. Treatment depends on the severity of disease. In mild and moderate disease, topical therapies should be used first line. Combination therapy has been shown to be particularly effective. In moderate to severe disease, there are a range of oral therapies available. It is important to counsel patients appropriately before starting isotretinoin.

🔑 Key learning points

Acne

- Topical therapies include:
  - Topical retinoids: these should be used for all patients unless contraindicated or taking oral isotretinoin.
  - Topical antibiotics: these are particularly useful for inflammatory acne.
  - Benzoyl peroxide.
- Topical therapies are particularly effective when used in combination.
- For more severe acne, there are a range of systemic treatments:
  - Oral antibiotics
  - Hormonal agents in women, such as the combined oral contraceptive pill
  - Oral isotretinoin: this is teratogenic and has a significant side-effect profile so patients must be counselled appropriately.

FURTHER READING

Useful guidelines for the management of acne are:

- Strauss JS, Krowchuk DP, Leyden JJ *et al.* (2007). Guidelines of care for acne vulgaris management. *J Am Acad Dermatol* 56: 651–63.
- Nast A, Dreno B, Bettoli V *et al.* (2012). European evidence-based (S3) guidelines for the treatment of acne. *J Eur Acad Dermatol Venereol* 26 (Suppl. 1): 1–29.

Two reviews of evidence in acne management are:

- Dawson AL, Dellavalle RP (2013). Acne vulgaris. *BMJ* 346: f2634.
- Williams HC, Dellavalle RP, Garner S (2012). Acne vulgaris. *Lancet* 379: 361–72.

Now visit **www.wileyessential.com/pharmacology** to test yourself on this chapter.

References

Arowojolu AO, Gallo MF, Lopez LM *et al.* (2009). Combined oral contraceptive pills for treatment of acne. *Cochrane Database Syst Rev* (3): CD004425.

Ashcroft DM, Dimmock P, Garside R *et al.* (2005). Efficacy and tolerability of topical pimecrolimus and tacrolimus in the treatment of atopic dermatitis: meta-analysis of randomised controlled trials. *BMJ* 330: 516–22.

Baron SE, Cohen SN, Archer CB (2012). Guidance on the diagnosis and clinical management of atopic eczema. (On behalf of the BAD and RCGP) *Clin Exp Dermatol* 37 (Suppl. 1): 7–12.

Bell-Syer SEM, Khan SM, Torgerson DJ (2012). Oral treatments for fungal infections of the skin of the foot. *Cochrane Database Syst Rev* (10): CD003584.

Berth-Jones J, Damstra RJ, Golsch S *et al.* (2003). Twice weekly fluticasone propionate added to emollient maintenance treatment to reduce risk of relapse in atopic dermatitis: randomised, double blind, parallel group study. *BMJ* 326: 1367–70.

Bieber T (2008). Atopic dermatitis. *N Engl J Med* 358: 1483–94.

British Association of Dermatologists (BAD) (2010). *Guidelines for the Management of Atopic*

Eczema. Available at: http://www.bad.org.uk/healthcare-professionals/clinical-standards/clinical-guidelines (accessed March 2016).

British Medical Association and Royal Pharmaceutical Society of Great Britain (BMA/RPS) (2015). *British National Formulary 69*, 69th edn. BMJ group and Pharmaceutical Press, London.

Chivot M (2005). Retinoid therapy for acne. A comparative review. *Am J Clin Dermatol* 6: 13–9.

Christophers E, Segaert S, Milligan G *et al.* (2013). Clinical improvement and satisfaction with biologic therapy in patients with severe plaque psoriasis: results of a European cross-sectional observational study. *J Dermatolog Treat* 24: 193–8.

Clinical Resource Efficiency Support Team (CREST) (2005). *Guidelines on the Management of Cellulitis in Adults*. Crest, Belfast. Available at: http://www.acutemed.co.uk/docs/Cellulitis%20guidelines,%20CREST,%2005.pdf (accessed Dec. 2015).

Crawford F, Hollis S (2007). Topical treatments for fungal infections of the skin and nails of the foot. *Cochrane Database Syst Rev* (3): CD001434.

Devaux S, Castela A, Archier E *et al.* (2012). Topical vitamin D analogues alone or in association with topical steroids in psoriasis: a systematic review. *J Eur Acad Dermatol Venereol* 26: 52–60.

Gamble R, Dunn J, Dawson A *et al.* (2012). Topical antimicrobial treatment of acne vulgaris: an evidence-based review. *Am J Clin Dermatol* 13: 141–52.

Gollnick H, Cunliffe W, Berson D *et al.* (2003). Management of acne: a report from a Global Alliance to Improve Outcomes in Acne. *J Am Acad Dermatol* 49 (1 Suppl.): S1–37.

Gupta AK, Drummond-Main C (2013). Meta-analysis of randomised controlled trials comparing particular doses of griseofulvin and terbinafine in the treatment of tinea capitis. *Pediat Dermatol* 30: 1–6.

Haider A, Shaw JC (2004). Treatment of acne vulgaris. *JAMA* 292: 726–35.

Hegyi Z, Zwicker S, Bureik D *et al.* (2013). Vitamin D analog calcipotriol suppresses the Th17 cytokine–induced proinflammatory S100

"alarmins" psoriasin (S100A7) and koebnerisin (S100A15) in psoriasis. *J Invest Dermatol* 132: 1416–24.

Hughes BR, Norris JF, Cunliffe WJ (1992). A double-blind evaluation of topical isotretinoin 0.05%, benzoyl peroxide gel 5% and placebo in patients with acne. *Clin Exp Dermatol* 17: 165–8.

James WD (2005). Clinical practice. Acne. *N Engl J Med* 352: 1463–72.

Kilburn S, Featherstone P, Higgins B *et al.* (2010). Interventions for cellulitis and erysipelas. *Cochrane Database Syst Rev* (6): CD004299.

Leyden JJ, Del Rosso JQ, Webster GF (2009). Clinical considerations in the treatment of acne vulgaris and other inflammatory skin disorders: a status report. *Dermatol Clin* 27: 1–15.

Mease PJ, Goffe BS, Metz J *et al.* (2000). Etanercept in the treatment of psoriatic arthritis and psoriasis: a randomized trial. *Lancet* 356: 385–90.

Moriarty B, Hay R, Morris-Jones R (2012). The diagnosis and management of tinea. *BMJ* 345: e4380.

Nast A, Dreno B, Bettoli V *et al.* (2012). European evidence-based (S3) guidelines for the treatment of acne. *J Eur Acad Dermatol Venereol* 26 (Suppl. 1): 1–29.

National Institute for Health and Care Excellence (NICE) (2007). *Management of Atopic Eczema in Children from Birth up to the Age of 12 Years*, CG57. Available at: www.nice.org.uk/guidelines/cg57 (accessed March 2013).

Newman MD, Bowe WP, Heughebaert C *et al.* (2011). Therapeutic considerations for severe nodular acne. *Am J Clin Dermatol* 12: 7–14.

Ozolins M, Eady EA, Avery AJ *et al.* (2004). Comparison of five antimicrobial regimens for treatment of mild to moderate inflammatory facial acne vulgaris in the community: randomised controlled trial. *Lancet* 364: 2188–95.

Reitamo S, Ortonne JP, Sand C *et al.* (2005). A multicentre, randomized, double-blind, controlled study of longterm treatment with 0.1% tacrolimus ointment in adults with moderate to severe atopic dermatitis. *Br J Dermatol* 152: 1282–9.

Sawyer L, Samarasekera EJ, Wonderling D *et al.* (2013). Topical therapies in the treatment of localised plaque psoriasis in primary care: a cost effectiveness analysis. *Br J Dermatol* 168: 1095–105.

Simonart T, Dramaix M, De Maertelaer V (2008). Efficacy of tetracyclines in the treatment of acne vulgaris. *Br J Dermatol* 158: 208–16.

Singh P, Gupta S, Abidi A *et al.* (2013). Comparative evaluation of topical calcipotriol versus coal tar and salicylic acid ointment in chronic plaque psoriasis. *J Drugs Dermatol* 12: 868–73.

Slutsky JB, Clark AF, Remedios AA *et al.* (2010). An evidencebased review of the efficacy of coal tar preparations in the treatment of psoriasis and atopic dermatitis. *J Drugs Dermatol* 9: 1258–64.

Svensson A, Chambers C, Ganemo A *et al.* (2011). A systematic review of tacrolimus ointment compared with corticosteroids in the treatment of atopic dermatitis. *Curr Med Res Opin* 27: 1395–406.

Tarr A, Iheanacho I (2009). Should we use bath emollients for atopic eczema? *BMJ* 339: b4273.

Thomas KS, Armstrong S, Avery S *et al.* (2002). Randomised controlled trial of short bursts of a potent topical corticosteroid versus prolonged use of a mild preparation for children with mild or moderate atopic eczema. *BMJ* 324: 768–71.

Tsuji S, Higashiyama M, Inaoka M *et al.* (2013). Effects of adalimumab therapy on musculoskeletal manifestations and health-related quality of life in patients with active psoriatic arthritis. *Modern Rheumatol* 23: 529–37.

Zaenglein AL, Shamban A, Webster G *et al.* (2013). A phase IV, open-label study evaluating the use of triple-combination therapy with minocycline HCl extended-release tablets, a topical antibiotic/retinoid preparation and benzoyl peroxide in patients with moderate to severe acne vulgaris. *J Drugs Dermatol* 12: 619–25.

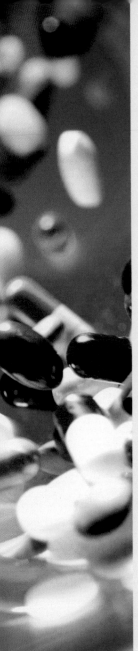

CHAPTER 14

Obstetrics and Gynaecology

Marie O'Sullivan

Key topics:

Learning objectives

By the end of this chapter you should…

- …be able to write a prescription for pregnant patients in a range of different situations taking into account relevant contraindications, cautions and side effects.
- …be able to talk about the mechanisms of action of the key drugs used in pregnancy.
- …be able to describe the physiological changes of pregnancy and how this will alter pharmacological mechanisms.

Essential Practical Prescribing, First Edition. Georgia Woodfield, Benedict Lyle Phillips, Victoria Taylor, Amy Hawkins and Andrew Stanton. © 2016 by John Wiley & Sons, Ltd. Published 2016 by John Wiley & Sons, Ltd.

Introduction

Obstetrics and gynaecology provides a uniquely challenging area for the prescribing practitioner; one must consider the physiological changes in the mother that affect drug absorption, distribution and metabolism (Table 14.1), as well as counselling the woman on the effect the drugs may have on the developing fetus. Close to the time of delivery the effect on the neonate must be understood, in addition to the effects if the mother chooses to breastfeed.

More than 80% of UK women (Headley *et al.*, 2004) take medications during pregnancy, so complete avoidance is neither necessary nor possible.

Table 14.1 Key changes in pregnancy (Stephens and Wilson, 2009; Koren, 2011; Giacoia and Mattison, 2009; Dawes *et al.*, 2001).

Change	Effects related to pharmacology
Increased progesterone	Promotes smooth muscle (gut, ureter, uterus) relaxation.
Increased oestrogen	Increased water retention.
Increased human placental lactogen	Structure and function similar to growth hormone. Alters metabolism increasing energy supply to fetus. Increases insulin secretion but dampens the peripheral effect of insulin.
Thyroid changes	Due to increased demand the maternal thyroid increases in size, increased renal clearance leaves the mother relatively deplete of iodide, this causes increased uptake by the thyroid gland. Thyroid binding globulin levels increase in the 1st trimester due to high oestrogen levels – this leads to a rise and then fall of free T3 and T4. *Iodine, antithyroid medications and antithyroid receptor antibodies can cross the placenta.*
Plasma volume	Expands throughout pregnancy to 30–50% above non-pregnant levels (1100–1600 mL at term).
White cell count	Rises, predominantly a neutrophilia. Although lymphocyte count remains almost constant; their function is depressed.
Platelets	Slight physiological decrease in pregnancy although function is unchanged.
Clotting	In preparation for labour, pregnancy is a hypercoaguable state, levels of most clotting factors increase.
Cardiovascular changes	Cardiac output increases (from 5 to 6.5L/min) due to increased stroke volume and pulse rate.
	Blood pressure should physiologically decrease due to decreased peripheral vascular resistance (thought to be due to increased prostaglandins).
Respiratory changes	Increased tidal volume due to the effect of progesterone on the respiratory centre. Pregnant women often feel breathless as their Pco_2 is set lower to allow fetal – maternal transfer of CO_2.
Renal changes	Kidneys increase in size and the eGFR increases in line with increased cardiac output. This leads to increased clearance of urea, creatinine and renally excreted drugs. (NB urea and creatinine in the 'normal range' may depict renal impairment in a pregnant woman.)
Gastrointestinal changes	Decreased tone of the oesophageal sphincter and upward displacement due to the growing fetus often lead to oesophageal reflux. There is delayed gastric emptying due to low gastric mobility and reduced gastric secretions.
	Pregnant women have a tendency for constipation due to decreased gut motility plus increased sodium and water reabsorption.

The obstetric and gynaecology teams will always be willing to give advice on prescribing in these special circumstances and the *British National Formulary* (BNF) (BMA/RPS, 2015) has appendices for prescribing in pregnancy and breastfeeding.

Common drugs to avoid in pregnancy are (Rubin and Ramsay, 2008):

- **Non- steroidal anti-inflammatory drugs:** cause premature closure of the ductus arteriosus
- **Warfarin:** teratogenic in first trimester
- **Antibiotics:** many antibiotics are advised to be used with caution in pregnancy. Avoid (amongst others) tetracyclines, quinolones, chloramphenicol and co-trimoxazole
- **Antihypertensives:** angiotensin-converting enzyme inhibitors (ACEi), angiotensin receptor blockers and diuretics
- **Statins:** all statins should be avoided
- **Antiepileptics:** all may have some fetal effects, but epilepsy in itself increases the risk of fetal malformations. Carbamazepine is the safest drug in pregnancy. Sodium valproate should be avoided if at all possible.

Pain in pregnancy

> **Miss Wendy Bright**
>
> **Age: 22**
>
> **Hospital number: 123456**

 Case study

Presenting complaint: *A 22-year-old primigravida (first pregnancy) who is 39/40 (39 weeks pregnant – 'term') self-refers to the delivery suite with a 2-hour history or painful contractions 1 : 10 (1 contraction every 10 minutes).*

Background: *She is fit and healthy with no medical history, no previous surgery and no hospital admissions.*

Allergies: *Nil known*

Examination (maternal): *HR 90, RR 16, BP 112/64, Temp 36.5. Abdomen soft and non-tender between contractions. Contractions 1 : 10 and palpable. Baby: long lie, cephalic (head down) presentation, head engaged in the pelvis. Cervix mid position, firm and 1 cm dilated.*

Examination (fetal): *cardiotocograph (CTG): baseline rate 125, variability >5 bpm, accelerations present, no decelerations; overall reassuring (Figure 14.1).*

Diagnosis

She is in early labour, but has not yet established. As she has no risk factors she can go home with analgesia, to return when her contractions are stronger and more frequent.

Initial measures

Assess maternal and fetal wellbeing – as has been done above. Remember that there are other causes for pain in pregnant women as well as labour; colicky pain can be caused by the bowel or renal colic. Suspect placental abruption (an emergency for mum and baby) when there is continuous pain with or without bleeding and a hard 'woody' tender uterus.

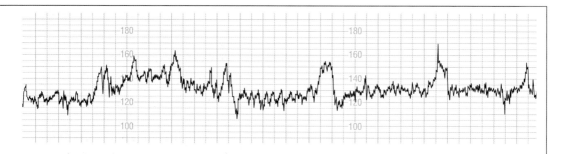

Figure 14.1 Section of cardiotocograph (CTG) to assess fetal wellbeing (normal CTG).

Prescribing for pain in pregnancy

Almost all simple analgesia is safe to be administered to the pregnant woman. The exception to this are NSAIDs as these can cause premature closure of the fetal ductus arteriosus.

In a situation such as this a combination of paracetamol and a weak opiate such as codeine would be suitable for her to take home until she establishes in labour.

For women that are progressing further in labour and who will be staying in the birth centre/delivery suite then the next step is often to try a stronger opiate such as pethidine.

AS REQUIRED MEDICATION						
DRUG PARACETAMOL					Date	
					Time	
Dose 1 g	Route PO	Frequency PRN QDS		Start date xx/xx/xx	Dose	
					Route	
Signature/Bleep A. Doctor		Max dose in 24 hrs 4 g/24 hr		Review	Given	
					Check	
Additional instructions						

DRUG CODEINE PHOSPHATE					Date	
					Time	
Dose 30–60 mg	Route PO	Frequency PRN QDS		Start date xx/xx/xx	Dose	
					Route	
Signature/Bleep A. Doctor		Max dose in 24 hrs 240 mg/24 hr		Review	Given	
					Check	
Additional instructions						

DRUG PETHIDINE					Date	
					Time	
Dose 50–100 mg	Route IM	Frequency PRN Repeat after 1-3 hrs		Start date xx/xx/xx	Dose	
					Route	
Signature/Bleep A. Doctor		Max dose in 24 hrs 400 mg/24 hr		Review	Given	
					Check	
Additional instructions						

Paracetamol: rationale and evidence

Paracetamol is used as the first-line analgesic and an antipyretic at all stages of pregnancy. When used as required and at normal, therapeutic doses it has not been associated with any fetal defects or compromise.

✓ DRUGS checklist for PARACETAMOL

Dose	1 g
Route	PO/IV/PR
Units	g
Given	When required, maximum 4 g/24 hours (4–6 hourly)
Special situations	Be cautious of dosing in young women, if body weight <50 kg. Paracetamol should be dosed by weight.

Paracetamol: essential pharmacology

The absorption, metabolism and renal clearance of paracetamol is similar in the pregnant and non-pregnant state. Paracetamol crosses the placenta but is not known to be harmful. Paracetamol overdose can be harmful to the mother and unborn child. When used as an antipyretic for intrapartum sepsis paracetamol can improve fetal outcomes.

Codeine phosphate: rationale and evidence

Despite some studies associating codeine with fetal malformations widespread use and experience means that codeine is thought to be safe in the first and second trimesters. Safety of third trimester use is uncertain; as with all opioid analgesics, frequent third trimester use can lead to neonatal dependence. Use during the later stages of labour can lead to neonatal respiratory depression.

✓ DRUGS checklist for CODEINE PHOSPHATE

Dose	30–60 mg
Route	PO
Units	mg
Given	When required, maximum 240 mg/24 hours
Special situations	Use with caution in renal impairment. Can cause dependence and withdrawal in the neonate if used for long periods antenatally. No longer recommended postnatally to breastfeeding mothers.

Codeine phosphate: essential pharmacology

Codeine is used in the same doses in pregnancy as outside of it and the metabolism is unchanged. Codeine is metabolised to the active ingredients of morphine and morphine-6-glucuronide. The enzymes responsible for this metabolism are genetically varied, meaning that some people ultrametabolise, creating higher doses in shorter time periods. In these women, if they are breastfeeding, toxic levels of morphine could reach the infant. Consequently, codeine is not recommended in breastfeeding. If strong pain relief is required an oral preparation of morphine is preferable, as the morphine received by the infant is more predictable.

Pethidine: rationale and evidence

Pethidine is a synthetic opioid analgesic – its use remains popular in labour due to its safety profile following decades of usage. The drug crosses the placenta and use close to the time of delivery can cause neonatal respiratory depression.

✓	DRUGS checklist for PETHIDINE	
Dose	50–100 mg	
Route	IM	
Units	mg	
Given	1–3 hours later if needed, max 400 mg/24 hours	
Special situations	Caution in hepatic or renal impairment.	
	Contraindicated in those with a history of epilepsy or convulsions.	
	Should be avoided (when possible) close to the time of delivery due to the possibility of respiratory distress in the newborn (effects reversed by naloxone).	

Pethidine: essential pharmacology

Pethidine works in a similar way to morphine and is an agonist of the μ opioid receptor.

Case outcome and discharge

As mum and baby are well and this woman is not in established labour she can be sent home with simple analgesia (paracetamol and codeine). She should return when the contractions are stronger or closer together, or sooner if the baby is not moving, she experiences bleeding or continuous pain.

DISCHARGE MEDICATION						
Date	Medication	Dose	Route	Frequency	Supply	GP to continue?
xx/xx/xx	PARACETAMOL	1 g (max 4 g/ 24 hours)	PO	As required, maximum 4 times a day	7 days	N
xx/xx/xx	CODEINE PHOSPHATE	15–30 mg	PO	As required, maximum 4 times a day	7 days	N

Notes to patient/GP:
Short-term pain relief for early labour. Return for assessment if increasing pain or any concerns (e.g. vaginal loss/bleeding or reduced foetal movements)

Common pitfalls

Women, especially in their first pregnancy, will be unsure what labour feels like and may be scared to leave the hospital. It is important to reassure them that they are safe to be at home when they are not in established labour.

Stay vigilant of other diagnoses – pregnant women can have all of the same problems as any other patient; not all pain will be pregnancy related.

Timing of analgesia is important also. If delivery is imminent some analgesia (such as pethidine) would be inappropriate as the newborn may experience respiratory distress. There will also be cases where drugs administered in labour can impact the newborn and so it is vital to handover this information to the paediatricians.

- Most analgesic options are suitable to be used in pregnancy with the exception of NSAIDs, which can cause premature closure of the ductus arteriosus.
- Analgesia can and should be given to pregnant women whether or not their pain is pregnancy related.

FURTHER READING

- Briggs G, Freeman R, Yaffe S (2005). *Drugs in Pregnancy and Lactation*, 7th edn. Lippincott Williams and Wilkins.
- GP Notebook. *Prescribing in Pregnancy*. Available at: www.gpnotebook.co.uk/simplepage.cfm?ID=1758462007 (accessed May 2015).
- Mattison D (2013). Clinical Pharmacology During Pregnancy. Elsevier.

Nausea and vomiting in pregnancy

Mrs Fatima Hassan

Age: 22

Hospital number: 123456

🔍 Case study

Presenting complaint: A 22-year-old woman presents to the emergency department with severe vomiting. She is 9 weeks pregnant.

Background: She is normally fit and well and lives with her husband. This is her first pregnancy and she has suffered with morning sickness from 4 weeks gestation. Over the last 2 days this has worsened and she is now unable to tolerate any oral fluids. No abdominal pain or PV bleeding.

PMH: Nil

DH: No known allergies, as per FP10

On examination:
Tired and pale with dry mucous membranes.
RR 14, Sats 99% (room air), BP 117/76, HR 105, Temp 37
Chest: expansion equal and adequate, vesicular breath sounds throughout, no added sounds
CVS: heart sounds normal, CRT <2 seconds, pulse regular and strong
Abdo: soft and non-tender

Urine dip: +++ *ketones, + leucocytes*

Bloods: *Hb 121, WCC 10.9, Plts 145, LFTs normal, Na 134, K 3.3, Ur 4.3, Cr 98*

Diagnosis
Hyperemesis gravidarum. This patient has severe vomiting in pregnancy that has led to derangement of her electrolytes (hypokalaemia) and ketosis. She needs admission for rehydration. Other medical and surgical diagnoses must

Case study (Continued)

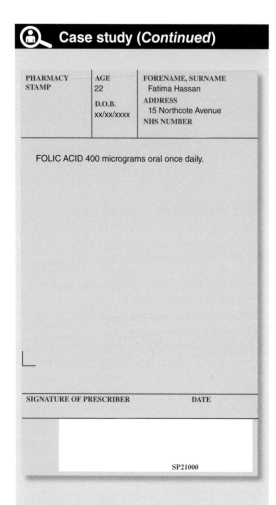

PHARMACY STAMP	AGE 22	FORENAME, SURNAME Fatima Hassan
	D.O.B. xx/xx/xxxx	ADDRESS 15 Northcote Avenue
		NHS NUMBER

FOLIC ACID 400 micrograms oral once daily.

SIGNATURE OF PRESCRIBER   DATE

SP21000

be considered (urinary tract infection [UTI], gastroenteritis, appendicitis).

Nausea and vomiting are common symptoms in pregnancy (affecting 70–80% of all pregnant women) but this severe form, which requires hospitalisation, occurs in only 1% of all pregnancies.

Initial measures

Management should follow the ABCDE approach; some women may be so dehydrated that they have become drowsy or unstable. Seek senior and obstetrics and gynaecology report early for the severely unwell woman. Site wide-bore IV access, send bloods for FBC, U&E, LFT and thyroid studies. Commence rapid IV rehydration.

Prescribing for nausea and vomiting in pregnancy

AS REQUIRED MEDICATION

DRUG CYCLIZINE				Date	
				Time	
Dose 50 mg	Route PO/IV/IM	Frequency PRN TDS	Start date xx/xx/xx	Dose	
Signature/Bleep A. Doctor		Max dose in 24 hrs 150 mg/24 hr	Review	Route	
				Given	
Additional instructions				Check	

DRUG METOCLOPRAMIDE				Date	
				Time	
Dose 10 mg	Route PO/IV/IM	Frequency PRN TDS	Start date xx/xx/xx	Dose	
Signature/Bleep A. Doctor		Max dose in 24 hrs 30 mg/24 hr	Review	Route	
				Given	
Additional instructions				Check	

DRUG ONDANSETRON				Date	
				Time	
Dose 4-8 mg	Route PO/IV/IM	Frequency PRN TDS	Start date xx/xx/xx	Dose	
Signature/Bleep A. Doctor		Max dose in 24 hrs 32 mg/24 hr	Review	Route	
				Given	
Additional instructions				Check	

Cyclizine: rationale and evidence

Cyclizine has been widely used in pregnancy and no conclusive evidence to suggest any risk of congenital abnormality. It is the first-line antiemetic at all stages of pregnancy.

✓ DRUGS checklist for CYCLIZINE

Dose	50 mg
Route	PO/IM/IV
Units	mg
Given	8 hourly (max 150 mg/24 hours)
Special situations	May cause drowsiness and should be avoided in severe heart failure.

Cyclizine: essential pharmacology

Cyclizine is a histamine H1 receptor antagonist, it acts centrally to reduce the feelings of nausea. The dosage used is the same as in the non-pregnant state.

Metoclopramide: rationale and evidence

There is less evidence available surrounding the use of metoclopramide in pregnancy but there is no evidence that it causes any adverse fetal effects.

✓ DRUGS checklist for METOCLOPRAMIDE	
Dose	10 mg
Route	PO/IM/IV
Units	mg
Given	8 hourly (max 30 mg/24 hours)
Special situations	Can cause extrapyramidal side effects in young people. Should be avoided or used at a reduced dose in severe renal failure. Contraindicated in gastrointestinal obstruction.

Metoclopramide: essential pharmacology

Metoclopramide is a prokinetic; it works as a dopaminergic blocker. Dosage given is the same as in the non-pregnant state. Metoclopramide stimulates prolactin release from the anterior pituitary and can therefore also be used to stimulate lactation; it does not appear to affect fetal prolactin levels.

Ondansetron: rationale and evidence

Ondansetron should be used as a third-line antiemetic as there is little data available on potential fetal toxicity. It should be considered for use where initial treatments have failed and the benefits outweigh the risks.

✓ DRUGS checklist for ONDANSETRON	
Dose	4–8 mg
Route	PO/IM/IV
Units	mg
Given	Stat where necessary followed by two further doses of 8 mg at 4-hourly intervals
Special situations	Contraindicated in congenital prolonged Q-T syndrome.

Ondansetron: essential pharmacology

Ondansetron is a serotonin 5HT receptor antagonist. It is not certain if the site of action of ondansetron is peripheral, central or both.

Other medications used in the management of hyperemesis gravidarum

- **Vitamin B supplementation – pyridoxine** (vitamin B_6) and **thiamine** (vitamin B_1): Nausea and vomiting in pregnancy can be caused by pyridoxine deficiency. Thiamine should be considered for any patients with severe hyperemesis to prevent Wernicke's encephalopathy.
- **Ranitidine:** Consider if there are also reflux symptoms or prolonged vomiting.
- **Steroids:** Sometimes used under senior guidance for intractable vomiting.

Further aspects of hyperemesis management

Complications of severe hyperemesis are:
- Mallory–Weiss tears
- Electrolyte imbalances/ hyponatraemia/ hypokalaemia
- Vitamin deficiencies
- Depression
- Weight loss
- Wernicke's encephalopathy:severe thiamine (vitamin B_1) deficiency (IV dextrose should be avoided for rehydration)
- Fetal complications: intrauterine growth restriction (IUGR), prematurity.

  If the patient has not yet had an ultrasound scan, arrange for them to have one in the next few days. Hyperemesis is more common when there is more trophoblastic tissue; this would be the case in multiple pregnancy and these patients need referral to consultant antenatal care. Equally, there is also more hyperemesis in cases of trophoblastic disease (hydatiform mole). Women who are discovered to have a molar pregnancy will need counselling that the pregnancy is not viable and the management thereafter.

Case outcome and discharge

After a 24-hour admission with antiemetics and IV rehydration the patient felt much better and was able to tolerate oral fluids and antiemetics. Retesting the urine found that there were no longer any ketones – a sign of better hydration. The patient was discharged with cyclizine as a to take away (TTA) medication, and with advice to return to her GP if she is unable to tolerate fluids again.

Common pitfalls

Hyperemesis gravidarum is a diagnosis of exclusion and one cannot attribute all vomiting in pregnancy to this; consider gastroenteritis, UTI, appendicitis and other differentials.

Ensure thyroid function tests are conducted, especially in those with recurrent intractable hyperemesis as pregnancy may exacerbate previously undiagnosed hyperthyroidism.

DISCHARGE MEDICATION						
Date	Medication	Dose	Route	Frequency	Supply	GP to continue?
xx/xx/xx	FOLIC ACID	400 micrograms	PO	Once daily	28 days	Y
xx/xx/xx	CYCLIZINE	50 mg	PO	As required, maximum 3 times a day	28 days	Y

Notes to patient/GP:
Folic acid to be continued until 12 weeks. Cyclizine for nausea (diagnosis; hyperemesis gravidarum) please continue for as long as required.

SUMMARY

- Nausea and vomiting are symptoms that affect a huge number of pregnant women (up to 80%).
- One percent of women develop the more serious hyperemesis gravidarum; a severe form of morning sickness that can lead to electrolyte, acid base and vitamin disturbances. They can be severely dehydrated and lose weight. Such women need rehydration and control of their vomiting with antiemetics.

FURTHER READING

- National Institute for Health and Care Excellence (NICE) (2013). *Nausea/Vomiting in Pregnancy*, Clinical Knowledge Summary. Available at: http://cks.nice.org.uk/nauseavomitingin-pregnancy#!topicsummary (accessed May 2015).
- National Institute for Health and Care Excellence (NICE). *Antenatal Care for Uncomplicated Pregnancies*, CG62, 2008. Available at: www.nice.org.uk/guidance/cg62 (accessed May 2015).
- NHS Choices (2014). *Severe Vomiting in Pregnancy*. Available at: www.nhs.uk/conditions/pregnancy-and-baby/pages/severe-vomiting-in-pregnancy-hyperemesis-gravidarum.aspx (accessed May 2015).
- Public Health England. *UK Teratology Information Service*. Available at: www.uktis.org (accessed Dec. 2015).

Hypertensive disease in pregnancy

Mrs Megan Smythe

Age: 33

Hospital number: 123456

 Case study

A 33-year-old woman in her second pregnancy attends her routine 36/40 midwife appointment. She has been experiencing frontal headaches and has had some visual floaters. The baby is moving well.

Examination: *HR 90, BP 150/97 (repeated 160/92), temp 37.1, reflexes are brisk. Fetal heart is heard 145–155 bpm with a fetal Doppler.*

Background: *This lady suffered with pre-eclampsia in her first pregnancy and was induced at 36/40.*

Investigations: *Urine dip: protein +++, U&Es, LFTs normal. Hb 110, WCC 7.2, Plts 165. CTG confirms fetal wellbeing.*

Diagnosis

This woman is displaying pre-eclampsia; gestational hypertension ≥140/90 mmHg on two occasions >4 hours apart, occurring *de novo* in a previously normotensive woman, associated with proteinuria (>300 mg in 24-hour urine collection). Symptoms include headache, visual disturbance, oedema and epigastric pain.

Initial measures

This woman is symptomatic of pre-eclampsia, she has signs consistent with the diagnosis (raised BP, proteinuria and brisk reflexes).

Her BP needs to be measured regularly. Bloods need to checked:

- FBC (Useful to know Hb if planning delivery, platelets can also drop in pre-eclampsia; this can impact regional anaesthetic options. Women can also develop HELLP (haemolysis elevated liver enzymes and low platelets).
- LFTs (can be abnormal in pre-eclampsia, especially the transaminases)

- U&Es (leakage of fluid into the extravascular space can make alter renal function)
- Clotting (can become deranged in pre-eclampsia)
- G&S if considering delivery.

Her urinalysis shows proteinuria but should also be sent for a protein creatinine ratio (PCR) or 24 hour collection to quantify the proteinuria.

Reducing her blood pressure is the initial step in treatment and this would usually be with a dose of labetalol (200 mg) and her BP checked 30 minutes later. This can be repeated once if the blood pressure does not respond. If she cannot tolerate labetalol (e.g. she is asthmatic) nifedipine MR can be used. Immediate release nifedipine is usually avoided antenatally as it can profoundly drop blood pressure, which can then lead to fetal distress.

Women who have a very high blood pressure (>160/100) and especially those that are symptomatic (headache, visual disturbances, oedema, epigastric pain) are at risk of eclampsia (seizures). Seizures carry the same risks as they do outside of pregnancy; when the blood pressure is high there is a risk of haemorrhagic stroke. The fetus will also become distressed as the mother will be hypoxic when seizing. The management of eclampsia should follow the guidance in the Box Emergency management of severe pre-eclampsia/eclampsia. In the case of severe pre-eclampsia or eclampsia seek immediate help from senior obstetricians and anaesthetists; this can be done by making an emergency call for the Obstetric Emergency Team.

Most obstetric units have a designated Eclampsia Box containing all of the drugs required for emergency management.

Emergency management of severe pre-eclampsia/eclampsia

In women with severe pre-eclampsia (BP ≥ 160/100 mmHg) who have or have had a seizure the emergency treatment is with magnesium sulphate.

- A loading dose of 4 g given intravenously over 5 minutes, followed by infusion of 1 g/h for 24 hours.
- A further dose of 2–4 g given over 5 minutes if the woman is having recurrent seizures (NICE, 2010).

Hypertensive disease in pregnancy is a spectrum, from pregnancy-induced hypertension (hypertension after 20/40 in the absence of proteinuria), to eclampsia (hypertension, proteinuria and seizures), with pre-eclampsia in the middle. Hypertensive disorders of pregnancy remain a leading cause of maternal mortality and morbidity in the UK.

There is no treatment for pre-eclampsia *per se,* except for delivery of the baby. The mechanism leading to pre-eclampsia is not fully understood but is believed to be related to insufficient invasion of the trophoblast, hence delivery of the baby and placenta reverses the hypertensive process.

Antihypertensives are used to reduce blood pressure to reduce the maternal risks of stroke and eclampsia. If blood pressure can be stabilised then the baby can be left *in utero* longer, giving time for antenatal steroids (for fetal lung maturation) to be administered if a preterm delivery is being considered due to pre-eclampsia.

Most modern antihypertensives are associated with teratogenicity – the safest ones are labetalol (beta-blocker), nifedipine (calcium channel blocker) and methyldopa (alpha adrenergic agonist).

Prescribing for hypertension in pregnancy

REGULAR PRESCRIPTIONS

DRUG LABETALOL				Circle/enter times below ↓	Day 1	Day 2	Day 3	Day 4
Dose 200 mg	Route PO	Freq BD	Start date xx/xx/xx	06				
				08				
				12				
Signature A. Doctor		Bleep	Review	16				
Additional instructions				18				
				22				

DRUG NIFEDIPINE MR					06				
Dose 20 mg	Route PO	Freq BD	Start date xx/xx/xx	08				
				12				
Signature A. Doctor		Bleep	Review	16				
Additional instructions				18				
				22				

DRUG METHYLDOPA					06				
Dose 500 mg	Route PO	Freq BD	Start date xx/xx/xx	08				
				12				
Signature A. Doctor		Bleep	Review	16				
Additional instructions				18				
				22				

Labetalol: rationale and evidence

Labetalol has been widely used in pregnancy for a long time and therefore has a good safety profile. There is no evidence of teratogenicity at any stage of pregnancy.

✓ **DRUGS checklist for LABETALOL**

Dose	200 mg
Route	PO (in severe cases can be given IV – different dosing)
Units	mg
Given	200 mg a stat oral dose, can be given regularly if needed, up to 2.4 g/24 hours in divided doses
Special situations	Contraindicated in asthmatics.

 Evidence

Aspirin for pre-eclampsia

A Cochrane review concluded that antiplatelet therapy, namely low-dose aspirin, had a moderate effect on reducing the development of pre-eclampsia and its complications (Duley *et al.*, 2007).

More research is needed to determine who should receive aspirin, when they should start and at what dose.

⊙ **Guidelines**

NICE recommends that all women are antenatally assessed to ascertain their pre-eclampsia risk (NICE, 2010). Those at high risk (i.e. primigravidas, multiple pregnancies, chronic hypertension) should be offered prophylactic aspirin (75 mg OD). Their treatment plan should be individualized.

Women with chronic hypertension must be counselled of the teratogenic side effects of angiotensin-converting enzyme inhibitors (ACEis) and angiotensin receptor blockers

(ARBs) and changed to safer antihypertensives preconceptually.

Providing that there is no contraindication, NICE recommends labetalol as the first-line treatment for gestational hypertension and pre-eclampsia.

Labetalol: essential pharmacology

Labetalol is a combined alpha/beta adrenoreceptor blocker. Clearance is more rapid in pregnant women; this can lead to the need for higher and more frequent dosing.

Nifedipine: rationale and evidence

Use of nifedipine in pregnancy has not shown any evidence of teratogenicity. It is the second-line antihypertensive (it is used first-line in asthmatic patients).

✓ DRUGS checklist for NIFEDIPINE	
Dose	10–20 mg
Route	PO
Units	mg
Given	As a stat dose, can be given regularly if needed, up to 80 mg/24 hours in divided doses
Special situations	Note that nifedipine comes as a modified release (MR)/sustained release (SR) preparation and as an immediate-release preparation. MR/SR is favoured antenatally as rapid hypotension can cause fetal distress due to sudden decreases in placental perfusion. Nifedipine also has a tocolytic effect (is used to halt preterm labour) and can therefore stop contractions if given intrapartum.

Nifedipine: essential pharmacology

Nifedipine is a calcium channel blocker, it reduces contractility of smooth muscle. This leads to a reduction of blood pressure and also allows usage as a tocolytic.

Nifedipine is manufactured as an immediate release and a sustained/modified release preparation. Sustained/modified release preparations are used antenatally as they reduce blood pressure gradually; a rapid drop in blood pressure can reduce placental perfusion and lead to fetal distress.

Methyldopa: rationale and evidence

Methyldopa has been used for many years as an antihypertensive in pregnancy; it is widely accepted as being safe to use.

✓ DRUGS checklist for METHYLDOPA	
Dose	500 mg–2 g
Route	PO
Units	mg
Given	500 mg–2 g in 2–4 divided doses
Special situations	Avoid in those with liver disease. Only used antenatally

Methyldopa: essential pharmacology

Methyldopa is an antiadrenergic drug, which acts centrally. It is the first-line drug for use in pregnancy for pre-existing essential hypertension, or hypertension that develops early in pregnancy.

It crosses the placenta but with no evidence of harm to the fetus and long-term follow-up of children whose mothers received methyldopa shown no adverse effects.

In the most severe cases of pre-eclampsia the next steps would be IV labetalol or hydralazine. To reduce the risk of seizures (or to stop eclamptic seizures) magnesium sulphate is administered IV, but this is beyond the scope of this book.

Case outcome and discharge

Outcomes for women with pre-eclampsia depends on the gestation at which they are diagnosed and the progression of the disease. The decision about timing delivery depends on balancing the risks of continuing the pregnancy versus preterm delivery of the baby. Women with milder pre-eclampsia with well-controlled blood pressure can be monitored in the community until the decision for delivery is made. If there is evidence of fetal compromise (such as IUGR) they may be delivered sooner. In cases of eclampsia the first step is to stabilise the mother and then to proceed to delivery.

In this case the woman would be admitted as she has a new diagnosis of pre-eclampsia that requires treatment. If her blood pressure remains high it is likely that she will be induced in the next few days.

REGULAR PRESCRIPTIONS

DRUG LABETALOL				Circle/enter times below ↓	Day 1	Day 2	Day 3
				06			
Dose 200 mg	Route PO	Freq BD	Start date xx/xx/xx	⑧			
				12			
Signature A. Doctor		Bleep	Review	16			
Additional instructions				⑱			
				22			

Common pitfalls

Be vigilant of pregnant women that you are seeing for other medical reasons; they should have their blood pressure recorded manually and regularly and their urine tested for protein. All doctors should be aware of the signs and symptoms of pre-eclampsia.

SUMMARY

- Pregnancy-induced hypertension and pre-eclampsia are common complications of pregnancy.
- The disease process is not fully understood and the only *treatment* is delivery of the baby.
- High blood pressure can be controlled pharmacologically and the older antihypertensives have the best safety profile for antenatal use.
- Severe pre-eclampsia/eclampsia is an obstetric emergency and needs prompt management with senior obstetricians and anaesthetists.

FURTHER READING

- National Institute for Health and Care Excellence (NICE). *Hypertension in Pregnancy: the Management of Hypertensive Disorders During Pregnancy*, CG107, 2010. Available at: www.nice.org.uk/guidance/cg107 (accessed May 2015).

Diabetic disease in pregnancy

Miss Sinead Riley

Age: 29

Hospital number: 123456

Case study

A 29-year-old woman is 29/40 in her first pregnancy. She had an oral glucose tolerance test (GTT) *at 28/40 because she had a raised BMI at booking (36). The results are:*

Fasting: 7.2 mmol/L

2-hour: 8.6 mmol/L

Ultrasound scan shows that the baby is continuing to grow along the 50th growth centile.

Diagnosis
These levels reach the diagnostic values for gestational diabetes according to the WHO

definition (fasting plasma venous glucose concentration greater than or equal to 7.0 mmol/L or 2-hour plasma venous glucose concentration greater than or equal to 7.8 mmol/L).

Initial measures

Women diagnosed with gestational diabetes should be taught to monitor their own blood sugars and keep a diary of the results. Women should be cared for in a multidisciplinary, consultant-led antenatal clinic. It is reasonable to manage women with gestational diabetes with dietary modifications in the first instance but oral antiglycaemics will be necessary if 1–2 weeks of dietary changes have not brought blood sugars to the target range. If there is evidence of fetal macrosomia at diagnosis then antiglycaemics should be commenced immediately.

Tight glycaemic control preconception and antenatally reduce the risks associated with diabetes in pregnancy.

Risks of diabetes in pregnancy

- Macrosomia
- Birth trauma (e.g. shoulder dystocia)
- Increased risk of stillbirth and neonatal death
- Increased risk of fetal anomalies.

Diabetes in pregnancy is becoming more common due to increasing diagnosis of type 2 diabetes in women of child bearing age, the increasing BMI of the population and pregnancy in older mothers.

None of the more recent antiglycaemics are licensed for use in pregnancy; all women with either pre-existing type 2 diabetes or newly diagnosed gestational diabetes mellitus (GDM) are managed with dietary modifications, metformin and, if required, insulin. Women with pre-existing type 1 diabetes who are already on insulin must carry it on throughout the pregnancy and increase the dose as the pregnancy progresses. All women with diabetes should be on high-dose folic acid (5 g rather than the usual 400 microgram) due to the increased risk of fetal anomaly.

Prescribing for diabetes in pregnancy

REGULAR PRESCRIPTIONS				Circle/enter times below ↓	⬇ Enter dates below			
					Day 1	Day 2	Day 3	Day 4
DRUG METFORMIN				06				
				08				
Dose 500 mg	Route PO	Freq BD	Start date xx/xx/xx	12				
Signature A. Doctor		Bleep	Review	16				
Additional instructions				18				
				22				

Metformin: rationale and evidence

Metformin is not known to be harmful if used at any stage of pregnancy, indeed it is used by the fertility team in some women when trying to conceive.

⊘ Guidelines

NICE recommends a target preconception HbA1c of 6.1% and advises that women with an HbA1c ≥10% avoid pregnancy until it is lowered (NICE, 2008).

Metformin is safe to use in pregnancy but all other oral antiglycaemic agents should be discontinued/ substituted. There is insufficient evidence to support the use of long-acting insulin analogues.

Women at risk of developing gestational diabetes (raised BMI, history of GDM, family history of diabetes or ethnic origin of known high diabetes prevalence) should be tested at around 28/40 for diabetes.

✓ DRUGS checklist for METFORMIN

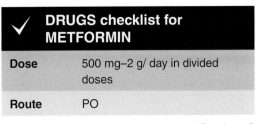

Dose	500 mg–2 g/ day in divided doses
Route	PO

(Continued)

✓ DRUGS checklist for METFORMIN (*Continued*)

Units	mg
Given	Usually BD
Special situations	Avoid in renal failure due to the risk of lactic acidosis

🔍 Evidence

Treatment for gestational diabetes
A Cochrane review concluded that treatment for gestational diabetes significantly reduced maternal and perinatal morbidity but that more research is required comparing dietary advice, oral medications and insulin (Alwan *et al.*, 2009).

Active management and surveillance of gestational diabetes does increase induction of labour rates.

Metformin: essential pharmacology

Metformin is an oral antihyperglycaemic drug, its mechanism of action is to improve insulin sensitivity. It is a biguanide, it increases peripheral uptake and utilisation of glucose while reducing intestinal absorption of glucose. It is also thought to decrease glucose production by the liver.

Case outcome and discharge

Despite dietary modification this lady's blood glucose levels remained high and therefore she was commenced on metformin. She was seen regularly in the multidisciplinary team (MDT) diabetes antenatal clinic for review of her glycaemic control and serial growth scans. Timing of delivery depends on all maternal and fetal factors, but women with diabetes are usually induced from 38/40 onwards.

As soon as a woman with diabetes in pregnancy delivers her baby she should return to her prepregnancy doses of medication (in the case of pre-existing diabetes) or have all medications stopped if she has gestational diabetes. If diabetes is thought to be gestational she should have a 6-week postnatal GTT to ensure her glycaemic control has normalised.

DISCHARGE MEDICATION						
Date	Medication	Dose	Route	Frequency	Supply	GP to continue?
xx/xx/xx	METFORMIN	500 mg	PO	Twice daily	28 days	Y

Notes to patient/GP:
Commenced on metformin for gestational diabetes.
Will be reviewed in Diabetes Antenatal Clinic.

Common pitfalls

It is important to identify women at risk of gestational diabetes and ensure that a GTT has been organised for them; women should be counselled as to why attending the test is so important. Women with persistent glycosuria should have a GTT and this should be repeated if the glycosuria continues.

SUMMARY

- Diabetes in pregnancy is associated with significant maternal and fetal morbidity and care must be taken not to miss it.
- Women with pre-existing diabetes should be counselled prepregnancy ideally.
- Pregnant women noted to have high blood sugars or persistent glycosuria should have a formal GTT and, if found to have diabetes, be referred promptly to a consultant antenatal clinic.

FURTHER READING

- National Institute for Health and Care Excellence (NICE). *Diabetes in Pregnancy*, CG63, 2008. Available at: www.nice.org.uk/guidance/cg63 (accessed May 2015).

Labour

> **Mrs Fern Miller**
>
> **Age: 25**
>
> **Hospital number: 123456**

🔍 Case study

A 25-year-old woman in her first pregnancy attends the labour ward for induction of labour (IOL). Her pregnancy has been uncomplicated but she has been counselled that IOL is recommended now that she is T+10 (term plus 10 days) due to the increased stillbirth rate with postmaturity.

Background: *Normally fit and well. No previous hospital admissions or operations.*

Allergies: *Penicillin – rash*

Examination (maternal): *HR 80, BP 120/70, RR 20, Temp 36.5. Abdomen soft, symphysis–fundal height 40 cm (= dates) Vaginal examination: cervix long, posterior and closed (unfavourable).*

Examination (fetal): *Long lie, cephalic. Head 3/5 palpable and fixed in the pelvis (engaged). CTG: baseline rate 150, accelerations present, no decelerations, variability >5 bpm. Occasional uterine activity but no palpable contractions.*

Diagnosis

This woman is not contracting regularly and her cervix is not dilating; she is not in labour.

Initial measures

After confirming maternal and fetal wellbeing the induction of labour can be started, if it is not possible to break the membranes (i.e. the cervix is not yet dilated) the cervix is ripened with prostaglandins inserted vaginally.

Analgesia in labour

Analgesia should be given in a stepwise approach – see Pain in Pregnancy Section for simple analgesics to use in early labour. Many women get relief from 'gas and air' (50% nitrous oxide, 50% oxygen). Some women also like to use non-medical and non-invasive methods such as warm water, TENS machines, hypnotherapy and aromatherapy.

If a caesarean section or instrumental birth in theatre is required, or if a woman wants further analgesia, the next step would be for an epidural or spinal anaesthetic. In emergency situations where there is not time to site regional analgesia or it is not providing adequate analgesia to perform a caesarean section, women may require a general anaesthetic.

Prescribing in labour

Induction of labour means starting the labour process artificially.

Augmenting labour means artificially increasing the frequency and/or intensity of contractions once labour has already started, but is not progressing adequately.

The lady in this case study has an 'unfavourable cervix'; the first step in induction is to 'ripen' the cervix – making it more favourable for labour to start. Cervical ripening is measured using the Bishop's Score (Table 14.2). The cervix can be ripened using vaginal prostaglandins (e.g. Propess or Prostin).

The higher the Bishop Score the 'riper' or more favourable the cervix is. The purpose of ripening the cervix is to be able to artificially rupture the amniotic

Table 14.2 Bishop's Score of cervical ripening (GP Notebook, 2015).

Score	0	1	2
Cervical dilatation (cm)	<1	<1–2	3–4
Length of cervix (cm)	>2	1–2	<1
Station of presenting part (cm)	Spines -3	Spines -2	Spines -1
Consistency	Firm	Medium	Soft
Position	Posterior	Central	Anterior

membranes (ARM); sometimes the membranes rupture spontaneously with cervical ripening.

Once the membranes have been ruptured, some women will start to have contractions spontaneously, others will require Syntocinon (synthetic oxytocin). This causes uterine contractions and can be titrated to achieve regular, strong contractions (no more that five contractions every 10 minutes).

Syntocinon: rationale and evidence

Syntocinon is a synthetic analogue of the hormone oxytocin. When Syntocinon is used it is mandatory that the fetus is continually monitored for any signs of distress. Uterine activity must be monitored to ensure that hyperstimulation does not occur.

✓	**DRUGS checklist for SYNTOCINON**
Dose	30 units diluted in 500 mL of normal saline (some units use different volumes, check your local policy)
Route	IV
Units	International units
Given	IV as a continuous infusion, titrated to the rate and strength of uterine contractions
Special situations	Syntocinon can be used to induce or augment labour; it should be used under senior guidance. Special caution must be exercised in multiparous women, women who have had a previous caesarean section, where there are signs of obstructed labour or fetal distress.

Syntocinon: essential pharmacology

Syntocinon stimulates oxytocin receptors in the uterine myometrium and causes muscular contraction by increasing intracellular calcium concentrations. The dose is titrated to how many contractions are initiating, thus allowing the normal process of labour to be recreated.

Oxytocin is released in a pulsatile manner from the posterior pituitary. Maximal release coincides with delivery. As above, oxytocin is known to stimulate myometrial contraction. Its exact role in the labour process remains uncertain. Historically, it was believed that oxytocin was the initiating factor for parturition but further studies, including animal studies where oxytocin levels are reduced, show that the labour process is more complicated than that, with a complex signalling process between the mother and fetus, and is still not fully understood (Blanks and Thornton, 2003).

FLUID CHART								
	Infusion fluid				Drug to be added		Signature	Print name
Date	Name and strength	Volume	Rate	Route	Approved name	Dose		
xx/xx/xx	NORMAL SALINE	500 ml	As per protocol	IV	SYNTOCINON	30 units	A. Doctor	A. Doctor

Managing the third stage of labour

The third stage of labour is the delivery of the placenta – this can be managed 'passively' (awaiting natural separation and delivery) or 'actively' (using medications to cause placental separation and delivery). Active management of the third stage has been shown to reduce the incidence of postpartum haemorrhage (PPH).

Syntometrine must be avoided in women with high blood pressure (either **pre-existing, pregnancy induced hypertension** or **pre-eclamptic toxaemia**) as the ergot component can cause a rapid and dangerous increase in maternal blood pressure.

Evidence

Management of the third stage
The third stage can be managed with a bolus dose (5 or 10 units) of syntocinon alone or with a dose of syntocinon combined with ergometrine (syntometrine 5 units). A Cochrane review showed that there is a small but statistically significant reduction in PPH rates when syntometrine is compared to syntocinon alone (McDonald *et al.*, 2004).

Labour is induced using a combination of prostaglandins and synthetic oxytocin. Labour is also augmented using synthetic oxytocin. Active management of the third stage of labour reduces the risk of PPH.

SUMMARY

FURTHER READING

- National Institute for Health and Care Excellence (NICE). *Intrapartum Care*, CG55, 2007. Available at: www.nice.org.uk/guidance/cg55 (accessed May 2015).
- McDonald S, Abbott JM, Higgins SP (2004). Prophylactic ergometrine-oxytocin versus oxytocin for the third stage of labour. *Cochrane Database Syst Rev* (1): CD000201.

Gynaecology – contraception

Miss Georgina Lewis

Age: 15

Hospital number: 123456

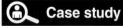 **Case study**

A 15-year-old girl attends her GP surgery enquiring about contraception. She has a 15-year-old boyfriend and she is thinking that they may soon want to start a sexual relationship.

Background: *She is normally fit and well. She has regular but heavy periods. She does not smoke. There is no family history of breast cancer or venous thromboembolic disease.*

Allergies: *Nil known*

Examination: *HR 65, BP 110/62, BMI 22.*

A note on UK law

Despite this girl being below the UK age of consent a doctor can still prescribe her contraception as long as they feel she displays "Fraser Competency." This means that you believe the girl is mature enough to make the decision that she wants to become sexually active. Other factors to consider are if the partner is a lot older than the patient you are seeing or if the partner is in a role of authority (e.g. a teacher). If you are in any way concerned you must discuss the case with a senior and/or your local safeguarding team.

- The Fraser Guidelines help doctors decide if a child has the capacity to decide about medical treatments:
- That the girl (although under the age of 16) can understand your advice
- That you cannot persuade her to tell her parents, or allow you to tell her parents
- That she is very likely to have sexual intercourse with or without your contraceptive advice
- That without contraceptive advice or treatment her physical or mental health or both are likely to suffer
- That it is in her best interests to receive contraceptive advice or treatment.

Prescribing for contraceptive purposes

Choice of contraception is a very individual decision. The failure rate and contraindications for the most common contraceptives are shown in Table 14.3. Points to consider are:

- How long is contraception desired for and how good is your patient at remembering a daily pill – would a long-acting reversible contraceptive (LARC) be appropriate?
- Does the patient want additional benefits from their contraception such as reducing menstrual flow or improving acne?
- It is always worth reiterating that **only** barrier methods protect against sexually transmitted

infections (STIs) and therefore should always be used in addition to other methods unless both partners have had sexual health screening.

- Most contraception will be prescribed in General Practice or by the Family Planning Service. The hospital practitioner must remember that women may miss their contraceptives if admitted to hospital – leaving them unprotected on discharge, or that new medications (such as antibiotics or liver enzyme inducers) may reduce the effect of their contraception.

A note on emergency contraception

There are three options for emergency contraception in the UK.

The Copper Coil (intrauterine contraceptive device) can be inserted 5 days from unprotected sexual intercourse (UPSI) or 5 days from the expected date of ovulation. There are two hormonal contraception options:

1. Levonorgestrel is licensed for use up to 72 hours after UPSI. Efficacy decreases the longer it is taken after UPSI.
2. Ulipristal acetate is licensed for use up to 120 hours after UPSI.

If a woman is using liver enzyme-inducing drugs the dose of levonorgestrel should be doubled and ulipristal acetate should be avoided.

The copper coil can be used after 4 weeks postpartum and is safe when breastfeeding. Levonorgestrel can be used in breastfeeding but ulipristal acetate cannot.

Assess whether the woman could already be pregnant and do not prescribe emergency contraception if they are. Explore risk of sexual transmitted disease and offer screening/treatment.

If the window for emergency contraception has passed or the woman is already pregnant and does not wish to proceed with the pregnancy, refer to the Pregnancy Advisory Service (PAS).

Table 14.3 Common contraceptives (Collins *et al.*, 2008; Guillebard, 2009).

Method	Mechanism of action	Failure rate	Benefits	Disadvantages/ contraindications
Natural rhythm method	Selective abstinence around the time of ovulation	2–6/100 women years dependent on use	Acceptable in many religions/ cultures that do not approve of contraception	Very dependent on the ability of partners maintain selective abstinence
Barrier methods (male/ female condoms)	Physical barrier to sperm	3.1–4.8/100 women years	Protection from STIs and no contraindications	Could interfere with intercourse and not deemed acceptable by some users, may affect sensitivity
Barrier methods + spermicide (female cap or diaphragm)	Physical barrier and antisperm	0.7–6/100 women years, improved efficacy when used for longer	Independent of intercourse and allows the woman to feel in control Neither partner feels loss of sensation	Some forward planning required to ensure it is in place before intercourse Can be perceived as messy (spermicide)
Combined oral contraceptive pill (COCP) e.g. Microgynon®, Yasmin®, Dianette®	Inhibit ovulation (negative feedback on the hypothalamus and pituitary) Thicken cervical mucous and thin the endometrium	0.2–0.3/100 woman years (with perfect use)	Regulates menstrual cycle and reduces menstrual loss Can reduce symptoms of PMS and endometriosis. Decreases risk of ovarian cancer. Improves acne.	Increases VTE, stroke and cardiovascular risk. Increases risk of cervical and breast cancer. Contraindicated if history of VTE, hypertension or diabetes. In those >35 who smoke or who have BMI >35; those who have migraine with aura, cardiovascular or hepatobiliary disorders or oestrogen-dependent tumours.
Progesterone only pill (POP, Mini Pill) e.g. Cerezette®	Alteration of cervical mucous and in some women it inhibits ovulation.	0.3–4.0/100 woman years	Can usually be used when the COCP is contraindicated.	Requires excellent compliance to ensure efficacy.
Depot injection	Prevents ovulation	0.3–1.0/100 women years	LARC – does not require daily pills. May reduce menstrual flow or cause amenorrhoea	May cause irregular bleeding/ patient may not want amenorrhoea. Patient must arrange to have injection every 12 weeks or risks pregnancy. Long-term use can reduce bone density.

(*Continued*)

Table 14.3 Common contraceptives (Collins *et al.*, 2008; Guillebard, 2009). (*Continued*)

Method	Mechanism of action	Failure rate	Benefits	Disadvantages/ contraindications
Implant (Nexplanon, Implanon)	Prevents ovulation and thickens cervical mucous	<0.1% failures at 1 year	LARC – does not require daily pills. May reduce menstrual flow or cause amenorrhoea. Can last 3 years.	May cause irregular bleeding/ patient may not want amenorrhoea.
Copper IUCD	Blocks fertilisation, copper is toxic to sperm and ova	0.2–2.0/100 women years	LARC – does not require daily pills. Can last 10 years	Increase risk of PID. Relative increase in risk of ectopic pregnancy. Can make periods heavier.
Mirena IUS	Local progesterone effects – endometrial suppression and alteration of cervical mucous	0.2/100 women years	LARC – does not require daily pills. Can last 5 years. May reduce menstrual flow or cause amenorrhoea.	Can perforate at the time of insertion (as can the copper coil) and can be expulsed.Most women have a changed bleeding pattern in the first 6 months, but for some women this does not settle to an acceptable pattern.
Sterilisation	Physical occlusion of fallopian tubes or vas deferens	1/200 years (female) 1/5000 years (male)	Permanent	Irreversible and may be regretted, especially if patients are young or if begin new relationships. Increased risk of ectopic pregnancy if a woman does become pregnant.

LARC, long-acting reversible contraceptive.

SUMMARY

- There are a huge variety of contraceptive methods available and each has their own pros and cons; the choice is based on what is right for that individual, combined with the consideration of any medical contraindications.
- Whilst the majority of contraception is prescribed in primary care it is the responsibility of all doctors to consider;
  - Any safeguarding issues with regards to children seeking contraception
  - The fact that only barrier contraceptives protect against STIs
  - That admission to hospital or new drug interactions may affect hormonal contraceptives.

FURTHER READING

- WHO (2015). *Medical Eligibility Criteria for Contraceptive Use*. Available at: www.who.int/reproductivehealth/publications/family_planning/MEC-5/en/ (accessed May 2015).
- Faculty of Sexual and Reproductive Healthcare of the Royal College of Obstetricians and Gynaecologists (2009). *UK Medical Eligibility Criteria for Contraceptive Use*. Available at: www.fsrh.org/pdfs/UKMEC2009.pdf (accessed May 2015).
- Faculty of Sexual and Reproductive Health of the Royal College of Obstetricians and Gynaecologists. *Clinical Guidelines*. Available at: www.fsrh.org/pages/clinical_guidance.asp (accessed May 2015).
- Sarris I, Bewley S, Agnihotri S (2009). *Training in Obstetrics and Gynaecology, the Essential Curriculum*. Oxford Specialty Training, Oxford.

Gynaecology – pain and bleeding in early pregnancy

Mrs Anna Mantle
Age: 40
Hospital number: 123456

🔍 Case study

A 40-year-old woman in her third pregnancy attends the Early Pregnancy Unit (EPU) with a 3-day history of central, period-like cramps and a small amount of fresh red bleeding.

Ultrasound scanning shows an intrauterine pregnancy equivalent to 9+3/40 but sadly no fetal heart pulsations are seen. This is consistent with a miscarriage. You offer your condolences.

Examination: *(not always necessary, unless appear unstable or are bleeding very heavily). Abdomen is soft and non-tender. HR 80, BP 120/70, Temp 37.1.*

Management

Each EPU will have their own protocols for the management of miscarriage. Unless you are working with the EPU/Gynaecology then your role as a doctor is to ensure the woman is safe (haemodynamically stable) and that symptoms such as pain are well controlled. Be aware that when women are miscarrying they can go into cervical shock – this is a vagal response caused by products of conception lodging within the open cervix. Women will become bradycardic and hypotensive – these women need to have a speculum examination so that products of conception can be removed.

Miscarriage is a very common occurrence (10–20% of all clinical pregnancies) but this does not belittle the emotional and physical trauma experienced by women, their partners and families. Management of miscarriage can be conservative, surgical or medical. The latest NICE guidance (NICE, 2012) recommends that where it is not contraindicated (signs of infection, heavy bleeding, suspicion of trophoblastic disease, vulnerable adults) all women should be recommended conservative management for at least 2 weeks. These women should be warned that they will experience pain and heavy bleeding. They should have a 24/7 helpline/ contact number or know that they can attend the Emergency Department if they cannot cope at home or are very unwell. Surgical management of miscarriage (also known as ERPC – evacuation of retained products of conception) involves suction curettage of the uterine cavity to remove the pregnancy tissue. Traditionally this is done under general anaesthetic but some units are now doing a similar procedure (MVA – manual vacuum aspiration) with local analgesia.

Medical management of miscarriage

For women who are <12/40 and well supported, some units now offer medical management of miscarriage on an outpatient basis.

An example regime (NICE, 2012) would be a single dose of misoprostol (e.g. 800 microgram) per vagina; this can be inserted by a health professional or put on top of a tampon and inserted by the patient herself. Some units use smaller doses but given repeatedly. Women need to be fully counselled that they will experience pain and bleeding and be told who and where they can go for help and advice. Women should also be provided with sufficient analgesia such as co-codamol and ibuprofen.

Misoprostol: rationale and evidence

Synthetic prostaglandin E1 causes uterine contraction and is therefore used in the medical management of miscarriage and also in termination of pregnancy. A reduced dose, under senior advice, is used in women who have had a previous caesarean section or uterine surgery due to the increased risk of uterine rupture.

✓	DRUGS checklist for MISOPROSTOL	
Dose	800 microgram (if one off dose)	
Route	PV/PR or SL	
Units	microgram	
Given	See your local units protocol	
Special situations	Avoid if any possibility of viable pregnancy (unless decision made and appropriate legal paperwork completed for a termination). Lower doses should be used in women who have had a previous caesarean section.	

Misoprostol: essential pharmacology

Prostaglandins cause contraction of myometrial cells.

Medical management of ectopic pregnancy

Ectopic pregnancy (pregnancy outside of the uterus) occurs in about 1/100 pregnancies. They remain notoriously difficult to diagnose due to their often atypical presentations. The findings of the Centre for Maternal and Child Enquiries (CEMACE) Saving Mothers' Lives remind us to consider ectopic pregnancies in all women of childbearing age with abdominal pain, unusual bleeding, collapse and diarrhoea and vomiting.

The safest management is surgery (salpingectomy or salpingotomy) but this is not the only management option.

In asymptomatic women, with a small ectopic and no evidence of rupture, a senior gynaecologist after they have reviewed the patient may consider expectant or conservative management. These women need to be monitored to ensure that their beta human chorionic gonadotropin (bHCG) levels return back to non-pregnant levels and be made aware that if they experience pain or bleeding they must seek help promptly. Conservative management can be successful if the pregnancy tissue has ceased growing; it will then be resorbed.

In correctly selected women it is possible to manage ectopic pregnancies medically with methotrexate.

Contraindications to methotrexate are:
- Haemodynamic instability (tachycardia, hypotension, faint or collapse)
- 'Free fluid' or haematoperitoneum on ultrasound scan
- Pain that requires more than paracetamol
- bHCG >3000 international units/L (unit protocols may vary)
- Live ectopic (fetal heartbeat) seen on ultrasound scan
- Liver dysfunction or blood dyscrasia.

Methotrexate essential pharmacology

Methotrexate is a cytotoxic drug which works by inhibiting folate metabolism. The decision to give it should only be made by a senior doctor.

✓	DRUGS checklist for METHOTREXATE
Dose	50 mg/m2
Route	IM
Units	mg
Given	One-off dose – may need repeating if there is not a sufficient fall in bHCG

Special situations	See safety contraindications above. FBC and LFTs need monitoring as methotrexate can affect these. Women need to be aware that the severe teratogenic effects mean that they must avoid another pregnancy for the next 3 months at least. Must be avoided if there is any doubt that the pregnancy is viable and intrauterine. Very rarely heterotopics (simultaneous ectopic and intrauterine pregnancies) can occur; methotrexate would not be suitable for these.

SUMMARY

- Pain and bleeding are common in early pregnancy. These symptoms can herald an ectopic pregnancy or a miscarriage (although often the pregnancy is fine and no cause for pain or bleeding is found).
- All women should have access to a specialist early pregnancy service, which can provide ultrasound scans and appropriate advice.
- Miscarriage and ectopic pregnancies can both be managed conservatively, medically or surgically. The correct choice of management is based up each woman's personal choice, her circumstances and any medical contraindications.
- For women being managed at home they must have access to a 24/7 helpline or know where they can access help.
- Most medications required are specialist obstetrics and gynaecology medications, but any doctor should remember that women miscarrying or with an ectopic pregnancy can become very unwell very quickly; management should follow ABCDE principles and have early senior and obstetrics and gynaecology input.

FURTHER READING

- National Institute for Health and Care Excellence (NICE). *Ectopic Pregnancy and Miscarriage*, CG154, 2012. Available at: www.nice.org.uk/guidance/cg154 (accessed May 2015).
- Royal College of Obstetricians and Gynaecologists (2004). Tubal Pregnancy,Management (Green-top Guideline No. 21). Available at: www.rcog.org.uk/en/guidelines-research-services/guidelines/gtg21/ (accessed May 2015).

Now visit **www.wileyessential.com/pharmacology**
to test yourself on this chapter.

References

Alwan N, Tuffnell DJ, West J (2009). Treatments for gestational diabetes. *Cochrane Database Syst Rev* (3): CD003395.

Blanks A, Thornton S (2003). The role of oxytocin in parturition. *BJOG* 110 (Suppl. 20): 46–51.

British Medical Association and Royal Pharmaceutical Society of Great Britain (2015). *British National Formulary 69*. 69th edn. BMJ group and Pharmaceutical Press, London.

Collins S, Arulkumaran S, Hayes K *et al.* (2008). *Oxford Handbook of Obstetrics and Gynaecology*, 2nd edn. Oxford University Press: Oxford.

Dawes M and Chowienczyk PJ (2001). Drugs in pregnancy. Pharmacokinetics in pregnancy. *Best Pract Res Clin Obstet Gynaecol* 15: 819–26.

Duley L, Henderson-Smart DJ, Meher S *et al.* (2007). Antiplatelet agents for preventing pre-eclampsia and its complications. *Cochrane Database Syst Rev* (2): CD004659.

Giacoia G, Mattison D (2009). *Obstetrics and Fetal Pharmacology*.Global Library of Women's Medicine. Available at: www.glowm.com/section_view/heading/Obstetric%20and%20Fetal%20Pharmacology/item/196 (accessed Dec. 2015).

GP Notebook (2015). *Bishop's Score*. Available at: www.gpnotebook.co.uk/simplepage.cfm?ID=899284994 (accessed Dec. 2015).

Guillebard J (2009). *Contraception: Your Questions Answered*, 5th edn. Churchill Livingston, Elsevier.

Headley JE, Northstone K, Simmons HM *et al.* (2004). Medication use during pregnancy: data from the Avon Longitudinal Study of Parents and Children. *Eur J Clin Pharmacol* 60: 355–61.

Koren G (2011). Pharmacokinetics in pregnancy; clinical significance. *J Popul Ther Clin Pharmacol* 18: e523–7.

McDonald S, Abbott JM, Higgins SP (2004). Prophylactic ergometrine-oxytocin versus oxytocin for the third stage of labour. *Cochrane Database Syst Rev* (1): CD000201.

National Institute for Health and Care Excellence (NICE) (2008). *Diabetes in Pregnancy: Management of Diabetes and its Complications from Pre-conception to the Postnatal Period*, CG63. Available at: www.nice.org.uk/guidance/cg63 (accessed May 2015).

National Institute for Health and Care Excellence (NICE) (2010). *Hypertension in Pregnancy*, CG107. Available at: www.nice.org.uk/guidance/cg107 (accessed May 2015).

National Institute for Health and Care Excellence (NICE) (2012). *Ectopic Pregnancy and Miscarriage*, CG154. Available at: www.nice.org.uk/guidance/cg154 (accessed May 2015).

Rubin P, Ramsay M (2008). *Prescribing in Pregnancy*, 4th edn. Blackwell.

Stephens S, Wilson G (2009). Prescribing in pregnant women: guide to general principles. *Prescriber* 20: 43–46. Available at:http://onlinelibrary.wiley.com/doi/10.1002/psb.578/pdf (accessed May 2015).

CHAPTER 15
Diabetes
Amy Hawkins

Key topics:

Learning objectives

By the end of this chapter, you should be able to…

- …write prescriptions for patients with diabetic ketoacidosis, hyperosmolar hyperglycaemic syndrome and hypoglycaemia, taking into account relevant cautions, contraindications and side effects.

- …evaluate the key drugs used in the management of the above conditions.

- …discuss the mechanisms of action of the drugs used to treat these conditions.

Essential Practical Prescribing, First Edition. Georgia Woodfield, Benedict Lyle Phillips, Victoria Taylor, Amy Hawkins and Andrew Stanton. © 2016 by John Wiley & Sons, Ltd. Published 2016 by John Wiley & Sons, Ltd.

Diabetic ketoacidosis

Billy Ullman
Age: 28
Hospital number: 123456

🔍 Case study

Presenting complaint: A 28-year-old man is brought to the emergency department by his friend with vomiting and drowsiness. He is known to have diabetes and his blood glucose in the ambulance is 27 mmol/L.

Background: He lives in a flat-share and works part time in a bar. He smokes 20 cigarettes per day and drinks 15–20 units of alcohol per week. He often works long hours and eats erratically.

PMH: Diabetes (diagnosed aged 7)

Allergies: none known

Examination:
Pulse 98, Sats 99% on air, RR 30

CVS: capillary refill time <2 seconds, pulse regular, no pitting oedema, HS I + II + 0

RS: equal expansion with air entry to both bases and no added sounds

Abdo: soft, mild generalised tenderness. No masses, bowel sounds present

Neuro: responding to voice, pupils equal and reactive

Urine ketones: 3+

VBG:
pH 7.15
Pco_2 4.7 kPa
Po_2 20.0 kPa
HCO_3 12.3 mmol/L
Na^+ 132 mmol/L
Cl^- 101 mmol/L
K^+ 5.3 mmol/L
Glucose 25 mmol/L

PHARMACY STAMP	AGE 28 D.O.B. xx/xx/xxxx	FORENAME, SURNAME Billy Ullman ADDRESS 57D Mayfield Road NHS NUMBER

NOVOMIX 30 INSULIN® 16 units twice daily.

SIGNATURE OF PRESCRIBER   DATE

SP21000

Diagnosis
Diabetic ketoacidosis.

Initial measures
Diabetic ketoacidosis (DKA) consists of the triad of hyperglycaemia (>13.9 mmol/L), ketonaemia and acidaemia (pH <7.30) (Kitabchi *et al.*, 2006, 2009). An initial 'ABCDE' approach will be required to resuscitate the patient. Seek senior support and advice from HDU/ITU early.

Prescribing for diabetic ketoacidosis

FLUID CHART						
Date	Fluid	Dose	Route	Rate	Signature	Print name
xx/xx/xx	0.9% SALINE	1 litre	IV	1 hour	A. Doctor	A. Doctor

The patient's weight is 70 kg and this was used to calculate the dose of Actrapid insulin.

FLUID CHART

Date	Infusion fluid			Drug to be added		Signature	Print name
	Name and strength	Volume	Rate	Approved name	Dose		
xx/xx/xx	NORMAL SALINE 0.9%	50 ml	7 units (7 ml) per hour (0.1 units/ kg/hour)	ACTRAPID INSULIN	50 units	A. Doctor	A. Doctor

Repeat VBG 1 hour later:

pH 7.22

P_{CO_2} 4.9 kPa

P_{O_2} 19.0 kPa

HCO_3 15 mmol/L

Na^+ 131 mmol/L

Cl^- 100 mmol/L

K^+ 5.2 mmol/L

Glucose 20 mmol/L

FLUID CHART

Date	Fluid	Dose	Route	Rate	Signature	Print name
xx/xx/xx	0.9% SALINE	1 litre	IV	2 hours	A. Doctor	A. Doctor
xx/xx/xx	0.9% SALINE with 40 mmol KCL	1 litre	IV	4 hours	A. Doctor	A. Doctor

Fluids: rationale and evidence

The most important initial step in the management of DKA is appropriate fluid replacement. This is then followed by insulin administration.

Evidence

Colloids versus crystalloids

There has been controversy regarding whether crystalloids or colloids are the most appropriate fluid for resuscitation purposes. A Cochrane review found no evidence to support the use of colloids in preference to crystalloids for fluid resuscitation (Perel et al., 2013). Moreover, a consensus statement suggests that colloids (such as Gelofusin) should be avoided in the resuscitation setting as their use leads to increased morbidity and mortality (Reinhart et al., 2013). Therefore, current guidelines for the management of DKA suggest that crystalloid fluids (such as 0.9% saline or Hartmann's) should be the initial fluid of choice (JBDS, 2013a).

Evidence

Which crystalloid?

Alongside the 'crystalloid versus colloid' debate, there has also been a lack of consensus as to which crystalloid fluid should be used (Dhatariya, 2007). The two most widely studied options are 0.9% saline and Hartmann's. Two randomized controlled trials have compared the use of these two fluids, and have found no evidence to suggest that one is superior to the other for use in DKA (Mahler et al., 2011; Van Zyl et al., 2012).

The key disadvantage of 0.9% saline is that it may cause hyperchloraemic metabolic acidosis. However, Hartmann's has insufficient potassium content for use in DKA and is not available with premixed potassium. Therefore, there are safety concerns regarding addition of potassium in ward environments. In light of this, current national guidelines suggest that 0.9% saline with premixed potassium chloride should be used as first choice due to its safety profile and widespread use.

In children and young adults, there have been concerns that rapid fluid replacement may lead to cerebral oedema. Therefore, fluid resuscitation should be undertaken cautiously in this group.

Patients with DKA commonly have prerenal acute kidney injury associated with dehydration; in these patients potassium should not be prescribed in the initial fluid resuscitation or whilst the serum potassium is >5.5 mmol/L.

✓ DRUGS checklist for 0.9% SALINE

Dose	1000 mL
Route	Intravenous
Units	mL
Given	According to individual patient assessment
Special situations	In patients with hyponatraemia requiring IV fluids (i.e. those who are clinically fluid depleted, replacement should be cautious (maximum 10 mmol/L rise in Na^+ over 24 hours) to prevent osmotic demyelination syndrome.

Fluids: essential pharmacology

Fluid depletion in DKA occurs predominantly through osmotic diuresis due to hyperglycaemia. In addition to this, patients often experience vomiting, which exacerbates fluid loss. Fluid resuscitation is required to restore the circulating volume, to correct electrolyte imbalances and aid clearance of ketones.

Typical fluid and electrolyte deficits in DKA are:

Water 100 mL/kg

Sodium 7–10 mmol/kg

Chloride 3–5 mmol/kg

Potassium 3–5 mmol/kg

Whilst the majority of patients will be potassium deplete, it is important to note that a normal or elevated serum potassium concentration may be seen due to the extracellular shift of potassium secondary to acidosis. Once insulin is given, the serum potassium will start to fall. Therefore, guidelines suggest that 0.9% sodium chloride solution with potassium 40 mmol/L is given if the serum potassium level is below 5.5 mmol/L and the patient is passing urine.

Fixed rate intravenous insulin infusion: rationale and evidence

Historically, patients with DKA were started on a 'sliding scale' for insulin replacement (JBDS-IP, 2014). However, evidence now favours the use of a fixed-rate intravenous insulin infusion rather than a variable rate insulin infusion ('sliding scale'). With a fixed-rate infusion, the insulin dose is calculated according to body weight. This increases the rate of ketone clearance and resolution of DKA (Savage *et al.*, 2011).

Evidence

How rapidly should plasma glucose be lowered?

There is a lack of recent evidence regarding the rate at which plasma glucose should be lowered in patients with DKA. The main theoretical risk of rapid glucose reduction is

that large osmotic shifts may cause cerebral oedema. Data from the 1970s suggested that low-dose insulin infusions (at a rate of 0.1 units/kg/h) reduced plasma glucose levels at approximately the same rate as high-dose insulin levels (JBDS, 2013a). This is the standard rate recommended by national guidelines.

✓ DRUGS checklist for fixed-rate INSULIN infusion

Dose	0.1 units/kg/h
Route	Intravenous
Units	Units
Given	As a continuous infusion
Special situations	If the ketones and glucose are not falling as expected, check that the pump is functioning correctly.

Fixed rate intravenous insulin infusion: essential pharmacology

Insulin is a peptide hormone that acts through a number of intracellular signalling pathways to promote glycogen production and inhibit gluconeogenesis in the liver. Insulin acts to promote uptake of glucose in fat and muscle and it inhibits lipogenesis and lipolysis in adipocytes. It is administered parenterally and is used in three main forms in clinical practice – as short-acting, long-acting (basal) or mixed insulin analogues.

A fixed-rate insulin infusion is given per kilogram of body weight and enables more rapid ketone clearance and resolution of acidosis compared with a 'sliding scale' insulin infusion.

According to guidelines, the recommended treatment targets for DKA are:

- Reduction of the blood ketone concentration by 0.5 mmol/L/h
- Increase the venous bicarbonate by 3.0 mmol/L/h
- Reduce capillary blood glucose by 3.0 mmol/L/h

- Maintain potassium between 4.0 and 5.5 mmol/L.

The insulin infusion rate will need to be altered according to these values.

Other aspects of management / treatments used in diabetic ketoacidosis

- It may be necessary to administer a **10% dextrose** infusion to avoid hypoglycaemia when the insulin infusion continues. This is recommended when the blood glucose value falls below 14.0 mmol/L and should be continued until the patient is eating and drinking normally.
- Current guidelines suggest that for patients prescribed **long-acting basal insulin** analogues (e.g. Levemir® and Lantus®), these drugs should be continued during the initial management of DKA. The aim of this is to avoid rebound hyperglycaemia when the insulin infusion is stopped, and to reduce patients' length of stay in hospital (Hsia *et al.*, 2012).
- Evidence suggests that the use of **bicarbonate** should not be required in DKA, as adequate fluid and insulin therapy will resolve the acidosis (Chua *et al.*, 2011). In fact, there is evidence to suggest that excessive bicarbonate use may delay the fall in plasma lactate compared with 0.9% saline infusion, and may also be implicated in causing cerebral oedema in children and young adults.
- Although DKA causes **phosphate** depletion, there is no evidence for the benefit of phosphate replacement in DKA.
- Ensure that you look for a precipitant for DKA, which may include poor compliance with insulin regimes, infection or intercurrent illness, and myocardial infarction (particularly in the elderly).
- DKA is a hypercoagulable state so venous thromboembolism (VTE) prophylaxis is mandatory unless there is a specific contraindication.

Case outcome and discharge

Mr Ullman was transferred to HDU from the Emergency Department. He received IV fluids with potassium replacement and a fixed-rate insulin infusion. Once he had stabilised he was reviewed by the inpatient diabetes team and the decision was made to switch to a 'basal bolus' regimen. This involves a long-acting insulin given at night, with a short-acting insulin given with each meal, depending on dietary intake. This will help him to achieve better glycaemic control whilst maintaining a flexible lifestyle. A follow-up appointment was booked with the diabetes specialist nurse.

DISCHARGE MEDICATION						
Date	Medication	Dose	Route	Frequency	Supply	GP to continue?
xx/xx/xx	HUMULIN S INSULIN	6–10 units	SC	With each meal, dose to vary according to dietary intake	14 days	Y
xx/xx/xx	LANTUS INSULIN	24 units	SC	At night	14 days	Y
Notes to patient/GP:						

Common pitfalls

- Remember to consider the underlying precipitant of DKA including intercurrent infection and non-compliance with insulin therapy.
- Diagnosis of DKA requires the following:
  - Ketonaemia > 3.0 mmol/L or significant ketonuria (more than 2+ on standard urine sticks)
  - Blood glucose > 11.0 mmol/L or known diabetes mellitus
  - Bicarbonate < 15.0 mmol/L and/or venous pH < 7.3.
- Occasionally, patients may have a relatively modest increase in blood glucose.
- Remember that long-acting insulin must be continued during the acute phase of treatment alongside IV insulin – failure to do this will make re-establishing good glycaemic control difficult.
- Patients should be reviewed by the inpatient diabetes team prior to discharge from hospital. This is an important opportunity to provide patient education regarding glycaemic control and insulin administration.

SUMMARY

Diabetic ketoacidosis is a potentially life-threatening emergency, which must be managed with early senior intervention and HDU support. Management includes fluid resuscitation, correction of electrolyte disturbances and insulin administration. Guidelines now suggest the use of a fixed-rate intravenous insulin infusion rather than the traditional 'sliding scale' method. Remember that DKA may be the first presentation of diabetes, so it is always important to consider the diagnosis in an acutely unwell patient presenting with the relevant features.

🔑 Key learning points

- DKA is a life-threatening emergency, which may be precipitated by intercurrent illness, infection or poor compliance with insulin therapy.
- Fluid resuscitation with an appropriate crystalloid fluid should commence as soon as possible.
- A fixed-rate insulin infusion should be administered and electrolyte disturbances corrected.
- Patients with DKA must receive follow-up from the diabetes team and a management plan must be devised to prevent further episodes.

FURTHER READING

- The Joint British Diabetes Societies Inpatient Care Group provides clear, comprehensive guidelines on the management of DKA.
- A useful review of evidence for the management of DKA is: Dhatariya KK (2007). Diabetic ketoacidosis. *BMJ* 334: 1284–5.

Hyperosmolar hyperglycaemic state

Judy Jones

Age: 75

Hospital number: 123456

👤 Case study

Presenting complaint: *A 75-year-old woman is brought to the emergency department by her* husband. *He reports that over the last week she has been weak and lethargic. He is particularly concerned as over the last 48 hours she has become drowsy and confused, which is not normal for her.*

Background: *She lives with her husband and is normally independent.*

PMH: *Hypertension, hypercholesterolaemia, obesity (BMI 30), left knee replacement 2 years ago. There is no history of ischaemic heart disease or cardiac failure.*

Allergies: *none known*

Examination:
Pulse 90, BP 148/88, Sats 97% on air, RR 18, temp 37.3

CVS: *capillary refill time 2 seconds, pulse regular, no pitting oedema, HS I + II + 0, clinically dry*

RS: *equal expansion with air entry to both bases and no added sounds*

Abdo: *soft and non-tender, no masses, bowel sounds present; no palpable bladder*

AMTS: *9/10*

Neurology: *no focal neurological deficit*

Blood glucose on BM stick testing: *34*

VBG:
pH 7.38
$P\text{CO}_2$ 5.0 kPa
$P\text{O}_2$ 8.0 kPa
HCO_3 22.2 mmol/L
Glucose 38 mmol/L

Blood results:
Na^+ 144 mmol/L
Cl^- 110 mmol/L
K^+ 4.9 mmol/L
Urea 14.2
Creatinine 142

Initial measures
In this case, there is no previous history of diabetes although there are risk factors in the history.

PHARMACY STAMP	AGE 75	FORENAME, SURNAME
		Judy Jones
	D.O.B. xx/xx/xxxx	ADDRESS Rose Cottage, Under Lane
		NHS NUMBER

RAMIPRIL 2.5 mg once daily.

SIMVASTATIN 40 mg once at night.

SIGNATURE OF PRESCRIBER　　　　DATE

SP21000

It is likely that this is a first presentation of type 2 diabetes. She also has renal impairment – without previous blood results for comparison it is difficult to say whether this is acute, chronic or acute on chronic.

Prescribing for hyperosmolar hyperglycaemic state

Hyperosmolar hyperglycaemic state (HHS) typically occurs in older patients, but it may occur in teenagers and young adults, and may be a first presentation of type 2 diabetes.

Compared with DKA, HHS often has a more subacute presentation over days rather than hours. For this reason, the extent of dehydration and metabolic disturbances seen may be more severe. Characteristically, hyperglycaemia is marked (>30 mmol/L), and significantly elevated ketones and acidosis are less prominent features. Plasma osmolality is usually >320 mosmol/kg.

Important complications of HHS may include vascular events such as myocardial infarction and stroke, venous thromboembolism and less commonly seizures and cerebral oedema. Rapid changes in plasma osmolality during treatment may precipitate central pontine myelinolysis.

Initial plasma osmolality is calculated as $2(\text{Na}^+\ \text{K}^+) + \text{glucose} + \text{urea}$:

$$2(144 + 4.9) + 38 + 14.2 = \textbf{350}\text{ mosmol/kg}$$

FLUID CHART						
Date	Fluid	Dose	Route	Rate	Signature	Print name
xx/xx/xx	0.9% SALINE	1 litre	IV	1 hour	A. Doctor	A. Doctor

Repeat bloods after 1 hour:
    Glucose 28 mmol/L
    Na^+ 147 mmol/L
    Cl^- 112 mmol/L
    K^+ 4.6 mmol/L
    Urea 12.2
    Creatinine 140
    Plasma osmolality after 1 hour:

$$2(147 + 4.6) + 28 + 12.2 = \textbf{343.4} \text{ mosmol/kg}$$

FLUID CHART						
Date	Fluid	Dose	Route	Rate	Signature	Print name
xx/xx/xx	0.9% SALINE	1 litre	IV	2 hours	A. Doctor	A. Doctor

Repeat bloods after a further 2 hours:
    Glucose 24 mmol/L
    Na^+ 143 mmol/L
    Cl^- 101 mmol/L
    K^+ 3.7 mmol/L
    Urea 11.2
    Creatinine 140
    Plasma osmolality after a further 2 hours:

$$2(143 + 3.7) + 24 + 11.2 = \textbf{328.6} \text{ mosmol/kg}$$

FLUID CHART						
Date	Fluid	Dose	Route	Rate	Signature	Print name
xx/xx/xx	0.9% SALINE	1 litre	IV	2 hours	A. Doctor	A. Doctor

Fluids: rationale and evidence

The rate of fluid resuscitation in HSS will depend upon the extent of dehydration and the comorbidities such as the presence of congestive cardiac failure. In the absence of congestive cardiac failure, current guidelines recommend relatively rapid fluid resuscitation in order to restore circulating volume and lower plasma glucose. In general, the aim of IV fluid therapy should be to obtain a positive balance of 3–6 litres by 12 hours.

Evidence

Which fluid to use?
As with DKA, there has been controversy over the years regarding which is the most appropriate fluid to use in patients with HHS. As mentioned with regards to DKA, a Cochrane review recommended the use of crystalloids rather than colloids in acutely unwell patients (Perel *et al.*, 2013). There is a lack of evidence regarding which crystalloid to use in patients with HHS (Milionis *et al.*, 2001, Kitabachi *et al.*, 2009). Current guidelines recommend the use of 0.9% saline with variable amounts of potassium added on the basis that the majority of losses in HHS are sodium, chloride and potassium. Hypotonic fluids such as 0.45% saline should be avoided in general terms to prevent rapid changes in plasma osmolality (see Guidelines; JBDS, 2012).

Guidelines

Joint British Diabetes Societies Inpatient Care Group. *The Management of Hyperosmolar Hyperglycaemic State in Adults* (JBDS, 2012).
- Guidelines suggest that plasma osmolality should be measured frequently to monitor the response to treatment.
- They advise that 0.9% saline should be used as the first-line fluid of choice, and it should be expected that the sodium may rise initially.
- Hypotonic fluids (such as 0.45% saline) should only be used if osmolality continues to rise despite a positive fluid balance.
- The **maximum rate of the fall in plasma sodium should be 10 mmol/24 h** to prevent central pontine myelinolysis (O'Malley *et al.*, 2008).
- Oral fluid intake should be encouraged as soon as it is safe to do so.

DRUGS checklist for 0.9% saline see checklist in Section Diabetic Ketoacidosis.

Fluids: essential pharmacology

As with DKA, in HHS fluid depletion occurs mainly due to osmotic diuresis resulting from hyperglycaemia. Compared with the deficits in DKA (Section Diabetic Ketoacidosis), water loss is often more profound, due to the marked hyperglycaemia seen in these patients.

Typical fluid and electrolyte deficits in HHS are:

Water 100–220 mL/kg

Sodium 5–13 mmol/kg

Chloride 5–15 mmol/kg

Potassium 4–6 mmol/kg

The aim of fluid therapy is to restore circulating volume and lower plasma osmolality. Compared with DKA, potassium replacement is less likely to be required. Patients with HHS are usually less acidotic than those with DKA so potassium shifts are less pronounced. In addition to this, the dose of insulin used is usually lower (see Section Fixed rate insulin infusion: rationale and evidence) and there may be coexisting renal impairment.

Fixed rate insulin infusion: rationale and evidence

Unlike in DKA, insulin should only be commenced once the blood glucose ceases to fall with IV fluids alone. The exception to this is if plasma or urinary ketones are present – in which case an insulin infusion should be started as would be the case in DKA (see Section Diabetic Ketoacidosis).

ⓘ Guidelines

Joint British Diabetes Societies Inpatient Care Group. *The Management of Hyperosmolar Hyperglycaemic State in Adults* (JBDS, 2012).

- Guidelines suggest that if there is significant ketonaemia, a fixed-rate insulin infusion should be commenced at a rate of 0.05 units/kg/h.
- If there is not significant ketonaemia, there is a risk of lowering the plasma osmolality too quickly. Unlike in DKA, fluid replacement alone is often sufficient to reduce the glucose and hence osmolality at the required rate.
- The target rate of decline of plasma glucose if an insulin infusion is required should be up to 5 mmol/L/h.

For patients commenced on a fixed-rate insulin infusion, this can be discontinued once oral intake is adequate. Patients should be reviewed by the diabetes team regarding ongoing management of their diabetes. It may be that oral hypoglycaemic agents or subcutaneous insulin are used; the choice will depend to some extent upon whether it is a first presentation of diabetes and which agents have been used previously.

DRUGS checklist for fixed-rate insulin infusion see checklist in Section Diabetic Ketoacidosis.

Fixed rate insulin infusion: essential pharmacology

See Section Diabetic Ketoacidosis.

Other treatments used in hyperosmolar hyperglycaemic state

- Although low magnesium and phosphate are common amongst patients with HHS, as in DKA there is no evidence for the use of IV phosphate replacement in acute HHS.
- Due to the increased risk of venous thromboembolism in patients with HHS, patients should receive **prophylactic low molecular weight heparin** unless contraindicated (Keenan *et al.*, 2007).
- Patients' feet should be checked regularly as they are at high risk of developing pressure ulcers (NICE, 2009).

Case outcome and discharge

Mrs Jones' HHS gradually resolved with IV fluid therapy and she did not require a fixed-rate insulin infusion. The biochemical abnormalities had largely resolved within 2–3 days. She was reviewed by the inpatient diabetes team and, in view of her obesity, was started on metformin as a first-line therapy (initially 500 mg once a day and titrated to 500 mg twice daily). She was discharged home with follow-up by the outpatient diabetes team. She was informed of the need to check her feet regularly and was enrolled in the retinal screening programme.

DISCHARGE MEDICATION						
Date	Medication	Dose	Route	Frequency	Supply	GP to continue?
xx/xx/xx	METFORMIN	500 mg	PO	Twice daily	14 days	Y
xx/xx/xx	RAMIPRIL	2.5 mg	PO	Once daily	14 days	Y
xx/xx/xx	SIMVASTATIN	40 mg	PO	Once at night	14 days	Y
Notes to patient/GP:						

Common pitfalls

- HHS has a higher mortality rate than DKA, and like DKA should be treated as a medical emergency.
- It is important to note that the patient's biochemistry may take up to 72 hours to normalise following an episode of HHS.

- Due to the increased risk of VTE in patients with HHS, a VTE risk assessment should be performed in all patients and the appropriate prophylaxis prescribed.
- Remember to consider the possible precipitants of HHS, assessing carefully for signs of sepsis.

SUMMARY

Hyperosmolar hyperglycaemic syndrome (HHS) has a high mortality and should be regarded as a medical emergency. The mainstay of therapy is IV fluid therapy, which should begin with 0.9% saline. For patients with significant ketonaemia or those whose blood sugar does not respond to IV fluid therapy alone, a fixed-rate insulin infusion should be commenced.

Key learning points

- Prompt assessment of patients with HHS should include assessment of fluid status and the presence of comorbidities such as cardiac failure.
- Remember that HHS may be the first presentation of diabetes so there may not always be a clear history of poor glucose control.
- Regular assessment of plasma osmolality should help guide the rate and choice of fluid therapy.
- All patients should be reviewed by the diabetes team prior to discharge and a plan made for glycaemic control and outpatient follow-up.

FURTHER READING

- The Joint British Diabetes Societies Inpatient Care Group provides clear, comprehensive guidelines on the management of DKA.

Hypoglycaemia

Edith Merchant

Age: 81

Hospital number: 123456

 Case study

Presenting complaint: *An 81-year-old woman is brought to the emergency department by her daughter. She was last seen well yesterday evening but was found by her daughter this morning to be drowsy and disorientated.*

Background: *She lives alone at home and mobilises independently. Her daughter does her weekly shopping and she has a cleaner once a week. She mobilises with a Zimmer frame. She does not smoke but drinks approximately three glasses of sherry per night.*

PMH: *type 2 diabetes diagnosed aged 45 years, hypertension, obesity, chronic venous leg ulceration.*

Allergies: *none known*

Examination: *Pulse 75, Sats 97% on air, RR 13, temp 37.4, BP 148/82*

CVS: *Capillary refill time <2 seconds, pulse regular, HS I + II + 0, chronic venous leg ulceration*

RS: *Equal chest expansion with good air entry throughout and no added sounds*

Abdo: *Abdomen soft and non-tender, bowel sounds present*

Neuro: *GCS 13 (E3 V4 M6). Pupils equal and reactive to light, cranial nerve, upper and lower limb examination NAD*

Capillary blood glucose: 1.9 mmol/L

Diagnosis
Hypoglycaemic episode.

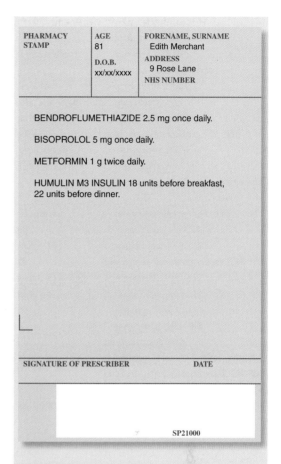

| PHARMACY STAMP | AGE 81 | FORENAME, SURNAME Edith Merchant |
| | D.O.B. xx/xx/xxxx | ADDRESS 9 Rose Lane NHS NUMBER |

BENDROFLUMETHIAZIDE 2.5 mg once daily.

BISOPROLOL 5 mg once daily.

METFORMIN 1 g twice daily.

HUMULIN M3 INSULIN 18 units before breakfast, 22 units before dinner.

SIGNATURE OF PRESCRIBER   DATE

SP21000

Initial measures

Risk factors for hypoglycaemia present in this case include long duration of diabetes, alcohol intake, and the fact that the patient is elderly. The initial priority is administration of a quick-acting carbohydrate to prevent permanent neurological deficits.

Prescribing in hypoglycaemia

Hypoglycaemia is the most common side effect of insulin therapy and some oral hypoglycaemic drugs (notably sulphonylureas) (Gerstein *et al.*, 2008). As part of the 'D for disability' of the ABCDE assessment of any acutely unwell patient, the capillary blood glucose should be measured. This is particularly important if a patient is known to have diabetes. Patients with diabetes may be unaware that they are having a 'hypo'; symptoms may include drowsiness, lethargy, aggressive behaviour or seizures. Autonomic features including sweating, palpitations and hunger may also be seen.

Current guidelines advise that any blood glucose value less than 4.0 mmol/L should be treated.

FLUID CHART						
Date	Fluid	Dose	Route	Frequency	Signature	Print name
xx/xx/xx	20% DEXTROSE	80 ml	IV	STAT	A. Doctor	A. Doctor

Oral glucose: rationale and evidence

The first group of patients consist of those who are conscious and able to swallow.

> ### ⚠ Guidelines
>
> Joint British Diabetes Societies Inpatient Care Group. *The Hospital Management of Hypoglycaemia in Adults with Diabetes Mellitus* (JBDS, 2013b).
> - Guidelines suggest that in patients who are conscious and able to swallow oral glucose should be given as soon as possible.
> - In those patients who are alert and orientated, 15–20 g of oral glucose should be given in the form of 150–200 mL of fruit juice, 90-120 mL of Lucozade® or 4–7 glucose tablets.
> - In patients who are confused and/ or aggressive but still able to swallow, guidelines suggest that 1.5–2 tubes of oral glucose gel such as GlucoGel® or Dextrogel® be used.
> - Capillary blood glucose measurement should be re-checked after 10–15 minutes, and if less than 4.0 mmol/L, further oral glucose should be administered.

If after three attempts at using oral glucose the capillary blood glucose remains <4.0 mmol/L,

intramuscular glucagon or intravenous glucose will be required (see Sections Glucagon: Rationale and Evidence and Intravenous Dextrose: Rationale and Evidence).

Once the patient has recovered from the episode and their capillary blood glucose is >4.0 mmol/L, a long-acting carbohydrate such as biscuits or toast should be given.

> ### ✓ DRUGS checklist for GLUCOGEL®
>
> | | |
> |---|---|
> | **Dose** | 1.5–2 tubes |
> | **Route** | Oral |
> | **Units** | Tubes |
> | **Given** | As required, when capillary blood glucose <4.0 mmol/L |
> | **Special situations** | Do not use in patients with reduced conscious level or in those who are unable to swallow safely. |

Oral glucose gel: essential pharmacology

Oral glucose gel such as Glucogel® is rapidly absorbed through buccal membranes to increase the plasma glucose level.

Glucagon: rationale and evidence

In patients who are unconscious or having seizures, either intramuscular glucagon or intravenous dextrose should be administered rather than oral preparations.

> ### ⚠ Guidelines
>
> Joint British Diabetes Societies Inpatient Care Group. *The Hospital Management of Hypoglycaemia in Adults with Diabetes Mellitus* (JBDS, 2013b).

- If intravenous access is available, intravenous dextrose should be used. This can either be used as 10% or 20% (see Evidence: Which concentration of intravenous dextrose?).
- Glucagon takes approximately 15 minutes to take effect, but is a useful option in patients without intravenous access. Of note, it may be less effective in patients with hypoglycaemia secondary to sulphonylurea therapy.

As before, once the patient has stabilised and the capillary blood glucose is >4.0 mmol/L, the patient should be given a long-acting carbohydrate.

DRUGS checklist for GLUCAGON

Dose	1 mg
Route	Intramuscular
Units	mg
Given	As required, when capillary blood glucose <4.0 mmol/L
Special situations	Glucagon may increase the anticoagulant effect of warfarin so careful monitoring is required.

Glucagon: essential pharmacology

Glucagon is an insulin antagonist, which acts by mobilising glycogen stores from the liver through accelerating glycogenolysis and gluconeogenesis. Therefore, it will be less effective in patients with malnutrition (including those with chronic liver disease). In these circumstances, intravenous dextrose should be used instead. The half life of IM glucagon is up to 18 minutes and the duration of action is up to 90 minutes.

Intravenous dextrose: rationale and evidence

 Evidence

Which concentration of intravenous dextrose?
Historically, 50% dextrose was widely used in the management of hypoglycaemia, but this has been associated with significant extravasation injuries (Wood, 2007). There is also evidence to suggest that use of 10% dextrose results in lower post-treatment glucose levels (Moore and Woollard, 2005).

(!) **Guidelines**

Joint British Diabetes Societies Inpatient Care Group. *The Hospital Management of Hypoglycaemia in Adults with Diabetes Mellitus* (JBDS, 2013b).
- For the reasons discussed in Evidence: Which concentration of intravenous dextrose?, 10% or 20% dextrose solutions are recommended instead of 50% dextrose.
- These guidelines recommend that all patients with diabetes should have IV dextrose prescribed on an 'as required' (PRN) basis.

It is important to note that the capillary blood glucose should be measured 10 minutes after intravenous dextrose is administered; if the value is <4.0 mmol/L, a further dose should be administered. As before, once the patient has stabilised and the capillary blood glucose is >4.0 mmol/L, the patient should be given a long-acting carbohydrate.

DRUGS checklist for intravenous DEXTROSE

Dose	Either 70–80 mL of 20% dextrose or 150–160 mL of 10% dextrose
Route	Intravenous

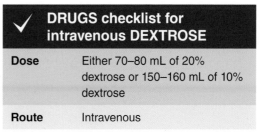

(Continued)

✓ DRUGS checklist for intravenous DEXTROSE (*Continued*)

Units	mL
Given	Over 10–15 minutes
Special situations	Repeated administration may be required if the capillary blood glucose fails to rise after an initial dose.

DISCHARGE MEDICATION

Date	Medication	Dose	Route	Frequency	Supply	GP to continue?
xx/xx/xx	BENDROFLU-METHIAZIDE	2.5 mg	PO	Once daily	14 days	Y
xx/xx/xx	BISOPROLOL	5 mg	PO	Once daily	14 days	Y
xx/xx/xx	METFORMIN	500 mg	PO	Twice daily	14 days	Y
xx/xx/xx	HUMULIN M3 INSULIN	12 units	SC	Twice daily (before breakfast and before dinner)	14 days	Y

Notes to patient/GP:

Intravenous dextrose: essential pharmacology

Intravenous dextrose is rapidly absorbed and is used and distributed by body tissues. It may also serve to minimise liver glycogen depletion. Intravenous dextrose undergoes metabolism to water and carbon dioxide.

Case outcome and discharge

Mrs Merchant was given IV dextrose and her GCS improved to 15/15. She was reviewed by the inpatient diabetes team and both the dose of metformin and Humulin M3 were reduced. Her capillary blood glucose levels on discharge were 12–15 mmol/L with no hypoglycaemic episodes. She was counselled about reducing her alcohol intake and the importance of regular blood glucose monitoring. Outpatient follow-up was arranged with her diabetes specialist nurse.

Common pitfalls

- Always check the capillary blood glucose in any acutely unwell patient.
- Regular monitoring of capillary blood glucose is essential once treatment has been commenced.
- It is not usually advisable to omit a patient's normal insulin, although review of a patient's diabetes regimen is likely to be required.
- If in doubt, specialist advice should be sought from the inpatient diabetes team.
- There is evidence that intensive therapy targeted at reducing HbA1c levels to <6.0% is associated with increased mortality without an associated reduction in cardiovascular events. Therefore, it is important to balance the risks of hypoglycaemic episodes with long-term glucose control.
- Capillary blood glucose can be falsely elevated in people who have been eating sweets (commercial confectionary contain some glucose as well as sucrose which may remain on the fingers).

SUMMARY

Current best practice recommends the use of 'hypo boxes' in a prominent place on the ward, such as on a resuscitation trolley. These contain all the equipment needed to manage hypoglycaemia in an emergency. Following an episode of hypoglycaemia, regular capillary blood glucose measurements should be taken and precipitants for the episode should be sought. The patient should be reviewed by the diabetes team and education and alteration in their diabetes regimen should be made as appropriate.

Key learning points

- Hypoglycaemia is a common problem, particularly amongst patients with type 1 diabetes, and may present with a range of non-specific symptoms.
- Once the initial episode has been managed, it is essential to consider appropriate long-term management of a patient's diabetes, including referral to the diabetes team.
- Precipitants for the episode of hypoglycaemia should be sought and patients and relatives should be educated to avoid future episodes.

FURTHER READING

- The Joint British Diabetes Societies Inpatient Care Group have a detailed guideline regarding the management of hypoglycaemia in adults.

Other aspects of prescribing in diabetes

Hyperglycaemia in the well diabetic patient

A common question encountered by junior doctors during 'on call' shifts is what to do about a well patient with high blood sugars. This may be in a patient with known diabetes or in a patient without a previous history of diabetes but with a concurrent medical issue (for example undergoing steroid treatment).

The key in this situation is to ensure that the patient is clinically well, and ascertain whether or not there is ketosis. In a scenario where the patient is well and there are no urinary ketones, there is no indication to administer fast-acting insulin such as Actrapid. Instead, a full assessment of the patient's diabetic regime should be carried out and their regular medications adjusted accordingly. Giving boluses of rapidly acting insulin leads to erratic blood glucose levels and risks the patient having a hypoglycaemic episode.

Types of insulin

A summary of some of the key types of insulin that are available is given in Table 15.1.

Table 15.1 Summary of some of the key types of insulin available.

Type of insulin	Examples	Uses
Rapid-acting analogue	Novorapid (insulin Aspart), Humalog (insulin Lispro), Apidra (insulin Glulisine)	Rapidly acting insulin analogues are often used as part of a 'basal bolus' regime with a long-acting analogue. This is particularly useful for those with erratic meal habits or those prone to hypoglycaemic episodes.
Short acting	Actrapid, Humulin S, Insuman Rapid	These soluble insulins have an onset of action at 30 minutes, peak at 2–3 hours and last for 8 hours.
Medium and long acting	Insulatard, Humulin I, Insuman Basal	These are usually used twice daily. They have an onset of action after approximately 2–4 hours, peak at 6–7 hours and last up to 20 hours.
Long-acting analogues	Lantus (insulin Glargine), Levemir (insulin Detemir)	Long-acting insulin analogues can be used once or twice daily. These have an onset of action after 1–3 hours, and last up to 24 hours.
Mixed insulins and analogue mixtures	Humulin M3, Humalog Mix 25/Mix 50, Novomix 30	Mixed insulins and analogue mixtures are usually used as part of a twice-daily regimen. They contain a mixture of rapid or short-acting insulin with a medium-acting insulin.

Newer diabetic agents

There are a wide range of drugs for diabetes, which have emerged in recent years. Table 15.2 provides a summary of oral hypoglycaemic agents used in diabetes along with the advantages and disadvantages of their use.

Table 15.2   Oral hypoglycaemic agents used in diabetes.

Hypoglycaemic agent	Indication(s)	Advantages	Disadvantages
Biguanides e.g. metformin	First-line drug for overweight patients when dietary control has failed	Reduces macrovascular complications and all-cause mortality, fewer hypoglycaemic episodes compared with sulphonylureas	Risk of lactic acidosis in patients with renal impairment, GI side effects at higher doses
Sulphonylureas e.g. gliclazide	Can be used in patients for whom metformin is not tolerated or is contraindicated	Reduces HbA1c	Significant risk of hypoglycaemic episodes, particularly in the elderly
Thiazolidinediones e.g. pioglitazone	Usually used in combination with metformin or gliclazide	Particularly effective in patients with insulin resistance when used in combination with metformin	Contraindicated in patients with heart failure; rare reports of liver failure have been documented; small increase in risk of fractures in women so should be avoided in those with risk factors for osteoporosis
Dipeptidyl peptidase-4 inhibitors e.g. sitagliptin, vildagliptin	Can be used alone or in combination with metformin, gliclazide or a thiozoladinedione	A useful 2nd or 3rd line adjunctive therapy	Hypersensitivity reactions including anaphylaxis may occur
Rapidly acting insulin secretogogues e.g. repaglinide and nateglinide	Rapaglinide is suitable for non-obese patients for whom metformin is contraindicated or not tolerated. Nateglinide is only licensed for use in combination with metformin	May be useful in patients with an erratic diet (short duration and rapid onset of action so given before meals)	Risk of hypoglycaemic episodes, although there is a limited evidence base
GLP-1 mimetics e.g. exenatide	A twice-daily subcutaneous injection used in combination with metformin or gliclazide	Has comparable efficacy to insulin, and is particularly useful in obese patients or HGV drivers who would lose their license if insulin were commenced	Nausea is common; may cause hypoglycaemic episodes; interact with warfarin so INR should be monitored closely
Acarbose	Usually only used in patients who cannot be prescribed other hypoglycaemic agents	Can be used in addition to metformin or gliclazide to improve glycaemic control	Significant GI side effects including diarrhoea and flatulence

Variable rate insulin infusions in patients without DKA

In diabetic patients who are due to be 'nil by mouth' prior to a procedure or operation and will miss more than one meal, or patients who are unable to eat and drink as normal (for example patients who are vomiting), it is usually necessary to set up a variable rate insulin infusion. This is often referred to as a 'sliding scale'.

Here, there is a grid available, which states the capillary blood glucose level in one column and subsequent columns for you to prescribe the appropriate dose of insulin for the patient. If the patient is prescribed regular insulin, you can calculate their 24-hour insulin requirement based on this information.

Table 15.3 gives examples of the appropriate insulin doses according to a patient's capillary blood glucose level.

Important safety points whilst a variable rate insulin infusion is running include to ensure that blood glucose is monitored hourly, to monitor fluid status, electrolytes and to regularly review the need for the infusion.

In general, long-acting insulin analogues should be continued during the variable rate infusion, and other types of insulin should be held. This will avoid rebound hyperglycaemia once the patient's usual insulin is restarted.

Table 15.3 Examples of the appropriate insulin doses to use for a variable rate insulin infusion according to a patient's capillary blood glucose level.

Capillary blood glucose (mmol/L)	Reduced rate for insulin-sensitive patients e.g. <24 units per day (mL/h)	Standard rate (first choice in most patients) (mL/h)	Increased rate for insulin-resistant patients e.g. >100 units per day (mL/h)
<4.0	0[a]	0[a]	0[a]
4.1–8.0	0.5	1	2
8.1–12.0	1	2	4
12.1–16.0	2	4	6
16.1–20.0	3	5	7
20.1–24.0	4	6	8
>24.1	6	8	10

[a]Treat hypoglycaemia and once capillary blood glucose >4.0 mmol/L, restart insulin infusion.

Now visit **www.wileyessential.com/pharmacology** to test yourself on this chapter.

References

Chua HR, Schneider A, Bellomo R (2011). Bicarbonate in diabetic ketoacidosis – a systematic review. *Ann Intensive Care* 1: 23.

Dhatariya KK (2007) Diabetic ketoacidosis. *BMJ* 334: 1284–5.

Gerstein HC, Miller ME, Byington RP *et al.* (2008). Effects of intensive glucose lowering in type 2 diabetes. *N Engl J Med* 358: 2545–59.

Hsia E, Seggelke S, Gibbs J *et al.* (2012) Subcutaneous administration of glargine to diabetic patients receiving insulin infusion prevents rebound hyperglycemia. *J Clin Endocrinol Metab* 97: 3132–7.

Joint British Diabetes Societies Inpatient Care Group (JBDS) (2012). *The Management of Hyperosmolar Hyperglycaemic State in Adults.* Available at: www.diabetes.org.uk/Documents/Position%20statements/JBDS-IP-HHS-Adults.pdf (accessed Oct. 2014).

Joint British Diabetes Societies Inpatient Care Group (JBDS) (2013a). *The Management of Diabetic Ketoacidosis in Adults.* Second edition. Available at: www.diabetes.org.uk/Documents/About%20Us/What%20we%20say/Management-of-DKA-241013.pdf (accessed Sept. 2014).

Joint British Diabetes Societies Inpatient Care Group (JBDS) (2013b). *The Hospital Management of Hypoglycaemia in Adults with Diabetes Mellitus.* Available at: https://www.diabetes.org.uk/Documents/About%20Us/Our%20views/Care%20recs/JBDS%20hypoglycaemia%20position%20(2013).pdf (accessed Dec. 2015).

Joint British Diabetes Societies for Inpatient Care (JBDS-IP) (2014). *Guideline for the Use of Variable Rate Insulin Infusion (VRII) in Medical Inpatients.* Available at www.diabetologists-abcd.org.uk/JBDS/JBDS_IP_VRIII.pdf (accessed May 2015).

Keenan CR, Murin S, White RH (2007). High risk for venous thromboembolism in diabetics with hyperosmolar state: comparison with other acute medical illnesses. *J Thromb Haemost* 5: 1185–90.

Kitabchi AE, Nyenwe EA (2006). Hyperglycemic crises in diabetes mellitus: DKA and hyperglycemic hyperosmolar state. *Endocrinol Metab Clin North Am* 35: 725–51.

Kitabchi AE, Umpierrez GE, Miles JM *et al.* (2009). Hyperglycemic crises in adult patients with diabetes. *Diabetes Care* 32: 1335–43.

Mahler SA, Conrad SA, Wang H *et al.* (2011). Resuscitation with balanced electrolyte solution prevents hyperchloremic metabolic acidosis in patients with diabetic ketoacidosis. *Am J Emerg Med* 29: 670–4.

Milionis HJ, Liamis G, Elisaf MS (2001). Appropriate treatment of hypernatraemia in diabetic hyperglycaemic hyperosmolar syndrome. *J Int Med* 249: 273–6.

Moore C, Woollard M (2005). Dextrose 10% or 50% in the treatment of hypoglycaemia out of hospital? A randomised controlled trial. *Emerg Med J* 22: 512–5.

National Institute of Health and Care Excellence (NICE) (2009). *Type 2 Diabetes: the Management of Type 2 Diabetes,* CG87. Available at: www.nice.org.uk/guidance/CG87 (accessed Dec. 2015).

O'Malley G, Moran C, Draman MS *et al.* (2008) Central pontine myelinolysis complicating treatment of the hyperglycaemic hyperosmolar state. *Ann Clin Biochem* 45: 440–3.

Perel P, Roberts I, Pearson M (2013) Colloids versus crystalloids for fluid resuscitation in critically ill patients. *Cochrane Database Syst Rev* (2): CD000567.

Reinhart K, Perner A, Sprung CL *et al.* (2013). Consensus statement of the ESICM task force on colloid volume therapy in critically ill patients. *Intensive Care Med* 38: 368–83.

Savage MW, Dhatariya KK, Kilvert A *et al.* (2011). Joint British Diabetes Societies guideline for the management of diabetic ketoacidosis. *Diabetic Med* 28: 508–15.

Van Zyl DG, Rheeder P, Delport E (2012). Fluid management in diabeticacidosis – Ringer's lactate versus normal saline: a randomized controlled trial. *Q J Med* 105: 337–43.

Wood SP (2007). Is D50 too much of a good thing? A reappraisal of the safety of 50% dextrose administration in patients with hypoglycaemia. *JEMS* 32: 103–6.

CHAPTER 16
Anticoagulation

Andrew Stanton

Key topics:

Learning objectives

By the end of this chapter, you should be able to…

- …understand the rationale behind therapeutic strategies combining low molecular weight heparin and warfarin in the initial days of management.
- …be aware of newer agent used in management of VTE and be able to prescribe them appropriately when recommended.
- …recognise and apply practical differences in an anticoagulation strategy in patients with atrial fibrillation.
- …understand the prescribing principles in considering reversal of anticoagulants.

Essential Practical Prescribing, First Edition. Georgia Woodfield, Benedict Lyle Phillips, Victoria Taylor, Amy Hawkins and Andrew Stanton. © 2016 by John Wiley & Sons, Ltd. Published 2016 by John Wiley & Sons, Ltd.

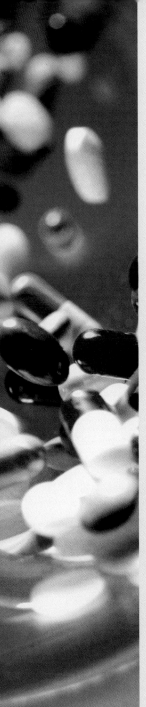

Venous thromboembolism

> ### Enid Robinson
> ### Age: 67
> ### Hospital number: 123456

 Case Study

Mrs Robinson is admitted with a 6-hour history of sudden onset shortness of breath, left sided pleuritic chest pain and haemoptysis. She was previously well and independent.

PMH: *Hypertension*

DH: *See FP10*

Allergies: *None*

Salient examination findings:

HR 110, BP 132/84, Sats 93% on air, RR 26, T 37.7
HS I+II +0
Chest clear
Abdo: soft, non-tender, no masses / organomegaly
Legs: No oedema/ sign of DVT

Investigations:
ABG (air) Po$_2$ 7.5, Pco$_2$ 18.6, pH 7.38, HCO$_3$ 18.6
ECG: Sinus tachycardia, normal axis, no other acute changes
CXR: Nil focal
FBC/ LFT normal. INR 1.1
Na 136, K 4.6, urea 6.5, creatinine 93
CTPA: occlusive thrombus seen in left main pulmonary artery and segmental arteries. Lungs clear otherwise, no sign of right heart strain

Diagnosis
Acute pulmonary embolism.

Initial measures
Oxygen must be prescribed to target saturations between 94 and 98%. The patient must be kept well hydrated with any concerns about oral intake addressed by providing supplemental IV fluids. Simple analgesics (paracetamol/ NSAIDs) should be provided for the pleuritic pain.

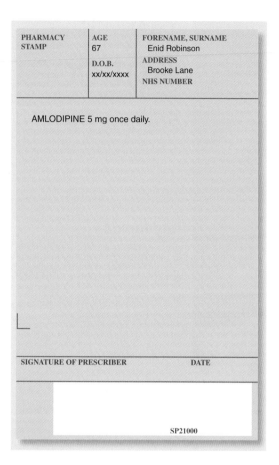

| PHARMACY STAMP | AGE 67 | FORENAME, SURNAME Enid Robinson |
| | D.O.B. xx/xx/xxxx | ADDRESS Brooke Lane NHS NUMBER |

AMLODIPINE 5 mg once daily.

SIGNATURE OF PRESCRIBER   DATE

SP21000

 Guidelines

The Scottish Intercollegiate Guidelines Network (SIGN) have produced the following guideline: *Antithrombotics: Indications and Management. A National Clinical Guideline*, SIGN 129, 2013. Available at:
  www.rcpsg.ac.uk/~/media/2D92925
http://www.sign.ac.uk/guidelines/fulltext/129/ (accessed February 2016).

Prescribing for venous thromboembolism (VTE)

Principles

Empirical anticoagulation is recommended before diagnostic confirmation of thromboembolic disease in patients with either high or moderate probability (either deep venous thrombosis [DVT] or pulmonary embolism[PE]) and the prescribing principles are no different for DVT or PE. Here systemic anticoagulation with low molecular weight heparin (LMWH) is the treatment of choice. This is superior to intravenous unfractionated heparin in the treatment of VTE and there are a number of agents licensed for use in this situation (e.g. dalteparin, tinzaparin, enoxaparin). There is no evidence any one is superior to others and the choice is usually guided by local hospital formulary availability/ guidelines. Once a diagnosis of VTE is confirmed, the patient needs to be commenced on formal oral anticoagulation. For decades, the only available treatment has been warfarin but there is now evidence of efficacy for newer oral anticoagulants, which do not require regular monitoring and ongoing dose adjustment. These drugs are not in uniform use and are not appropriate in all cases and so the situation of warfarinisation will be considered first.

Before commencing anticoagulation, care must be taken to ensure there are no contraindications to this treatment and the patient counselled about potential side effects/ interactions (see DRUGS checklist and Essential Pharmacology for Warfarin). The principle contraindication is either active or high risk of bleeding, especially in the CNS or GI tract. In patients who have had a previous significant bleeding event it still may be safe to initiate anticoagulation treatment but the decision will depend on time since bleed, type of bleed and whether any therapy has been employed to minimise the chance of recurrence, and senior (and often multidisciplinary) opinion would be needed.

Most hospitals will have a specific section in the drug chart for warfarin given its variability in its daily dosing, and some may also have a specific anticoagulation section where all forms of anticoagulation needs to be prescribed.

Contraindications to anticoagulation are (see BNF [BMA/RPS, 2015]):

- Haemorrhagic stroke.
- Bleeding disorders, such as:
  - Uncorrected major bleeding – avoid using warfarin until the bleeding has stopped and the cause healed.
  - Uncorrected major bleeding disorder, for example thrombocytopenia, haemophilia, liver failure and renal failure.
- Potential bleeding lesions, for example active peptic ulcer; oesophageal varices; aneurysm; proliferative retinopathy; recent organ biopsy; recent trauma or surgery to head, orbit, or spine; recent stroke; confirmed intracranial or intraspinal bleed; or within 72 hours of major surgery with risk of severe bleeding, or within 48 hours postpartum.
- Uncontrolled severe hypertension, for example systolic blood pressure greater than 200 mmHg or diastolic pressure greater than 120 mmHg.

The patient's weight was 80 kg and the drug doses were calculated accordingly.

ONCE ONLY PRESCRIPTIONS					Prescriber	
Date	Time to be given	DRUG	Dose	Route	Signature	Bleep
xx/xx/xx	20:00	PARACETAMOL	1 g	PO	A. Doctor	
xx/xx/xx	20:00	DALTEPARIN	15000 units	SC	A. Doctor	

REGULAR PRESCRIPTIONS

					Circle/enter times below ↓	Enter dates below			
						Day 1	Day 2	Day 3	Day 4
DRUG DALTEPARIN					06				
					08				
Dose 15000 units	Route SC	Freq	Start date xx/xx/xx		12				
Signature A. Doctor		Bleep	Review		16				
Additional instructions					(20)				
					22				
DRUG AMLODIPINE					06				
					(08)				
Dose 5 mg	Route PO	Freq	Start date xx/xx/xx		12				
Signature A. Doctor		Bleep	Review		16				
Additional instructions					18				
					22				

AS REQUIRED MEDICATION

DRUG PARACETAMOL				Date		
				Time		
Dose 1 g	Route PO	Max freq QDS	Start date xx/xx/xx	Dose		
Signature/Bleep A. Doctor		Max dose in 24 hrs 4 g	Review	Route		
				Given		
Additional instructions				Check		

VARIABLE DOSE ANTICOAGULANT					
Anticoagulant	WARFARIN		Therapeutic range 2-3		Duration of therapy 3 months
Indication for anticoagulation	PTE		Prescriber's signature A. Doctor		Date xx/xx/xx
FOR ADVICE PLEASE CONTACT THE ANTICOAGULATION CLINIC ON EXTENSION **** OR BLEEP ****					
New to warfarin? (Y)/N	Previous dose (if known warfarin patient)		Pre-treatment INR 1.1		Pre-treatment FBC/LFTs checked? Y / N

Date	First dose xx/xx/xx				
INR	1.1	First test			
Warfarin dose (mg)	10 mg				
Doctor or Practitioner (initials)	A. D.				
Given by (give @ 6pm)	A. D.				

Low molecular weight heparins: rationale and evidence

Numerous trials have shown that various LMWH are as efficacious as, or superior to, unfractionated heparin in the treatment of venous thromboembolism (van Dongen *et al.*, 2004). In addition, they have demonstrated a lower risk of bleeding (Cossette *et al.*, 2010) and heparin-induced thrombocytopenia (Stein *et al.*, 2009) than unfractionated IV heparin. Anticoagulation with LMWH in the context of thromboembolism provides rapid anticoagulation but the effect can be delayed if the dose is not sufficient to overcome the lower initial bioavailability (up to 60 minutes). In comparison, unfractionated intravenous heparin will always have an immediate onset of action (Hirsh *et al.*, 2001). This is generally not of significant clinical concern, but in obese patients or in patients more critically unwell some clinicians give an immediate dose of unfractionated IV heparin (of 5000 units) alongside the subcutaneous LMWH dose to mitigate against this. If warfarin is prescribed as the oral anticoagulant,

LMWH must be continued for **at least 5 days** irrespective of the patients INR. Failure to do so leaves the patient at risk of paradoxical increased risk of recurrent thromboembolism even if the INR is therapeutic in the early stage, as warfarin depletes protein C levels in the first few days of administration. Studies confirming benefit of LMWH also used therapy for at least 5, and in many as long as 10 days.

There are four LMWHs licensed in the UK for the treatment of DVT and PE – Enoxaparin, Dalteparin, Tinzaparin and also Fondaparinux.

🔍 Evidence

LMWH in VTE

A Cochrane review (van Dongen *et al.*, 2004) examined 22 randomised controlled trials (RCTs) comparing LMWH versus unfractionated heparin in the treatment of venous thromboembolism. Studies varied in the specific thromboembolic entity studied (either proximal/ distal DVT and/or PE), and timeframe, but a consistent message was demonstrated. Improved outcomes with LMWH included incidence of recurrent thromboembolism during treatment and follow up phases (up to 6 months in some studies) and major bleeding. In the 16 studies where mortality was included as an (albeit secondary) outcome measure, LMWH was found overall to be superior to unfractionated heparin. An important practical take-home message that needs to be translated into practice from this meta-analysis is that all studies gave LMWH for at least 5 days.

✓ DRUGS checklist for LMWHs in VTE

	Dalteparin	Enoxaparin	Tinzaparin	Fondaparinux
Dose (by weight)	40–45 kg 7500 units, 46–56 kg 10 000 units, 57–68 kg 12 500 units, 69–82 kg 15 000 units, >83 kg 18 000 units	1.5 mg/kg (150 units/kg)	175 units/kg	<50 kg 5 mg, 50–100 kg 7.5 mg, >100 kg 10 mg
Route	SC	SC	SC	SC

Units	Units	Units	Units	Units
Given	Once daily	Once daily	Once daily	Once daily
Special situations				
Pregnancy	Given twice daily with different dose/weight (early pregnancy based) regime to above (see BNF[BMA/RPS, 2015])	As per dalteparin – twice daily weight based regime as per BNF	Once daily regimen based on early pregnancy weight	Not recommended
Renal impairment	Caution if creatinine clearance (CrCl) <30 mL/min	Reduce dose if CrCl <30 mL/min	Monitor anti-Xa if CrCl <30 mL/min, dose reduction if CrCl <20 mL/min	Caution if CrCl 30–50 mL/min, avoid if <30 mL/min
Malignancy	Dose reduced after 30 days (see BNF)			

Low molecular weight heparins: essential pharmacology

Please see Chapter 7, Section Heparin and Pentasaccharide Preparations for VTE Prophylaxis: Essential Pharmacology and Chapter 3, Section Fondaparinux: Essential Pharmacology.

DRUGS checklist for HEPARIN in VTE

Dose	5000 units
Route	IV (can be given SC for VTE prophylaxis)
Units	Units
Given	Stat, then as continuous infusion of 18 units/kg/h
Special situations	Monitor using activated partial thromboplastin time (APTT) after 6 hours and then daily. Change IV infusion rate according to local nomogram if available.

Warfarin: rationale and evidence

Warfarin has been the standard oral anticoagulant of choice in venous thromboembolism since the latter half of the 20th century. In a great example of how vast numbers of patients are not required in an RCT when a treatment effect is so pronounced (in contrast with requirements of many modern day RCTs), Barritt and Jordan (1960) showed that heparin plus warfarin dramatically reduced mortality at 1 year (0% vs. 26%, number needed to treat (NNT) = 4, confidence interval (CI) 2–16) in 35 patients with clinical diagnosis of PE (with autopsy confirmation in those who died).

DRUGS checklist for WARFARIN

Dose	Initial loading regime depends on age

Subsequent doses depend on the INR (see Table 16.1) |
Route	PO
Units	mg
Given	Once daily
Special situations	Causes bleeding and has numerous interactions with any drugs that use cytochrome p450 pathway. This is important as drug interactions can cause the INR to be unexpectedly high or low.

Practical prescribing points

A number of initiation nomograms are available for warfarin initiation in the context of acute thrombo-embolic disease. Those using a 5 mg initiation dose rather than 10 mg report less excessive over-anticoagulation but with slower time to target INR (Harrison *et al.*, 1997; Garcia *et al.*, 2013). There is no evidence a 10 mg loading dose is any more superior in terms of reducing risk of recurrent thromboembolic events, but elderly patients may be less likely to develop high INRs early in treatment with lower dose initiation (Keeling *et al.*, 2011) and so a lower starting dose in the elderly is recommended.

From a practical point of view to make sure appropriate anticoagulant effect is obtained efficiently and safely, there are several principles that should be adhered to:

- Use a nomogram – they have been developed carefully on account of the fact that there are a variety of factors that influence sensitivity to warfarin (age, genetic factors, other drugs, diet and various disease states, e.g. low body weight, heart failure, liver failure) and are there to avoid prescribers randomly 'thinking of a number' when prescribing the next warfarin dose (Table 16.1). Try to resist the oft employed '10/10/5' initiation regimen (i.e. 10 mg day 1, 10 mg day 2 and 5 mg day 3) without checking the INR in between.

- Measure the INR before you give any warfarin and measure it daily, **especially** after dose 2 and 3 – in most nomograms the INR on day 4 (after the third dose) predicts the initial baseline warfarin dose. Without knowledge of previous INRs and continued loading doses prescribed accordingly, it is essentially guesswork and the patient is more likely to take longer to reach a steady state of INR.

- Review ongoing and regular prescription of other drugs – consider any short-term prescriptions that may adversely affect INR and make immediate judgements about predicted maintenance warfarin dose difficult. For example a patient on a short course of clarithromycin my need less warfarin initially but more once the antibiotic is finished.

Table 16.1 Example of warfarin initiation nomogram. Source: This table is reproduced from SIGN 2013 (Antithrombotics: indications and management. A national clinical guideline. SIGN 129) by kind permission of the Scottish Intercollegiate Guidelines Network.

DAY	INR	Dose for age (mg)			
		≤50 years	51–65 years	66–80 years	>80 years
1	< 1.4	10	9	7.5	6
2	<1.6	10	9	7.5	6
	≥1.6	0.5	0.5	0.5	0.5
3	<1.8	10	9	7.5	6
	1.8–2.5	4–5	3.5–4.5	3–4	2.5–3
	2.6–3.0	2.5–3.5	2.5–3.5	2–2.5	1.5–2
	3.1 –3.5	1–2	1–2	0.5–1.5	0.5–1.5
	3.6–4.0	0.5	0.5	0.5	0.5
	>4	0	0	0	0
4	< 1.6	10–15	9–13	7.5–11	6–9
	1.6–1.9	6–8	5.5–7	4.5–6	3.5–5
	2.0–2.6	4.5–5.5	4–5	3.5–4.5	2.5–3.5
	2.7–3.5	3.5–4	3–3.5	2.5–3	2–2.5
	3.6–4.0	3	2.5	2	1.5
	4.1–4.5	Omit next day's dose then:			
		1–2	0.5–1.5	0.5–1.5	0.5–1.5
	>4.5	Withhold warfarin until INR back between 2.0–3.0 (then restart on 0.5–1 mg)			

It is recommended that INR is checked every 2–3 days after day 4 unless the patient has been transferred to an ongoing INR monitoring service as continuing refinements in the INR may be required.

Warfarin: essential pharmacology

Warfarin inhibits the vitamin K-dependant formation of the active forms of the clotting factors II, VII, IX and X. Although warfarin is readily absorbed from the GI tract its peak pharmacological effect is not manifested until approximately 48 hours later, once preformed clotting factors have been eliminated. Warfarin also causes a decrease in protein C levels during the first 36 hours of therapy, which causes a potentially hypercoagulable state (Harrison *et al.*, 1997). This is the rationale for the advice within British Society of Haematology and European Society of Cardiology guidelines (Keeling *et al.*, 2011; Konstantinides *et al.*, 2014) to prescribe LMWH for 5 days at least, **and** until the patient's INR is therapeutic (between 2 and 3), whichever is the longer.

The anticoagulant effect of warfarin is measured by the INR, which is the product of the patient's prothrombin time ratio and the 'International Sensitivity Index' of the thromboplastin (which has high variability) used by an individual laboratory.

Warfarin interacts with multiple other medications, with some potentiating and some lessening effect.

Drugs can potentiate the effect of warfarin through:

- Inhibiting its hepatic metabolism (e.g. ciprofloxacin, metronidazole, amiodarone)
- Displacing its binding from albumin (e.g. some NSAIDs), inhibition of reduction of vitamin K (e.g. cephalosporins)
- Decreasing the availability of vitamin K by alteration of gut flora (e.g. broad-spectrum antibiotics).

Drugs that inhibit platelet function include aspirin. NSAIDs increase the risk of bleeding on warfarin but do not necessarily increase its anticoagulant effect. Warfarin also interacts with a number of over-the-counter medications and dietary supplements, including green tea (Holbrook *et al.*, 2005). Even drugs usually considered safe can cause interactions, with paracetamol reported to increase INR (Mahé *et al.*, 2006).

Drugs may lessen the effect of warfarin by reducing absorption (e.g. cholestyramine) or by inducing the cytochrome P450 system (e.g. rifampicin). Excessive alcohol does not necessarily increase INR but variability in alcohol consumption, in particular a decrease in intake, can (Penning-van Beest *et al.*, 2002).

Prescribing in VTE: special situations

Caution needs to be exercised in renal failure where the dose may need to be reduced as LMWH is cleared from the circulation more slowly than higher molecular weight species (Hirsh *et al.*, 2001). Unlike heparin, the APTT is not prolonged and routine monitoring is not required. In certain circumstances where there is increased risk of bleeding (renal impairment/ underweight/ overweight) monitoring of anti-factor Xa activity may be required and the dose adjusted accordingly. If required, measure peak levels 4 hours after dose and the trough just before next dose is due (seek haematology advice). In renal failure use of unfractionated heparin may be preferable. Heparins (including LMWH) do not cross the placenta and so these are the treatment of choice in VTE associated with pregnancy. LMWH are eliminated more rapidly in pregnancy, however, and so dosage is increased, given usually in twice-daily regimens (see BNF[BMA/RPS, 2015] and product literature).

Malignancy

A number of studies have shown that LMWH (enoxaparin [Deitcher *et al.*, 2006]; tinzaparin [Hull *et al.*, 2006]; dalteparin [Lee *et al.*, 2003]) is superior to warfarin in reducing risk of thromboembolic events in patients with active cancer. A Cochrane meta-analysis has confirmed these findings (Akl *et al.*, 2014) and so LWMH is recommended for 6 months (in the UK only dalteparin is licensed for this indication). In practice, most clinicians will extend the treatment indefinitely when active malignancy remains at 6 months, due to its ongoing presence as a risk factor for thromboembolic disease, supported within recent ESC guidelines, (Konstantinides *et al.*, 2014). The decision to do this should be made on a case by case basis following discussion of presumed risks and benefits with the patient. There are no data to support the use of fondaparinux or novel oral anticoagulants (NOACs) in the treatment of VTE associated with malignancy.

Novel oral anticoagulants: rationale, evidence and pharmacology

There are a number of newer drugs available and licensed for the management of thromboembolic disease that do not require regular monitoring and dose adjustment in the way warfarin does. These drugs act at a specific part of the coagulation cascade and have more predictable effects on coagulation at fixed doses. Rivaroxaban, apixaban and edoxaban are selective inhibitors of factor Xa. They inhibit both free and clot-bound factor Xa and prothrombinase. They indirectly inhibit platelet aggregation induced by thrombin but have no direct effect on platelet aggregation. Accordingly, thrombin generation and thrombus development are decreased. A similar effect is found with dabigatran which, by directly inhibiting thrombin, reduces the conversion of fibrinogen to fibrin. It inhibits both free and fibrin-bound thrombin and also platelet aggregation induced by thrombin. Currently licensed NOACs in the UK for treatment of DVT/PE are rivaroxaban, apixaban and dabigatran.

These drugs have been approved on the basis of RCTs showing non-inferiority to warfarin. A common theme of trials with all agents is that the risk of severe or life-threatening bleeding appears to be less with these drugs than with warfarin. For example in the EINSTEIN-PE trial of rivaroxaban (Buller *et al.*, 2012), major bleeding was twice as frequent in the warfarin group compared to rivaroxaban, largely related to dramatically less intracranial (10 patients vs. 1 patient) and retroperitoneal bleeding (7 patients vs. 1 patient).

Depending on how the clinical trials were conducted, different NOACs have different directions for prescription timing in relation to LMWH (see DRUGS checklist) to ensure adequate (and not excessive) anticoagulation is achieved. Rivaroxaban, for example, requires higher dosage in the initial weeks of therapy to lead to an earlier steady state, higher trough levels and better thrombus regression (Mueck *et al.*, 2011).

Currently, there are no specific antidotes available for any of the NOACs to improve outcomes in the event of significant bleeding and so treatment in that event is essentially supportive. Dabigatran (but not rivaroxaban or apixaban) is dialysable but this is not a routinely recommended way of managing bleeding complications. Haematology advice should be sought and in some circumstances prothrombin complex concentrate may be recommended. This was found in a small study of 12 healthy patients to reverse the anticoagulant effect of rivaroxaban, but not dabigatran (Eerenberg *et al.*, 2011). Specific antidotes are in development and in clinical trial stages for dabigatran (idarucizumab) and rivaroxaban/apixaban (andexanet alfa).

Only a minority of patients in the clinical trials for all drugs had active cancer and so NOACs are not currently recommended for VTE associated with active malignancy. It is also worth noting that patients who underwent thrombolytic therapy in the trials for all three agents were excluded and so although there is no theoretical reason why the drugs should not be effective in such patients, some clinicians will have anxiety in prescribing them in these situations. There are also limited data on long-term efficacy for these agents (past 1 year), and although apixaban and dabigatran have licences for treatment of recurrent VTE at the time of writing, most clinicians would currently commence warfarin for a patient presenting with recurrent VTE.

✓ DRUGS checklist for NOACs in VTE			
	Rivaroxaban	**Dabigatran**	**Apixaban**
Dose	15 mg initial phase then 20 mg	150 mg	10 mg initial phase then 5 mg
Route	Oral	Oral	Oral
Units	mg	mg	mg

Given	BD for 21 days (15 mg) then OD (20 mg dose) for remaining term	BD		BD 10 mg dose for 7 days then 5 mg thereafter
Special situations	Avoid in renal impairment with creatinine clearance (CrCl) <30 mL/min. Prescribe first dose 2 hours before patient due to have next dose of LMWH then stop LMWH.	Avoid in renal impairment with CrCl <30 mL/min, reduce dose to 110 mg BD if CrCl 30–50 mL/min. Reduce dose to 110 mg BD if >80 years or on verapamil. Patients should have at least 5 days LMWH before switch. Prescribe first dose 0–2 hours before patient due to have next dose of LMWH then stop LMWH.		Avoid in renal impairment with CrCl <15 mL/min, caution advised if CrCl 15–30 mL/min. Prescribe first dose to be taken at time next dose of LMWH due.

Other medications used in VTE

The biggest question regularly posed in the management of PE is whether thrombolytic therapy is appropriate. Thrombolysis in PE has been shown to improve angiographic appearances and initial haemodynamic parameters (especially cardiac index) in patients with PE but this has not translated into consistently improved clinical outcomes in general cohorts of patients presenting with acute PE. It has been accepted for some time, and it is recommended in current guidelines, that patients who present with acute PE who have evidence of shock or persistent haemodynamic instability, despite initial therapy, should be considered for thrombolytic therapy. The issue surrounding patients who are not haemodynamically unstable but who are at higher risk of adverse outcome has been hotly debated for decades, in particular patients who have evidence of acute right heart dysfunction. There is controversy surrounding aspects of study protocols and end points used, resulting in a lack of a definitive answer. An often quoted study (Konstantinides *et al.*, 2002) showed that patients who were randomised to thrombolysis (using alteplase) versus placebo had lower risk of treatment failure, a composite end-point consisting of death and 'clinical deterioration requiring escalation of treatment'. This 'escalation' included the use of 'rescue thrombolysis', which was given for reasons that could be

argued were vague (e.g. including 'worsening clinical symptoms'), and so ultimately did not in many eyes provide the answer to the clinical conundrum. More recently, the PETHIO study (Meyer *et al.*, 2014) showed that patients in this group were less at risk of the composite end-point of death and haemodynamic deterioration with thrombolysis using tenecteplase, but this was offset by a significant risk of major bleeding.

For the time being, the recommendation from current guidelines is that thrombolysis should not be routinely offered to patients without haemodynamic instability (ESC guidelines [Konstantinides *et al.*, 2014]). There are occasionally difficult situations that do not have reference in large RCTs where thrombolysis may be considered after careful senior discussion, for example patients with profound life-threatening hypoxia or worsening other organ dysfunction despite initial therapy.

Currently in the UK, streptokinase, urokinase and alteplase are licensed for use in pulmonary embolism.

Further aspects of VTE management

Risk assessment

Haemodynamically stable patients with a confirmed diagnosis of PE should have a risk assessment performed to guide management and need for any additional investigations. This should be performed using the Pulmonary Embolism Severity Index (PESI) score (Table 16.2) (Aujesky et al., 2005). Patients at low risk (30-day mortality 0–3.5% PESI class I/II) can be considered for immediate discharge and home-initiated and supervised anticoagulation. A simplified PESI has also been validated for identification of low-risk patients but this has not been used in any randomised study of home versus hospital treatment for VTE. Patients with intermediate risk (PESI class III and above) should have further evaluation by means of cardiac troponin measurement and echocardiography to determine if there is evidence of right heart dysfunction or early pulmonary hypertension. These patients are not suitable for home treatment (although the group with low–intermediate risk with normal echocardiography/troponin may be, but this has not been evaluated in any prospective clinical trial). These patients should be admitted until they have reached stable INR if being warfarinised. For these intermediate-risk patients commenced on a NOAC who achieve effective anticoagulation quicker compared to having been commenced on warfarin, it is not wholly clear what the minimum duration of hospital observation should be, and this remains down to clinical judgement. Patients who have evidence of right heart dysfunction at presentation require repeated investigations at follow up to ensure resolution before any consideration is given to cessation of anticoagulation.

Table 16.2 Pulmonary Embolism Severity Index (PESI).

Parameter	Points allocated	Classification and interpretation, including 30-day mortality risk
Age	Age in years	Class I ≤ 65 points 0–1.6%
Male gender	+ 10 points	
Active cancer	+ 30 points	
Chronic Heart Failure	+ 10 points	Class II 66–85 points 1.7–3.5%
Chronic Respiratory Disease	+ 10 points	
Pulse rate ≥ 110 bpm	+ 20 points	Class III 86–105 points 3.2–7.1%
Systolic BP < 100 mmHg	+ 30 points	
Respiratory rate > 30	+ 20 points	
Temperature < 36°C	+ 20 points	Class IV 106–125 points 4.0–11.4%
Altered mental status	+ 60 points	
Spo$_2$ < 90% (room air)	+ 20 points	Class V > 125 points 10.24.5%

A simplified PESI has also been validated in identification of low-risk patients but this has not been used in any randomised study of home versus hospital treatment for VTE (Jiminez *et al.*, 2010).

Length of anticoagulation

Any patient who has a venous thromboembolic event is at higher risk of having a further event compared to anyone who has never had VTE. However, in patients where there is a clear and reversible risk factor, the likelihood of further events (assuming the risk factor is removed, e.g. transient immobilisation after orthopaedic surgery) is much lower compared to patients without an obvious risk factor ('unprovoked VTE'). In provoked PE, there is little justification for continuing anticoagulation further than an initial 3 months, unless patients have had a prior history of VTE. The optimal length of anticoagulation in unprovoked PE is, however, an often debated area. The annual risk of recurrent VTE following an unprovoked event varies in different studies but is probably higher in the first 2 years (up to 10%) and approximates 3–4% per year thereafter, with a case-fatality rate quoted of 12%. Continued anticoagulation does reduce that risk but at the expense of increased bleeding risk. Annual risks of major bleeding range from 2 to 12% in controlled studies, with case fatality rates of 10–33% (Bounameaux and Perrier, 2008). On balance, most patients will be offered 3 months' anticoagulation for a single episode of unprovoked VTE (see ESC guidelines, Konstantinides *et al.*, 2014).

As above, patients with active cancer should have a minimum of 6 months' anticoagulation and it should only be stopped at that point if the cancer is considered cured.

Thrombophilia screening

There is no justification for routine thrombophilia screening in patients presenting with unprovoked VTE. The prevalence of thrombophilias that appreciably increases an individual's risk of further thrombosis is low, with the factor V Leiden mutation the most common (3–7% of the population). While the presence of an inherited defect does increase the risk of a first thrombosis, it does not significantly predict for the risk of recurrence in unselected VTE patients.

There is also no justification in screening for thrombophilia in patients where anticoagulation is going to be continued for whatever reason. Recommendations are to perform the following investigations in patients with *unprovoked* VTE in whom anticoagulation is to be stopped, but if positive would prompt ongoing anticoagulation:

- Antiphospholipid antibodies (all patients)
- Full thrombophilia testing in patients with a first-degree relative history of VTE.

Investigation for underlying malignancy

In patients with unprovoked VTE, and whose basic initial investigations (routine biochemistry, haematology, chest X-ray, urinalysis) are normal, the risk of subsequent presentation with a malignancy is low (NICE, 2012) and wide-ranging investigation in these patients is largely unrevealing. NICE guidance states to 'consider' investigating patients over the age of 40 with an unprovoked episode of VTE with CT abdomen and pelvis and mammogram (women). Further investigation (e.g. other tumour markers) is not recommended. Although it is likely more cancers will be found, the impact of this strategy on overall mortality is not clear. One RCT (Piccioli *et al.*, 2004) involving extensive screening of 99 patients with VTE identified a cancer prevalence of 13.1%, which were at an earlier stage than the cancers subsequently presenting in 9.8% of the control group of 102 patients, but there was no clear improvement in cancer-related mortality in the screened group.

Case outcome and discharge

Following the CTPA result confirming VTE, Mrs Robinson was classed as intermediate risk on the basis of her PESI score of 87. Both troponin and echocardiography were normal. Discussion was undertaken with Mrs Robinson about the options around anticoagulation and she was not keen on the requirement for regular INR checks required with warfarin and so was commenced on rivaroxaban. She was still referred to the anticoagulant clinic to make sure she dropped down to the once-daily dosing regimen at 21 days. Her tachycardia resolved and her oxygen saturations improved over the next 48 hours and after 3 days she was fully independent and without requirement for supplemental oxygen. She was discharged with plans for review in the respiratory clinic in 3 months time to ensure she was well and that no further investigation for possible pulmonary hypertension was required.

Common pitfalls

- Not adhering to a warfarin dosing nomogram, and not checking INR daily during warfarin initiation.
- Failing to recognise potential for interactions with warfarin and existing medications, and to

DISCHARGE MEDICATION

Date	Medication	Dose	Route	Frequency	Supply	GP to continue?
xx/xx/xx	RIVAROXABAN	15 mg	PO	Twice daily	19 days	See note
xx/xx/xx	AMLODIPINE	5 mg	PO	Once daily	28 days	Y

Notes to patient/GP:
Patient to attend anticoagulation clinic after 21 days on therapy (2 days given in hospital) to change RIVAROXABAN dose to 20 mg once daily. Please arrange for maintenance prescription from then to reflect this dose.

consider whether any short-term prescriptions may, on cessation, impact on warfarin control.
- Not prescribing a minimum of 5 days' LMWH irrespective of the patients INR with warfarin.
- Experience with NOACs is limited but accumulating; make sure you get the timing right for initiation with respect to LMWH; make sure you **stop** LMWH after the first NOAC dose and make sure the dose adjustment 7–21 days later (depending on the NOAC used) is arranged.

SUMMARY

VTE is a commonly encountered medical emergency. Prescribing for this consists of initially empirical low molecular weight heparin until the diagnosis is established and then commencement of either warfarin or, increasingly, novel oral anticoagulants. Thrombolysis is rarely indicated except in the case of primarily haemodynamic instability.

Key learning points

- When commencing warfarin for confimed PTE/DVT, be sure to continue low molecular weight heparin for at least 5 days irrespective of the patient's INR.
- In the initiation phase with warfarin, follow a recognised dosing schedule to include daily INR checks so that a reliable predicted maintenance dose is reached by the fourth day of warfarin prescription.
- Thrombolysis for PE is employed in cases of haemodynamic instability, not on the basis of imaging findings.

- Novel oral anticoagulants (NOACs) are increasingly being used in the treatment of VTE and appear to be associated with less risk of bleeding, but at present there are no commercially available antidotes.
- Once a NOAC is commenced, LMWH mus be discontinued, and dosage of all agents requires reduction at various levels of renal immpairent.

FURTHER READING

■ The European Society of Cardiology guidelines, endorsed by the European Reparatory Society (Konstantinides *et al.*, 2014) is a very readable document and contains valuable summary of evidence in relation to all the key issues discussed above. Other papers and guideline statements are listed in the References.

Anticoagulation in atrial fibrillation

The decision to anticoagulate patients with atrial fibrillation (AF) is made on the basis of their risk of systemic embolism. Patients with valvular AF (e.g. mitral regurgitation) are generally at higher risk of systemic embolism than those without valvular heart disease (non-valvular AF) and are routinely offered anticoagulation unless the risk of bleeding is felt to outweigh benefit. Only warfarin is licensed in this situation. For patients with non-valvular AF, there are a number of scoring systems available, with the CHA_2DS_2-VASc score currently recommended by NICE (see Table 16.3) (NICE, 2014). Men with a score of 1 or more or women with a score of 2 or more should be considered for anticoagulation, taking account of the risk of bleeding. Aspirin is no longer recommended in this situation.

Factor		Points
History of hypertension		1
Previous TIA/ stroke/ thromboembolism		2
History of vascular disease		1
Diabetes		1

Warfarin and the NOACs (discussed in Section Novel Oral Anticoagulants: Rationale, Evidence and Pharmacology) are all licensed for use in this situation, although there is a requirement for patients to have one or more specific risk factors for stroke. There are subtle differences between the NOACs in the precise definition of these specific risk factors (NICE, 2014) but common to all are:

■ Previous stroke or TIA
■ Left ventricular ejection fraction <40%
■ Symptomatic heart failure
■ Age ≥75 years
■ Diabetes (if ≥65 years for dabigatran)
■ Hypertension (if ≥65 years for dabigatran).

Most patients with AF who require anticoagulation do not require this urgently. Accordingly, these patients do not require LMWH, in the manner described for acute venous thromboembolism, and the majority are commenced on this treatment as outpatients. The nomogram detailed in Table 16.1 is not necessary, and often impractical given the nature of daily INR checking that is required. Current guidelines (SIGN, 2013) recommend a lower-intensity regimen such as that in Table 16.4, assuming baseline INR <1.4 (Tait and Sefcick, 1998).

Table 16.3 Calculation of CAD_2-DS_2-VASc score.		
Factor		Points
Age	< 65	0
	65–74	1
	≥ 75	2
Gender	Male	0
	Female	1
History of CCF		1

Table 16.4   Warfarin induction regimen for outpatient anticoagulation in patients with atrial fibrillation. Source: Tait and Sefcick, 1998. Reproduced with permission of Wiley.

d5 INR	dose (for d5-7)	d8 INR	dose (from d8)
≤1.7	5 mg	≤1.7	6 mg
		1.8–2.4	5 mg
		2.5–3.0	4 mg
		>3.0	3 mg for 4 days
1.8–2.2	4 mg	≤1.7	5 mg
		1.8–2.4	4 mg
		2.5–3.0	3.5 mg
		3.1–3.5	3 mg for 4 days
		>3.5	2.5 mg for 4 days
2.3–2.7	3 mg	≤1.7	4 mg
		1.8–2.4	3.5 mg
		2.5–3.0	3 mg
		3.1–3.5	2.5 mg for 4 days
		>3.5	2 mg for 4 days
2.8–3.2	2 mg	≤1.7	3 mg
		1.8–2.4	2.5 mg
		2.5–3.0	2 mg
		3.1–3.5	1.5 mg for 4 days
		>3.5	1 mg for 4 days
3.3–3.7	1 mg	≤1.7	2 mg
		1.8–2.4	1.5 mg
		2.5–3.0	1 mg
		3.1–3.5	0.5 mg for 4 days
		>3.5	omit for 4 days
>3.7	0 mg	< 2.0	1.5 mg for 4 days
		2.0–2.9	1 mg for 4 days
		3.0–3.5	0.5 mg for 4 days

At day 15 (or day 12) check INR and make fine dose adjustment as appropriate

✓ DRUGS checklist for NOACs in atrial fibrillation

	Rivaroxaban	Dabigatran	Apixaban
Dose	20 mg	150 mg	5 mg
Route	Oral	Oral	Oral
Units	mg	mg	mg
Given	OD	BD	BD
Special situations	Reduce dose to 15 mg if creatinine clearance (CrCl) 15–50 mL/min. Avoid in renal impairment with CrCl <15 mL/min.	Avoid in renal impairment with CrCl <30 mL/min; reduce dose to 110 mg BD if CrCl 30–50 mL/min. Reduce dose to 110 mg BD if age >80 years or on verapamil.	Avoid in renal impairment with CrCl <15 mL/min; caution advised if CrCl 15–30 mL/min. Reduce dose to 2.5 mg if age >80 years or body weight <60 kg.

Anticoagulation reversal

The risk of bleeding with anticoagulation is the most serious and life-threatening complication of therapy. All patients should be made aware of the risk of bleeding and to seek medical attention in its event. The specific management of an individual case will depend on the site, degree and clinical consequences of bleeding and so only general principles in relation to prescribing are discussed here. All patients should obviously have full clinical assessment (ABCDE approach), be appropriately resuscitated and monitored and managed in the clinical environment most appropriate to their situation.

The administration of prothrombin complex concentrate (PCC) (e.g. Beriplex, Octaplex, which include factors II, VII, IX and X) and/or fresh frozen plasma (FFP) will rarely be possible without discussion with and agreement from the local haematology team. During such discussions they will advise on the amount/volume to be prescribed in any individual situation.

Excess anticoagulation and bleeding on warfarin

As discussed in Section Warfarin: Rationale and Evidence, Practical Prescribing Points, patients commenced on warfarin for acute VTE should have their INR measured daily in the initial phase. By contrast, patients who are on warfarin for longer-term treatment (e.g. AF) and who achieve stable INRs may not have their INR measured more often than every 12 weeks. The presence of excess anticoagulation as evident by a high INR may only become evident during an INR check, and bleeding can occur irrespective of the INR. The amount of intervention depends on the INR and whether bleeding is major (limb or life-threatening e.g. intracranial, gastrointestinal haemorrhage, haemodynamic instability) or minor (e.g. superficial skin bleeding, minor epistaxis, no haemodynamic instability). The following is detailed within the BNF (BMA/RPS, 2015) and is based on national haematology guidelines (Keeling *et al.*, 2011) (Table 16.5). In major bleeding, administration of PCCs will completely reverse warfarin-induced anticoagulation within 10 minutes but the half-life is a short as 6 hours (factor VII), hence the recommendation that vitamin K is also given, but remember the effect of vitamin K will not be evident for up to 6–8 hours. Try to clarify why the bleeding and/or high INR has occurred, for example (e.g. Has the liver function changed? Have new drugs with warfarin interactions been prescribed and will they be continued?). This will help determine whether subsequent dose adjustment is required.

Table 16.5 Summary of guidance for managing excessive anticoagulation, as detailed in *British National Formulary* (BMA/RPS, 2015).

INR	None	Minor	Major
		Bleeding	
3–4.9	Reduce warfarin dose	Reduce warfarin dose	
5.0–8.0	Omit warfarin for 1–2 days and reduce subsequent dose	Stop warfarin Give vitamin K 1–3 mg IV stat Restart warfarin when INR <5.0	Stop warfarin Give vitamin K 5mg IV Give PCC 25–50 units/kg
>8.0	Stop warfarin Give vitamin K 1–5 mg orally (use IV preparation). Repeat if INR still high after 24 hours Restart warfarin once INR <5.0	Stop warfarin Give vitamin K 1–3 mg IV stat Repeat IV vitamin K if INR still too high after 24 hours Restart warfarin when INR <5.0	If PCC not available give FFP 15 mL/kg (NB FFP is less effective than PCC)

FFP, fresh frozen plasma; PCC, prothrombin complex concentrate.

There is often the concern that giving vitamin K will result in resistance to warfarin and difficulty in re-establishing a therapeutic INR once warfarin is reintroduced. This is unlikely at the doses recommended for the clinical situations described here. In situations where oral vitamin K is required, in general, the higher the INR, the higher the dose of vitamin K that is required, with one study using 2.5 mg orally when INR was between 8 and 12 and 5 mg when INR was above 12 (Baker *et al.*, 2006). In this study, over-correction did not occur.

Bleeding on heparin

Unfractionated heparin can be neutralised by giving protamine sulphate. This binds to heparin and the resulting stable ion pair has no anticoagulant activity. This complex is then removed by the reticuloendothelial system. Low-molecular weight heparins, however, are not as effectively neutralised by protamine as they have reduced and variable sulphate charge density, with tinzaparin likely to be most neutralisable, followed by dalteparin then enoxaparin (Crowther *et al.*, 2002). Protamine 1 mg neutralises approximately 100 mg of heparin and so the dose of protamine relates to amount of heparin that has been administered.

✓ DRUGS checklist for PROTAMINE SULPHATE

Dose	Up to 50 mg depending on situation and amount of heparin requiring neutralisation
Route	IV
Units	mg
Given	By IV injection not exceeding 5 mg/min
Special situations	To reverse IV injection of unfractionated heparin (UFH) • 1 mg per 100 units UFH given (less if reversal required greater than 15 minutes post injection; if 30–60 minutes have elapsed since heparin was injected intravenously, 0.5–0.75 mg protamine sulphate per 100 units of heparin is recommended. If 2 hours or more have elapsed, 0.25–0.375 mg per 100 units of heparin should be administered, up to maximum dose of 50 mg.

> **To reverse IV infusion of UFH**
> - 25–50 mg once infusion stopped.
>
> **To reverse SC injection of LMWH**
> - 1 mg per 100 units UFH given, maximum 50 mg.

Bleeding on NOACs

As discussed in Section Novel Oral Anticoagulants: Rationale, Evidence And Pharmacology, there are currently no commercially available antidotes for reversal of rivaroxaban, apixaban or dabigatran. Advice from haematology should be sought but the generally recommended treatment is supportive.

Anticoagulation prescribing in the perioperative situation

Warfarin should be stopped for 5 days before planned surgery, with INR checked preoperatively (ideally 1 day before surgery). If INR is ≥1.5, oral vitamin K 1–5 mg orally (see Section Excess Anticoagulation and Bleeding on Warfarin) is recommended. Usually, warfarin can be restarted on the evening of surgery or the next day.

In patients where there is felt to be a high risk of thromboembolism (e.g. VTE within previous 3 months, AF with recent stroke) where surgery cannot be deferred, cover with 'treatment dose' of a LMWH in the days when warfarin is not being taken is recommended. The last dose of LMWH should be ≥24 hours prior to surgery and can be restarted once haemostasis is adequate, unless surgery carries a high risk of bleeding, in which case waiting 48 hours would be advised.

The half-lives of NOACs in the presence of normal renal function are approximately 12–14 hours (although for rivaroxaban it is shorter in younger patients) and manufacturers of all these drugs advise discontinuation at least 24 hours prior to surgery, but earlier cessation is advised in renal impairment and/or if surgery carries a higher risk of bleeding. They can be restarted generally once haemostasis achieved.

Now visit **www.wileyessential.com/pharmacology** to test yourself on this chapter.

References

Akl EA, Kahale L, Barba *et al.* (2014). Anticoagulation for the long-term treatment of venous thromboembolism in patients with cancer. *Cochrane Database Syst Rev* (7): CD006650.

Aujesky D, Obrosky DS, Stone RA et al. (2005). Derivation and validation of a prognostic model for pulmonary embolism. *Am J Respir Crit Care Med* 172: 1041–6.

Baker P, Gleghorn A, Tripp T *et al.* (2006). Reversal of asymptomatic over-anticoagulation by orally administered vitamin K. *Br J Haematol* 133: 331–6.

Barritt DW, Jordan SC (1960). Anticoagulant drugs in the treatment of pulmonary embolism: a controlled trial. *Lancet* 1: 1309–12.

Bounameaux H, Perrier A (2008). Duration of anticoagulation therapy for venous thromboembolism. *Hematology Am Soc Hematol Educ Program*: 252–8.

British Medical Association and Royal Pharmaceutical Society of Great Britain. (BMA/RPS) (2015). *British National Formulary 69*. 69th edn. BMJ group and Pharmaceutical Press, London.

Buller HR, Prins MH, Lensin AW *et al.* (2012). Oral rivaroxaban for the treatment of symptomatic pulmonary embolism. *N Engl J Med* 366: 1287–97.

Cossette B, Pelletier ME, Carrier N, *et al.* (2010). Evaluation of bleeding risk in patients exposed to therapeutic unfractionated or low-molecular-weight heparin: a cohort study in the context of a quality improvement initiative. *Ann Pharmacother* 44: 994–1002.

Crowther MA, Berry LR, Monagle PT *et al.* (2002). Mechanisms responsible for the failure of protamine to inactivate low-molecular-weight heparin. *Br J Haematol* 116: 178–86.

Deitcher SR, Kessler CM, Merli G *et al.* (2006). Secondary prevention of venous thromboembolic events in patients with active cancer: enoxaparin alone versus initial enoxaparin followed by warfarin for a 180-day period. *Clin Appl Thromb Hemost* 12: 389–96.

Eerenberg ES, Kamphuisen PW, Sijpkens MK *et al.* (2011). Reversal of rivaroxaban and dabigatran by prothrombin complex concentrate: a randomized, placebo-controlled, crossover study in healthy subjects. *Circulation* 124: 1573–9.

Garcia P, Ruiz W, Loza Munarriz C (2013). Warfarin initiation nomograms for venous thromboembolism. *Cochrane Database Syst Rev* (7): CD007699

Harrison L, Johnston M, Massicotte MP *et al.* (1997). Comparison of 5-mg and 10-mg loading doses in initiation of warfarin therapy. *Ann Intern Med* 126: 133–6.

Hirsh J, Warkentin TE, Shaughnessy SG *et al.* (2001). Heparin and low-molecular-weight heparin - mechanisms of action, pharmacokinetics, dosing, monitoring, efficacy, and safety. *Chest* 119: 64S–94S.

Holbrook AM, Pereira JA, Labiris R *et al.* (2005). Systematic overview of warfarin and its drug and food interactions. *Arch Intern Med* 165: 1095–106.

Hull RD, Pineo GF, Brant RF *et al.* (2006). Long-term low-molecular-weight heparin versus usual care in proximal-vein thrombosis patients with cancer. *Am J Med* 119: 1062–72.

Jimenez D, Aujesky D, Moores L *et al.* (2010). Simplification of the pulmonary embolism severity index for prognostication in patients with acute symptomatic pulmonary embolism. *Arch Intern Med* 170: 1383–9.

Keeling D, Baglin T, Tait C *et al.* (2011). Guidelines on oral anticoagulation with warfarin – fourth edition. *Br J Haematol* 154: 311–24.

Konstantinides S, Geibel A, Heusel G *et al.* (2002). Heparin plus alteplase compared with heparin alone in patients with submassive pulmonary embolism. *N Engl J Med* 347: 1143–50.

Konstantinides SV, Torbicki A, Agnelli G *et al.* (2014). 2014 ESC Guidelines on the diagnosis and management of acute pulmonary embolism. *Eur Heart J* 35: 3033–69.

Lee AY, Levine MN, Baker RI *et al.* (2003). Low-molecular-weight heparin versus a coumadin for the prevention of recurrent venous thromboembolism in patients with cancer. *N Engl J Med* 349: 146–53.

Mahé I, Bertrand N, Drouet L *et al.* (2006). Interaction between paracetamol and warfarin in patients: A double-blind, placebo-controlled, randomized study. *Haematologica* 91: 1621–7.

Meyer G, Vicaut E, Danays T *et al.* (2014). Fibrinolysis for patients with intermediate-risk pulmonary embolism. *N Engl J Med* 370: 1402–11.

Mueck W, Lensing AW, Agnelli G *et al.* (2011). Rivaroxaban: population pharmacokinetic analyses in patients treated for acute deep-vein thrombosis and exposure simulations in patients with atrial fibrillation treated for stroke prevention. *Clin Pharmacokinet* 50: 675–86.

National Institute for Health and Care Excellence (NICE) (2012). *Venous Thromboembolic Diseases: Diagnosis Management and Thrombophilia Testing*, CG144. Available at: www.nice.org.uk/guidance/cg144 (accessed May 2015).

National Institute for Health and Care Excellence (NICE) (2014). *Atrial Fibrillation: Management*, CG180. Available at: www.nice.org.uk/guidance/cg180 (accessed May 2015).

Penning-van Beest FJ, Geleijnse JM, van Meegen E *et al.* (2002). Lifestyle and diet as risk factors for overanticoagulation. *J Clin Epidemiol* 55: 411–7.

Piccioli A, Lensing AW, Prins MH *et al.* (2004). Extensive screening for occult malignant disease in idiopathic venous thromboembolism: a prospective randomized clinical trial. *J Thromb Haemost* 2: 884–9.

Scottish Intercollegiate Guidelines Network (SIGN) (2013). Antithrombotics: indications and management. A national clinical guideline. *SIGN 129*. Available at: www.rcpsg.ac.uk/~/media/2D92925EEE144AF2857AFBA8E-002F7EF.ashx (accessed May 2015).

Stein PD, Hull RD, Matta F *et al.* (2009). Incidence of thrombocytopenia in hospitalized patients with venous thromboembolism. *Am J Med* 122: 919–930.

Tait RC, Sefcick A (1998). A warfarin induction regimen for out-patient anticoagulation in patients with atrial fibrillation. *Br J Haematol* 101: 450–4.

van Dongen CJ, van den Belt AG, Prins MH *et al.* (2004). Fixed dose subcutaneous low molecular weight heparins vs. adjusted dose unfractionated heparin for venous thromboembolism. *Cochrane Database Syst Rev* (4): CD001100.

Index

Page numbers in *italic* refer to figures.
Page numbers in **bold** refer to tables.

Essential Practical Prescribing, First Edition. Georgia Woodfield, Benedict Lyle Phillips, Victoria Taylor, Amy
Hawkins and Andrew Stanton. © 2016 by John Wiley & Sons, Ltd. Published 2016 by John Wiley & Sons, Ltd.